ORAL MICROBIOLOGY and IMMUNOLOGY

MICHAEL G. NEWMAN, D.D.S., F.A.C.D.

Section of Periodontics
School of Dentistry and Dental Research Institute
University of California
Los Angeles, California

RUSSELL NISENGARD, D.D.S., Ph.D.

Department of Periodontology and Department of Microbiology
School of Dental Medicine and School of Medicine
State University of New York at Buffalo
Buffalo, New York

1988
W. B. SAUNDERS COMPANY
Harcourt Brace Jovanovich, Inc.
Philadelphia ■ London ■ Toronto
Montreal ■ Sydney ■ Tokyo

W. B. SAUNDERS COMPANY
Harcourt Brace Jovanovich, Inc.

The Curtis Center
Independence Square West
Philadelphia, PA 19106

Library of Congress Cataloging-in-Publication Data

Oral mircobiology and immunology/[edited by] Michael G. Newman, Russell Nisengard.

p. cm.

Includes index.

1. Mouth—Microbiology.   2. Mouth—Immunology.
I. Newman, Michael G.   II. Nisengard, Russell J.
[DNLM: 1. Mouth—immunology.   2. Mouth—microbiology.   3. Mouth Diseases—immunology.
4. Mouth Diseases—microbiology. QW 65 0618]

QR47.068 1988 617'.522—dc19

DNLM/DLC
for Library of Congress   88–15846
                                                                CIP

ISBN 0–7216–2420–0

Editor: Darlene Pedersen
Developmental Editor: Linda Mills
Designer: Karen O'Keefe
Production Manager: Pete Faber
Manuscript Editor: Ann Houska
Illustration Coordinator: Brett MacNaughton
Indexer: Nancy Newman

Oral Microbiology and Immunology   ISBN 0–7216–2420–0

Last digit is the print number: 9   8   7   6   5   4   3   2   1

Dedication

Dentistry is demanding for both students and teachers. As dental educators, we recognize our own continuous need for learning. This book is dedicated to our wives and children, who have accepted our commitment to dentistry and have provided love, support, and encouragement, and to our teachers and students, who stimulated our interest in microbiology and immunology.

Acknowledgment

The conceptual development of this textbook was a result of input from many individuals. The editors wish to single out Dr. Joseph Zambon, our colleague and contributor, who made significant contributions to this text.

Contributors

MICHAEL A. APICELLA, M.D.
Professor of Medicine and Microbiology, School of Medicine, State University of New York at Buffalo; Erie County Medical Center, Buffalo Veterans Administration Hospital, Buffalo General Hospital, Buffalo, New York
Neisseria

CYNTHIA G. BLOOMQUIST, B.A.
Associate Scientist, School of Dentistry, University of Minnesota, Minneapolis, Minnesota
Normal Microbial Flora of the Human Body

SEBASTIAN G. CIANCIO, D.D.S.
Professor and Chairman, Department of Periodontology; Clinical Professor of Pharmacology, School of Dental Medicine, State University of New York at Buffalo; Consultant, Erie County Medical Center, Veterans Administration Medical Center, Buffalo, New York
Control and Prevention of Periodontal Disease; Antimicrobials and Antibiotics

JEFFREY L. EBERSOLE, Ph.D.
Associate Professor, Department of Periodontics, Dental School, University of Texas Health Science Center at San Antonio, Texas
Host Resistance and Immune Function

RICHARD P. ELLEN, D.D.S.
Professor of Dentistry and Microbiology; Head, Department of Periodontics, Faculty of Dentistry, University of Toronto, Toronto, Ontario
Genus Actinomyces *and Other Filamentous Bacteria*

RICHARD T. EVANS, Ph.D.
Associate Professor of Oral Biology and Microbiology, School of Dental Medicine, State University of New York at Buffalo, Buffalo, New York
Oral Infection and Immunity

SYDNEY M. FINEGOLD, M.D.
Professor of Medicine, Professor of Microbiology and Immunology, School of Medicine, University of California, Los Angeles; Associate Chief of Staff for Research and Development, VAMC, West Los Angeles, California
Bacillus and Clostridium

COLIN K. FRANKER, Ph.D.
Professor of Microbiology, School of Dentistry, University of California, Los Angeles, California
Oral Mycology

ANTHONY D. GOODMAN, D.D.S., M.Sc.D.*
Periapical Infections

EUGENE A. GORZYNSKI, Ph.D.
Professor of Microbiology, School of Medicine and Biomedical Sciences, State University of New York at Buffalo; Chief Microbiologist, Laboratory Service, Veterans Administration Medical Center, Buffalo, New York
Enterobacteriaceae and Vibrionaceae

STANLEY C. HOLT, Ph.D.
Department of Periodontics, Dental School, University of Texas Health Science Center at San Antonio, Texas
General Microbiology, Metabolism, and Genetics

KENNETH S. KORNMAN, D.D.S., Ph.D.
Professor and Chairman, Department of Periodontics, Dental School, University of Texas Health Science Center at San Antonio, Texas
Bacteroides

WILLIAM F. LILJEMARK, D.D.S., Ph.D.
Professor, School of Dentistry, University of Minnesota, Minneapolis, Minnesota
Normal Microbial Flora of the Human Body

WALTER J. LOESCHE, D.M.D., Ph.D.
Professor of Dentistry, School of Dentistry; Professor of Microbiology, School of Medicine, University of Michigan, Ann Arbor, Michigan
The Spirochetes; Ecology of the Oral Flora

PHILIP T. LoVERDE, Ph.D.
Associate Professor, Department of Microbiology, School of Medicine, State University of New York at Buffalo, New York
Parasitology

BERNARD J. MONCLA, B.S., M.S., Ph.D.
Research Assistant Professor, Departments of Periodontics and Oral Biology, School of Dentistry, University of Washington, Seattle, Washington
Pseudomonadaceae

MICHAEL G. NEWMAN, D.D.S.
Section of Periodontics, School of Dentistry, University of California, Los Angeles, California
Dental Plaque and Calculus; Periodontal Disease; Medical Infections of Interest; Diagnostic Microbiology and Immunology

RUSSELL J. NISENGARD, D.D.S., Ph.D.
Department of Periodontics, Schools of Dental Medicine and Medicine, Departments of Periodontology and Microbiology, State University of New York at Buffalo, New York
Periodontal Disease; Control and Prevention of Periodontal Disease; Periapical Infections; Medical Infections of Interest; Diagnostic Microbiology and Immunology

JOAN OTOMO-CORGEL, D.D.S., M.P.H.
Adjunct Assistant Professor, Department of Periodontics, School of Dentistry, University of California, Los Angeles; Staff Periodontist, VAMC, West Los Angeles—Wadsworth Division; Staff Periodontist, Rancho Los Amigos Hospital, Los Angeles, California
Legionella

---

*Deceased

NO-HEE PARK, D.M.D., Ph.D.
Professor, School of Dentistry, University of California, Los Angeles; Associate
Director, UCLA Dental Research Institute, Los Angeles, California
Virology

T. V. POTTS, D.D.S., Ph.D.
Associate Professor, Departments of Oral Biology and Operative Dentistry,
School of Dental Medicine, State University of New York at Buffalo, New York
Haemophilus and Pasteurella

ANN PROGULSKE, Ph.D.
University of Florida, Gainesville, Florida
General Microbiology, Metabolism, and Genetics

W. EUGENE RATHBUN, D.D.S., Ph.D.
Professor of Periodontics, School of Dentistry, Loma Linda University, Loma
Linda, California
Sterilization and Asepsis

BURTON ROSAN, D.D.S., M.Sc.
Professor of Microbiology, University of Pennsylvania School of Dental Medi-
cine, Philadelphia, Pennsylvania
The Streptococci; The Staphylococci

MARIANO SANZ, M.D., D.D.S.
Visiting Assistant Professor, UCLA School of Dentistry; Associate Professor,
School of Stomatology, University of Madrid, Spain
Dental Plaque and Calculus

BENJAMIN SCHEIN, D.D.S., M.Sc.D.
Assistant Professor, Department of Restorative Dentistry, University of Califor-
nia, San Francisco, California
Periapical Infections

JØRGEN SLOTS, D.M.D., M.D., Ph.D.
Professor of Periodontics and Director for Microbiology Testing Service, School
of Dental Medicine, University of Pennsylvania, Philadelphia, Pennsylvania
Actinobacillus Actinomycetemcomitans

NORTON S. TAICHMAN, D.D.S., Ph.D.
School of Dental Medicine, University of Pennsylvania, Philadelphia,
Pennsylvania
Actinobacillus Actinomycetemcomitans

L. E. WOLINSKY, Ph.D., D.M.D.
Associate Professor of Oral Biology, University of California, Los Angeles,
California
Caries and Cariology

JOSEPH J. ZAMBON, D.D.S., Ph.D.
Associate Professor of Periodontology and Oral Biology; Director of Graduate
Periodontology, School of Dental Medicine, State University of New York at
Buffalo; Consultant in Periodontology, Veterans Administration Medical Cen-
ter, Batavia, New York
*Bacterial Classification; Corynebacterium and Mycobacterium; Brucella, Yersinia, and
Francisella; Veillonella, Wolinella, and Campylobacter; Mycoplasmas, Chlamydiae,
and Rickettsiae; Periodontal Disease; Medical Infections of Interest*

Preface

Rapid expansion in the fields of microbiology and immunology during the past two decades has provided new insights into the etiology, diagnosis, and treatment of microbial and immunologic diseases. In particular, the study of oral microbiology and immunology has entered a new era. There is now a greater recognition of the complexity and diversity of factors within the oral cavity. Their importance to modern medical microbiology and immunology and to clinical dentistry has become increasingly clear. Early in the development of this book, we recognized that a multicontributor text was the best approach to provide the expertise necessary to properly cover the broad subject base. The contributors are all recognized authorities in their field, and they provide insight into and relevance to their individual topics.

This book is intended for students and practitioners of dentistry and other health-related fields. It provides an up-to-date survey with emphasis on basic principles of microbial and immunologic diseases of oral origin or diseases with secondary oral manifestations. Where applicable, the chapters include specific dental applications. Most references are review articles and other key references. The rate of advances in oral microbiology and immunology is very rapid, and thus revisions in this text will be made regularly.

Concepts concerning the bacterial and host interactions in caries and periodontal disease, two of the most common diseases of man, have had pronounced effects on health care delivery. Importantly, the association of specific bacteria in the pathogenesis of these diseases has been critical. Caries is known to result from three factors: specific bacteria, susceptible teeth, and environmental factors such as diet and oral hygiene. Specific knowledge regarding the influences of these factors has led to a significant reduction in the prevalence of caries in the United States and elsewhere.

Inflammatory periodontal disease, once considered to result from a non-specific, quantitative increase in plaque, is now recognized to result from increases in specific periodontopathic bacteria. The association of specific bacteria with gingival health and with various periodontal diseases, including gingivitis, periodontitis, rapidly advancing periodontitis, localized juvenile periodontitis, and acute necrotizing ulcerative gingivitis, has allowed more effective treatment to be directed toward the elimination of specific bacteria. Mechanical methods, originally the mainstay of clinical treatment, have been supplemented with chemotherapeutic agents. In the future, more specific antiplaque agents as well as agents that modulate host responsiveness may prove useful.

In addition to caries and periodontal disease, there are other microbiologically and immunologically associated diseases and conditions. These include those of viral, fungal, and autoimmune etiologies.

In order to have a thorough and complete source of information, this book is divided into five sections:

Section I—General Principles. This section includes oral infection and immunity, host resistance and immune function, bacteriology, and bacterial classification.

Section II—General Bacteriology. The most important bacteria in medicine and dentistry are discussed, often with examples related to dental practice.

Section III—Virology and Parasitology. This section provides in-depth, clearly written, relevant information for all oral health care workers. The increased awareness of virology, mycology, and parasitology by dental health care professionals and their patients is of utmost importance.

Section IV—Oral Health and Disease. This section includes ecology of the oral flora, dental plaque and calculus, caries and cariology, periodontal disease, control and prevention of periodontal disease, periapical infections, and medical infections of interest.

Section V—Applied Microbiology and Immunology. This section includes sterilization and asepsis, antimicrobials and antibiotics, diagnostic microbiology, and immunology.

Contents

section 1

General principles

chapter 1

Oral infection and immunity

Richard T. Evans, Ph. D.

Developments in understanding the role of infectious agents in the oral cavity closely parallel findings in medical microbiology, and, indeed, several key initial observations and descriptions of medical importance were made while describing an oral condition. Of equal importance were the technical advances made during these studies, which allowed an understanding of basic principles of oral infection and immunity and which in turn suggested methods of control. Examples are the early descriptions of bacterial forms found in the mouth by van Leeuwenhoek, studies of oral bacteria by W. D. Miller and G. V. Black, caries studies using gnotobiotic animals, and the occurrence of secretory antibody in oral secretions.

Origin, Development, and History of Infections

Epidemic diseases were well known among ancient peoples and civilizations. While the nature or source of the infection was unknown, the need for quarantine and hygiene was accepted. Disease transmission by contact was understood, but transmission by other means was not. Generally, disease was ascribed either to a natural occurrence such as the appearance of a comet or to a mystical event that would displease a deity.

The Old Testament contains references to laws to avoid disease. The Book of Leviticus contains detailed descriptions of leprosy:

. . . if the hairs in it have turned white and the sore appears to be deeper than the surrounding skin it is the dreaded skin disease [leprosy] . . . but if the sore is white and does not appear deeper than the skin around it and the hairs have not turned white, the priest shall isolate him for seven days [the concept of quarantine].

In Hebrew, the word for "dreaded skin disease [leprosy]" and "mildew" are the same, suggesting the ancients associated mildew and leprosy:

. . . if the mildew has spread, the object [in this case cloth] is unclean. The priest shall burn it, because it is a spreading mildew which must be destroyed by fire.

Preventive measures to be instituted, personal hygiene, and cleaning or removal of mildew from the home environment were also dealt with.

Hippocrates, a Greek physician, codified concepts of disease that influenced thinking well into the Middle Ages. He believed disease required two components: (1) intrinsic factors that could be equated with the host and the host's condition, and (2) extrinsic factors, or "miasms." While the extrinsic factor did not equate with an infectious agent, it embodied the concept that an influence outside the body could induce a disease. It remained for an Italian, Girolamo Fracastoro,

3

in 1546, to define contagion as occurring in one of three ways: (1) by contact, (2) through fomites or objects, and (3) from a distance (airborne). Fracastoro (or Fracastorius in the Latinized form of his name) also used the term "seminaria," or seeds, to denote an infectious agent. It is not clear whether he considered "seminaria" as living or not.

During the 17th century the first direct observations of living bacteria were made by Antony van Leeuwenhoek. The microscope had been used in its rudimentary form from around 1600 to describe fibers and small worms. Van Leeuwenhoek perfected a lens of sufficient quality to observe objects the size of bacteria. Since he studied living organisms whose refractive index is close to that of water, and the objects were generally smaller than the resolving power of his lens, it is believed that he used a form of darkfield illumination to achieve the contrast and magnification required. To determine the size of the "little animalcules," he made comparative estimates based on larger objects such as strands of hair or grains of sand. Using these reference points he was able to give remarkably accurate estimates of size.

Van Leeuwenhoek's letters to the Royal Society in London in 1683 and again in 1695 give a clear description of bacteria found in the mouth. These letters were illustrated with accurate drawings of the three morphologic shapes—rods, cocci, and spiral forms—used to describe bacteria today (Fig. 1–1). He also described motility of the rod-shaped "ani-

malcules" as "a very strong and swift motion and shot through the spittle like a pike through the water." He estimated that "there are more animals in the scum on the teeth in a man's mouth than there are men in the whole kingdom." He tried to kill them by rinsing his mouth with a strong wine vinegar but afterward found as many of them as before.

The observations of van Leeuwenhoek and of later microscopists raised questions as to the role of these unseen animals in disease. Without experimental evidence, Benjamin Marten, a London physician, wrote in 1720 that

certain species of animalcules may . . . (be) capable of existing in our juices and vessels . . . may by their spontaneous motion and injurious parts . . . cause . . . obstruction, inflammation, exulceration and all other phenomena and deplorable symptoms of disease.

Marten's writings, however, did not reflect the popular thinking of the day. The fermentation process, as well as the debate over spontaneous generation, held most of the attention of observers.

Since the processes of putrefaction and decay were readily seen, there was great interest as to how they occurred. Early speculation centered around the development of insects in putrefying meat. Francesco Redi in the late 17th century demonstrated that flies were attracted to decaying food, where they deposited their eggs and also found nourishment. In other experiments, he covered vessels containing meat with lids that allowed exchange of air but excluded flies. Naturally, no maggots or adult flies developed. These experiments helped lay to rest the concept of spontaneous generation for macroscopic organisms but did not eliminate this concept for microscopic animals. In 1776, approximately 100 years after Redi, another Italian furthered the demise of the theory. Lazzaro Spallanzani observed that heating meat infusions prevented finding "animalcules." He concluded that the organisms were airborne and the exclusion of air kept the infusions free of organisms for long periods of time. Still the debate continued, primarily because the experimental methods, while effective, could be attacked since so many of the underlying principles and variables were not well understood. Even so, practical applications were made. In the early 1800s Nicolas Appert proposed an early form of canning that preserved food by heating.

Finally, in 1860 Louis Pasteur performed his classic experiments, which totally dis-

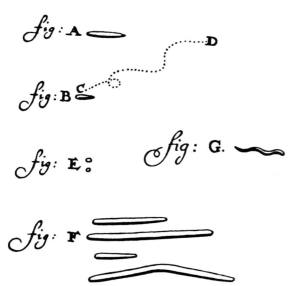

Figure 1–1 ■ Drawings of bacterial forms seen by Antony van Leeuwenhoek (1695).

proved spontaneous generation. Following the lead of an earlier investigator, Theodor Schwann (1837), he prepared a series of flasks containing growth media that was sterilized by boiling. The necks of the flasks had curved elbows, which allowed air to enter but excluded particles. Other flasks were sealed after similar treatment. If left undisturbed the flasks remained growth free. If, however, the flasks were opened the media soon became overgrown. Other similar experiments confirmed these results. While Pasteur's results were definitive, those of John Tyndall (1881) also contributed to our knowledge in this field. Tyndall removed particles from the air in a closed chamber by burning them in a flame. Media placed in the chamber remained uncontaminated as long as the particles were excluded from the chamber.

Fermentation of bread, wine, and beer was originally thought to be a chemical process rather than a biologic one. With the production of gases and acids, chemists formed most of the early theories. Charles Cagniard-Latour (1836) and Schwann (1837) independently discovered the yeast cell in wine and beer, respectively. Despite their descriptions of these cells and their presumed role in fermentation, chemical theories continued to dominate. Pasteur, a chemist, entered his studies into this debate on fermentation. Although Pasteur's ideas may not have been original, his experimental methods were definitive, giving him the credit for placing fermentation on a sound biologic basis. From 1857 onward, Pasteur produced a large volume of work devoted to descriptions of the fermentative processes. In his view, fermentation was essentially life without the presence of oxygen. How this occurred remained for others to describe.

Pasteur also studied the role of microorganisms in diseases of humans and animals. In 1880 he discovered that attenuated bacteria conferred protection in chicken cholera, and in 1884 he reported that attenuated virus was protective against rabies. These and studies of others introduced animal experimentation to microbiology, which led to many fundamental observations in medical and dental science. Among the earliest studies regarding infectivity and disease induction by microorganisms are those of Devaine (1863) and Koch (1877). Devaine, using blood from animals infected with anthrax, transmitted infections to healthy mice, sheep, and cattle. Normal blood was unable to induce disease. Filtration of the infected blood on clay filters removed the organisms from the filtrate so it would not induce disease while the deposit on the filter would. Devaine and coworkers also showed that organisms found in pustules could transmit the disease. These experiments showed the association of organisms with the disease. The classic experiment of Robert Koch (1877) described the formation of resistant spores in anthrax, cultivation of the organism in vitro, and the reintroduction of the disease by injection of the pure culture.

Staining procedures and isolation culture techniques allowed the study of individual organisms. While others attempted to stain bacteria with varied results, Koch in 1877 was the first to use crystal violet with consistent success on the anthrax bacilli. Paul Ehrlich used methylene blue and F. Ziehl and F. Neelsen developed the use of acid staining, which allowed Koch to visualize the tubercle bacilli. One of the most widely used stains in medicine is the gram-modification of Ehrlich's aniline stain. Developed by Christian Gram in 1884, it remains one of the most powerful diagnostic procedures employed in microbiology today. Culturing of bacteria had its beginnings with liquid media. Usually this consisted of either meat infusions or yeast byproducts with added sugar. The results on such media were highly variable and depended on the skill of the investigator for reproducibility. One of the first studies into the composition of media was made by Carl von Nageli, who in 1882 described the effects of sugars, complex carbohydrates, and peptones on the growth of bacteria. This work was soon followed by the use of meat extracts as a nitrogen source. Solid media was used as early as 1872 by Joseph Schroeter, who employed potato slices, bread, coagulated egg albumin, meat, and starch pastes to isolate his organisms. As a result, Schroeter was the first investigator to work with pure bacterial cultures.

While ingenious, these methods were limited to pigmented organisms and were laborious to perform, producing erratic results. The fundamental importance of pure cultures, however, was clearly established. Oscar Brefeld, a mycologist of the time, extended this concept indicating that inoculation of media should be from one spore and that the culture should be protected from contamination. Working with pure cultures of waterborne bacteria, Koch developed the pour plate, in which the water samples were incorporated into gelatin as the plates were poured. The use of agar-containing medium was also introduced in Koch's laboratory. This major step allowed the use of solid medium at temperatures at which gelatin would melt. Koch also pioneered the use of coagulated serum media for culturing tuberculosis bacteria.

Robert Koch's accomplishments in the field of microbiology are numerous and varied. He identified the tubercle bacillus, described the differences between the human and bovine forms of the disease, and was the first to isolate the causative bacteria of anthrax and Asiatic cholera. Koch provided criteria for identifying an organism as the causative agent of a disease. While working with Jacob Henle early in his career, he became exposed to Henle's views that an organism must be isolated from the disease and studied in pure culture. To this, Koch added that the organism grown in pure culture must produce the disease in an experimental animal, and in turn must be reisolated from the infected experimental animal in pure culture. These rigorous criteria were applied by Koch in all of his studies of human and animal diseases. Although they have been restated and modified many times, they stand today as the definitive criteria and are known as the Koch-Henle postulates.

HISTORY OF ORAL INFECTION

One of Koch's students was an American, Willoughby D. Miller, who obtained his D.D.S. from the University of Pennsylvania and continued his studies at the University of Berlin. His major work, published in 1890, was entitled "The Microorganisms of the Human Mouth." He proposed that carbohydrates from food were broken down by oral bacteria and the resulting acids caused dissolution of the enamel. He further stated that bacteria from plaque could enter the initial lesion and continue to damage the underlying tooth structures. Because of the staining and pure culture methods available to him in Koch's laboratory, Miller was able to isolate and describe many of the oral forms. Contemporary with Miller, another American dentist working with less formal training was also describing the oral flora and speculating on its effects in the mouth. Greene V. Black from Jacksonville, Illinois, taught himself both dentistry and microbiology. Fully aware of Miller's work, he speculated in 1883 in his book, *The Formation of Poisons by Microorganisms*, that "all life including microorganisms produce injurious waste and they were responsible for disease including dental caries." In a description of his work published in 1886, "Microorganisms of the Oral Cavity," Black wrote in the following manner regarding the oral streptococci, which he refers to as the caries fungus (Fig. 1–2):

We have found the product of the caries fungus to be lactic acid . . . . you saw the gelatine formed by the microorganisms . . . in a crevice or anywhere a lodgement can be obtained this fungus begins its growth . . . growing against the side of the tooth it will form this gelatine and protect itself until it works its way through. . . .

This description of the bacterial attack on the tooth by the organisms found in the mouth is still accurate today.

Miller isolated organisms from saliva and decayed teeth, which produced acid when grown with carbohydrates. Generally, it was felt that the oral acid-producing bacteria alone could cause caries. Many dentists had observed a salivary drop in pH following meals with a gradual return to normal some hours later. It was also observed that some individuals were more prone to decay than others. A search was begun to identify specific organisms associated with caries. Lac-

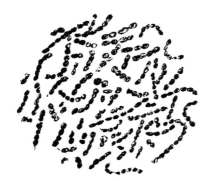

Figure 1–2 ■ Drawing by G. V. Black (1886) of streptococci grown in broth from a carious lesion.

Streptococcus Media (Fungus of Dental Caries).

tobacilli, which predominate in saliva, were considered, as were several other acid formers.

In 1924 J. K. Clark identified a coccus from a caries lesion, which he named *Streptococcus mutans*. This organism was present in higher numbers in the caries lesion, adhered to the tooth, and was acidogenic. At that time, other investigators were not able to reproduce his findings. However, it was believed that a variety of streptococci in plaque and lactobacilli in saliva produced sufficient acid to cause enamel caries. Animal experiments of the time did not help clarify the situation. Organisms similar to those found orally in humans could be isolated orally from rodents. When placed on "cariogenic" diets some animals developed caries, but not in all instances, even among the same strains of animals.

During the 1930s and 1940s, lactobacilli were thought to be the principal acid-producing oral bacteria, even though the streptococci were numerically superior. A conceptual change regarding bacteria found in plaque began with the work of Robert Stephan. He measured the plaque pH with special antimony electrodes and found that within minutes following a glucose rinse the pH fell in the plaque of all subjects, but more markedly in plaque from caries-active subjects than from caries-free or caries-inactive subjects (Fig. 1–3). Moreover, the pH in the plaque of caries-active individuals fell to levels necessary for enamel dissolution. Stephan believed there must be qualitative differences in the plaque bacteria from the subject groups. Stephan and his coworkers further confirmed the specific nature of the caries-

inducing bacteria by treating rats with antibiotics. Those rats receiving penicillin, an antibiotic most effective against gram-positive bacteria, had a greater than 90 percent reduction in caries.

In 1960 investigators working with caries-prone animals demonstrated that caries infections were transmissible. Paul Keyes treated hamsters with either penicillin or erythromycin to prevent caries. Offspring of antibiotic-treated animals did not develop caries, while offspring of the untreated animals did. When offspring of the antibiotic-treated animals were caged with the caries-active animals, they also developed caries. Feces from caries-prone animals added to the drinking water of offspring from antibiotic-treated animals also induced caries, demonstrating the transmission of the infectious agent. Thus began the search for the specific bacteria responsible for these observations, culminating in the rediscovery of *S. mutans* (described further in Chapter 6).

The early descriptions of periodontal disease frequently mentioned deposits surrounding the teeth involved in disease. Pierre Fauchard in 1745 described tartar and soft viscous deposits (plaque) in what appeared to be acute periodontal disease. The description, however, leads one to believe he considered the deposits diseases rather than the initiator of the disease. In his "Natural History of the Teeth," John Hunter (1773), the famous British physician, described gingivitis and pyorrhea and accurately stated that these diseases could serve as sources of infection elsewhere in the body. As mentioned earlier, W. D. Miller, in 1890, described the bacteria associated with soft tissue disease. He could

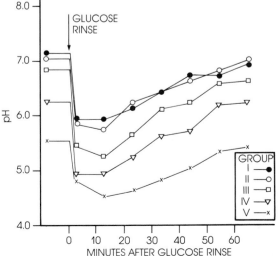

Figure 1–3 ■ pH Curves showing increase in acid production following a glucose rinse. Group I = caries free; groups II through IV = increasing levels of caries activity; group V = extreme caries activity. (From Stephan, R.M.: Intraoral hydrogen-ion concentrations associated with dental caries activity. J Dent Res 23:257, 1944, with permission.)

not ascribe a specific bacterium as the cause of periodontal disease and thus he felt that these conditions were multifactorial. He stated:

> . . . as far as we know there is no bacterium which, inoculated under the gums, is able to provoke the disease in healthy persons . . . and . . . according to this conception, pyorrhea alveolaris is not caused by any specific bacterium.

Nevertheless, continued study of diseases of soft tissue revealed associations of certain bacteria with given conditions. Plaut in 1894 and Vincent in 1896 published accurate, detailed descriptions of fusiform bacteria and spirochetes and related them to an acute disease of oral soft tissues. Although anaerobic bacteria were known prior to this time, the work of H. A. Gins (1934) was first to reveal the anaerobic nature of many of the bacteria found in the mouth and recovered from oral infections. Gins' study discusses the increase in numbers and types of anaerobic bacteria found in the mouth with increasing age and disease. He isolated *Leptothrix*, *Streptobacillus*, *Actinomyces*, and *Spirillum* species, as well as anaerobic cocci. He also noted the frequent finding of *Bacterium (Bacteroides) melaninogenicum* associated with his isolates. As discussed in Chapter 16, black-pigmented *Bacteroides* species are often associated with forms of human periodontal disease.

Lack of information regarding a specific bacterium associated with periodontal disease led to several groups of organisms being implicated. During the 1920s and 1930s ameba and spirochetes were thought to be involved, since they were commonly found in material taken from periodontal pockets. Their numbers and motility undoubtedly influenced investigators. Because of their numbers and ease of isolation, streptococci were also considered to be involved. Most investigators at that time used only aerobic culturing techniques and were thus unable to study the majority of microorganisms. Failure to culture specific organisms associated with disease led to the "nonspecific plaque" hypothesis, which considered most bacteria found in plaque to be possible instigators. Interest waned in isolating plaque bacteria and identifying their role in periodontal disease.

Renewed interest occurred, however, when MacDonald and colleagues (1956) described mixed infections, which included *Bacteroides* species. These studies, while not identifying a specific organism, were notable for several reasons. First, anaerobic methods were routinely employed. Second, the products of organisms were recognized as playing a role in disease pathogenesis. Last, spirochetes, fusiforms, and anaerobic streptococci were no longer considered as pathogens. Knowledge obtained with the advent of improved cultural methods, and with sophisticated biochemical and serologic identification methods, has led to the conclusion that specific bacteria are responsible for adult and juvenile periodontitis (see Chapter 28).

Studies in Immunity

The field of immunology developed from the early studies in bacteriology, although some immunologic practices predated an understanding of the infectious process. The Chinese, Brahmins of India, and Persians during the Middle Ages practiced a form of immunization, called variolation, against smallpox. The technique consisted of deliberately exposing susceptible (unscarred) individuals to dried crusts taken from lesions of patients recovering from the disease. This form of immunization was not widely accepted, however, because of its danger. In 1776, Edward Jenner, a British physician, recognized that milkmaids recovering from cowpox were protected against smallpox. With this observation, Jenner introduced the practice of active immunization, using an antigen to evoke protection against a subsequent infection. In this case, he deliberately exposed patients to a milder disease to protect them against the more virulent smallpox.

Approximately 100 years later, the concept of active immunization was extended by Pasteur, who observed that chicken cholera could be prevented by injecting bacteria that had been aged in culture to weaken their virulence. Pasteur developed this method of protecting against disease with attenuated cultures and prepared protective vaccines against anthrax, swine erysipelas, and rabies. In 1886, Theobald Smith and others showed that killed bacteria could protect against living infectious agents. Finally, von Behring and Kitasato (1890) showed that toxins of tetanus and diphtheria, free of bacteria, also induced protection. Shortly thereafter, antitoxins were used for passive immunization. The field of immunology was early divided into that which studied practical therapeutic and preventive uses for immunizations and that which studied theoretical and basic principles.

While interest in serum effects on microorganisms continued, the host's cellular reaction to infection was also studied. The classic example of cell-mediated immunity was the original observation by Koch that intradermal injections of tuberculin, an antigen derived from the tuberculosis organism, elicited delayed inflammatory responses in humans and animals previously exposed to the organism. This reaction could not be transferred by serum, but could be transferred by cells. Elie Metchnikoff (1884) observed that leukocytes took up bacteria (phagocytosis) and destroyed them by intracellular digestion. Metchnikoff proposed that cellular immunity acted as the principal host-protective defense against disease mechanism. His ideas, however, were not widely accepted. It was not until the studies of contact allergy by Landsteiner and Chase in the 1940s that cell-mediated immunity was fully recognized as a major immune mechanism.

Early attempts were made to control periodontal disease by immunologic means. Joseph Head in 1914 reported at the first annual meeting of the American Association of Immunologists on the use of either autogenous or stock bacterial vaccines, usually consisting of staphylococci and streptococci, as treatment combined with oral hygiene. Although many dental investigators felt encouraged, it soon was apparent that results obtained from such therapy were mixed, and the practice was soon discarded.

Of particular interest in oral microbiology and immunology is the description of the secretory immune system. Experiments of Kiyoshi Shiga (1908) examined the feeding of killed bacteria to rabbits, which were later challenged with an intravenous injection of toxin taken from the same bacteria. The animals were protected from the intestinal effects of the toxin even though no agglutinating activity was found in the serum. Similar experiments were performed throughout the ensuing two decades. In 1927, A. Besredka at the Pasteur Institute published a monograph entitled "Local Immunization," in which he asked the question " . . . will animals resist a fatal dose of virus (i.e., bacteria) after previous preparation by the buccal route?" Repeating and extending the previous work of Shiga, he concluded that "ingestion of heated cultures confers an immunity against a fatal dose of dysentery virus when inoculated intravenously." He further stated " . . . . the plan in artificial vaccination therefore is to follow the route which the virus takes in its penetration into the body." Burrows, in 1948, working with Asiatic cholera in guinea pigs, demonstrated the protective role of coproantibody. The concept of local protective immunity became clear when Fazekas de St. Groth in the 1950s demonstrated the presence of experimentally induced local antibody to influenza on the respiratory membranes of mice following stimulation by aerosols of the antigen. The stage was thus set for Heremans' descriptions in the 1960s of the IgA class of antibody in serum and for Tomasi's work on the predominance of this class of antibody in a variety of secretions such as saliva and colostrum. Today the secretory immune system is recognized as playing a major protective role against diseases which are acquired via the respiratory and oral routes. As will be seen in Chapter 27, the role of secretory immunity against caries and other oral diseases is currently an active field of investigation.

REFERENCES

Black, G. V.: Microorganisms of the Oral Cavity. Journal Illinois Dental Soc., pp. 180–208, 1886.

Bulloch, W.: The History of Bacteriology. Oxford Press, London, 1938.

Conant, J. B.: Pasteur's and Tyndall's Study of Spontaneous Generation. Harvard University Press, Cambridge, 1953.

Dayton, D. H., Small, P. A., Jr., Chanock, R. M., Kaufmann, H. E., and Tomasi, T. B. (eds.): The Secretory Immune System. U.S. Government Printing Office, Washington, D.C., 1970.

Dobell, C.: Antony van Leeuwenhoek and His "Little Animals." Staples Press, London, 1932.

Fouchard, P.: The Surgeon Dentist, or Treatise on the Teeth. Trans. Lindsay, L. from ed. 2, 1746. Milford House, New York, 1969.

Gins, H. A.: Die nichtversporenden Anaerobier der Mundhöhle und der Zähne. Zentralbl. f. Bakt. Parasit. u. Infekt. 132:129–145, 1934.

Head, J.: Society reports: American Association of Immunologists. Medical Record 86:942–946, 1914.

Keyes, P. H.: The infectious nature and transmissible nature of experimental dental caries. Arch. Oral Biol. 1:304–320, 1960.

Kobler, J.: The Reluctant Surgeon, A Biography of John Hunter. Doubleday, New York, 1960.

MacDonald, J. B., Sutton, R. M., Knoll, M. C., Madliner, E. M., and Grainger, R. M.: The pathogenic components of an experimental fusospirochetal infection. J. Infect. Dis. 98:15–20, 1956.

Miller, W. D.: The Microorganisms of the Human Mouth. S. S. White Dental Mfg. Co., Philadelphia, 1890.

Pappas, C. N.: The Life and Times of G. V. Black. Quintessence Publishing, Chicago, 1983.

Ring, M. E.: Dentistry—An Illustrated History. C. V. Mosby, St. Louis, 1985.

Stephan, R. M.: Intraoral hydrogen-ion concentrations associated with dental caries activity. J. Dent. Res. 23:257–266, 1944.

Vallery-Radot, R.: The Life of Pasteur. Doran and Co., New York, 1928.

Wilson, G., Miles, A., and Parker, M. T.: Principles of Bacteriology, Virology, and Immunity, ed. 7. Williams and Wilkins, Baltimore, 1983.

chapter 2

Host resistance and immune function

Jeffrey L. Ebersole, Ph. D.

Inflammation

The inflammatory response, whether acute, chronic, or granulomatous, constitutes a common host response to injury and a primary internal defense mechanism. The protective effect of the inflammatory process is dramatically revealed by the finding that anti-inflammatory agents such as corticosteroids markedly reduce resistance to infectious agents. It must be noted, however, that whereas the early inflammatory responses are protective, when inflammation persists and extensive necrosis occurs, there may be increased susceptibility to infection.

TYPES

Acute inflammatory responses involve a rapid local vessel dilation and an influx of plasma proteins and phagocytic cells (polymorphonuclear leukocytes, or PMNs) into the tissue spaces. Accompanying this is a local release of mediators, which exacerbate the responses. If the acute response eliminates the agent, repair and regeneration ensues. If unsuccessful, the continued influx of PMNs and serum leads to cell death and, in some cases, an abscess.

Continuing acute inflammation may lead to *chronic inflammatory responses*, which are characterized by different cellular and soluble-protein constituents. Chronic inflammatory responses include an infiltration of lymphocytes and cells of the monocyte-macrophage lineage. This is in response to infectious agents that have a capsule or cell wall antigens, making them resistant to phagocytosis and to killing by PMNs. In these situations, increased vascular permeability, allowing passage of plasma into the affected tissue, becomes a critical asset in the host defense. The plasma may contain antibody, which by itself promotes phagocytosis of the agent, and complement, which together with specific antibody further promotes phagocytosis. In addition, the plasma contains a number of antimicrobial substances (i.e., transferrin). Also, soluble chemotactic substances produced by leukocytes promote the accumulation of additional phagocytic leukocytes into the tissue. Generally, these responses provide antibacterial capabilities.

In certain types of infection (e.g., *Mycobacterium tuberculosis*), macrophages tend to accumulate in large numbers at the site of the infection, forming a nodule. Although lymphocytes and neutrophils also occur, macrophages predominate. The macrophages can nonspecifically affect the course of infection favorably, owing to their cellular activation and enormous numbers. This granulomatous response is characteristic of tuberculosis, for example, and is known as *granulomatous inflammation*.

CELLS—CHARACTERISTICS AND FUNCTION

Polymorphonuclear leukocytes (granulocytes) are produced in the bone marrow at a rate of approximately 1.5 million per second and are short lived (2 to 3 days). The PMNs, representing 60 to 70 percent of the total blood leukocytes, can adhere to and penetrate the endothelial cell junctions lining the blood vessels and infiltrate into the tissue. They are subdivided into neutrophils, eosinophils, and basophils. The predominant function of the PMNs is phagocytosis, and their central role in protection is demonstrated by the extreme susceptibility to infections in people with PMN dysfunction.

Neutrophils comprise more than 90 percent of the circulating granulocytes and are the major cellular elements in most acute inflammations. These cells are distinguished by their large numbers, mobility to chemotactic stimuli, short lifespan, rapid metabolism during cell stimulation, extensive phagocytic capacity, and variety of digestive enzymes and oxidative metabolites that kill and degrade microorganisms and tissue debris.

Neutrophils possess two main types of granules. The primary granules, or lysosomes, contain acid hydrolases, myeloperoxidase, lysozyme, elastase, and collagenase, while the specific or secondary granules contain lactoferrin, lysozyme, and collagenase. Ingested microorganisms are contained within vacuoles termed *phagosomes*, which fuse with the enzyme-containing granules to form phagolysosomes. It is within the phagolysosomes that the neutrophils perform their intracellular cytocidal (cell-killing) functions. Release of their granule enzymes is primarily in response to a heavy phagocytic challenge. In general, the release of enzymes from specific granules is high compared with the release of primary granule enzymes. Most changes seen in activated neutrophils

involve cellular or membrane movement associated with binding of ligands to the cell surface. The neutrophils have specific receptors on their surface for IgG, complement components (C3b, C5a, C3a), formyl-methionyl-leucyl-phenylalanine (FMLP, a homologue of bacterial substances), and leukotriene B_4 (LTB_4), allowing them to respond to a wide variety of surface stimuli and accounting for their continual presence in sites of inflammatory and immune responses.

Eosinophils comprise 2 to 5 percent of blood leukocytes in normal healthy individuals. Similar to neutrophils, these cells are capable of phagocytosing and killing microorganisms, although this is not their primary function. Eosinophils can be triggered to degranulate by appropriate membrane-active stimuli. These cells contain surface receptors for IgG, IgE, and numerous complement components (C3b, C4, C1s, C3a, C5a) that provide recognition sites for cellular activation and the release of granule contents. Eosinophils are attracted by soluble products of T lymphocytes, mast cells, and basophils. The eosinophils may also have a role as modulators of inflammation. The cells contain histaminase and aryl sulfatase, which can inactivate the mast cell products, histamine and slow-reacting substance of anaphylaxis (SRS-A).

Basophils and mast cells are found in very small numbers in the circulation (<0.2 percent). These cells are similar in that they both contain granules that stain deep violet-blue with basic dyes as a consequence of large amounts of acidic proteoglycans. The granules contain histamine, heparin, SRS-A, and eosinophil chemotactic factor of anaphylaxis (ECF-A). Mast cells and basophils are the cellular mediators in immediate hypersensitivity responses of the anaphylactic type. The mast cells and basophils may also play a role in cell-mediated delayed inflammatory responses. These reactions, termed *cutaneous basophil hypersensitivity* (Jones-Mote reaction), are primarily erythematous and skin associated.

Platelets, myeloid-derived, circulating, nonreplicating cells, arise by shedding from megakaryocytes in the bone marrow. Although their primary function is in blood clotting, platelets may undergo activation during inflammatory immune reactions. Following endothelial injury, platelets adhere to and aggregate at the endothelial surface, releasing mediators that increase the permeability and activate complement components that attract leukocytes. The leukocytes are then trapped and help produce vascular occlusion. In addition, activated platelets may release clotting and growth factors, vasoactive amines and lipids, and various hydrolases that further contribute to inflammatory responses.

26/4/2002

MEDIATORS

Hydrolases, including cathepsins, fucosidases, hexoxidases, and phosphatases, are primarily produced and stored in azurophilic granules of the neutrophils. In addition to antibacterial functions, these enzymes are involved in kinin generation, chronic inflammation, coagulation, thrombin formation, fibrinolysis (digesting clots), and plasminogen activation.

Myeloperoxidase is a hemoprotein present in azurophilic granules of neutrophils and monocytes. This enzyme exhibits toxicity microorganisms, tumor cells, erythrocytes, platelets, and other leukocytes. Oxidation products of the myeloperoxidase system can release vasoactive amines from platelets and mast cells and can inactivate chemotactic peptides.

Lysozyme is a prominent neutrophil enzyme that causes lysis of bacteria by affecting the bacterial wall constituents. The enzyme cleaves glycosyl bonds, thus breaking down the peptidoglycan cell wall of many microorganisms.

Neutral proteases, including cathepsin G, elastase, and collagenase, are also major components of the neutrophil azurophilic granules. Cathepsin G generates angiotensin from plasma, which constricts blood vessels, increases blood pressure, and may be involved in chronic granulomatous inflammation. Elastase and collagenase degrade elastin and collagen, respectively, and this affects the tissue matrix at the site of inflammation. In addition, elastase and collagenase affect complement, which acts as an amplification signal for inflammation.

Cationic proteins from neutrophil granules have trypsin-like activities. They potentiate the release of vasoactive amines, including histamine from mast cells, and produce irreversible aggregation of platelets.

Lactoferrin is a neutrophil-specific granule protein that binds iron and is bacteriostatic.

Major basic protein (MBP) is the primary component of eosinophil granules. This mediator is cytotoxic for parasites. It may also be involved in neutralizing heparin or DNA,

in stabilizing the binding of eosinophils to parasites, and in clotting or fibrinolysis.

Heparin and other proteoglycans are present in large quantities in mast cells. Heparin interferes with thrombin and a variety of other serum proteins involved in clotting. Heparin also has broad effects on inflammation.

Histamine, a dibasic vasoactive amine produced and localized largely in mast cells and basophils, is a principal mediator of immediate hypersensitivity. Histamine induces contraction of tracheobronchial and intestinal smooth muscle and increases vascular permeability of the skin and elsewhere, stimulates acid secretion in the stomach, and increases contractility and rate of heart function.

Serotonin is a major component of platelets and mast cell granules. Serotonin, to a weaker extent than histamine, affects vascular permeability and smooth muscle contraction. It also enhances delayed-type hypersensitivity skin reactions by promoting the emigration of sensitized lymphocytes through the vascular endothelium.

Complement fragments are produced during activation of the complement and coagulation systems and amplify the inflammatory response. They release histamine from mast cells and basophils, are spasmogenic for smooth muscle, increase the permeability of small blood vessels, and attract leukocytes.

Kinins are small basic peptides that alter vascular tone and permeability, decrease blood pressure, initiate or potentiate mediator release from leukocytes, and affect leukocyte motility. Bradykinin is one of the most active kinins and is as potent as histamine in increasing vascular permeability. The formation of bradykinin is related to three factors of coagulation [Hageman factor (factor XII), prekallikrein, and kininogen] that comprise the first step in the coagulation and fibrinolytic pathways. In addition, activated neutrophils release kinin-generating enzymes. The local injection of bradykinin produces pain, swelling, and inflammation. Many of the activities of bradykinin appear to be mediated through prostaglandin production.

Arachidonate metabolites are products of arachidonic acid metabolism in mammalian cells. LTC_4, LTD_4, and LTE_4 are the slow-reacting substances of anaphylaxis (SRS-A) and are produced by neutrophils, eosinophils, basophils, mast cells, and some monocytes. SRS is released from the cells by both immunologic (i.e., IgE on mast cells) and nonimmunologic (FMLP, cobra venom, zymosan) stimuli. The primary biologic activity of SRS is its spasmogenic action on smooth muscle. LTB_4 has potent chemokinetic and enzyme-releasing activities (i.e., neutrophil lysozomes). The major sources of LTB_4 are mast cells, basophils, neutrophils, and eosinophils. It is active in stimulating chemokinetic and chemotactic migration of neutrophils. 5-Hydroxyeicosatetranoate (5-HETE) product is the major lipoxygenase product from leukocytes and mast cells. These products are less potent than SRS and LTB_4 in their biologic activities. Biologically important cyclooxygenase products include prostaglandin D, E, and F (PGD_2, PGE_2, PGF_2), prostacyclin (PGI_2), and thromboxane A_2 (TXA_2). Leukocytes show marked differences in their ability to produce prostaglandins:

1. Macrophages and monocytes make large amounts of PGE_2 and PGF_2 and little PGD_2
2. Neutrophils make moderate amounts of PGE_2 and little PGF_2 or PGD_2
3. Mast cells and basophils make large amounts of PGD_2 and little PGE_2 or PGF_2

These mediators affect blood vessel tone, promote smooth muscle contraction or relaxation, and induce differentiation of immature lymphocytes and increased collagenase secretion by monocytes. Generally, PGE_2 is inhibitory for mature lymphocyte functions, release of inflammatory mediators from granulocytes, and platelet aggregation. TXA_2 (TXB_2) is primarily derived from platelets, macrophages, and monocytes. This mediator is a very potent vasoconstrictor causing constriction of tracheal and bronchial smooth muscle. The primary function of TXA_2 is to promote platelet aggregation. It may similarly have a role in neutrophil adherence as an important step in migration of the cells into inflammatory tissue sites. PGI_2 is primarily formed by vascular endothelium. This mediator is a potent vasodilator, inhibits platelet aggregation, and may act as a control agent for TXA_2. PGI_2 also potentiates the increased vascular permeability caused by other inflammatory mediators and is a potent inducer of pain.

Platelet-activating factor (PAF) is a family of lipids produced by basophils, mast cells, neutrophils, macrophage/monocytes, and platelets. PAF can be generated by both nonimmunologic and immunologic stimuli. In addition to platelet aggregation, PAF affects neutrophil aggregation and secretion, vascular permeability, and smooth muscle contraction. PAF is substantially more potent than histamine in producing acute inflammatory wheal and flare reactions.

Toxic metabolites of oxygen are produced by neutrophils, macrophage/monocytes, mast cells, basophils, and eosinophils. The reactive metabolites [superoxide $(O_2)^•$, H_2O_2, hydroxy radical $(OH^•)$] are capable of damaging microorganisms or tissues either directly or in combination with other components of neutrophils (i.e., myeloperoxidase). In neutrophils, the production of these metabolites is essential for microbicidal reactions. These metabolites may also contribute to inflammation by inactivating serum alpha-1-antitrypsin, which is an important factor for inactivation of leukocyte proteases.

Immune Response Systems

Vertebrates possess an immune system that recognizes and specifically protects against infectious microbial agents (bacteria, fungi, viruses, and parasites) in the environment. The immune system is divided into *innate* immune mechanisms, which provide a first line of defense, and *adaptive* immune mechanisms. Innate immunity is composed primarily of nonspecific inflammatory responses. If innate immunity is unsuccessful in eliminating pathogenic agents, the adaptive immune system produces a specific reaction to each agent. The adaptive immune system consists of various cells and molecules that are distributed throughout the body.

SYSTEMIC AND SECRETORY IMMUNE SYSTEMS—GENERAL

The adaptive immune response can be separated into reactions occurring in the internal secretions (i.e., serum, synovial fluid, gingival crevicular fluid) and those in the external secretions (i.e., saliva, colostrum, tears). The mucosal surfaces of the body provide an extensive surface on which pathogenic microorganisms make their initial contact. A variety of nonimmune and immune factors have evolved in this autonomous immune system to prevent colonization, invasion, and local disease. However, if this first line of adaptive immune responses is unable to eliminate the pathogen, the systemic immune system usually maintains host homeostasis.

SYSTEMIC IMMUNITY

Systemic immune protection maintains two basic defenses against foreign invaders:

cellular and humoral. Both respond specifically to most foreign substances, although one response generally is favored. The *cellular* immune response is primarily effective against intracellular viruses, fungi, parasites, neoplastic cells, and foreign tissue. The *humoral* immune response is active against the extracellular stages of bacterial and viral infections. The cellular immune reactions reside in cells of the lymphoid system, while the humoral immune reactions are associated with the fluid phase of blood (plasma or serum). The dual nature of the immune system is a consequence of two populations of lymphocytes. Individual lymphocytes recognize and respond to one or a few related foreign substances. In addition to lymphocytes, the immune system includes accessory cells, which trap foreign substances for presentation to lymphocytes and scavenge invaders.

Tissue and Structure

Cells responsible for immune responses are organized into the lymphoid system of tissues and organs. The lymphoid system is composed of lymphocytes and epithelial and stromal cells in discrete encapsulated organs or diffuse lymphoid tissue. Lymphocytes are derived from undifferentiated hematolymphoid precursor stem cells. They are first detected in the embryonic yolk sac and eventually lodge in the bone marrow.

The lymphoid organs, which contain lymphocytes at various development stages, are the central (primary) lymphoid organs and the peripheral (secondary) lymphoid organs. The central lymphoid organs are the major source of lymphopoiesis, the process by which lymphocytes differentiate from stem cells, proliferate, and mature. In mammals, the central lymphoid organs include the thymus, fetal liver and fetal bone marrow. Peripheral lymphoid organs provide the environment for lymphocyte-lymphocyte and lymphocyte-antigen interactions, as well as for dissemination of immune components. These organs include lymph nodes, the spleen, and mucosal-associated tissue (i.e., Peyer's patches of the gut).

Thymus ▪ The thymus, a bilobed organ located in the thorax, originates with cellular movement from the embryonic endoderm into the mesoderm. The thymic rudiment initially collects T-lymphocyte precursors from the blood and, throughout life, the hematopoietic tissues of the bone marrow provide a low level of thymic precursors. The

developed thymus has three layers associated with lymphocyte maturation. In the outer cortex, lymphoblasts interact with specialized epithelial cells to promote lymphoblast renewal and maturation of other thymic and T-cell subpopulations. The deep cortex mainly contains the lymphoblast progeny, which are nondividing, small thymic lymphocytes associated with dendritic cortical epithelial cells. The inner medulla comprises predominantly medium-sized, thymic lymphocytes, which interact with medullary epithelial cells and interdigitating dendritic cells. The dendritic cells appear to be important in the process of learning to recognize self-antigens. The thymic cortex in conjunction with a subpopulation of medullary T (thymus-derived) cells yield thymus cells with properties of antigen recognition, cell interaction capabilities, homing receptors for T-cell domains, and the primary immune functions of mature T lymphocytes. These T cells emigrate to the peripheral lymphoid tissues.

Bone marrow ▪ Hematopoietic cells in the fetal liver and bone marrow and adult bone marrow form B lymphocytes. The maturation of B cells from stem cells to small lymphocytes is initially controlled by antigen-independent inductive forces in the bone marrow. B-cell maturation is complete when they express surface immunoglobulin, major histocompatibility complex structures, and receptors for directed homing to secondary lymphoid tissues. In addition, the bone marrow contains a minor subset of pre-T lymphocytes, which provide a reservoir throughout life.

Lymph nodes and lymphatics ▪ The formation of lymphocytes in central lymphoid organs and their migration to peripheral organs is accomplished by two circulatory networks—the blood and lymphatic systems—which parallel each other throughout the body. Lymphocytes make up 70 to 80 percent of the nucleated cells in the blood and more than 99 percent of the nucleated cells in the lymphatic fluid (lymph). The lymphoid system has three principal functions:

1. To concentrate antigens into distinct structures

2. To circulate lymphocytes through tissues

3. To carry the products of the immune responses to the bloodstream and tissues

Antigens in the intercellular tissue spaces enter the lymphatic system and are carried to lymph nodes.

The typical lymph node is a bean-shaped organ consisting of an outer layer (cortex)

and an inner core (medulla). The cortex contains a sinus, which lies beneath the capsule of the lymph node and communicates with the sinuses of the medulla. The lymphatic vessels drain into the cortical sinus that is lined with phagocytic cells (macrophages), which sample and present antigen to lymphocytes. The cortex is densely packed with lymphocytes and is primarily the B-cell portion of the node. The paracortex underlying the cortex is the T-cell portion of the lymph node. Within the cortex are scattered, dense lymphocyte aggregations, termed *lymphoid follicles.* In an immune reaction, some follicles have foci of intense mitotic activity called *germinal centers* (secondary follicles). These contain dendritic antigen-presenting cells, some macrophages, a few T cells, and natural killer cells. These, together with specialized sinus macrophages, play a role in the development of B-cell responses and B-cell memory. The medullary portion of the node surrounds the hilus (blood supply and efferent lymphatics). The efferent lymphatics fuse into ducts that empty into the venous system.

Spleen ■ The spleen is a bright-red organ that lies at the upper left quadrant of the abdominal cavity behind the stomach and close to the diaphragm. There are two main types of spleen tissue: the red and white pulp. The red pulp removes and destroys dead erythrocytes, and the white pulp containing the lymphoid tissue provides an important (although not indispensable) element in the immune system. The lymphocyte passage through the spleen is via blood circulation. The splenic arterioles are surrounded by a pale mass of lymphoid tissue (white pulp) composed of T-and B-cell areas. The T cells are around the arterioles, and the B cells are further away. The B cells are localized in primary or secondary (stimulated) follicles, which possess a germinal center. Dendritic reticular cells and phagocytic macrophages are also in the germinal center. The dendritic cells and the specialized macrophages are critical for antigen presentation to the B cells. Some lymphocytes, especially maturing plasmacytes, pass from the white pulp into the red pulp where they enter the venous circulation.

Thus, the lymphocytes of the immune system migrate from primary to secondary lymphoid tissues. Once in the secondary tissues, the lymphocytes move from one lymphoid organ to another through the blood and lymphatics (Fig. 2–1). All lymphocytes return to the circulation from the lymph nodes via the efferent lymphatics which pass through the thoracic duct into the left subclavian vein. Lymphocytes also enter nonencapsulated lymphoid tissues (i.e., tonsils, Peyer's patches) and pass into the afferent lymphatics of the draining nodes. The lymphocytes enter the spleen via capillaries in the marginal zone and exit into the splenic veins.

Cells

All cells of the immune system arise from pluripotential stem cells through (1) the lymphoid lineage (lymphocytes) or (2) the myeloid lineage (phagocytes and other cells). Two major kinds of lymphocytes, T cells and B cells, provide different functions. There also appears to be a third lymphocyte type—the "null cells"—which do not correspond to either T or B cells. The three lymphocyte types can be separated functionally; however, morphologically the T and B cells are quite similar. The null cells can be distinguished by their numerous intracytoplasmic granules.

The lymphocytes are produced in the thymus and adult bone marrow at a very high rate. Some migrate via the circulation, where they constitute 20 percent of the total white blood cells, into secondary lymphoid tissues. Many mature lymphoid cells persist as memory cells for several years.

T Cells ■ In vertebrate embryos, the yolk sac followed by the fetal liver are the major sites of hematopoiesis. Cells from both sites migrate into the thymus. The immunocompetent T cells appear first in the thymus and later in the peripheral lymphoid organs. The T cells then migrate into the bloodstream, where they constitute about 60 percent of the peripheral blood lymphocytes. The T cells recirculate from blood to lymph node to thoracic duct and back to the blood. In the lymph nodes, the T lymphocytes reside in the deep cortex and areas between germinal centers (thymic-dependent areas). Some T cells considered to be a pool of long-lived cells also migrate from the blood to the spleen and back to the blood, and smaller numbers recirculate back to the bone marrow. The lymphoid cells must be continually renewed throughout adult life. This is accomplished by bone marrow stem cells capable of giving rise to T cells, and long-lived mature T cells. Adult bone marrow cells migrate to or are influenced by the thymus and mature into thymocytes with distinctive surface phenotypes and functional capabilities.

T-cell subsets ■ The T-cell population of

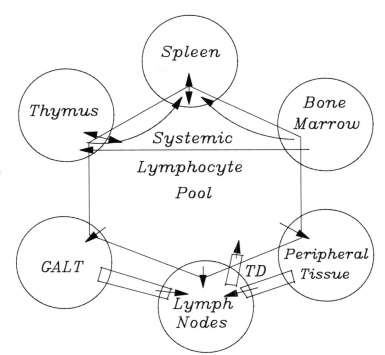

Figure 2–1 ■ Migration and pattern of lymphocyte flow.

mice, humans, rats, and other mammalian species have been separated into subsets based upon functional and phenotypic characteristics. T11 subsets have specific receptors that allow antigen recognition, not unlike immunoglobulin receptors on B lymphocytes. In addition, T cells require certain histocompatibility antigens in order to generate immune responses to the foreign antigens.

The T cells demonstrate phenotypic characteristics associated specifically with the T-cell surface or cytoplasm. Examples are TL (thymic leukemia) in mice; T6, T3, and T11 in humans; and OX7 in rats.

T-HELPER CELLS ■ These cells are involved in the activation of effector cells. They proliferate in response to foreign antigen and specific self-antigens (Ia) on accessory cells (i.e., macrophages). These cells induce both proliferation and maturation of B cells into antibody-secreting cells. Some T cells also secrete soluble factors (i.e., IL-2, T-cell replacing factor) that activate or help activate T and B cells. These cells may also induce delayed-type hypersensitivity reactions. T-helper cells are identified by certain phenotypic surface antigens. Examples are Ly1 and L3T4 cells in mice, T4 or Leu3a in humans, and W3/25 in rats.

T-INDUCER CELLS ■ Some T cells induce other T cells to become suppressor T cells

and appear to be involved in regulation of the immune response. In mice, they induce Ly1,2 T cells to become Ly2 suppressor cells. T-inducer cells (Ts1) can also be activated by immunization schedules that induce tolerance. These cells have common phenotypic characteristics. Examples are Ly1a and Ly2 cells in mice.

T-SUPPRESSOR CELLS ■ Several T-suppressor cells have been described. Suppressor-effector T cells bind antigen and release factors that inactivate T-helper cells. T-suppressor cells can (1) suppress delayed-type hypersensitivity reactions, (2) prevent proliferation and antibody secretion by antigen-binding B cells, and (3) suppress antibody secretion by some types of B cells. Examples are Ly2,3 in mice, T8 or Leu2a in humans, and OX8 in rats.

T-CYTOTOXIC CELLS ■ These cells recognize certain histocompatibility antigens and are capable of killing foreign cells (i.e., virus) and altered self-cells (i.e., tumor antigens). T-cytotoxic cells are important in the cytotoxicity of graft reactions and graft-versus-host reactions. Cytolysis requires direct contact between the T-cytotoxic cell and the target cell, which occurs as a result of antigen-specific receptors on the T cell.

T-CONTRASUPPRESSOR CELLS ■ These cells prevent the inactivation of T-helper and T-inducer cells by the action of suppressor-effector T cells. They are antigen specific and may be important in immunologic memory. Examples are Ly1 and L1,2 cells in mice.

T-CELL ACTIVATION ■ Following interaction of T cells with specific antigens or with mitogenic substances that stimulate most T cells nonspecifically, the T lymphocytes express their function and additional phenotypes. These phenotypes include Ia in mice and HLA-DR and TAC in humans.

B cells ■ B lymphocytes represent 5 to 15 percent of circulating lymphoid cells and are primarily defined by surface immunoglobulins. The B lymphocytes are common in areas of antibody production, such as the germinal centers of lymph nodes and diffuse lymphoid tissue of the gastrointestinal and respiratory tracts. They are less common in the blood, rare in the lymph and thoracic duct, and virtually absent from the thymus. Resting B lymphocytes, commonly found in the peripheral blood, are physically indistinguishable from T lymphocytes. T-lymphocyte development and maturation results in the formation of plasma cells, the antibody-producing cells of the body.

B-lymphocyte development ■ The early stages of B-lymphocyte development are identical with T-cell ontogeny. The pluripotent mesenchymal stem cells migrate to the yolk sac and differentiate along erythroid and myeloid pathways. Stem cell differentiation along the B-cell pathway begins later, with migration into special inductive microenvironments. Throughout life, the bone marrow remains the major repository of stem cells for B lymphocytes. There are two classes of lymphocytes with surface immunoglobulins, based upon their circulation and cell-turnover patterns. One class is primarily found in solid lymphoid tissue and is continuously and rapidly renewed every 2 to 3 days throughout adult life. These are mature, immunocompetent B cells that have not yet encountered antigen. When mature B cells are antigenically stimulated to divide, some revert back to small lymphocytes (the second class of B cells) and do not differentiate into plasma cells. These are relatively long-lived in the circulation, where they are easily triggered on subsequent encounters with the same antigen. These are termed *memory cells* and are responsible for the prompt, heightened antibody responses following secondary exposure to an antigen.

The differentiation of B cells is a multistage event defined by specific intracellular and surface changes. B stem cells in bone marrow differentiate into pre-B cells that eventually express IgM immunoglobulin on their surface and are termed immature B cells. These B cells then migrate from the marrow to peripheral lymphoid tissue, express surface IgD, and become fully mature, antigen-responsive B lymphocytes. Further differentiation into plasma cells requires interaction with antigen and generally T-cell help. This process leads to a gradual loss of surface immunoglobulin and conversion from synthesis of membrane-associated immunoglobulins to secreted immunoglobulins. The plasma cells produce and secrete several thousand immunoglobulin molecules per second; however, they seldom divide, and have a lifespan of 2 to 3 days. The bone marrow of most adult mammals contains B lymphocytes in various stages of development; however, the advanced stages of B cell development take place in the spleen and lymph nodes.

B-cell receptors and phenotypic markers

SURFACE IMMUNOGLOBULIN ■ Although B cells seem to be functionally homogeneous compared with T cells, various subpopulations can be defined based on surface markers. The principal B-lymphocyte marker is surface immunoglobulin. These molecules, synthesized by the B lymphocytes, are inserted into the surface membrane, where they act as specific antigen receptors. The majority of human peripheral blood B lymphocytes express both surface IgM and IgD antibodies. Very few cells express surface IgG, IgA, or IgE, although at specific locations in the body large numbers of B cells express these surface immunoglobulins. At maturity, each B cell secretes only one class of immunoglobulin that expresses a single antigenic specificity.

Specific antigens activate specific B-cell clones (cells from a single progenitor); however, the mode of antigen presentation is critical for successful B-cell responses. Some methods of presentation can even turn off B cells (i.e., tolerance). Thus, it appears that B cells require two signals for efficient triggering: a required *specific signal* (antigen receptor) and a *nonspecific signal* that aids in cell activation, differentiation, and proliferation (i.e., adjuvants).

To produce antibodies to most substances, B lymphocytes require help from T lymphocytes. However, a few antigens, called *thymus-independent antigens*, can trigger B cells directly. Such antigens are composed of repetitive subunits and probably function by cross-linking large numbers of surface immunoglobulin receptors. The T-independent antigens at low concentrations generally trigger IgM responses in B cells and do not usually promote production of memory B cells. Many T-independent antigens at higher concentrations are also mitogenic (nonspecific activators) for B cells and have been called *polyclonal B-cell activators.*

MITOGEN RECEPTORS ■ Mitogens are substances that induce cells to divide and, in the case of B cells, to secrete immunoglobulin nonspecifically. Some mitogens stimulate both T and B cells, while others only stimulate B lymphocytes (Table 2–1). The biochemical nature of the polyclonal B cell activator receptor is not known. Not all B cells can respond to each mitogen, and those that do, respond at different times during ontogeny. It appears that all B cells have receptors for LPS or dextran sulfate, or both. While the physiologic role of the polyclonal B-cell activators is unknown, since several are derived from bacterial cell walls, these responses may be important in host immunity.

T-CELL FACTOR RECEPTORS ■ Soluble factors produced by T cells can effect B-cell growth and differentiation. These include T-cell–replacing factor (TRF) and B-cell–differentiation factors (BCDF).

FC RECEPTORS ■ Certain cells bind immunoglobulin molecules by virtue of receptors specific for determinants located on the Fc (nonantigen, complement-binding) portion of immunoglobulin. Immunoglobulin binding occurs via a membrane receptor called the Fc receptor. Fc receptors primarily bind subclasses of IgG; however, some bind IgM. The primary role for the Fc receptors is thought to be the regulation of humoral immune responses.

COMPLEMENT RECEPTORS ■ Complement receptors have been identified in some but not all B cells from most mammals. Many memory B cells lack these receptors, and B cells lose them when they terminally differentiate into plasma cells. The function of the complement receptor is not completely understood; however, these receptors are thought to be important in concentration of antigen on B cells, enhancement of cell cooperation, receipt of the second signal in B-cell activation, and facilitation of cell-cell interaction.

MAJOR HISTOCOMPATIBILITY (MHC) ANTIGENS ■ One of the most important surface components expressed by B cells is a representative of the MHC complex (see section on histocompatibility systems, further on) termed Ia (murine) and HLA-DR (human). These serve as recognition elements in the interaction with antigen-activated T cells and antigen-presenting cells. They are generally expressed on precursor B cells and mature B cells and are lost during plasma cell differentiation.

OTHER ANTIGENS ■ The Ly1 (mouse) and T1 (human) antigens are primarily markers

Table 2–1 ■ Mitogens and polyclonal activators (PA)

Mitogen/Polyclonal Activator*	Target Cell	Source
Phytohemagglutinin (PHA)	T_H	*Phaseolus vulgaris* (red kidney bean)
Concanavalin A (ConA)	T_s	*Canavalia ensiformis* (jack bean)
Pokeweed mitogen (PWM)	T & B	*Phytolaca americana*
LPS	B	Gram-negative bacteria
Dextran	B	*Streptococcus mutans* & *Streptococcus sanguis* (synthetic)
Levan	B	*A. viscosus*
T-independent antigens	B	Pneumococcal polysaccharide (SIII), polyvinylpyrollidone (PVP)
Lipoprotein (LP)	B	Gram-negative bacteria
Nocardia water-soluble mitogen	B	*Nocardia*
Polynucleotides	B	Synthetic
Purified protein derivative (PPD)	B	*Mycobacterium tuberculosis*
Dextran sulfate	B	Synthetic
Epstein-Barr virus (EBV)	B	—
Protein A (PrA)	B	*Staphylococcus aureus*
A. actinomycetemcomitans	B	—
Polymeric flagellin	B	*Salmonella spp.*

*Mitogen is any substance capable of inducing a cell to begin DNA synthesis and cell division. Polyclonal activators are substances that activate large numbers of different lymphocytes, independent of their antigenic specificity. PBAs trigger B cells to a state of immunoglobulin secretion.

for T cells but are also present on a subpopulation of B lymphocytes. In addition, a subpopulation of human B cells has receptors for mouse erythrocytes (ME-R). The presence of ME-R and T1 defines immature B cells and their identification aids in the diagnosis of various immune disorders.

Monocyte series ■ Bone marrow–derived myeloid progenitors give rise to the cells of the mononuclear phagocyte system. This system includes the phagocytic macrophages, which remove particulate antigens, and the antigen-presenting cells, which present antigen to specific antigen-sensitive lymphocytes. Thus, these cells participate (1) in host defense against microorganisms, particularly obligate intracellular microorganisms; (2) as scavengers to remove damaged, dying cells and sequestered, nonmetabolizable inorganic materials; (3) in cellular interactions with lymphocytes; (4) as secretory cells involved in the production of biologic materials that regulate cellular functions; and (5) in control of neoplasms.

Monocyte development ■ The mononuclear phagocytes are composed of a number of functionally and morphologically distinct cell types including the bone marrow monoblast to the tissue macrophage. Monoblasts are normally seen outside the bone marrow only in monocytic leukemias. Promonocytes of the bone marrow are adherent, large, rapidly dividing and poorly phagocytic. In contrast, the monocyte is smaller and is found in the blood. The monocyte has a high rate of DNA synthesis and morphologically is difficult to differentiate from larger lymphocytes. These cells have lysosomes and often a characteristic horseshoe-shaped nucleus. They are also phagocytic with an activity between promonocytes and macrophages. The blood monocytes migrate into peripheral tissues where they enlarge up to 10 times and differentiate into macrophages or histiocytes. The term macrophage is generally applied to the cells found free in body cavities while histiocyte is applied to cells found fixed in tissues, especially the lymph nodes, spleen and liver. The macrophages are avidly adherent, have abundant cytoplasm filled with hydrolytic granules and are highly specialized for phagocytosis. The mature macrophage loses its ability to divide and is therefore a terminal cell.

Kupffer, Langerhans, and dendritic cells ■ Several populations of tissue macrophages develop which have some distinctive phenotypic and biologic characteristics.

Epithelioid cells, found in granulomas, arise from antigen-activated blood monocytes and are generally less phagocytic than macrophages.

Multinucleated giant cells are formed by the fusion of macrophages and have been characterized as either Langhans types with relatively few nuclei arranged in the periphery of the cytoplasm, or foreign body types with many nuclei dispersed throughout the cytoplasm.

Kupffer cells are long-lived resident liver macrophages situated at the interface with the bloodstream. This location affords first contact with immunogens arising in the intestinal lumen. They primarily ingest and degrade materials in portal blood and also clear the blood of a variety of toxic materials including bacterial endotoxins, microorganisms, activated clotting factors, and soluble immune complexes.

Alveolar macrophages line the alveoli and encounter inhaled pathogens. These cells have been shown to be effective in antigen presentation to T cells.

Dendritic cells are characterized by numerous long, slender processes and by irregularly shaped nuclei. These cells show little or no phagocytic activity but appear to be very effective in antigen presentation to T and/or B lymphocytes. Types of dendritic cells include lymphoid, follicular, and interdigitating cells.

Langerhans' cells, located in the epidermis, have a dendritic cell morphology and a Birbeck granule similar to interdigitating cells. They seem to interact preferentially with T cells and function in antigen presentation.

Monocyte series phenotypic characteristics

PHAGOCYTOSIS/PINOCYTOSIS ■ The ability of cells to contact, adhere to, and ingest particulate foreign materials is termed *phagocytosis*. Monocytes and macrophage/histiocytes are all capable of phagocytosis, while members of the dendritic cell type are nonphagocytic. The ability to ingest soluble materials, termed pinocytosis, is a function common to all these cell types.

FC RECEPTORS ■ Receptors for the Fc portion of IgG are detected on the surface of blood monocytes, macrophages, most tissue histiocytes, lymphoid and follicular dendritic cells, and Langerhans' cells. The veiled cells and interdigitating dendritic cells lack Fc. These receptors are involved in the phagocytic capability of these cells by enhancing contact between antigen and the phagocytes after IgG binding to the antigen. Some monocytes/macrophages also display an Fc receptor for IgE.

COMPLEMENT RECEPTORS ■ Receptors for complement component C3 are also found on monocytes, macrophages/histiocytes, lymphoid and follicular dendritic cells, and Langerhans' cells. The complement receptors, in conjunction with the Fc receptors, are important in the adherence and phagocytosis of microorganisms.

MAJOR HISTOCOMPATIBILITY (MHC) ANTIGENS ■ Ia (HLA-DR) antigens are generally present on most monocytes and macrophages. This antigen is critical for the antigen-presenting capacity of these cells.

ENZYME MARKERS ■ The presence of the cytoplasmic enzyme, nonspecific esterase, is one of the best markers for mononuclear phagocytes. Peroxidase is also an important marker of phagocytes and helps delineate different developmental stages of monoblasts, promonocytes, monocytes, and tissue (exudate) macrophages. In addition, a number of enzymes (5'-nucleotidase, leucine aminopeptidase) increase with activation of the cells.

BIOLOGIC FACTOR RECEPTORS ■ A variety of lymphocyte factors act on members of the mononuclear phagocyte series. These include interferon, macrophage migration inhibition factor, and macrophage activation factor. These factors and the macrophage response are thought to be important components of host immunity.

Lymphoid cell mediators ■ A variety of soluble mediators are produced by mononuclear lymphoid and myeloid cells. Principal mediators produced by B lymphocytes are immunoglobulins, which are secreted by a terminally differentiated B lymphocyte, the plasma cell. Members of the T-lymphocyte pathway produce lymphokines, which can activate B lymphocytes, macrophages, and other T lymphocytes. In addition, macrophage/monocyte cells release soluble factors called *monokines*. These substances have been shown to primarily affect T-cell functions.

Immunoglobulins ■ Immunoglobulins, or antibodies, are glycoproteins present in the serum and tissue fluids of all mammals. Their major function is to bind specifically to foreign or nonself molecules (antigens) such as microorganisms, parasites, and toxins and to affect their inactivation or removal from the body or both. They are induced when the host's lymphoid system contacts immunogenic (immune-stimulating) foreign molecules. To achieve this, the host has the capacity to produce a vast array of structurally similar, yet individually unique immunoglobulins. The immunoglobulins are part of the

adaptive immune system. Functionally, immunoglobulins interact selectively with the particular antigen that induced their production. Structurally, antibodies in their monomeric form are four-chain macromolecules containing two identical heavy (H) chains and two identical light (L) chains per molecule (see Fig. 2–2). The four chains are covalently linked by disulfide bonds. Each chain is made up of a variable (V) region and a constant (C) region. There are two domains in light chains (one variable region and one constant region) and four or five in heavy chains, depending on the class of heavy chain. The variable regions of the immunoglobulin molecules are the antigen-combining sites (Fab), and the constant regions (Fc) carry unique portions of the immunoglobulin molecule as well as important functional aspects. Five distinct classes of immunoglobulin molecules are recognized in most higher mammals, namely IgG, IgA, IgM, IgD, and IgE. These are differentiated by size, charge, amino acid composition, and carbohydrate content with structural differences in heavy chains. In contrast, all immunoglobulin classes have the same two forms of light chains (kappa or lambda).

ANTIGEN-ANTIBODY INTERACTIONS ■ The binding of antigens to antibodies results from multiple noncovalent bonds similar to interactions of enzymes with their substrates. Thus, while individual noncovalent bonds are weak, the multiple bonds produce considerable binding energy. These noncovalent interactions include hydrogen bonds, electrostatic interactions, Van der Waals bonds (i.e., dipole interactions of electron clouds), and hydrophobic bonds. The critical parameter is the requirement for minimal distances between the antigen and the antibody. Thus, the combination of these reactants requires suitable atomic grouping and a good structural fit so that several noncovalent bonds can form at once.

Antigens are molecular or cellular substances that can be bound by an antibody or an immune lymphocyte. Because of the limited area of an antigen-combining site on an antibody, only a small portion of the antigen actually interacts with the antibody. These discrete portions of the antigen that bind to the antibody's antigen-combining site are called *epitopes*. An *immunogen* is a material that has the ability to elicit an immune response. While all immunogens are antigens, not all antigens are immunogens. For example, low molecular weight materials called *haptens* cannot induce antibodies unless they

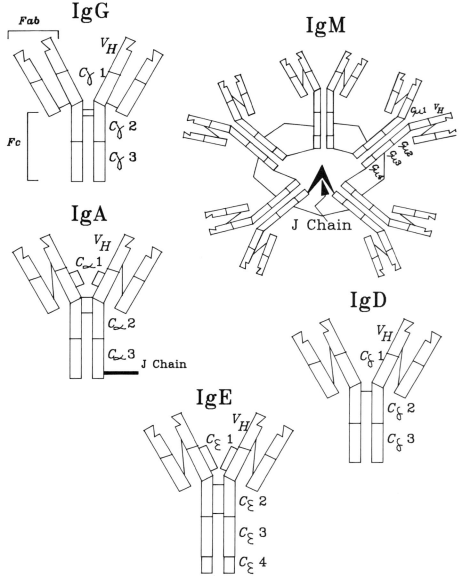

Figure 2–2 ■ Schematic diagram of IgG, IgM, IgA, IgD, and IgE structures.

are attached to carrier materials; however, they can bind to previously induced antibody.

Antibody valence describes the maximum number of antigen molecules that can be bound to each antibody molecule. Thus, IgG with two Fab sites has a valence of 2, secretory IgA (s-IgA) comprising two monomeric units has a valence of 4, and pentameric IgM has a valence up to 10. The valence of the antibody is important, when a single antibody molecule can bind multiple sites on the same antigen, thereby increasing the antibody-binding capacity for the antigen.

The *affinity* of an antibody is determined by the strength of a single antibody-antigen bond. The result of the interactions that take place between a multivalent antigen and a multivalent antibody is termed *avidity*. Therefore, the avidity of an antibody is dependent on the individual affinities of each antigen combining site and is generally greater than the sum of these affinities. The affinity and/or avidity of antibody increases during the maturation of an immune response to a particular antigen. This is accomplished by a switch from the initial IgM response to IgG production. In addition, there appears to be selective expansion of clones of high-affinity antibody producing cells during an immune response, presumably because of a greater ability of these cells to bind (high-affinity receptors) the decreasing amounts of antigen in the host.

A remarkable feature of antigen-antibody interactions is their *specificity*. Even minor structural differences in antigens are easily detected by antibody molecules. It is thought that the low cross-reactivity in antibody populations is a result of the enormous diversity of biologic molecules toward which the immune system responds. Antibodies produced by the immune system arise from the germline of the cells and are generated independent of antigen instruction. Contact with antigen simply selects and expands those cells that have the ability to bind that particular antigen.

A further feature of the immune response is that antibodies to an exceptionally large number of antigens can be produced. Also, synthesized compounds, which never before existed, stimulate specific antibody responses. This facet of the antibody response is described as *antibody diversity.* This diversity is accounted for by the fact that the genetic information necessary to code for antibodies is present in all B cells prior to contact with antigen. Thus, a rearrangement of the germline takes place in a single clone, producing a specific antibody.

A characteristic feature of the immune system is its ability to exhibit a more vigorous response upon second contact with an antigen. This is defined as *immunologic memory,* or the presence of a secondary (booster) response. Memory lasting up to 10 years can be generated to almost any antigen and is found for both humoral and cell-mediated immune responses. Immunologic memory can be explained by clonal expansion after primary antigen contact. Thus, upon a secondary challenge there exists a larger population of cells to respond to the antigen so that this memory exhibits three main features:

1. A shorter lag time until an immune response is detected

2. A higher level of immune reactivity to the antigen

3. A longer duration of immune response

TYPES OF ANTIGEN-ANTIBODY REACTIONS ■ A number of techniques can be used to examine the interactions between antibodies and antigens. Many of these procedures, while originally developed for immunologic investigations, are now used in many biologic fields. As a result of antibody specificity, these procedures can identify and discriminate among antigenic molecules.

Precipitin Reactions ■ Among the earliest observed properties of antibody molecules was their ability to form an insoluble complex with antigens. This precipitate is a result of formation of a cross-linked antigen-antibody "lattice" network. Precipitation studies performed in solution showed three zones of antigen-antibody reactivity. When there is more antibody than antigen (antibody excess) a precipitate is formed, but free antibody is still detectable. As more antigen is added, more antibody is incorporated into the precipitate, until a "zone of equivalence" is reached where no antibody or antigen remains in solution. With further addition of antigen, all antibody is bound, but a lattice (precipitate) is not formed and soluble immune complexes exist. This precipitin reaction has been modified by use of agarose gels to immobilize the precipitate.

Ouchterlony or double immunodiffusion uses a procedure where wells are cut into a shallow layer of agarose. Antiserum is added to one well and antigen to another well. As the materials diffuse radially through the agarose, a zone of equivalence is reached and a precipitin band formed. Where there are multiple antigen-antibody systems, multiple bands can be visualized. The antigenic relationship between various antigens can also be assessed using this procedure (Fig. 2–3). Following formation of the precipitin bands, one of three relationships will be observed:

1. *Identity*—If the arcs from two antigens fuse, the antisera is detecting identical epitopes on the two antigens.

2. *Nonidentity*—If the arcs from two antigens intersect and cross, the antiserum is detecting different antigenic epitopes on each antigen.

3. *Partial identity*—If the arc of one antigen fuses but the arc from the second antigen intersects, the antiserum is detecting a similar epitope on both antigens and a unique epitope on the second antigen.

Immunoelectrophoresis is another application of the precipitin reaction. This procedure incorporates immunodiffusion with the physical separation of antigens on the basis of charge in an electrophoretic field. The antigens are placed into wells cut in an agarose layer. An electric current is transferred through the gel, and the antigens move along the axis of the applied current (Fig. 2–3). Following electrophoresis, antiserum is added to a trough cut along the axis and the

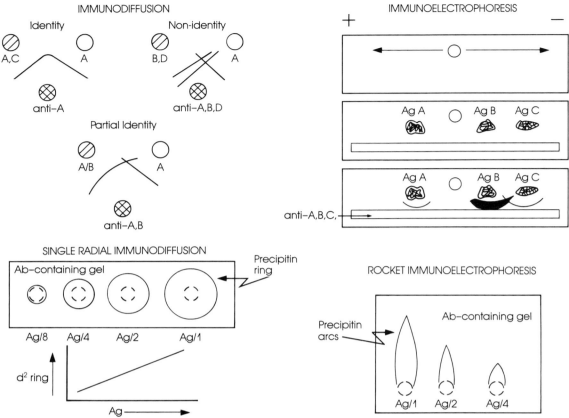

Figure 2–3 ■ Schematic diagram of ouchterlony double immunodiffusion (ID), immunoelectrophoresis (IEP), single radial immunodiffusion (SRID), and rocket immunoelectrophoresis (RIEP).

antigens and antibody diffuse until reaching a zone of equivalence where a precipitin arc is formed. Generally, this assay is not used as a quantitation of antigens but allows comparison of complicated mixtures of antigens, such as those in serum.

Single radial immunodiffusion is a method that utilizes a precipitin reaction to quantitate antigen in a sample. In this procedure, antibody to a specific antigen is incorporated into an agarose layer. The antigens are placed into wells and allowed to diffuse radially into the antibody-containing agarose. A precipitin ring is formed at the zone of equivalence and the diameter squared if the circle is proportional to the antigen concentration (Fig. 2–3). Absolute amount of antigen in unknown samples is determined by comparison to a standard curve from known antigen levels.

Rocket electrophoresis uses antibodies incorporated in agarose gel under pH conditions, rendering them immobile, while antigens added to wells migrate in an electric field. Based upon the concentration of the antigen, a zone of equivalence will be reached and a rocket shape formed (Fig. 2–3). This proce-

dure is used primarily to quantitate the amount of antigen in a sample using a monospecific antibody.

Two-dimensional immunoelectrophoresis incorporates both immunoelectrophoresis and rocket electrophoresis with antibody incorporated into an agarose layer. In this procedure, antigen is electrophoresed in one dimension in agarose. This strip is melded to a second agarose slab containing antiserum. The antigens are electrophoresed in a second dimension into the antibody-containing agarose. As zones of equivalence are reached for individual antigen moieties, an arc is formed based upon the electrophoretic mobility and concentration of the antigens. This procedure is qualitative for characterizing complex antigen or antibody populations.

Solid Phase Reactions ■ These techniques are exquisitely sensitive for quantitating antigens and antibodies. Generally, two types of solid phase assays are in common use: *radioimmunoassay (RIA)* and *enzyme-linked immunosorbent assay (ELISA)*. Many modifications of these procedures have been developed for specific uses; however, the standard procedure is designed such that an antigen is coated onto a solid phase material (i.e., polystyrene, polyvinyl, insoluble beads). An antibody (i.e., rabbit antiserum)–containing sample is then added to the bound antigen and specific antibody binds to the solid phase. The amount of antibody is determined by incubation with either a radiolabeled (RIA) or an enzyme-conjugated (ELISA) second antibody (i.e., goat antirabbit IgG) (Fig. 2–4). The radioactivity bound can be counted or a colorimetric enzyme substrate added so that the count or intensity of color is proportional to the antibody in the original sample.

Complement Fixation (CF) Test ■ The CF test is used to detect and estimate specific antibodies in serum. Since it is dependent upon complement fixation by the antibody, it can only measure IgM and IgG antibody. In this text, the known antigen is reacted with serum, followed by the addition of a standard amount of complement. If antigen-antibody complexes have formed, the complement is activated and consumed. The supernatant from this reaction mixture is then added to an indicator system composed of antibody-coated erythrocytes that lyse in the presence of complement. If antibody is absent in the test serum, the complement is available and will lyse in the indicator erythrocytes. Thus, the amount of lysis is proportional to the concentration of specific antibody.

Western Immunoblotting Assays ■ Another technique for analyzing the interaction between antigens and antibodies takes advantage of the ability of polyacrylamide gels to separate antigens based upon their molecular weight. Antigens are treated with sodium dodecyl sulphate (SDS), causing them to form as individual globular units. They are then subjected to an electric current through a slab of polyacrylamide which is termed *polyacrylamide gel electrophoresis* (PAGE). The antigens migrate in the gel according to their molecular weight with the smallest weight materials migrating farthest into the gel. A sheet of nitrocellulose is then placed against the gel and an electric current applied across the gel-sheet interface (Western electroblotting). In this manner, the antigens are transferred to the nitrocellulose sheets. Serum containing antibodies to the antigens is then layered onto the sheets and incubated. The antibodies will bind to the immobilized antigens on the sheets. The binding of antibody can be detected by incubation with either a radiolabeled or an enzyme-labeled anti-antibody probe. The antigen-antibody reactions are visualized on the sheets as individual bands. Generally, this procedure is used to identify individual antigens in complex mixtures or to describe the complexity of antibody specificities in a serum.

Reaction of Antibodies with Cells ■ The ability of antibody molecules to clump cells in suspension is called *agglutination*. Agglutin-

ELISA

1. Ag bound to plates

2. Add 1° Ab

3. Add enzyme conjugated 2° Ab

4. Add substrate

5. Spectrophotometric detection of color

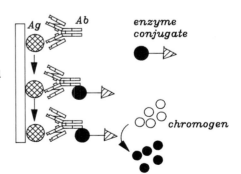

Figure 2–4 ■ Schematic of enzyme-linked immunosorbent assay (ELISA) and radioimmunoassay (RIA).

RIA

1. Ag bound to plates

2. Add 1° Ab

3. Add radiolabeled 2° Ab

4. Count radioactivity bound

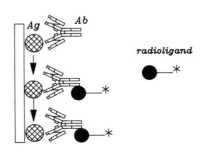

ation is a phenomenon of antibody binding to surface antigens of almost any cell. Similar to precipitin reactions, a lattice is formed between the antibodies and the multivalent particulate antigens. This procedure can provide an estimate of the level of antibody to a particular antigen. A more sensitive method of agglutination, *hemagglutination,* utilizes the ability of antigens to bind to the surface of erythrocytes. Specific antibodies reacting with the antigen coat agglutinates the erythrocytes. This procedure also provides a semiquantitative value for antibodies in serum.

The binding of antibody to living cells can also be assessed by their ability to kill the cells causing *cytolytic reactions*. This generally assays IgM and IgG antibodies. The assay can be designed so that the antigens are coated onto erythrocytes, and if there is antibody binding and complement activation, the erythrocytes are lysed. There are also assays in which antibody levels are determined by the ability of antibody and complement to cause lysis or death of gram-negative bacteria or to enhance phagocytosis and killing of gram-positive bacteria.

Antibody binding to cellular antigens can also be assessed using fluorochrome dyes or compounds that fluoresce under ultraviolet light. These compounds can be conjugated to antibodies and are especially useful for detecting autoantibodies and antibodies to tissue and cellular antigens. By *direct immunofluorescence,* the primary antibody is conjugated with the fluorochrome and added to the specimen. The *indirect immunofluorescence* test uses conjugates of a secondary antibody that is directed to the primary antibody (i.e., anti-Ig). Each of these procedures can be used to estimate the levels of antibody. These procedures are especially useful in detecting antibodies to different antigens primarily by differences in their cellular location. This procedure can also identify live cells in a suspension that carry a particular antigen. Extension of the fluorescence techniques has now become automated using fluorescence-activated cell sorters (FACS).

ISOTYPES, ALLOTYPES, AND IDIOTYPES ■ Antibodies are complex glycoprotein molecules that can also act as antigens. Thus, antiserum can distinguish among subsets of these molecules serologically. Isotypes are present in all normal members of a species. For example, genes necessary for coding for gamma, mu, alpha, delta, and epsilon immunoglobulin heavy chains are present in the human genome and are thus isotypic

(Fig. 2–5). Allotypes, on the other hand, are allelic variants at a specific locus for immunoglobulin polypeptide chains and are not found in all members of a species. Allotypes occur mostly as variants of heavy chain constant regions and generally are attributable to amino acid substitutions (Fig. 2–5). Idiotypes are antigenic determinants expressed in the variable region domain of immunoglobulin molecules (Fig. 2–5). Idiotypes are usually specific for a clone-derived antibody population (private idiotypes) or are shared among antibody clones with similar antigenic specificity (public idiotypes).

Anti-Idiotypes and Networking ■ In the immune system, networking involves a group of interconnected elements that regulate the system. The immune system must be capable of negative regulation so that responses to antigens or infectious agents do not proceed unchecked. Otherwise, the immune apparatus would be unable to respond to other stimuli, or the response could generate tissue destruction. Methods of this "down-regulation" in response to antigen include antigen elimination, generation of T-suppressor cells, and idiotype–anti-idiotype networks. In addition, the immune response must also be regulated to discrimate between self and nonself antigens. The conceptual basis of this regulation is by

1. Clonal deletion (e.g., during differentiation, contact with self-antigen eliminates self-reactive clones)

2. Generation of T-suppressor cells

3. Idiotype–anti-idiotype networks

The idiotype network functions by antibody acting directly on clones of other antibody producing cells. Thus, antibody (Ab1) formed to a particular antigen demonstrates a characteristic idiotype defined by the structure of the variable regions of the molecule. Other antibody clones respond to this idiotype of Ab1 and produce anti-idiotype (Ab2). This cascade can continue with the production of Ab3 (anti-anti-idiotype), and so forth. In this case the anti-idiotype antibody acts on the cells producing the idiotype antibody and down-regulates the synthesis of Ab1. Therefore, there are numerous avenues of regulating the immune response and this regulation is critical to host survival.

IgG and Subclasses ■ IgG is the predominant immunoglobulin in serum of higher vertebrates, composing 70 to 75 percent of the total immunoglobulin pool. IgG monomers have a molecular weight of approximately 150,000 and are composed of two light

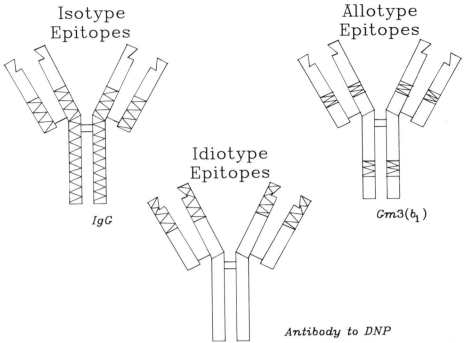

Figure 2–5 ■ Schematic diagram of immunoglobulin structure for isotype (i.e., IgG), allotype (i.e., Gm3[b$_1$]), and idiotype (i.e., antibody to DNP) determinants.

chains, either kappa or lambda, and two gamma heavy chains. The polypeptide chains are covalently bound to each other by disulfide bonds (Fig. 2–2). The light chains of the immunoglobulin molecule are composed of a constant region (C_L) and a variable region (V_L). The heavy chains of the immunoglobulin molecule are composed of a variable region (V_H) and three constant regions (C_H1, C_H2, C_H3). The V_H plus V_L regions comprise the antigen-combining portion of the Ig molecules. The C_H1 and C_H2 regions of IgG bind complement components. The structure of the C_H2 regions controls the catabolic rate of the immunoglobulin molecules. Binding to Fc receptors of macrophages and monocytes is related to the structure of the C_H3 region. The structural conformation of the C_H2 and C_H3 regions provides binding capabilities for staphylococcal protein A and Fc receptors on the placenta, neutrophils, and K cells. In all cases, these functional characteristics of the immunoglobulin domains are critical for the protective aspects of the antibody molecules.

There are four subclasses of human IgG: IgG$_1$, IgG$_2$, IgG$_3$, and IgG$_4$. These differences are attributable to the existence of distinct antigen epitopes on the heavy chains of the molecules, which are dictated by differences in the amino acid sequence of the chains. In

addition, the IgG$_3$ subclass has a longer heavy chain with an additional domain termed C_H4. The linkage of the light chains of IgG$_1$ also differs from the other IgG subclasses (Fig. 2–2). The subclasses of human IgG occur in serum in a proportion of approximately 65, 24, 7, and 4 percent, respectively. There are functional differences in the IgG subclasses resulting from the structural differences. IgG$_3$ is the most effective molecule for complement activation, while IgG$_4$ does not fix complement. All subclasses except IgG$_2$ can cross the placenta. IgG$_1$ and IgG$_3$ bind to the Fc receptors of monocytes and, as such, are effective opsonins, as well as being involved in antibody-dependent cellular cytotoxicity (ADCC) reactions. IgG$_2$ and IgG$_4$ subclasses can also bind to phagocytic cells when they are aggregated after binding to complex antigens. While responses to most antigens involve all four subclasses, it has been shown that the primary response to polysaccharide antigens is IgG$_2$. In contrast, IgG$_1$ and IgG$_3$ are the principal responders to protein antigens. IgG$_4$ antibodies have been associated with responses to allergenic types of antigen molecules.

Allotypes have been well defined for human IgG immunoglobulins of all four subclasses and are designated as G1m, G2m, G3m, or G4m, followed by a specific allelic type [i.e., G3m(5)]. In addition, human kappa light chains present as one of three allotypes [i.e., Km(1)]. Allotypes have not yet been identified for human IgA₁, IgD, IgE, or lambda light chains. Heavy chain allotype markers of the different isotypes are usually inherited together as a closely linked cluster referred to as a *haplotype*.

During the early portion of a primary immune response, relatively low levels of IgG are produced; however, IgG is the major antibody formed during secondary immune responses. IgG provides one of the principal defenses against bacterial infections in mammals. Its antibodies are effective neutralizers of toxins and viruses in the bloodstream and tissue spaces, and by complement activation can recruit phagocytic cells to a site of infection. IgG is normally distributed equally in the circulation and extravascular tissue fluids. IgG antibody has also been shown to be the exclusive isotype of antitoxin responses. This immunoglobulin isotype is also important in the neonate because it is the only isotype to cross the placenta and provide protection during the first few months of life.

IgM ■ IgM is the first immunoglobulin class to appear in the immune response, being the dominant form of antibody in the serum during the first week after an infection or immunization. IgM is the first antibody formed by the neonate and is incapable of crossing the placenta. Monomeric forms of this immunoglobulin function as antigen receptors on the surface of mature B lymphocytes. Serum IgM exists as a pentamer, having five monomeric units arranged radially with the Fc portions in the center and a molecular weight of 950,000 (Fig. 2–2). Each pentameric IgM molecule has associated with it one J (joining) chain, which is a glycopeptide (molecular weight 15,000) and which is produced by plasma cells synthesizing IgM. Two of the monomers are attached to the J chain, while the remaining three units are connected via disulfide bonds. IgM molecules also have an additional constant region domain on their heavy chains (C_H4), but lack a hinge region. The pentameric nature of the IgM antibody provides for a binding valence of 10 (i.e., number of Fab) and yields a molecule that is an exceptionally good antigen agglutinator compared with other immunoglobulins. IgM is also potent in complement fixation due to the ability of the early complement components to bind to several Fc regions simultaneously. IgM is

thus a critical immune component in combating bacterial diseases.

IgA and Subclasses ■ IgA composes 10 to 15 percent of normal human serum immunoglobulins, while it is the predominant immunoglobulin isotype in external secretions. In serum, IgA exists primarily as a monomer, but also may exist as various-sized polymers comprised of two or more monomeric units. Monomeric IgA has a structure similar to IgG, with two heavy and two light chains. Polymeric serum IgA contains a J chain, identical to IgM (Fig. 2–2). Serum IgA antibody responses have been identified to both protein and carbohydrate antigens, but the functional significance of the serum IgA antibody response is unclear. In contrast, the biologically important form of IgA is the dimeric form present in external secretions as secretory IgA (s-IgA).

In human beings, two isotypes (subclasses) of IgA have been identified in normal individuals, IgA₁ and IgA₂. IgA₁ is the major subclass found in serum, comprising 90 percent of the IgA molecules. Neither subclass fixes complement or functions efficiently as opsonizing antibodies. The hinge region linking the Fab to the Fc portions and providing a locus of flexibility between the regions in immunoglobulin molecules has been found to differ significantly between IgA₁ and IgA₂ molecules. IgA₂ molecules have a 13 amino acid deletion in this region of the heavy chain. A proteolytic enzyme produced by a number of microorganisms including *Streptococcus sanguis, Neisseria gonorrhoeae, N. meningitidis, Haemophilus influenzae,* and *Bacteroides* species has specificity for this hinge region sequence and is termed an *IgA₁ protease*. This enzyme has unique specificity for the IgA₁ molecule and may provide a pathogenic potential to these microorganisms.

No allotypes for IgA₁ have been identified; however, there are two allotypic forms of IgA₂—the A2m(1) and A2m(2) allotypes. Thus, individuals have either one or the other of these allotype markers.

IgD ■ IgD is a trace immunoglobulin in normal human serum (less than 1 percent). IgD is unique in its extreme susceptibility to proteolysis and even undergoes spontaneous degradation. The molecule is composed of two heavy and light chains with three constant domains on the heavy chains (Fig. 2–2). IgD appears to play a small role as an immune component in the serum. However, like monomeric IgM, IgD is found on the surface of a high proportion of B lymphocytes, especially in newborns. In addition, some B cells bear both surface IgM and IgD with the same idiotypic determinants. Thus, IgD appears to act as an antigen receptor on the membrane and is necessary for activation and maturation of B cells.

IgD does not bind complement, cross the placenta, or bind to phagocytic cells, owing to a lack of Fc receptors for IgD on cell surfaces.

IgE ■ IgE is found in extremely low concentrations in normal human serum, but dramatically increases in highly allergic ("atopic") individuals. This reflects the biologic importance of IgE in anaphylactic immediate hypersensitivity. This molecule has also been identified as the "reaginic antibody" in allergic reactions. It may also be important in protection from parasitic infections. The molecule is composed of two heavy and two light chains (Fig. 2–2). It lacks a hinge region, and the heavy chains contain an extra domain C_H4. The IgE molecule has a molecular weight of 190,000, is heat labile, and is extremely susceptible to disulfide-reducing agents. IgE does not cross the placenta and is unable to fix complement.

IgE is the major immunoglobulin involved in arming mast cells and basophils for their role in allergic reactions. The unique biologic functions of the IgE antibodies are localized in their Fc region. The IgE antibodies bind to the cell surface via specific receptors for the Fc portion of the molecule. Upon cross-linking of several IgE molecules by antigen, the mast cell or basophil releases vasoactive amines and other pharmacologic substances. The IgE molecule in serum has a short half-life of approximately 2 days. However, IgE bound to the cell surfaces lasts for longer periods of time and can result in prolonged hypersensitivity.

Complement ■ The classical complement system includes a complex group of 11 interacting blood proteins and glycoproteins found in all vertebrates. The alternative pathway comprises six serum components that are important in the initiation and control of this pathway (Fig. 2–6). The primary functions of these components are the production of inflammation, opsonization of foreign materials for phagocytosis, and direct toxicity against various cells and microorganisms.

CLASSICAL PATHWAY ■ The classical pathway of activation can be separated into recognition, enzymatic activation, and mem-

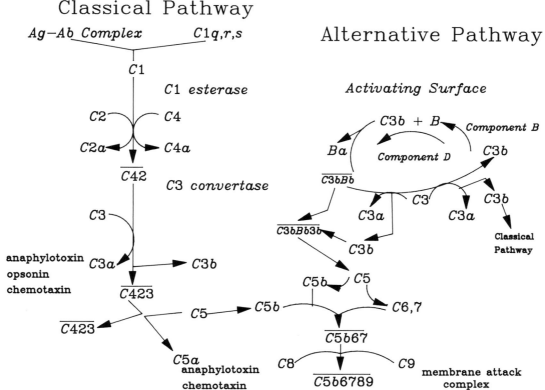

Figure 2–6 ■ Schematic diagram of the classical and alternative complement activation cascade.

brane attack sequences. The initiation is accomplished by recognition and binding of C1 to an antigen-antibody complex and the activation of the bound C1. The binding and activation of C1 leads to the generation of an enzyme—C1 esterase—that cleaves C4 into C4a and C4b. This step is a major amplification portion of complement activation, since a single C1 molecule can activate hundreds to thousands of C4 molecules. C4a is released, which can stimulate an anaphylactic reaction ("anaphylotoxin"). The C4b remains bound to the antigen-antibody-C1 complex. Numerous phagocytic cell types contain receptors for C4b and can actively phagocytize this complex. C4b also binds the C2 component, which is cleaved by activated C1 in the complex. C2a remains bound to the C4b fragment, and together they comprise an enzyme termed the *C3 convertase.* C3 is present in plasma in the largest quantities and fixation of C3 is the major reaction of the complement sequence. C3 is cleaved into C3a and C3b, the latter remaining bound to the complex. C3b also allows soluble and cellular immune complexes to bind to phagocytic cells bearing C3b receptors. This enhancement of phagocytosis is termed *immune adherence.* The C423 complex acts as an enzyme, C5 convertase, that has C5 as its substrate. C5 is cleaved, liberating C5a with C5b remaining bound to the complex and providing a site for binding of C6. C5bC6 is a stable complex in serum and can interact with nonsensitized cells leading to a phenomenon termed *reactive lysis.* C7 binds rapidly to C5b6 and is stable when membrane-bound for interaction with one molecule of C8. The C5678 complex can bind 8 to 11 molecules of C9, representing the "membrane attack complex" of complement activation. The C5678 complex polymerizes C9 to form a tubule that is highly amphiphilic, inserts into the lipid bilayer, and traverses the membrane. This activated complex can damage a wide range of membranes, including bacterial (gram-negative), mammalian, and synthetic lipid bilayers. This process leads to osmotic lysis and death of the affected cells.

Various cleavage products are major biologic molecules released by complement activation. C3a and C5a are termed *anaphylotoxins* because they cause histamine release from mast cells, resulting in smooth muscle contraction and vasodilation. C5a is 10 to 20 times more active than C3a in this process and possesses additional biologic functions. C5a is a major *chemotactic factor* for neutrophils, activates bactericidal capabilities of the neutrophils, and enhances neutrophil production of leukotrienes, thus prolonging the inflammatory response. C3a and C5a also effect immunoglobulin secretion, apparently interacting via the T cell. The complement cascade is also linked with proteins that initiate clotting and generate kinins, which are involved in the initiation and control of the "nonspecific inflammatory response."

ALTERNATIVE PATHWAY ■ The alternative pathway of complement activation is initiated without the participation of antibody or other elements of the immune system. It is not antigen specific and does not require an inductive period prior to its actions. The components of the alternative pathway collaborate to cause various immunologic responses, such as inflammation and phagocytosis, through the activation of C3. The activation of this pathway begins by an apparently random deposition of C3b on the surface of a cell or bacterium. The C3b will bind component B or C3 proactivator, which is synthesized by macrophages and lymphocytes. The C3b.B complex is inactive; however, in the presence of component D (C3 proactivator convertase), the complex is converted to C3b.Bb, which is similar to the C3 convertase (C142) of the classical pathway. This convertase cleaves C3 into C3a and C3b, which can interact further with components B and D, enter the classical pathway, or form an amplification C5 convertase (C3b.Bb.C3b). This convertase generates additional anaphylactic activity through C5a, as well as leading to the C5b-9 attack complex.

Three other proteins are critical to the regulation of this pathway: properdin (component P), component H, and component I. Component P enhances the alternative pathway by stabilizing the C3b.Bb complex. Component H down-regulates the system by impairing binding of B to C3b, by accelerating dissociation of Bb from C3b, and by facilitating conversion of C3b to an inactive form by component I.

The primary distinction between the classical and alternative pathways is that deposition of C3b is a random event (alternative) and does not require specific target recognition. Thus, host contact with a pathogen can immediately initiate the alternative pathway to provide protection, while specific immune responses are being developed to activate the classical pathway.

Lymphokines ■ Lymphokines are lymphocyte-derived soluble mediators released by both T and B lymphocytes. These can affect a variety of cells, including other lymphocytes, phagocytic cells, fibroblasts, and osteoclasts. Evidence suggests that only certain subsets of lymphocytes release particular lymphokines; however, the data are not conclusive. A summary of these different factors is presented in Table 2–2. These molecules are important in amplifying immune responses and protection against both infectious agents and abnormal host cell changes (neoplasia). Specifics on a few of the lymphokines follow:

1. *Interleukin-2 (IL-2):* IL-2 (originally called T-cell growth factor) is produced by activated, mature T lymphocytes, primarily of the T4 (helper) subset, and causes proliferation of all subsets of T lymphocytes. IL-2-stimulated T cells also secrete a variety of lymphokines, including interferon (IFN_γ), tumor necrosis factor (TNF_β), B-cell growth factor (BCGF), and B-cell differentiation factor (BCDF). The cytotoxic capability of the T cells can also be enhanced by IL-2. IL-2 also causes proliferation of large granular lymphocytes (LGL) with natural killer (NK) cell activity.

2. *Interferon (IFN):* IFN comprises peptides that promote nonspecific antiviral activities by making cells resistant to all viruses. The IFN also promotes cellular differentiation,

regulates immune reactivity, and inhibits cellular proliferation. There are three types of IFN: that which is nonimmunologically produced by T lymphocytes (IFN_α), that produced by virus-stimulated fibroblasts (IFN_β), and that produced by mitogen-activated or antigen-activated T-helper and T-suppressor lymphocytes (IFN_γ). The IFN molecules degrade viral RNA and inhibit viral protein synthesis. IFN also affects macrophage functions by increasing their antigen-presenting capacity, by increasing bactericidal and tumoricidal activity, and by decreasing their immunosuppressive capabilities. IFN can also suppress or augment cellular and humoral immune responses.

3. *T-Cell Replacing Factor (TRF):* TRF, primarily produced by T-helper cells, nonspecifically activates B lymphocytes, causing their differentiation. It also supplants the genetic restriction for T-B cell cooperation that normally exists.

4. *B-Cell Growth Factor (BCGF):* BCGF is a nonspecific factor, which is released by T-helper cells in the presence of macrophages and which synergizes with IL-1 to cause B-cell activation.

5. *T-Helper Factor (T_HF) and T-Suppressor Factor (T_SF):* These are antigen-specific T-helper and T-suppressor factors. The T_HF is produced by T-helper cells, target macro-

Table 2–2 ■ Lymphokines and monokines

Factor	Function
Monokines	
Interleukin-1 (IL-1)	T lymphocyte activation
	Fibroblast proliferation
Interferon α ($IFN\alpha$)	Virus inhibition
Angiogenesis (AF)	Microvasculature proliferation
Colony-stimulating (CSF)	Granulocyte, erythrocyte, megakaryocyte
B-cell differentiatiion (BCDF)	B lymphocytes
Tumor necrosis α ($TNF\alpha$)	Tumor cell killing
Genetically related (GRF)	Antigen specific T-helper cell activation
Ia-containing complex (IAC)	Binds to antigen specific T cells (proliferation)
Lymphokines	
Interleukin-2 (IL-2)	Killer cell activation
	T-lymphocyte activation
Interleukin-3 (IL-3)	T-lymphocyte activation
Interferon α & γ ($IFN\alpha$, $IFN\gamma$)	Virus inhibition
Allogeneic effect (AEF)	T-lymphocyte activation
T-cell replacing (TRF)	B-lymphocyte activation
Skin reactive (SKF)	Inflammation and mononuclear cell infiltration
Migration inhibition (MIF)	Macrophage movement
Macrophage activation (MAF)	Macrophage activation
Chemotactic (CFM)	Macrophage migration
Colony stimulating (CSF)	Macrophages & other tissues
Osteoclast activating (OAF)	Osteoclast activation
Lymphotoxin (LTF)	
Tumor necrosis β ($TNF\beta$)	Destruction of tissue cells

phages, and B lymphocytes resulting in B-cell differentiation (i.e., BCDF). T_sF is released by antigen stimulated T suppressor cells and suppress T cell function.

6. *Macrophage Inhibitory Factor (MIF), Macrophage Activation Factor (MAF), and Chemotactic Factor for Macrophages (CFM):* MIF is produced primarily by T-helper cells and maintains macrophages at the site of antigen. MAF is probably identical to IFN_γ and activates macrophages to enhance killing of intracellular microorganisms. CFM is also produced by antigen-stimulated T-helper lymphocytes and is responsible for recruiting macrophages into sites of antigen deposition. These lymphocytes can also produce the chemotactic factor that attracts neutrophils.

7. *Colony-Stimulating Factor (CSF):* CSF is produced by antigen- and mitogen-activated T lymphocytes. It stimulates growth and proliferation of granulopoietic cells and fibroblasts.

8. *Osteoclast Activating Factor (OAF):* OAF is produced primarily by T-helper lymphocytes. This factor activates osteoclasts, leading to enhanced bone resorption. Recently, extensive structural homology has been shown between OAF and IL-1.

9. *Tumor Necrosis Factor (TNF):* TNF_β, originally called lymphotoxin, is produced by cytotoxic T lymphocytes. This factor is released by both antigen- and mitogen-stimulated T cells and nonspecifically affects other cells. In vitro TNF_β kills tumor cells and can be toxic for other adjoining cells (i.e., fibroblasts). Its in vivo significance has not yet been determined.

Monokines ■ Monokines are products of macrophages involved in antigen processing and presentation. These monokines are soluble protein factors that modulate immunologic and inflammatory responses by regulating growth, mobility, and differentiation of numerous cell types (Table 2–2). Representative monokines are described here:

1. *Interleukin-1* (IL-1): IL-1, previously called lymphocyte activating factor (LAF) or thymocyte activating factor (TAF), is produced by a variety of cells including macrophages in response to specific antigen-processing and nonspecific agents (i.e., LPS). IL-1 provides the "second signal" necessary for T_H activation and allows the T_H cells to interact with B lymphocytes. IL-1 also enhances immune responses by promoting other T-cell functions, such as stimulating B lymphocytes to increase surface immunoglobulin receptors and to increase production and secretion of antibody, promoting the specific toxic effects of cytotoxic T lymphocytes, and enhancing nonspecific killing of tumor cells. IL-1 is chemotactic for neutrophils and increases neutrophil activity following their mobilization to the antigen site. IL-1 stimulates both proliferation and the production of collagenase by fibroblasts, thus providing an influence on inflammatory fibrosis and wound healing. Finally, IL-1 can also promote bone resorption and may be homologous to OAF.

2. *Tumor Necrosis Factor* (TNF_α): TNF_α is a glycoprotein produced by activated macrophages, which causes extensive hemorrhagic necrosis of tumors in vivo without damaging normal cells and, which may play a role in tumor immunity.

Macrophages also produce a variety of other monokines including angiogenesis factors, colony-stimulating factors for granulocytes and macrophages, IFN_α, and factors that suppress T- and B-lymphocyte function.

SECRETORY IMMUNITY

Shortly after birth, the mucosal surfaces of the upper respiratory tract, the intestinal tract, and the genital tract become colonized by a variety of microorganisms. Most become established as the indigenous or normal microflora. In health, all of the mucosal surfaces contain remarkable barriers against attachment, colonization, and disease by invading bacterial pathogens. When these protective mechanisms are compromised, pathogenic microorganisms quickly produce disease by invading deeper tissues or excreting toxins that damage tissues. Predominant among the immune components are antibodies in the secretions that bathe the mucosal surfaces of the body. These secretory antibodies play an essential biologic role because they interact with a large variety of viable and nonviable materials deposited on mucous membranes. Thus, the mucosal immune system provides a "first line of defense."

Tissues and Structure

Oral lymphoid tissues and tonsils ■ The group of lymph nodes including the tonsils and adenoids in the oropharyngeal area is called Waldeyer's ring of lymphoid tissue. Both extraoral lymph nodes and intraoral lymphoid tissue aggregates are associated with the oral cavity. The extraoral lymph nodes are crucial for drainage of the materials from the gums, teeth, and oral mucosa. The lymphatics drain into various lymph nodes, including cervical, submandibular, and pharyngeal.

While the intraoral lymphoid tissue is not well organized, there are four types of aggregates of lymphoid tissue in the oral cavity.

1. The "palatine tonsils," "lingual tonsils," and "adenoids" (pharyngeal tonsils) are important components in defense against orally ingested microorganisms. Microorganisms are trapped in the tonsils, where they elicit an immune response prior to penetration of the body. These structures contain organized lymphoid follicles that contain mature B lymphocytes.

2. "Scattered submucosal lymphoid cells" beneath the mucosa may be stimulated to proliferate into discrete lymphoid tissue.

3. "Salivary gland lymphoid tissue," mainly B cells and IgA plasma cells, includes both major (parotid, submandibular, sublingual) and minor salivary glands.

4. "Gingival lymphoid tissue" results from host responses to accumulations of bacteria in plaque. As the plaque increases to induce gingivitis, the neutrophils increase and lymphocytes (primarily T cells) appear in the local tissues. Further development of the disease process is accompanied by B-cell and plasma-cell infiltration.

Peyer's patches ■ In addition to the major lymphoid tissues and organs described for the systemic immune system, there are also aggregates of nonencapsulated lymphoid tissue, especially in the submucosal areas of the respiratory, gastrointestinal, and genitourinary tracts. These areas range from loose clusters of a few cells in the lamina propria, to organized lymphoid follicles, to more complex aggregates like the appendix, tonsils, and Peyer's patches. These lymphoid structures normally provide the main portal of entry into the body for foreign microorganisms.

Peyer's patches are compact nodes of lymphoid cells in the outer wall of the intestine with a discrete T and B cell–dependent area, lymphoid follicles, and germinal centers. The Peyer's patches primarily give rise to B lymphocytes committed to IgA synthesis, which migrate to mucoepithelial surfaces of the body. The lamina propria of the gut also contains B cells, plasma cells, T-helper cells, and cytotoxic cells and macrophages. Intraepithelial lymphoid cells are primarily large granular lymphocytes that can be involved in both ADCC and NK activities.

Salivary (secretory glands) ■ In addition to the plasma cells critical to production of IgA antibodies in salivary secretions, these glandular tissues also contain T-helper and -suppressor cells; mature B cells of the IgA, IgG, and IgM isotypes; and macrophages. Therefore, the salivary glands, as representative tissues of secretory immunity, appear to provide all of the cellular mechanisms necessary to mount a local immune response following antigen challenge.

Homing and cellular migration in the mucosal system ■ A mechanism for controlling and focusing IgA responses in the mucosal immune system involves the migration and homing of IgA B cells to mucosal sites. In this system, following antigen stimulation, local B cells differentiate to s-IgA-bearing cells that are precursors to mature IgA B cells and plasma cells secreting IgA. Few IgA plasma cells are found in the Peyer's patches, however, owing to the antigen-initiated rapid emigration of the IgA precursor cells. The cells pass into the local draining lymph nodes (mesenteric lymph nodes), differentiate and mature into IgA blast cells, and migrate through the lymphatics and thoracic duct into the blood. From this point, the IgA cells home to mucosal tissues and develop into IgA plasma cells. The effect of this migration is to distribute sensitized cells to other mucosal sites where they can interact with the sensitizing antigen (Fig. 2–7). In addition to the generalized migration of cells throughout the mucosal system, there is also some tissue localization. Thus, cells sensitized in the bronchi have a predilection for the respiratory lamina propria. T cells also have been shown to migrate out of the mucosal follicles and specifically home to other mucosal sites.

Various mechanisms for this homing phenomenon have been suggested:

1. Specific receptors on the homing cells (i.e., s-IgA)

2. Selective proliferation of cells at mucosal sites

3. Differential distribution of antigen at mucosal sites

4. Recognition sites on endothelial cells that are necessary for cellular localization and passage into the tissues

Recognition sites on the endothelial cells appear critical for binding of migrating cells and passage of the cells into the tissues. While the initial entry of cells into the mucosal tissues is antigen-independent, trapping and proliferation of the cells in the tissues appears to be antigen-directed.

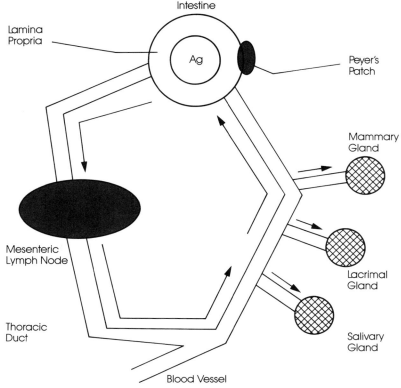

Figure 2–7 ■ IgA cellular homing and schematic of common mucosal immune system.

Nonspecific Defenses at Mucosal Surfaces

Specific and nonspecific defenses at mucosal surfaces interact with potential pathogens. The nonspecific defenses are represented by the flushing and cleansing mechanisms of secretions and luminal contents. The desquamation of the cells with attached bacteria also eliminates bacteria from mucosal surfaces. Mucus, a viscous fluid secreted by goblet cells and mucous glands, forms a protective coating over the entire mucosal surface. It can cover receptors for bacteria on epithelial cells and prevent their adhesion.

Immunoglobulin Defenses at Mucosal Surfaces

Secretory IgA (s-IgA) ■ The predominant immunoglobulin in external secretions including mammary secretions, saliva, tears, perspiration, and gastrointestinal, genitourinary and respiratory secretions is secretory IgA. Plasma cells in or near the epithelial cells of the mucosal surfaces secrete dimeric IgA composed of two IgA monomers attached by a J chain (Fig. 2–8A). This J chain is necessary for polymerization of both IgA

and IgM and is produced by the plasma cells. The secreted dimeric IgA attaches to the basal epithelial cell surface through interaction of the J chain with a special receptor termed the *secretory component* (SC). SC is a normal constituent of s-IgA molecules and is also found free in secretions. SC is a glycoprotein (molecular weight 70,000) synthesized by epithelial cells as an integral membrane protein. After binding dimeric IgA, SC is endocytosed in a membrane vesicle that migrates to the luminal surface of the epithelial cell. The transmembrane SC is then cleaved by proteolysis with a fragment of the SC precursor remaining covalently bound to the IgA dimer (Fig. 2–8B). The intact s-IgA molecule in secretions has a molecular weight of approximately 380,000. The SC not only provides a mechanism for transport of the IgA into the external secretions but also helps provide increased resistance to proteolytic degradation of the s-IgA in the secretions.

s-IgA$_1$ and s-IgA$_2$ are present in nearly equal quantities in external secretions. Similar to serum IgA, the secretory immunoglobulin does not fix complement and is a poor opsonin. s-IgA has antibody activity to bacteria, viruses, and fungi that colonize mucosal surfaces, and provides protection

SIgA

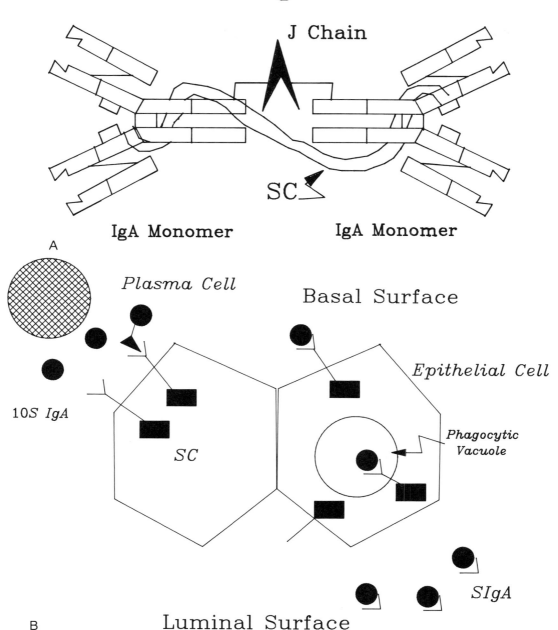

Figure 2–8 ■ *A*, Structure of SIgA, and *B*, transport mechanism.

against diseases caused by *Streptococcus mutans*, *Vibrio cholerae*, *Shigella dysenteriae*, poliovirus, influenzae viruses, and rhinoviruses. This protection occurs by "blocking" the ability of the organisms to adhere and colonize mucosal surfaces. Also, s-IgA blocks absorption of antigenic molecules across the gastrointestinal tract and may function in limiting allergic responses to common food antigens.

IgG, IgM, and IgE in secretions ■ IgM is synthesized locally in several secretory tissues, as indicated by the predominance of IgM versus IgG plasma cells in the tissues, and high IgM concentrations relative to IgG in certain exocrine fluids. Generally more than 75 percent of IgM remains in the circulatory system, while more than 50 percent of IgG is found extravascularly in the body; thus, the IgM must be selectively transported out of serum, or a mechanism of local synthesis is required. In addition, IgM binds secretory component and presumably can be selectively transported into secretions by a mechanism analogous to IgA. This capability is especially important in selective IgA deficiency where there is a predominance of IgM in secretions and IgM plasma cells in secretory tissues. This provides protection at mucosal surfaces and has been termed *compensatory immunity*.

IgG is a quantitatively important component in many secretions, and in systems such as bovine colostrum, immunoglobulins other than IgG are barely detectable. Mucosal immune responses to viral antigens in the upper respiratory tract often involve high IgG antibody titers from local synthesis and transport of serum into the local sites.

IgE plasma cells are rare in lymphoid tissues. However, large numbers of IgE cells occur in the lamina propria of the respiratory and gastrointestinal mucosa. This suggests that IgE is synthesized primarily in secretory sites, and while the IgE concentration in saliva is lower than other immunoglobulins, the ratio of salivary to serum IgE is the greatest.

Host Responses

All vertebrates possess an immune system that protects the host from pathogenic microorganisms and parasites and from neoplasms. The immune system recognizes and selectively eliminates foreign materials from the host. To survive in a relatively hostile environment, the host has developed a variety of nonspecific and specific mechanisms for elimination of pathogenic microorganisms.

BENEFICIAL RESPONSES

Antibacterial

Nonspecific antibacterial effects ■ The nonimmunologic methods of host resistance, sometimes termed "innate" or "natural" immunity, can be anatomic or systemic:

1. The low skin surface pH and its general dryness inhibit bacterial growth.
2. Epithelial desquamation, mucus barrier, ciliary activity, pH of the lumen, and fluid flow of the mucous membranes limit bacterial colonization.
3. Lysozyme, a basic peptide in high concentrations in many secretions, including saliva, hydrolizes the mucopeptide of bacterial walls and is bactericidal.
4. Lactoferrin—a blood protein that binds iron, which is necessary for the growth of many microorganisms—is a nonspecific bacteriostatic agent.
5. Salivary glycolipids compete with bacteria for attachment to host tissues.
6. A variety of fatty acids in secretions cause osmotic lysis of some microorganisms.
7. Beta lysin, a cationic platelet protein, is lytic for gram-positive bacteria.
8. Leukin and plakin, basic polypeptides produced by neutrophils and platelets, respectively, are general bactericidal agents.
9. NK cells provide a bridge between innate (natural) immunity and acquired immunity.

Chemotaxis, diapedesis, and phagocytosis ■ The most important element in host resistance to infectious disease is phagocytosis. Phagocytosis, a specialized form of pinocytosis, is mediated principally by polymorphonuclear leukocytes (neutrophils) and macrophages. Both are attracted to infections by a variety of soluble chemotactic factors.

Chemotaxis is the process of attraction of phagocytes to sites of inflammation. The phagocytes actively migrate toward chemoattractant molecules. Chemotactic agents are both bacterial derived, such as N-formyl-methionyl-leucyl-phenylalanine (FMLP), and host derived, such as C5a resulting from complement activation. The chemotactic peptides diffuse into the adjacent capillaries and induce adherence of passing phagocytes to the endothelium.

Following adherence, phagocytes insert pseudopods between the endothelial cells, dissolve the basement membrane and traverse the blood vessel wall, a process termed *diapedesis*.

The phagocytes then pass out of the blood vessel and move along the chemotactic gradient toward the site of inflammation. Once there, the phagocytes must recognize and form stable contacts with particles to be ingested. Stable contacts result from the trapping of the particles against other cells (*contact phagocytosis*). A second and most efficient method of enhancing a stable contact is by *opsonization*, whereby the particle is bound to the phagocyte surface by macromolecular interactions. Nonspecific receptors have been identified on the surface of phagocytes that will bind bacteria and enhance contact. Certain microorganisms also activate the alternative complement pathway, resulting in attachment of complement components, which then enhance contact. By far the most efficient opsonins are antibodies that specifically bind to bacterial surfaces and then attach to Fc receptors on the phagocyte surface.

The next step in phagocytosis after stable contact is ingestion of the particle. The phagocytes are highly motile cells and binding of the foreign material to the cell surface causes a temporary immobilization of a portion of the plasma membrane. The adjacent membrane continues to move, resulting in an outward movement of the membrane and formation of a phagocytic vacuole or *phagosome*. After the phagosome detaches from the plasma membrane it moves into the interior of the phagocyte and fuses with a lysosomal granule, forming a *phagolysosome*. The lysosomal contents are thus available to initiate microbial destruction.

Specific antibacterial effects ■ When bacteria enter host tissues, the immunologic mechanisms activated depend upon the nature of the microorganisms and the disease caused (Table 2–3). The pathogenicity of certain noninvasive infections on mucosal and epithelial surfaces is dependent upon the release of soluble protein factors called *toxins* ("toxigenic infection"). Bacterial toxins are generally highly immunogenic and the primary immune defense involves neutralization of the toxins by antibody. Antibodies may also inhibit epithelial adhesion or act as

Table 2–3 ■ Types of bacterial, viral, fungal, and parasitic infections and host protective response

Infection	Pathogenesis	Host Defense
Bacterial		
Toxigenic	Toxin	Neutralizing Antibody
Corynebacterium diphtheriae		Antibody blocks adherence
Vibrio cholerae		
Acute		
Neisseria meningitidis	Bacteremia	Opsonizing antibody and complement lysis,
Staphylococcus aureus	Tissue inflammation	opsonizing antibody, complement, and killed by phagocytes
Chronic		
Mycobacterium tuberculosis	Invasive and locally toxic	Macrophage activation by T cells
Viral		
Cytolytic		
Rhinovirus	Cell lysis	Systemic and secretory antibody
Enterovirus (polio virus)		
Vaccinia (smallpox)		
Steady-State (Latent):		
Herpes simplex	Intracellular replication	Cell-mediated immunity
Varicella-zoster	Budding of virus	Systemic antibody
Rubella	Cell death	
Rubeola		
Integrated		
DNA viruses		
Polyoma	Viral antigens on host cells	Cell-mediated immunity
SV-40		
EBV		
Parasitic		
Intracellular		
Leishmania spp.	Destruction of tissue cells	Cell-mediated immunity
Toxoplasma gondii		
Plasmodium spp.		Antibody blocks invasion, opsonins for phagocytosis
Blood and Intracellular		
Trypanosoma cruzi	Destruction of tissue cells	Cell-mediated immunity, antibody vs blood stage
Blood		
Trypanosoma gambiense	Tissue inflammation	Antibody and complement
Trypanosoma rhoesiense		Lysis; antibody opsonins for phagocytosis
Intestinal		
Entamoeba histolytica	Local and systemic tissue damage	Secretory antibody

opsonins for increased bacterial phagocytosis and killing. Various bacteria exhibit this type of pathogenicity, including *Staphylococcus aureus* (skin infection, food poisoning, toxic shock syndrome), *Vibrio cholerae* (intestinal infection), *Corynebacterium diphtheriae* (pharyngitis), and *Clostridium botulinum* (toxin inhibits neuromuscular communication).

Acute or pyogenic infections are caused by invasive microorganisms so that immunity to the bacteria requires that it be killed. Gram-negative bacteria such as *Neisseria meningitidis*, *N. gonorrhoeae*, and *Hemophilus influenzae* can be killed by specific antibody with complement activation. In contrast, gram-positive microorganisms such as streptococci and staphylococci are refractory to complement-mediated lysis as a result of their cell walls. The major defense against these microorganisms is phagocytosis potentiated by opsonic antibody and complement. Generally, infections by these bacteria attract large numbers of phagocytic cells. However, these bacteria are relatively resistant to phagocytosis, so that pus can accumulate at the foci of infection (i.e., pyogenic, or pus-generating).

Chronic or intracellular infections such as tuberculosis and leprosy are caused by bacteria that are resistant to killing by polymorphonuclear leukocytes and macrophages and elicit poor antibody responses. The principal mechanism of immunity in these diseases is by T-cell–mediated inflammatory reactions. The T cells are activated by bacteria or bacterial antigens on the surface of infected macrophages to release lymphokines that enhance the macrophages' ability to kill the intracellular parasite. An undesirable side effect is local tissue damage, as in tuberculosis. Another group of intracellular bacterial parasites are the *Chlamydiae*. These microorganisms can be phagocytosed by host cells and are capable of destroying the ingesting cells. However, in the presence of opsonizing antibody, the phagocytes are able to kill the bacteria.

Antiviral

Immunity to viral infections is primarily a result of specific neutralizing antibody which binds to extracellular viruses (Table 2–3). This neutralization can take place at mucosal surfaces via s-IgA antibody or in the circulation via IgG and IgM antibody. A "latent infection" such as a herpes infection occurs when a virus enters a cell, remains dormant, and then is later reactivated. With the sustained intracellular and extracellular phases, both antibody and cell-mediated responses appear operative in immunity. In addition, a combination of the two pathways of response may be critical in immunity to certain viral infections. This process, termed *antibody-dependent cellular cytotoxicity*, is controlled by antibody binding to viral-infected cells and subsequent killing of the cells by K (killer) cells. "Integrated" viral infections are those in which the viral genome becomes part of the host genetic apparatus. Generally, viral particles are not released in these infections, but both viral-specific antigens or modified host antigens can be expressed on the cell's surface. Immunity to this type of viral infection (i.e., polyoma, SV40, Epstein-Barr) is generally associated with cell-mediated immune responses by functioning T lymphocytes and macrophages.

Interferons produced by many cell types in response to viral infections inhibit viral infection of healthy cells, thus limiting the infection.

Antifungal

The precise immune mechanisms in fungal infections are not well understood but appear to be similar to antibacterial immunity. Human fungal infections are divided into three types:

1. "Superficial mycoses" are usually restricted to the nonliving keratinized portions of skin, hair, and nails. Recovery is generally not immunologically mediated but rather a result of treatment with topical antifungal agents.

2. "Subcutaneous mycoses" cause chronic nodules or ulcers in the subcutaneous tissues, generally following trauma. These are usually self-limiting infections with some resistance based upon cell-mediated immunity.

3. "Respiratory mycoses" produce subclinical or acute lung infections and rarely disseminate. Resistance appears to be T-cell mediated because of the presence of delayed hypersensitivity reactions to fungal antigens and the ability to transfer resistance with immune T cells. It has been suggested that activated T cells secrete lymphokines that activate macrophages to phagocytize and kill the fungi.

Candida albicans is a commensal microorganism that can cause superficial infections of the skin and mucous membranes. This fungus exerts its primary pathogenicity in situations in which the T-cell–mediated immune capacity is undermined or the normal microflora is disrupted, as with antibiotics.

However, as with the other fungal infections, the cell-mediated arm of the immune system appears to be critical in host resistance.

Antiparasitic

Parasitic infections are a major health problem in most parts of the world. The major parasite-induced diseases of human beings are listed in Table 2–3. These parasites typically stimulate more than one immunologic defense mechanism. In addition, important nonimmunologic factors may be critical in resistance to certain parasites (see Chapter 24).

DESTRUCTIVE HYPERSENSITIVITY REACTIONS

Under certain circumstances, exposure to antigen can result in complex immunologic events that are deleterious to the host. These reactions which take place in an exaggerated or inappropriate manner and may involve both lymphocytes and antibodies are termed *hypersensitivity reactions*. The tissue damage from hypersensitivity reactions is primarily due to inflammation, which, if not exaggerated, would be beneficial. Hypersensitivity reactions can be separated into two types: *immediate hypersensitivities* that are mediated by antibodies and *delayed hypersensitivities* that are mediated by T lymphocytes. There is little difference between immunity and hypersensitivity other than a qualitative one.

Immediate-type hypersensitivities ■ Immediate hypersensitivity reactions result from the indirect effects of antigen-antibody interactions. The symptoms result from the release or activation of mediators in inflammation by the antigen-antibody combination. Three types of immediate hypersensitivity have been described: type I (anaphylactic), type II (cytotoxic), and type III (immune complex).

Anaphylactic (Type I) ■ Type I hypersensitivity, or allergy, occurs when an IgE antibody response is formed against frequently innocuous antigens (i.e., pollen). During initial exposure to antigens, IgE antibodies may be produced in addition to other immunoglobulins (Fig. 2–9). Normally, IgE is produced in high levels only in parasitic infections. However, certain individuals have a genetically determined propensity for IgE production and are termed *atopic*. They have high IgE levels and show clinical features of asthma, eczema, hay fever, and urticaria, as well as demonstrating wheal and flare skin reactions in 15 to 30 minutes after exposure to commonly inhaled antigens. Depending on the animal, IgG and IgE may both initiate systemic anaphylactic reactions, but IgE is generally more potent.

IgE antibodies are cytophilic for mast cells and basophils and bind to these cells via Fc receptors. This binding leaves the antigen-combining sites of the IgE antibody available. Following new exposure to antigen (allergen), the IgE molecules are cross-linked through the antigen, and degranulation of the cells into the intercellular spaces ensues. The pharmacologic mediators released that result in the inflammatory reactions include histamine, serotonin, SRS-A, platelet-activating factor, the prostaglandins and leukotrienes, and chemotactic factors for eosinophils, neutrophils, basophils, and monocytes. These mediators cause inflammatory infiltration, vasodilation and vascular permeability, microthrombi, proteolytic activation of C3, edema, bronchial smooth muscle contraction, mucosal edema, and mucus secretion. IgE hypersensitivity in humans can be either localized or systemic.

Local allergic reactions include *hay fever* (allergic rhinitis) in response to plant pollens, industrial chemicals, microbial spores, and insects contained in household dust. *Asthma*, a complex condition that sometimes has an immunological basis, is generally directed toward similar allergens as hay fever. *Allergic dermatitis* may be secondary to hay fever or asthma and is represented by eruptions on the skin and face that resemble eczema.

Systemic allergic reactions (termed *anaphylaxis*) result from the allergen reaching the blood or lymph circulations. The ensuing reaction involves several organs and may be triggered by insect venoms, drugs, or even certain foods. Each of these allergic reactions can have severe consequences.

Cytotoxic (Type II) ■ This type of hypersensitivity is characterized by antibody to cell surface or tissue antigens. Binding of IgM or IgG antibody to the antigens on the cell surface activates the classical complement pathway leading to cytolysis. The release of complement components can trigger the influx of phagocytic cells. The interactions among the target cell, antibody, and effector cells is antibody-dependent cellular cytotoxicity, which has been mentioned earlier. The effector cells can be neutrophils, eosinophils, mononuclear phagocytes, and K cells, which all contain surface Fc receptors (Fig. 2–9). The mechanism of phagocytic damage to cells

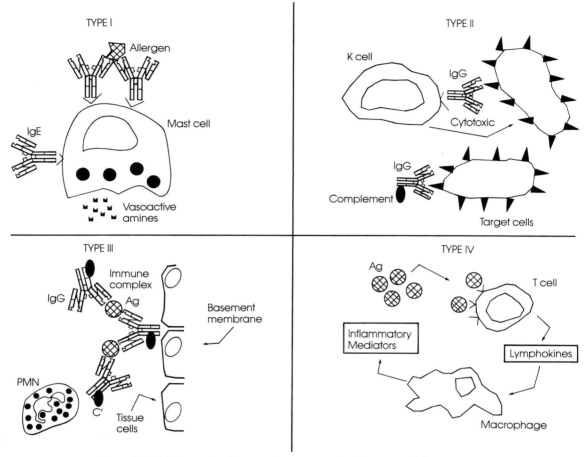

Figure 2–9 ■ Schematic diagram of components of hypersensitivity reactions.

is similar to the manner by which phagocytes deal with infectious pathogens. The antibody-coated cells can be phagocytized and internally destroyed by the phagocyte enzymes. In addition, if the phagocytes cannot adequately engulf large substances, the granule and lysosomal enzymes are exocytosed into intercellular spaces and damage the host tissues.

Several human syndromes have been associated with cytotoxic hypersensitivity. *Transfusion reactions* to various blood group antigens on erythrocytes arise from antibody directed to surface antigens on the red blood cells. *Hemolytic disease of the newborn* is a cytotoxic hypersensitivity whereby antibody from the maternal circulation is directed to incompatible Rh antigens on the fetal erythrocytes. *Autoimmune hemolytic anemias* take place when patients produce antibodies to their own erythrocytes. *Drug-induced reactions* are provoked by drugs eliciting an allergic reaction against erythrocytes or platelets. These result from the drug or its metabolites

adsorbing to the cell surface and antibodies reacting with the altered cell (thrombocytopenic purpura, lysis of platelets). Also, a drug may induce autoantibodies to erythrocyte surface antigens, and cytotoxic hypersensitivity ensues. *Hyperacute graft rejection* results when the recipient has preformed antibodies to antigens on the graft. *Goodpasture's syndrome* results from antibody directed to both glomerular and lung basement membranes, which causes nephritis and lung hemorrhage. Patients with *myasthenia gravis* demonstrate antibodies to the acetylcholine receptor on the surface of muscle membranes. The binding of IgG and complement to these receptors causes an increased rate of receptor turnover and can block acetylcholine binding and transduction of the muscle impulse. In *thyroiditis and diabetes* antibodies occur that are directed to thyroid cells and pancreatic islet cells. Whether thyroid and islet cell antibodies cause the disease or are formed as a consequence of the disease process is unknown.

Complex-mediated (Type III) ■ Immune-complex disorders are a type of hypersensitivity initiated by antigen-antibody complexes that form in solution rather than on a cell surface (Fig. 2–9). Immune complexes are produced each time antibody reacts with antigen, but since the concentration of antigen in the circulation is usually low, these are usually effectively removed by the reticuloendothelial system. However, under certain circumstances, the antigen-antibody complexes persist in high concentrations and cause tissue damage by sticking to the walls of capillary vessels or depositing on basement membranes, or both. The complexes bind complement and release both C3a and C5a, which are chemotactic for polymorphonuclear leukocytes. The attracted cells phagocytize the complexes and release hydrolytic enzymes into the intercellular spaces, resulting in tissue destruction, inflammation, and sometimes local hemorrhage and organ dysfunction.

Disease resulting from immune-complex hypersensitivity can be separated into three major categories:

1. Persistent infection with microbial antigens

2. Autoimmune reactions to self-antigens

3. Responses to extrinsic environmental antigens

Persistent infection with viridans streptococci or staphylococci, viral hepatitis, or parasites *(Plasmodium spp.)* can induce chronic immune complex formation and damage to the infected organs and to the kidney. Immune-complex hypersensitivity often occurs as a complication of autoimmune diseases in which continued presence of antibody and host or self-antigen overloads the reticuloendothelial system and results in tissue deposition of immune complexes in kidneys, joints, arteries, and skin. Systemic lupus erythematosus (SLE) and polyarteritis nodosa are two examples of this type of hypersensitivity. Immune complexes can also form at mucosal surfaces following repeated contact with antigens. Inhalation of antigens from molds, plants, or animals can elicit circulating IgG antibody and result in tissue damage in the lung (i.e., farmer's lung disease and pigeon fancier's disease in response to environmental fungi).

There are experimental models for complex-mediated hypersensitivities. "Serum sickness" is now uncommon, but was a consequence of earlier-used serum therapy for control of various microbial diseases. In this, the host produces antibody to the foreign serum proteins (i.e., horse) with deposition of antigen-antibody complexes. A strain of mouse (NZW/NZB) develops an "autoimmune disease" similar to human SLE with production of autoantibodies to erythrocytes, cell nuclei, and DNA. Resulting immune complexes are deposited in the kidney glomeruli and cause tissue destruction. The "Arthus reaction" takes place in walls of small blood vessels in the skin when circulating IgG antibody contacts extrinsically administered antigen with subsequent complement activation. Neutrophils infiltrate the area and local clumping of platelets ensues. Vascular occlusion and necrosis can occur in severe cases. The inflammatory response usually peaks by approximately 4 to 10 hours and subsides by 48 hours.

Delayed-type (Type IV) ■ This cell-mediated hypersensitivity is initiated by lymphocytes rather than antibody (Fig. 2–9). As such, it cannot be transferred by serum but can be by T lymphocytes. The T cells involved have been sensitized by previous contact with the antigen. Although these sensitized T cells are critical in producing delayed type reactions, a major portion of the reaction involves nonsensitized cells that are recruited by the antigen-specific T lymphocytes. The prototype reaction is the detection of challenge with *M. tuberculosis*, which is elicited by intradermal injection of the microorganism, or more commonly by antigens from the mycobacteria (i.e., purified protein derivative, or PPD). Approximately 8 to 10 hours after the challenge, leukocytes infiltrate the site and are composed primarily of lymphocytes and macrophages. The extent of cellular infiltration increases to a maximum in 24 to 48 hours. Characteristics are:

1. Many local cells blast and thus are synthesizing DNA.

2. The lymphocytes migrate via the bloodstream rather than through the lymphatics, and are sensitized in the draining nodes.

3. The majority of lymphocytes are attracted nonspecifically.

4. The site shows erythema (reddening) and induration (hardening) due to the lymphocyte infiltrate.

5. Severe responses can lead to tissue necrosis.

6. T cells do not cause the tissue damage directly, but the release of lymphokines attracts mononuclear and polymorphonuclear leukocytes that can release tissue-destructive enzymes.

While the tuberculin response is a classic manifestation of delayed hypersensitivity reactions, there are four main types. *Jones-Mote hypersensitivity*, or cutaneous basophil hypersensitivity, is a local response to intradermal administration of soluble antigens characterized by a primary basophil infiltrate approximately 24 hours postchallenge. *Contact hypersensitivity* is maximal about 48 hours after contact with the allergen and manifests as eczema in humans. Allergens that commonly cause contact hypersensitivity are nickel, a variety of chemicals, poison ivy, and poison oak. These are generally considered haptens that elicit the immune response after binding to normal host proteins, which act as immunogenic carriers. Langerhans' cells, which are specialized antigen-presenting cells in the skin, are critical to this response, and as a consequence, the reaction is limited to the epidermis. *Tuberculin-type hypersensitivity* is characterized by a dermal infiltration of lymphocytes and monocytes leading to induration and swelling at the site of antigen challenge. Soluble antigens from many microorganisms (*M. tuberculosis, M. leprae, Leishmania spp.*) elicit this response in individuals with previous exposure to these pathogens. If antigen persists in the tissues, *granulomatous hypersensitivity* can develop and result in much of the pathology of diseases that provoke cell-mediated immune responses. Granulomatous hypersensitivity is induced by microorganisms, noninfectious antigens (i.e., sarcoidosis, zirconium, beryllium) or nonantigenic stimulants (i.e., talc). In all cases, the macrophages phagocytize but are unable to digest or destroy the internalized material. Granulomatous reactions are characterized by epithelioid cells (elevated endoplasmic reticulum), lymphocytes, macrophages, and Langhans' giant cells (multinucleated). The effect of this reaction is to wall off the foreign material from the host.

Numerous chronic diseases elicit delayed hypersensitivity such as mycobacteria (i.e., tuberculosis, leprosy), bacteria (i.e., listeriosis), fungi (i.e., blastomycosis), and parasites (i.e., leishmaniasis, schistosomiasis). In all of these infections, the agent provides a persistent, chronic antigenic stimulation to the host.

Immunologic Tolerance and Autoimmunity

Immunologic tolerance is the inability to respond to a specific antigen. This differs from immunosuppression, in which there is a general diminution or elimination of *all* immune response capabilities. Antigen-specific tolerance can be induced in both B and T cells and requires previous exposure to the antigen.

B-cell tolerance can be induced by multiple mechanisms dependent upon the type of antigen and maturity of the B cell. Low concentrations of multivalent antigens react with immature B cells to induce "clonal abortion." Repetitive challenge with T-independent antigens stimulates mature B cells to undergo terminal differentiation into short-lived plasma cells without formation of memory B cells necessary for responding to a subsequent challenge. A state of "clonal exhaustion" is therefore attained. T-helper cells are required for normal B-cell responses to T-dependent antigens. If T_H activity is absent, the mature B cells respond abnormally to the antigen and are "functionally deleted." Similarly, the binding of excess levels or nonimmunogenic forms of T-independent antigens to mature B cells can lead to specific functional deletion. Finally, high levels of T-independent antigens can tolerize by binding to the surface of plasma cells and interfering with antibody secretion.

T-cell tolerance can be similar to B-lymphocyte tolerance, including clonal abortion and functional deletion. T-suppressor cells are elicited as antigen-specific cells and directly suppress both B and T cells. The tolerance associated with the induction of the T_S is maintained only in the presence of these cells.

The ability to tolerize T and B lymphocytes is dependent on a number of factors for induction and maintenance. In general, high doses of antigen are effective as tolerogens; however, "low-zone tolerance" can be induced by small antigen doses, which elicit T_S cells. Another requisite for maintenance of tolerance is persistence of the antigen. Also, the tolerant state has been shown to exist for individual antigenic determinants (epitopes) rather than for the whole antigen molecule. If tolerance is due to clonal deletion, its duration is maintained until mature cells develop from the stem pool. In contrast, tolerance initiated by high levels of antigen binding to the cell surface is rapidly reversed if the antigen is removed.

Immune response to self-antigens, or autoimmunity, usually does not occur. However, since the immune system has such a diverse repertoire of antigenic specificities, it is possible for some responses to be to self-components. The host has developed extensive mechanisms for maintaining immunologic tolerance to self-antigens. This regulation is required because self-reactive T cells, B cells, and autoantigens are available in the circulation. Under normal circumstances, T_H cells specific for self-antigens are absent and autoantibodies are therefore not produced. This lack of T_H cells results from either clonal abortion (early in development these cells are eliminated because of the presence of large amounts of self-antigens), or by the presence and activity of T_S that abrogate the T_H functions. The T_S cells may also act directly on B cells that produce self-reacting antibody. In this scheme, autoimmunity arises as an alteration in the host that bypasses this critical regulatory step. This bypass occurs by direct activation of the T_H cells or activation of a T-contrasuppressor cell, which makes the T_H refractory to suppression. Finally, autoantigens could directly induce activation of functional T-effector cells, or B lymphocytes, which differentiate into antibody-producing plasmacytes.

Autoimmune diseases of humans are quite varied. In some cases the abnormal responses are directed to antigens with limited distribution and the destruction is organ specific. In other cases, abnormal responses occur to widely distributed antigens and the destructive consequences are disseminated (Table 2–4). In some patients, multiple types of autoimmune phenomena exist with both organ- and nonorgan-specific symptoms. Finally, there is strong evidence delineating a genetic basis for various autoimmune diseases, as well as an apparent genetic predisposition to multiple forms of autoimmunity within a family.

Immunogenetics

GENERAL OVERVIEW

Vertebrates have systems of genes ("histocompatibility genes") and gene products ("histocompatibility antigens") that determine whether tissues or cells grafted or transferred from one animal to another will be immunologically compatible and survive in the new environment. These histocompatibility systems have been defined at the genetic level for at least 20 different vertebrate organisms, including humans.

HISTOCOMPATIBILITY SYSTEMS

The earliest studies of the mammalian histocompatibility system were performed in mice, in which a major histocompatibility complex, H-2, was identified. The H-2 complex functions were accounted for by only two loci (K and D), which coded for all of the known H-2–associated antigenic specificities. In addition, it appears that the K and D loci have genetic material (Ir-1) separating them and that this complex is actually a group of alleles of various H-2–related genetic loci, termed a *haplotype*. At present, in the mouse 30 to 40 different histocompatibil-

Table 2–4 ■ Human autoimmune diseases	
Disease	**Target Tissue**
Hashimoto's thyroiditis	Thyroid
Thyrotoxicosis	Thyroid
Primary myxedema	Thyroid
Addison's disease	Adrenal
Goodpasture's syndrome	Lung and kidney
Pernicious anemia	Intrinsic factor (RBC)
Juvenile diabetes	Islet cells (pancreas)
Multiple sclerosis	Brain
Pemphigus vulgaris	Epidermis
Pemphigoid	Skin (basement membrane)
Myasthenia gravis	Muscle (acetylcholine receptor)
Autoimmune hemolytic anemia	Erythrocytes
Ulcerative colitis	Colon
Idiopathic thrombocytopenic purpura	Platelets
Sjögren's syndrome	Salivary gland
Rheumatoid arthritis	IgG
Dermatomyositis	Nuclear (muscle)
Scleroderma	Nuclear (skin)
Systemic lupus erythematosus (SLE)	DNA
Idiopathic leukopenia	Leukocytes

ity genes have been identified and mapped which code for cell surface antigens that lead to graft rejection. The H-2 complex is assigned to chromosome 17.

The major histocompatibility complex (MHC) in all mammals contains genes coding for class I antigens that are expressed on the surface of almost every cell in the body. "Class I antigens" are the major antigens recognized by the immune system during rejection of a foreign transplant. A second class of genes and antigens has been described that are associated with the MHC. These antigens, the "class II antigens," are principally on surfaces of lymphocytes and reticular cells and regulate the antibody response to specific antigens.

The MHC in humans, homologous to H-2 in the mouse, is the HLA system. The principal mode of analysis of the HLA system has been the genetic and serologic analysis of families and populations. The antibodies to the gene products coded for by components of the HLA complex have been obtained. These include:

1. Sera from multiparous women, which have antibodies directed to the HLA alleles of the father that are present in the fetus

2. Sera from patients who have received blood transfusions

3. Sera from individuals who have volunteered to undergo planned immunizations (by lymphocyte transfusion) to produce anti-HLA antibodies of restricted specificity

4. Mouse monoclonal antibodies to HLA antigens

The HLA antigens identified by these serologic tests fit into two distinct multiallele groups defined by the genes HLA-A and HLA-B (Fig. 2–10). These appear to correlate with the mouse class I MHC products, H-2K and H-2D. In addition, a third gene coding for cell surface alloantigens has been identified: HLA-C. Finally, a D region of the HLA complex has been defined by cellular products that stimulate mixed lymphocyte reactions (MLR). Recently, the D gene has been divided into subregions HLA-DP, HLA-DQ, and HLA-DR. The products of these loci are glycoproteins that are present on nucleated cells and have a distribution similar to the class II MHC products in the mouse.

TRANSPLANTATION

The technical transplant of healthy tissue for replacement of defective organs has been developed and perfected during the past decade. However, it was early noted that the technical success did not ensure the retention and functioning of the tissue. Failure of tissue survival has an immunologic basis. Therefore, major advances have been those to limit the host rejection of the tissues. Various types of transplants have been used in studying tissue rejection:

1. *Xenograft*—graft between xenogeneic individuals (individuals of different species)

2. *Allograft*—graft between allogeneic individuals of the same species

3. *Isograft*—graft between syngeneic individuals, such as identical twins or inbred strains of mice

4. *Autograft*—tissue grafted back onto the original donor tissue

The specificity of the antigens involved in graft rejection is under genetic control. In

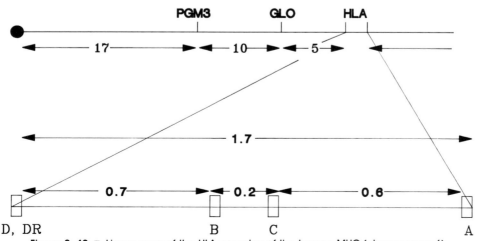

Figure 2–10 ■ Linear map of the HLA complex of the human MHC (chromosome 6).

humans there is one dominant group of antigens that provokes strong reactions, and these are under the control of the MHC (i.e., HLA) system. In addition, the ABO blood group provides strong transplantation antigens. Tissue rejection is an unfortunate side effect of a system that has evolved to recognize and destroy virally altered or neoplastic cells.

Only sites in the recipient that are accessible to the immune system are susceptible to the graft rejection phenomenon; thus, there are certain "privileged" sites in the body where allografts can survive indefinitely.

Rejection Mechanisms

Transplants of cells, tissues, or organs will be uniformly rejected if the donor and recipient differ by one or more histocompatibility genes. These genes code for cell surface histocompatibility antigens, which are detected and responded to principally by the cell-mediated (T-cell) arm of the immune system. The most extensively studied form of graft rejection is the allograft reaction, which occurs when tissues are exchanged between two members of the same species displaying different alleles of at least one histocompatibility antigen.

Certain characteristics of allograft rejection have been clearly elucidated:

1. Transplants in either direction between two allogeneic individuals are rejected.

2. When two parents are completely homozygous for all histocompatibility loci, the F_1 (first generation) progeny are uniformly heterozygous for the loci and will permanently accept a graft from either parent.

3. Tissues from F_1 will be rejected by either parent, owing to the presence on the F_1 cells of antigens from the other parent.

4. Rejection is most rapid if donor and recipient differ by genes in the MHC.

Skin allografts, when there is an MHC incompatibility, are rejected in 10 to 14 days. When the MHC is matched but differences in minor loci are present, graft rejection occurs from 2 weeks to several months. This latter type of reaction has been noted when male tissues are transplanted to female mice, who reject the tissues because of the antigens coded for by the Y gene of the male mouse.

A second graft from the same or a genetically identical donor will be rejected much more quickly than the first graft. This accelerated, or "second-set," rejection results from the cell-mediated rejection of the primary allograft increasing both the frequency of responsive cells and rapidity of response to the antigenic challenge.

The first stages of tissue rejection take place after the vascularization of the graft and the circulation of recipient blood cells throughout the donor graft. This cellular infiltrate comprises all types of lymphoid cells. However, it has not been determined whether the recipient cells are sensitized in the graft or whether donor antigens from the graft sensitize recipient cells in draining lymph nodes. In approximately 7 days the graft shows signs of rejection as sensitized host lymphocytes destroy the graft's blood vessels. The congested blood accumulates in the graft, which becomes indurated, separates from the graft bed, and is sloughed in 10 to 14 days when there are major MHC incompatibilities. In graft rejection reactions, donor leukocytes may be the primary cells in eliciting graft rejection.

Tissues vary considerably in their immunogenicity, and the site of implantation also affects the eventual survival of the tissues. "Privileged sites" with minimal adverse transplantation effects include the brain and the cornea, which lack lymphatic drainage. The success of corneal transplants is directly related to the tissue's lack of vascularization and its isolation from the recipient's immune system.

T-cell–mediated rejection ■ In skin allograft rejection, cytotoxic T cells and T cells that secrete lymphokines are the primary effector immune cells. This has been substantiated by the fact that:

1. Serum from a primary rejection animal does not accelerate graft rejection, while transfer of lymphoid cells leads to a second-set rejection.

2. The histology of the early rejection reaction shows infiltration of mononuclear cells with few neutrophils or plasma cells.

3. Increased survival of allografts occurs in thymic deficient children, thymectomized animals, and nude (thymic aplasia) mice.

4. Cells that mediate graft rejection in the mouse bear the Thy-1 marker of the T lymphocyte.

Antibody-mediated rejection ■ While cell-mediated immunity is the major effector in primary graft rejection, antibodies are involved in recipients previously sensitized to donor antigens. The effects of antibody are most frequently seen in grafts directly connected to the host's blood supply, as in kidney transplants. The primary rejection of kidney allografts results from deposition of antigen-antibody complexes in the glomerular blood vessels and subsequent binding of complement components that lead to vascular lesions. Hyperacute graft rejection is caused entirely by cytotoxic antibodies directed to ABO blood group antigens or to class I MHC antigens.

Antibodies may also protect an allograft from detection and/or destruction by the immune system. This phenomenon, termed *enhancement*, takes place by binding antibody to the histocompatibility antigens of the donor tissue and by blocking access of sensitized cytotoxic T cells.

Graft-Versus-Host Reaction

The events following injection of immunocompetent allogeneic lymphocytes into an immunocompromised recipient is called graft-versus-host (GVH) reaction. The GVH reaction is initiated by the reactivity of grafted immunocompetent cells toward the histocompatibility antigens of the recipient. The GVH reaction depends upon viable small, nondividing, donor T lymphocytes.

While donor lymphocytes in GVH only undergo a limited proliferation, their most important role is secretion of lymphokines. These lymphokines stimulate the proliferation of recipient cells, attract recipient cells and induce localized destruction of the recipient tissues. Class II antigens of recipient lymphoid cells also play a role in producing symptoms of GVH reaction by providing the principal antigenic stimulus to sensitize donor T cells. Finally, because recipient lymphoid cells contain the highest distribution of MHC determinants, they are particularly susceptible to damage by sensitized donor T cells.

Although MHC disparities are the most potent stimulators of GVH reactions, there are other histocompatibility loci that also elicit this reaction. There remains approximately a 50 percent failure rate even in the best cases of allogeneic matched donor-recipient grants. The condition is frequently fatal and GVH disease is a major impediment for bone marrow transplantation in human beings even when the donor is an HLA-identical sibling.

Immunosuppression

The success of any allograft is often due to immunosuppressive measures. The strategy for suppressing the host response is divided into two phases. Immediately after implantation of the graft, initial acute phase rejection is blocked by preventing sensitization of pre-existing T lymphocytes that are capable of recognizing the graft. After this, a cumulative unresponsiveness to the graft must be instituted since the recipient is continually exposed to donor MHC. This stable state depends upon the development of antigen-specific T_S cells. These immunosuppressive tactics may be antigen nonspecific or antigen specific.

Antigen nonspecific measures include immunosuppressive drugs and other methods that reduce T-cell function. Most immunosuppressive, cytotoxic drugs primarily affect dividing cells and therefore have some specificity for lymphoid cells that are activated to divide by donor antigens. However, the use of these drugs is limited since they also damage other rapidly dividing tissues such as the gut epithelium. Corticosteroids are also routinely used as anti-inflammatory agents, in conjunction with the cytotoxic drugs. Antilymphocyte and antithymocyte sera have been used, but their broad-based nonspecific immunosuppressive capacity and effects on other metabolic systems requires secondary treatment of the complications. Recently, cyclosporin A, a drug derived from a decapeptide secreted by the fungus *Trichoderma polysporum*, has shown great promise in organ transplantation. Cyclosporin A primarily prevents activation of T_H and T-cytotoxic cells and has minimal effect on T_S and other cells of the immune system. While these materials have been used successfully in preventing rejection the recipient is more susceptible to infection. If an infection ensues, the immunosuppression is usually suspended, at which time rejection reactions frequently develop.

Another strategy under intensive study is to create a situation where immunologic tolerance can develop toward the donor organ. This strategy of *antigen-specific immunosuppression* has taken various forms:

1. Selective elimination of class II antigen-bearing cells prior to transplantation. Class I antigens may be tolerogenic in the absence of class II antigens.

2. Total lymphoid irradiation with small, cumulative doses of irradiation that induce long-term depressed T-cell function as a result of antigen-specific T-suppressor cells.

3. Induction or transfer of antibodies to graft alloantigens. This has been termed *enhancement* and may function by removing donor passenger cells or recipient T_H cells, or by shielding the graft antigens from the responsive recipient cells.

4. Induction of anti-idiotypic antibodies to the T cells, which recognize the graft and block the recognition of the MHC antigens on the graft.

5. Blood transfusions in kidney transplants to prolong survival apparently by removing antigen-presenting cells or donor-specific T_H cells.

IMMUNE RESPONSE GENES

There are many mechanisms by which genetic factors could play a role in the generation of an immune response. MHC-linked immune response (Ir) genes act in an antigen-specific fashion, but not all the immune response genes are linked to the MHC. Most of the immune response genes that are not linked to MHC appear to have a lower degree of antigen specificity than the MHC-linked Ir genes.

Ir genes control antigen presentation between macrophages and the T cells, and regulate T/B cooperation. MHC-linked Ir gene control is very specific, and small changes in the antigen structure dramatically affect responsiveness. It is likely that the Ir genes play a role in determining the level of response to any T-dependent antigen.

IMMUNODEFICIENCIES

Immunodeficiency diseases are generally separated into primary (congenital) and secondary (acquired) deficiencies (Fig. 2–11).

Congenital immunodeficiencies are present at birth, although they may not be noted for several months and usually represent genetically determined lesions that occur during ontogeny of the immune system. A high proportion of these lesions are linked to the X chromosome with a propensity for expression in male offspring.

Acquired immune disorders, occurring later in life, may represent a lag in expression of a genetically linked immune dysfunction, or may accompany a malfunction of some portion of the immune system secondary to a nonimmunologic disease.

An abnormally high frequency of neoplastic changes and autoreactive antibodies, which may be associated with autoimmune disease, has been documented in patients with immunodeficiencies.

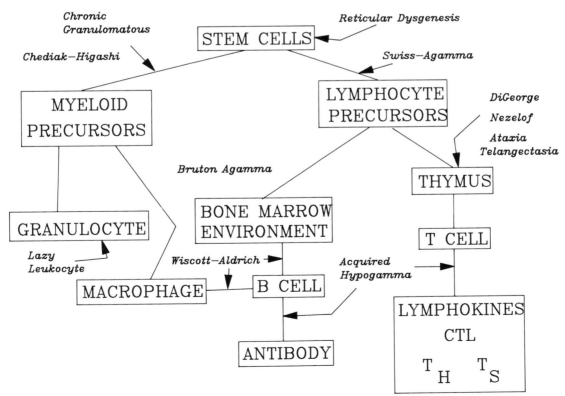

Figure 2–11 ■ Description of affected developments in human immunodeficiencies.

Congenital Immunodeficiency

The primary immunodeficiency syndromes can be grouped into four groups.

Dysfunctions primarily affecting the ability to produce normal quantities of serum immunoglobulins

Bruton's agammaglobulinemia ■ This is usually detected when maternal antibodies begin to deplete toward the end of the first year of life. It is characterized by low or nonexistent levels of serum immunoglobulins, atrophic B-cell regions in lymphoid tissues (i.e., germinal centers), and a virtual absence of plasma cells. There is also a selective IgA deficiency, which is often characterized by circulating antibodies to IgA. These patients have repeated infections by a wide range of microorganisms, including *Staphylococcus aureus*, *Streptococcus pyogenes* and *pneumoniae*, *Neisseria meningitidis*, *Hemophilus influenzae*, and protozoans (i.e., *Pneumocystis carinii*).

Common-variable immunodeficiency (late-onset hypogammaglobulinemia) ■ This is the most common immunodeficiency. Patients have low or absent circulating B cells with surface immunoglobulins. In many cases the B cells cannot differentiate into plasma cells or produce antibody. It is sometimes treated with periodic administration of pooled human serum gamma globulin, which contains antibodies to most common microorganisms.

Dysfunctions affecting normal delayed hypersensitivity and graft rejection reactions

DiGeorge's syndrome and Nezelof's syndrome ■ These disorders are characterized by antibody production to common bacteria being relatively unaffected by levels of plasma cells within normal ranges. The small lymphocytes in the blood are drastically reduced and the "thymus-dependent" areas of lymph nodes are depleted of cells. The selective T-cell suppression can also arise from a deficiency in *purine nucleoside phosphorylase*, an enzyme necessary for cell functions. These patients have poor T-cell responses but normal B-cell immunity.

Ataxia-telangiectasia ■ This is characterized by depressed cell-mediated immunity, concomitant lack of IgE and IgA responses, and an increased incidence of upper respiratory infections.

Wiskott-Aldrich syndrome ■ Thrombocytopenia and eczema characterize this syndrome. Because of a vestigial or congenitally aplastic thymus, cell-mediated immunity is depressed and there is a low IgM and poor antibody response to bacterial polysaccharide antigen. As a result, there is increased susceptibility to viral infections and depressed resistance to commensal fungal microorganisms. There has been some success in treatment with transplantation of neonatal thymus tissue or use of the transfer factor.

Dysfunctions with broad effects, termed "combined immunodeficiency diseases" or stem cell deficiencies

Swiss-type agammaglobulinemia ■ This is an autosomal-linked recessive genetic defect that includes symptoms of both B- and T-cell deficiencies. It results from rudimentary or aplastic development of all lymphoid organs. Subjects are virtually defenseless and rarely survive beyond the first year or two of life. Treatment with limited success has centered on bone marrow transplantation.

Reticular dysgenesis ■ This is a rapidly fatal form of severe combined immunodeficiency, in which there is also a lack of myeloid cell precursors.

Genetically controlled dysfunctions in innate immunity

These dysfunctions are reflected in the inability of the phagocytic cells to perform normal phagocytosis, chemotactic functions, or bacterial killing functions.

Chronic granulomatous disease ■ This disease is characterized by the inability of monocytes and neutrophils to produce H_2O_2 owing to a defect in an enzyme activated by phagocytosis. Thus, the cells can phagocytize microorganisms coated with antibody but are unable to kill them.

Chédiak-Higashi disease ■ Abnormal structure and function of the lysosomes characterizes this disease. As a consequence, patients suffer from severe pyogenic bacterial infections.

Myeloperoxidase deficiency ■ This deficiency is associated with a susceptibility to systemic candidiasis.

Lazy leukocyte syndrome ■ In this syndrome, there is a chemotactic defect in the neutrophils with an increased susceptibility to bacterial infections.

Localized juvenile periodontitis ■ This condition is characterized by a neutrophil chemotactic defect (see Chapter 28). This defect results from a decrease in receptors for both bacterial and host chemoattractants on the surface of neutrophils.

Acquired Immunodeficiency

The ability to mount effective immune responses against infection or neoplasia can also be depressed nonspecifically by numerous secondary phenomena. Malnutrition has a major effect on cell-mediated and secretory immune capabilities. In particular, decreased blood iron depresses the cell-mediated immune system.

Infectious agents, particularly viruses, are also immunosuppressive. The measles virus has a direct cytotoxic effect on lymphocytes. The human immunodeficiency virus (HIV) which causes AIDS (acquired immunodeficiency syndrome) and its secondary manifestations (i.e., susceptibility to infections *[Pneumocystis carinii]*, development of Kaposi's sarcoma) are a direct result of the virus's ability to infect and kill helper T lymphocytes.

Many substances used for nonimmunologic reasons can also dramatically and nonspecifically affect the immune system. These include radiographs, various cytotoxic drugs, and anti-inflammatory steroids.

Finally, numerous neoplastic changes associated with B-lymphocyte development have been identified, including various forms of leukemia, multiple myeloma, and Waldenström's macroglobulinemia. In each case, neoplastic transformations result in a defective antibody response and in substantially increased frequency and severity of pyogenic bacterial infections. In contrast, Hodgkin's disease and the leukemias that affect the T-cell arm of the immune response will often compromise cell-mediated immunity and result in increased bacterial, viral, and fungal infections.

Tumor Immunology

Neoplastic cells have two general characteristics: (1) qualitative differences in the DNA of the cells possibly related to the presence of certain "oncogenes," and (2) phenotypic changes in the plasma membrane components resulting from the DNA changes. These membrane changes result in immunologically recognizable changes and are the basis for immunologic interference with neoplastic development.

ETIOLOGY

Early experiments used the "carcinogenic" property of organic chemicals to elicit neoplastic changes in experimental models. These chemicals are structurally diverse and include methylcholanthrene (MCA), benz-

pyrene (BP), and dimethylbenzanthracene (DMBA). Although the host would mount an immune response to antigens of these tumors, little antigenic cross-reactivity was detectable between tumors induced in the same or different animals with the same chemical. Thus, tumor-specific transplantation antigens (TSTA) were identified, although their molecular nature is unknown. It has been suggested that the carcinogens act directly on DNA, leading to formation of new antigens which are altered normal membrane molecules.

A range of DNA and RNA viruses can cause neoplastic changes in animals with antigens expressed by the transformed cells that are characteristic of a particular virus. These virus-specific transplantation antigens (VSTA) are detectable on tumors caused by the same virus in different species of animals and are usually encoded by the viral genome. Also, oncogenic virus-transformed cells can express new host-derived antigens that result from alteration in the host genome.

Spontaneous neoplasia may also result from altered control over naturally occurring oncogenes in mammalian cells. This explanation is consistent with increased neoplasia that accompanies the aging process whereby numerous host control mechanisms are gradually compromised. The antigens in these types of tumors are not well defined, and it has been suggested that they are weakly immunogenic, which allows them to escape detection and destruction by the host's immune apparatus.

Therefore, there are a variety of antigens associated with neoplastic changes. One type of antigen is restricted to a single tumor. A second major type is detected on the same type of tumor from different individuals, as well as on a subset of normal cells, and it probably represents differentiation antigens. Other antigens are expressed on a broad range of normal and malignant cells and are represented by autologous tumor antigens. "Oncofetal antigens" are antigens that are normally expressed on fetal cells, that are generally absent on normal adult cells, but that are re-expressed on certain neoplasms (i.e., alpha-fetoprotein, carcinoembryonic antigen).

HOST RESPONSES

Host resistance to neoplastic development has been termed *immunosurveillance*. This process involves numerous specific and nonspecific mechanisms and copes with the constant aberrations during normal cell differentiation, proliferation, and maturation that result in a malignancy.

Cell-mediated

Specific cellular immunity to tumors is similar to T-cell responses to other cell-surface antigens, including transplantation and autoimmune antigens. The activation of T cells results in the elicitation of helper, suppressor, and cytotoxic T cells. The T_C cells can interact directly with the tumor cells, leading to cell death. Activation of T_H can lead to B-cell cooperation, with subsequent antibody production, and to lymphokine production that activates and recruits other immune cells. A variety of lymphokines have been suggested to be involved in tumor resistance. Three of these factors could substantially enhance immunity to the tumor by recruiting macrophages into the site (chemotactic factor for macrophages), by immobilizing the phagocytes at the tumor site (macrophage migration inhibition factor), and by activating the cells for enhanced killing capacity (macrophage activating factor; IFNγ). The lymphotoxin ($TNF_β$) secreted by the activated T cells can act directly on the tumor and cause cell lysis. Interferon gamma (IFNγ), secreted by tumor antigen–stimulated T cells, can modulate the production of antibody and the expression of cell-surface antigens and can stimulate both natural killer (NK) cell and macrophage activity. Finally, numerous mitogenic factors are released by the activated T cells, especially IL-2 which is antigenically nonspecific and stimulates other T cells to proliferate. In addition, IL-2 can stimulate the differentiation and activation of NK cells and can stimulate the formation of cytotoxic T cells (lymphokine-activated killer [LAK] cells).

The cytotoxic T lymphocytes (CTLs), NK cells, and macrophages appear to be critical to neoplastic development both in natural and in adaptive immunity. The CTLs function by both direct killing and production of TNFa. The NK cells constitute a portion of the large granular lymphocyte (LGL) populations of humans and rodents. In general, the NK cells are phenotypically different from T and B cells. These cells are present at 2 to 5 percent of human peripheral blood mononuclear cells and decline with aging. The NK cells require no time for specific activation, so that they provide an immediate nonspecific response to the malignancy. The

NK cells can also be activated by products of immune T cells, including IFNγ and IL-2. Macrophages overlap as effectors of both natural and adaptive immunity. In general, macrophages are most effective following activation by T-cell–derived lymphokines. Once activated, the macrophages demonstrate nonspecific cytotoxicity for tumor cells presenting foreign antigens. This killing activity results from both direct contact and secretion of cytolytic factors, including $TNF_β$.

Although cell-mediated responses appear to provide the major mechanism for antitumor immunity, antibodies against neoplastic antigens are demonstrable in many tumor/host systems. These antibodies may activate complement and cause direct lysis of the tumor cells. The binding of antibody to the tumor cells may opsonize the cells for enhanced phagocytosis by granulocytes and macrophages. Also, it has been shown that these antibodies participate in a unique form of immunity, mentioned earlier, called *antibody-dependent cellular cytotoxicity* (ADCC). This immunity requires production of antibody isotypes for which specific Fc receptors are present on cytotoxic cells. These have been termed *killer* (K) cells and are present in the LGL population of cells. NK and K cells in human peripheral blood are generally distinct. Although NK cells also have Fc receptors, they are not involved in cell lysis; while the Fc receptor is necessary for K-cell function. Additionally, K-cell activity is minimally affected by modulators that augment NK activity.

The concept of "immunologic escape" attempts to describe the inconsistency between the immunogenic nature of neoplasia and the neoplastic cell's ability to grow in the host. This capacity to elude host destructive immunity probably represents a balance between tumor cell factors that enhance its survival and host immunity attempting to destroy the foreign cells. Numerous activities have been described that can affect this immunologic escape mechanism:

1. *Kinetics of tumor growth*—The initial slow growth of the tumor may allow it to sneak through the host immune armamentarium and go unrecognized until it is established.

2. *Tolerance*—Early acquisition of viruses or viral transformed cells can induce a state of tolerance to this foreign antigen and allow the neoplasia to proliferate.

3. *Genetics*—The haplotype of certain hosts appears to provide a genetically based nonresponsiveness to certain types of tumor antigens.

4. *Tumor products*—Various tumors produce factors that can down-regulate the activity of NK and K cells, inhibit inflammation, minimize chemotaxis and complement activation, and induce angiogenesis (enhance blood supply to the tumor).

5. *Growth factors*—Tumor inhibition of critical factors for immune development (i.e., IL-2, IL-1) can minimize the host protective response.

6. *Antigen masking, shedding, modulation, and blocking*—Various tumors have the ability to alter surface tumor-specific antigens by endocytosing and redistributing the antigens (modulation), by shedding the antigen into the local microenvironment and short-circuiting the immune system, and by enhancing attachment of normal host components that "mask" the tumor-specific antigens. Also, the shedding of tumor cell antigens can bind specifically to host antibody, and the resulting complexes interact either with the cytotoxic T cells to prevent cell contact or with T_H cells, thus preventing the induction of cytotoxic T cells.

Immunization/Vaccination

GENERAL PRINCIPLES AND BACKGROUND

The use of vaccines, or "immunoprophylaxis," developed as it became clear that individuals who recovered from specific infectious diseases were resistant to future challenges with the infecting microorganism. The use of vaccines is based upon the stimulation of immunity within the host (active immunization) or the transfer of preformed immune components to a host (passive immunization). Thus, vaccination involves the use of an immunizing agent, which elicits protection by the formation of neutralizing antibodies or cytotoxic cells against a biologically active material (bacteria, virus, or toxin). The immunizing agent may be composed of the intact organism or an extract of the agent that specifically elicits neutralizing

activity. The effectiveness or efficacy of a vaccine is determined by the degree of protection induced in the immunized host following challenge with the infectious agent. This effectiveness is dependent upon numerous host and parasite factors.

SPECIFIC REQUIREMENTS (Table 2–5)

To use vaccines, "a knowledge of the pathogenesis of the disease under study is essential." Infections may be divided into two groups: (1) localized, in which protection is best at the portal of entry by affecting local replication and inflammatory changes; and (2) generalized, in which the protection is effective following dissemination of the organisms or their toxic products after a limited local replication.

A second consideration for vaccination is the antigenic epitopes. The identification of antigens was not a necessity in the early days of vaccination because either whole intact microorganisms were used, in an attenuated or inactivated form, or the relevant antigen was obvious (i.e., diphtheria and tetanus toxin). However, there may be undesirable effects with these complex antigens. In addition, the majority of protozoan and helminthic infections have complex life cycles and do not produce these types of toxins. Numerous viruses, bacteria, and parasites can also alter their cell-surface antigens as a method of evading host defenses. Therefore, "a clear understanding of the stability of antigens and the virulence mechanisms of the infectious agents is required for vaccine development."

The immune system provides two different functions in connection with infectious disease: (1) elimination of the infection and (2) establishment of immunity that prevents reinfection with the same pathogen. Immune protection may be mediated by humoral or cellular aspects of the immune system, or both. In general, most currently used vaccines are effective at antibody induction. However, immunization against isolated mucosal infections has not as yet been extremely successful.

Finally, "an assessment of the benefit/risk ratio is necessary in the development and use of a particular vaccine." In this regard, the more severe or contagious a disease, the higher the benefit for effectively eliminating it. However, vaccination may present an inherent risk to the host. Several pathogens, including bacteria, viruses, and parasites,

Table 2–5 ■ Requirements for vaccine development
1. Identification of etiologic agent in disease
2. Identification of critical virulence factors of the agent
3. Definition of natural host resistance to the agent
4. Assessment of benefit/risk ratio for the vaccine

share antigens with their host. Consequently, the host may either not develop an immune response, thus allowing infection to occur, or respond with destruction of its own tissues. In addition, attenuated vaccines or toxins can exhibit some pathogenicity in compromised hosts, such as those with immunodeficiencies or those immunosuppressed by other infections. Certain vaccines may also exacerbate immunopathology associated with the disease or induce immunopathology as a result of immune complexes. Thus, a purified antigen vaccine may be best. Other considerations for vaccines include immunogenicity, availability, and delivery of the vaccine.

PRESENT-DAY VACCINES

The objective of vaccination is to provide long-term effective immunity. This is accomplished by eliciting adequate humoral or cellular immune responses and inducing a primed population of immune cells that can rapidly expand upon secondary contact with the antigen. Various methods have been used to prepare vaccines (Table 2–6).

Toxoids

Exotoxins, the principal pathogenic mechanism for some microorganisms, can be detoxified to form toxoids. Immunization with the toxoids produces antibody that neutralizes the toxin and protects the host. Vaccines using this approach include the diphtheria and the tetanus toxoids.

Killed Organisms

Dead bacteria and viruses can provide a safe vaccine preparation. These have been used for typhoid, cholera, and polio (Salk) vaccines. However, in many cases the killed vaccines are not as effective in sustaining immunity when compared with the response to a natural infection. This presumably results from a larger and more sustained antigen dosage than with the killed vaccine.

Attenuated Organisms

Attenuation is the process of weakening the capacity of an organism to cause disease. The attenuation of pathogenic microorganisms for vaccines is a long-established alternative to the use of killed organisms or their products. Microorganisms ideally attenuated for vaccines (1) must be capable of establishing an infection following artificial administration; (2) should have lost the capacity to produce anything but the mildest of disease symptoms and should be free of any undesirable secondary characteristics (i.e., malignancies, latent infections); (3) should have a low propensity for spreading to others and disseminating through the population; and (4) should be genetically stable and incapable of reverting to a virulent form. Various attenuated vaccines are currently in use, including measles, polio (Sabin), and the bacillus of Calmette and Guérin (BCG) for tuberculosis.

A variety of vaccines are currently in use for bacteria, viruses, and parasitic worms (Table 2–6). Because of vaccines, various infectious or communicable diseases have diminished in their incidence and importance.

Table 2–6 ■ Present-day vaccines

Inactivated (killed) Vaccines	
Whole Microorganisms	
Bacteria	*B. pertussis, S. typhosa, S. paratyphi, V. cholerae, B. abortus, B. anthracis*
Viruses	Rabies, influenza, polio, foot-and-mouth disease, animal parvoviruses, feline leukemia
Subunit Vaccines	
Toxoid (formalin-fixed toxin)	*C. tetani, C. diphtheriae*
Components	Hepatitis B surface Ag, adenovirus, influenza hemagglutinin
Live Vaccines	
Bacteria	*M. tuberculosis* (BCG), *B. abortus*
Viruses	
Natural	Vaccinia, rubella (German measles), Newcastle disease, Marek's disease
Attenuated	Mumps, measles, polio, yellow fever
Genetically manipulated	Influenza, rotavirus

However, concomitantly new diseases, caused by other pathogens, are replacing them, thus requiring new vaccines and strategies. Therefore, recent developments in our conceptual approach to understanding the significant antigens of the pathogens and induction of protective immunity have added a new dimension to this aspect of immunology.

The production of killed vaccines has revolved around three primary strategies:

1. *Expression of protective antigens in prokaryotic or eukaryotic host cells.* These antigens include those of influenza, polio, herpes, and hepatitis B viruses.

2. *Synthetic peptides as immunogens.* This strategy represents antigenic sequences of protective antigens and has been used for foot-and-mouth disease, polio, and hepatitis B viruses.

3. *Mimicking antigenic sites with anti-idiotypic antibodies.* This is based on the hypothesis that a portion of the idiotypic determinants of an antibody contains the antigen-binding site. Antibodies directed toward these idiotypic determinants (anti-idiotype) can mimic the original antigen configuration and can thus be used as a vaccine to induce antibodies to the original antigen.

The production of live vaccines has included four strategies:

1. *Attenuation by genetic reassortment.* This method involves intermolecular recombination of selected regions from different parental viruses. This has been used for influenza and polio viruses.

2. *Attentuation by gene deletion.* This approach is directed toward specific elimination of sequences of the microorganisms genome that codes for pathogenic molecules and has been investigated in a herpes simplex virus model.

3. *Attenuated virus vectors that carry foreign genes.* This work has involved the replacement of portions of the vaccinia virus genome with foreign genes without affecting its ability to grow in tissue-culture cells or animals. These recombinant viruses are generally less virulent and can protect against the foreign genes' parental virus.

4. *Bacterial vectors that carry foreign genes.* This has been a particularly interesting approach for vaccines to induce mucosal immunity. The direction has been to use an avirulent mutant of *Salmonella typhimurium* that can express gene products of foreign pathogens.

Vaccination strategies have provided dramatic success in eliminating smallpox, providing successful treatment of rabies, diphtheria, tetanus, whooping cough, and poliomyelitis and in minimizing the extent and severity of meningococcal, pneumococcal, and tuberculosis diseases. However, the control of numerous infectious diseases, in particular tropical diseases, by vaccination has still not been accomplished. In addition, the possible use of vaccines in the major diseases of the oral cavity (i.e., caries, periodontitis) remains to be elucidated.

REFERENCES

Burnet, F. M.: The Clonal Selection Theory of Acquired Immunity. Cambridge University Press, London, 1959.

Dausset, J.: The major histocompatibility complex in man. Science 213:1469, 1981.

Dick, G.: Immunological Aspects of Infectious Diseases. University of Pennsylvania Press, Baltimore, 1979.

Gottlieb, P. D.: Immunoglobulin genes. Molec Immunol 17:1423, 1980.

Herberman, R. B.: Basic and Clinical Tumor Immunology. Martinus Nijhoff, Boston, 1983.

Honjo, T.: Immunoglobulin genes. Ann Rev Immunol 1:499, 1983.

Kabat, E. A.: Structural Concepts in Immunology and Immunochemistry. Holt, Rinehart and Winston, New York, 1978.

Klein, J.: Immunology: The Science of Self-Nonself Discrimination. New York, Wiley, 1982.

Klinman, N., Wylie, D., and Teale, J.: B cell development. Immunol Today 2:12, 1981.

Lachmann, P. J.: Complement. In Sela, M. (ed.): The Antigens, vol. V. Academic Press, New York, 1979.

Lachmann, P. J., and Peters, D. K.: Clinical Aspects of Immunology, ed. 4. Blackwell Scientific, Oxford, 1981.

McConnell, I., Munro, A., and Waldmann, H.: The Immune System, ed. 2. Blackwell Scientific, Oxford, 1981.

Nisonoff, A.: Introduction to Molecular Immunology. Blackwell Scientific Publications, Oxford, 1982.

Roitt, I. M.: Essential Immunology, ed. 5. Blackwell Scientific, Oxford, 1984.

Sites, D. P., Stubo, J. D., Fudenberg, H. H., and Wels, J. V.: Basic and Clinical Immunology, ed. 5, Lange Medical Publications, Los Altos, CA, 1984.

Wall, R., and Kuehl, M.: Biosynthesis and regulation of immunoglobulin. Ann Rev Immunol 1:343, 1983.

Weir, D. M.: Handbook of Experimental Immunology, vols. I and II, ed. 4. Blackwell Scientific, Oxford, 1985.

chapter 3

General microbiology, metabolism, and genetics

Stanley C. Holt □ Ann Progulske

It was almost 350 years ago that the first observations of the presence of bacteria were made by Anton van Leeuwenhoek. In addition to the numerous microscopic animals and plants that he observed, he also saw the three basic morphologic types of what we now call bacteria: rods, spheres, and spirals. With the development of improved light microscopic optics, techniques of staining cells, and the development of the electron microscope, bacteria were soon observed to consist of a variety of cell structures (Fig. 3–1a), including a cytoplasm containing ribosomes, nucleic acid, and, under certain physiologic conditions, storage products. Most bacteria are surrounded by a cell wall, under which lies a close-fitting cytoplasmic membrane. In addition, some bacteria contain capsules on their surface, flagella for motility, and some form of heat- and chemical-resistant endospores; others form sheaths, cysts, and specialized holdfast appendages that anchor them to surfaces in their environment.

The development of the electron microscope, and its associated methods of preserving cells, revolutionized our concepts of cell structure. In fact, it was the results of electron microscopy, combined with intuition, that argued for recognition of fundamental differences in the anatomy of bacterial cells and those constituting the remainder of the biologic world. This resulted in the naming of two cell types: the *prokaryotes* and the *eukaryotes*. The prokaryotes are represented by the bacteria (Fig. 3–1a) and are those cells that lack both a nuclear membrane and the large number of membrane-limited organelles that abound in eukaryotic cells. Eukaryotic cells (Fig. 3–1b) include the plants, animal cells, protozoa, algae, and fungi. Table 3–1 describes the major differences between prokaryotes and eukaryotes. The major feature separating prokaryotes from eukaryotes is a "true" nucleus (surrounded by a nuclear membrane) in the latter. In addition, eukaryotes contain numerous organelles, many of which are membrane bound. These include mitochondria, Golgi bodies, and an extensive endoplasmic reticulum. Interestingly, the mitochondrion also contains genetic information similar to that of the nucleus. However, the mitochondrion is very small and contains only enough genetic information for the synthesis of no more than 13 proteins. The genetic information for the other proteins required for mitochondrial function is found in the nucleus. In contrast to the complex anatomy of eukaryotic cells, that of the

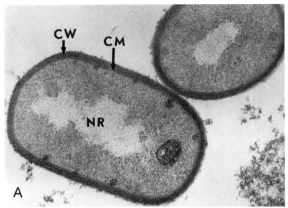
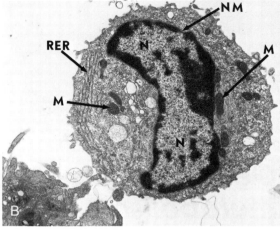

Figure 3–1 ■ Electron photomicrographs of (A) prokaryotic cell and (B) eukaryotic cell. A, Bacillus fastidiosus consists of a cytoplasmic region, which contains a central fibrous nuclear region (NR), surrounded by electron dense particulate ribosome (R). The cell is surrounded by a cell wall (CW) and an inner cytoplasmic membrane (CM). B, In contrast, the platelet consists of numerous membrane bound organelles. The large central nucleus (N) is surrounded by a nuclear membrane (NM). M = mitochondria; REF = rough endoplasmic reticulum.

Table 3–1 ■ Distinguishing characteristics of prokaryotic and eukaryotic cells

	Prokaryotic Cells	Eukaryotic Cells
Major Groups	Bacteria	Algae, fungi, protozoa, plants, animals
Size (approximate)	1 × 3 μm	>5 μm
Cellular Structures		
Cell wall peptidoglycan	+	−
Membrane composition	Sterols absent from most bacterial membranes	Sterols abundant
Mitochondria	−	+
Chloroplasts	−	Present in photosynthetic organisms
Gas vesicles	±	−
Nuclei		
Nuclear membrane	−	+
Chromosome number	1	1+
Mitotic apparatus	−	+
Nucleolus	−	+
Histones	±	+
Golgi apparatus	−	+
Microtubules	−	+
Ribosomes (sedimentation coefficient)	70S	Cytoplasmic ribosomes 80S; chloroplast, mitochondrial ribosomes 70S
Glycocalyx	±	±
Movement		
Cytoplasmic streaming	−	±
Amoeboid movement	−	±
Flagella	If present, simple	If present, 9 + 2
Metabolism		
Oxidative phosphorylation	Membranes	Mitochondria
Photosynthetic structure	Intracytoplasmic membranes or vesicles	Chloroplasts
Reduced inorganic compounds as energy source	±	−
Nonglycolytic anaerobic energy generation	±	−
Poly B-hydroxybutyrate reserve storage material	±	−
Nitrogen fixation	±	−
Peptidoglycan synthesis	+	−
Exo- and endocytosis	−	±
DNA base ratios (Mol% G + C)	20–70	Approx 40

+ = present; − = absent; ± = may occur in some cells.

prokaryotic cell can be considered relatively simple.

While there are significant chemical and morphologic differences between prokaryotes and eukaryotes, the two cell types share a basic commonality. Both, for example, have a common or universal genetic code and overall chemical composition. They also have very similar mechanisms for the replication, transcription, and translation of their genetic information into a viable and functional cell. The high degree of similarity in the genetic information suggests a common evolution of these two cell types, separating at some time in the distant past while yet maintaining a common thread to the basic mechanism for producing and transferring information into a functional cell.

Macroscopic Morphology

SIZE

Prokaryotic cells (i.e., bacteria) are the smallest of the unicellular organisms. They are, for the most part, approximately 1 to 1.5 μm wide and 2 to 6 μm long. The most studied of the bacteria, the enteric microorganism (e.g., *Escherichia coli*), is approximately 1 μm in diameter. The smallest are the wall-less mycoplasmas, which are approximately 0.1 μm in length, while the largest are the sulfur-utilizing *Beggiatoa*, such as *Beggiatoa gigantea*, which may be as long as 26 to 60 μm.

Although it is not clear why bacteria range from the very small to the very large, it appears that the lower limit of their size is determined by the space required in their cytoplasm to contain all of the required "machinery" for independent growth and development. Large bacteria have an apparent upper size limit for the necessary surface-to-volume ratios required for the efficient movement of nutrients into the cell and the products of metabolism out of the cell.

SHAPE

The various bacterial shapes are seen in Figure 3–2. In addition to the three basic bacterial shapes (rods, spheres, and spirals), some bacteria are square, others exist as long filaments, and a large number produce buds, similar to those of a budding tree. Others, either because of the age of the culture or environmental conditions, are very irregularly shaped, or pleomorphic. These "morphotypes" compose the general group of bacteria referred to as the *eubacteria*, or "true bacteria." The rod or cylindrical bacteria are routinely referred to as bacilli (distinguished from the genus *Bacillus*), the spheres are referred to as cocci, while spirals are referred to as spirilla. The spirilla are characteristic of members of the genus *Vibrio* and have a single wave form, while multiple spirillum wave forms are referred to as spirochetes. Other eubacteria are members of the actinomycetes, which are a very large group of primarily branching filaments.

Cocci

These spherical bacteria vary in diameter between 0.5 and 2 μm. The general morphology of various cocci is seen in Figure 3–3. They occur as single cells (**micrococci**), as pairs of cocci (**diplococci**), as chains (**streptococci**), or as packets of cells (**staphylococci**). Cube-shaped cellular packets are referred to as **sarcinae**, and are typical of the genus *Sarcina*. Characteristic of the cocci are the members of the genus *Streptococcus* (*S. mutans, S. sanguis, S. pneumoniae*). While these latter streptococci are spherical, they tend more toward being pear-shaped. *S. pneumoniae* is lancet-shaped, while the *Neisseria* (*N. gonorrhoeae, N. meningitidis*) are bean-shaped.

Bacilli

This morphotype consists of cylindrical cells, which are either large or small rods with almost parallel sides, or rods with rounded, square, or tapered ends. The bacilli are usually 0.2 to 1 μm in diameter, with lengths of approximately 10 μm being common. The majority of the bacilli are members of the genus *Bacillus* and require air for growth (aerobic). However, the bacilli of the genus *Clostridium* grow in the complete absence of air; that is, they are **anaerobic.** The numerous subtle variations of this morphology are discussed in other chapters.

Spirilla and Related Forms

In reality, the spirilla are bacilli twisted into a helix. The rigid spirilla are surrounded by a cell wall (p. 65) and are represented by the genera *Spirillum* and *Vibrio*. The flexible spirilla (which also contain a cell wall) with more than one wave are typical of the spirochetes, represented by the genera *Treponema, Spirochaeta, Leptospira, Borrelia,* and

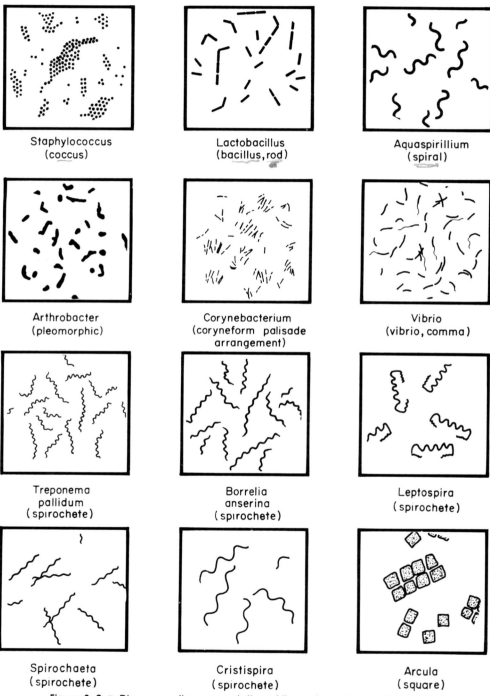

Staphylococcus
(coccus)

Lactobacillus
(bacillus, rod)

Aquaspirillium
(spiral)

Arthrobacter
(pleomorphic)

Corynebacterium
(coryneform palisade
arrangement)

Vibrio
(vibrio, comma)

Treponema
pallidum
(spirochete)

Borrelia
anserina
(spirochete)

Leptospira
(spirochete)

Spirochaeta
(spirochete)

Cristispira
(spirochete)

Arcula
(square)

Figure 3–2 ■ Diagrammatic representation of the various shapes of bacteria.

A. Diplococci (double cells):

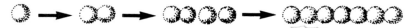

B. Streptococci: (cells in chains):

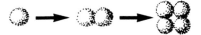

C. Tetrads: (cells in fours):

D. Staphylococci: (cells in clusters):

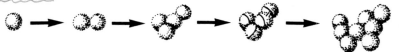

E. Sarcinae: (cells in cubes):

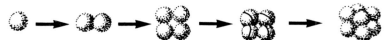

Figure 3–3 ■ Various morphologies of cocci. The spherical cells can exist as single cocci, as diplococci, as arrangements of four cells (tetrads), as irregular clusters (staphylococci), or as cubes (sarcinae).

Cristispira. *Treponema* are very tightly coiled, while the coils of *Borrelia* are larger and looser. *Leptospira* have very regular tight coils in the central region of the cell, with either one or both ends of the cell bent into a characteristic hook.

The Structure and Chemistry of Bacterial Cells

Figure 3–4 depicts an idealized prokaryotic cell composed of all of its associated structures. We will describe first those components that are associated with the cell surface, that is, with the cell wall, and then those that occupy the interior, or cytoplasmic region, of the cell.

FLAGELLA AND MOTILITY

Flagella (sing. flagellum) are organelles of motility (Fig. 3–5a). Eukaryotes also contain

flagella as organelles of motility; however, they will not be described here. The bacterial flagellum (Fig. 3–5b, c) is constructed of three distinct regions: a basal body, which is embedded in the cytoplasmic membrane and portions of the cell wall (or outer membrane in gram-negative bacteria; see page 61); and a hook region, which connects the basal body to the distal portion of the flagellum, or filament. The basal body itself consists of a series of discs or rings, which connect the proximal end of the filament through the hook to the cytoplasmic membrane and cell wall. The number of rings varies with the genus of bacterium and group; gram-negative cells possess four rings, while gram-positive bacteria have only two rings. The body contains the machinery for flagellar rotation, and the fact that they are embedded in the cytoplasmic membrane permits them to obtain the necessary energy (as ATP from the electron transport system in the cytoplasmic membrane; see page 83) for their rotation. Chemically, the basal bodies, hook, and filament all consist of specific polypep-

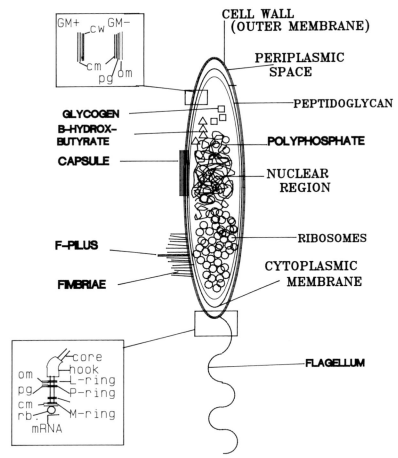

Figure 3–4 ■ Diagram of a typical prokaryotic (bacterial) cell (see also Table 3–1). The structures designated in **boldface** are not found in all bacterial cells, nor are they required for cell viability. All other structures are routinely found in prokaryotes. The boxed areas are enlargements of the gram-positive cell wall and gram-negative cell envelope (see Fig. 3–9), and flagellum (see Fig. 3–5).

tides. The filament polypeptides comprise a bundle of at least three parallel or intertwined protein fibers, known as *flagellin*.

While all of the prokaryotic flagellar filament proteins belong to the same general class of flagellins, the flagellin structure of each bacterial species is sufficiently unique to confer immunologic specificity (see Chapter 2). This immunologic specificity, or "type" specificity, provides the cell with its immunologic uniqueness, and is especially useful in microbiological identification of specific microorganisms and their diseases (i.e., *Vibrio cholerae, Pseudomonas aeruginosa*). The number and arrangement of the flagella over the bacterial surface also vary among bacteria (Fig. 3–6). The genera *Pseudomonas* and *Vibrio*, for example, are unipolarly flagellated cells and hence **monotrichous,** while *Salmonella typhi, Escherichia coli* and *Proteus vulgaris* have flagella distributed over their entire cell surface, and so are **peritrichously** flagellated.

PILI AND FIMBRIAE

Both pili (sing. pilus) and fimbriae (sing. fimbria) are attached to the outermost surface of the cell (Fig. 3–7*a, b*). They are confined to the gram-negative bacteria and to selected gram-positive bacteria (i.e., *Streptococcus, Actinomyces*). They range in thickness between 0.0085 μm and 0.003 μm, and are of variable length, with lengths of 20 μm or more being common. They number approximately 150 and are arranged peritrichously around the cell. The pili are distinguished from flagella in being approximately one-half their diameter as well as in being distinctively straight or "stiff" in appearance. Pili consist of essentially one protein, termed *pilin.* Small amounts of carbohydrate have also been found to be associated with pili, suggesting that they may be glycoproteins in chemical composition.

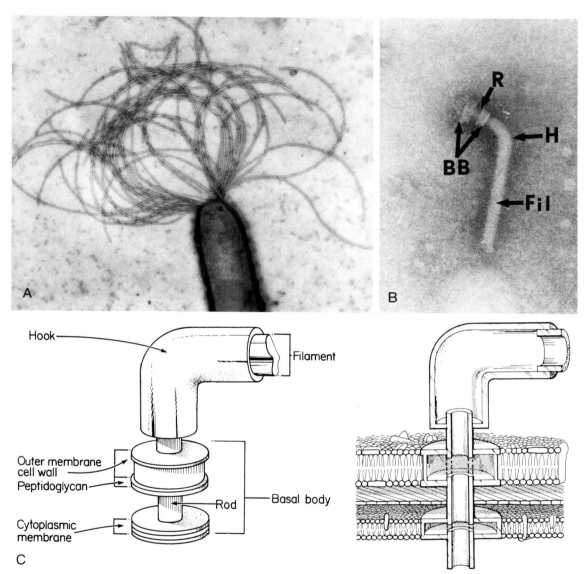

Figure 3–5 ■ The prokaryotic flagellum. *A,* The flagella tuft emerges from the pole of *Aquaspirillum serpens,* strain "straight Rhodes." The central rod (R) connects the disks. *B,* The apical portion of a flagellum is seen. The filament (FiL) has been torn, and the basal body (BB) is intact. Note the hooked (H) region of the flagellum, as well as the fan disks of the basal body. *C,* The flagellum and its relationship with the cytoplasmic membrane is represented in diagrammatic form. The disks of the basal body insert into the cytoplasmic and outer membrane of the gram-negative bacterial cell envelope. (Parts *B* and *C* courtesy of Dr. R. G. E. Murray.)

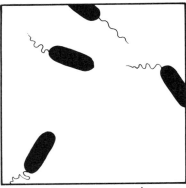

Pseudomonas aeruginosa
(Monotrichous; single
polar flagellum)

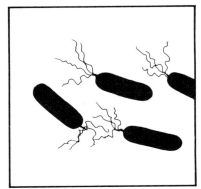

Pseudomonas fluorescens
(Lophotrichous; cluster
of polar flagella)

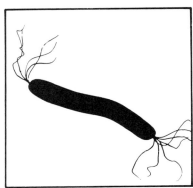

Aquaspirillum serpens
(Amphitrichous; flagella at both
poles, either single or in clusters)

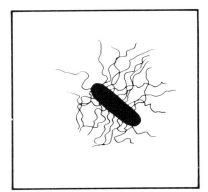

Salmonella typhi
(Peritrichous; cell
encircled by
lateral flagella)

Figure 3–6 ■ Various flagella arrangements in bacterial cells.

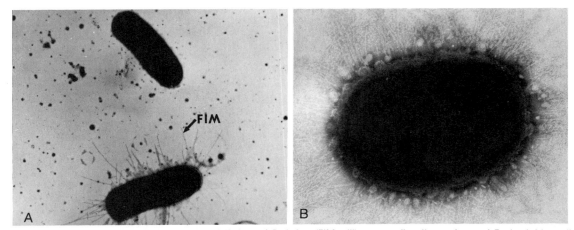

Figure 3–7 ■ Electron photomicrograph of *(A)* type 1 fimbriae (FIM; pili) surrounding the surface of *Escherichia coli*. The nonfimbriated cell in *A* is representative of a cell in which fimbriae synthesis has been "switched-off." In *B*, *Bacteroides gingivalis* numerous long fimbriae cover the cell surface and extend out of it in a tangled array of fibers.

Functions of Pili and Fimbriae

These structures function primarily in the transfer of genetic material between bacteria, as well as in adherence (i.e., **adhesins**). When functioning in the transfer of genetic material, the pili are referred to as F or *sex* pili. The F pili form physical bridges between donor and recipient cells (see page 107), known as conjugation bridges. This conjugation bridge permits the transfer of DNA between these two cell types. The pili are also bacteriophage (bacterial virus) receptors. Specific bacteriophage will adsorb to the tips of the F pili, which are then retracted into the cell. This retraction results in the virus being brought into close contact with the bacterial cell surface, where a second receptor in the outer membrane functions to transfer the virus into the cell cytoplasm.

Pili are also adherence structures; they are referred to as either type-specific pili or fimbriae. Their adherence specificity for certain bacterial cells gives them their type-specific character. The fimbriae are irregularly distributed over the surface of the cell and are sometimes collectively referred to as a "fuzzy coat."

The type-specific fimbriae are also involved in cell-cell agglutination (type 1 fimbriae), as antigens, as well as in the agglutination of erythrocytes. The type 1 fimbriae are able to agglutinate both chicken and guinea pig erythrocytes in the absence of D-mannose; they are, however, unable to do so in the presence of this sugar. Hence, type 1 fimbriae are "mannose-sensitive." Type 3 fimbriae are only capable of agglutinating animal red blood cells if the erythrocytes have been treated with tannic acid. Type 2 fimbriae do not hemagglutinate red blood cells, and since they resemble type 1 fimbriae structurally and antigenically, they are considered to be structural variants of the type 1 fimbriae. This hemagglutination appears to be the result of surface electrical charge interactions with specific adhesin molecules, which are firmly attached to the tips of the fimbriae.

Importantly, the ability of several of the gram-negative pathogens to express their virulence in a susceptible host is regulated by the presence or absence of fimbriae. *Neisseria gonorrhoeae*, for example, when cultured in vitro on solid agar quickly lose their fimbriae and become nonpathogenic (i.e., avirulent). These avirulent *N. gonorrhoeae* are also unable to infect humans since they are unable to adhere to host tissue. The adherence of *E. coli* to gastric mucosa and to erythrocytes and leukocytes, as well as the adherence of *Pseudomonas aeruginosa* to alveolar tissue, is mediated by type-specific fimbriae. *Streptococcus pyogenes* also requires fimbriae in order to adhere to the epithelial mucosa of the throat and to cause streptococcal sore throat.

CAPSULES, SLIMES, AND OTHER SURFACE-ASSOCIATED COVERINGS

The outer layer of all cells is responsible for the ultimate survival and interaction of the cell with its environment, because it is this layer that is in direct contact with the influences of the environment. Bacteria, especially those that interact with cells, are usually surrounded by a slimy, gummy, or mucilaginous layer, various forms of which are seen in Figure 3–8a through e. Depending upon the overall consistency of this material, this layer is referred to as either a **capsule** or a **slime layer.** The capsule is usually of uniform consistency and integrity; slime layers, on the other hand, are ill-defined and loosely formed. The oral streptococci, *Streptococcus salivarius* and *S. mutans,* form large capsules consisting of glucan (dextran) or fructan (levan), depending upon the carbon source on which or in which they are grown. In the case of the streptococcal capsules, they are synthesized by specific polysaccharide synthesis enzymes at the cytoplasmic membrane and are transported to the bacterial cell surface through pores in the cell wall by specific transferases (glucosyl and fructosyl transferases) (see following section on chemical composition).

Chemical Composition of Capsules

Capsules are composed of either carbohydrate or protein, with their composition varying depending on the species, the carbon and nitrogen source, as well as the gaseous environment in which the cells are grown. Capsules have been identified that contain pectin (homopolymer of D-galacturonic acid), cellulose, and mixed carbohydrate polymers. As discussed earlier, the oral streptococci, *Streptococcus mutans* and *S. salivarius,* can form dextran and levan capsules, while *S. pneumoniae*, which forms several different chemical types of capsules (see further on), forms a capsule consisting of glucose polymers and is referred to as a type 2 capsule. The type 3 capsular polymers of *S. pneumoniae* are more complex, consisting of glucose

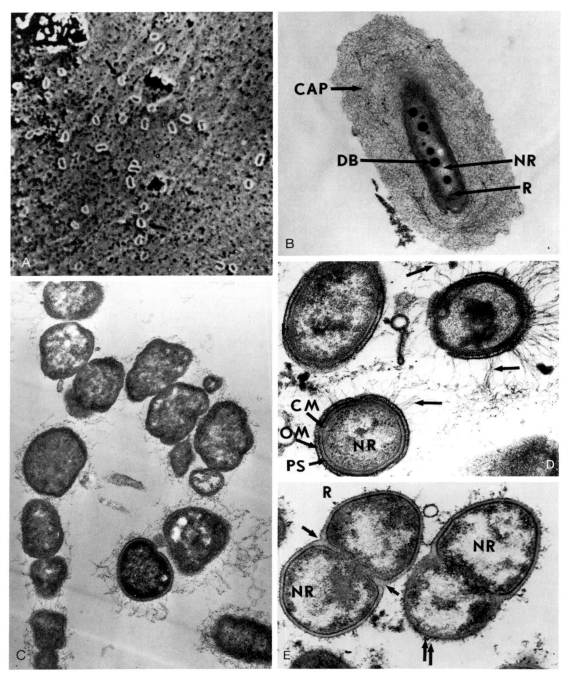

Figure 3–8 ■ Electron photomicrographs of bacterial capsules. *A,* India ink smear of *Bacteroides gingivalis* showing thick capsule. *B,* The thick alginic acid capsule of *Pseudomonas aeruginosa* surrounds the bacterial cell. *C,* The capsule of *Streptococcus mutans* is a loosely adherent structure that adheres very closely to the thick cell wall. *D,* The capsule of a *B. capillus* consists of a loosely adherent fibrous layer *(arrows). E,* The loosely adherent capsule of *B. gingivalis* attaches numerous cells into an adherent cell wall. The *single arrows* in *E* indicate the ingrowing division septum, while the *double arrows* indicate loosely adherent capsular material. Note in *E* the concentration of ribosomes in the division plane of the dividing streptococci. CAP = capsular; DB = dense storage body; NR = nuclear region; R = ribosomes; PS = periplasmic space; OM = outer membrane; CM = cytoplasmic membrane.

and glucuronic acid subunits. *Bacillus anthracis,* the microorganism causing anthrax, produces a polypeptide capsule of polyglutamic acid. This polyglutamyl polypeptide is produced only in the presence of CO_2 and functions as a virulence factor in anthrax.

Several of the bacterial capsules have been formulated into effective vaccines. For example, the numerous pneumoniae capsular types have been combined into a vaccine that is effective against pneumococcal diseases, while the capsular polysaccharide from *Neisseria meningitidis* is protective against meningitis for infants younger than 6 months of age. The capsule of *Mycobacterium tuberculosis* has been used with some success in Europe to immunize against tuberculosis; however, because it cannot be completely separated from the nucleic acid of *M. tuberculosis,* its use is not permitted in the United States. A potential capsular vaccine has been produced from *Streptococcus mutans* that may be effective against dental caries.

Function of Capsules

Capsules are important in permitting bacteria to express their virulence capabilities, as well as providing them with the ability to survive the numerous host defense mechanisms with which animals and plants are endowed. Capsules also provide an immunologic specificity. Encapsulated bacteria produce smooth (S) colonies and are immunologically characterized as "S-type" colonies, while bacteria that have had their capsules removed by either genetic or chemical means are immunologically termed "R-type" cells. The S-type colonial morphology is associated with the virulence of pathogenic bacteria, with the capsules protecting them from the defense mechanisms of infected animals, especially from phagocytosis. The immunologic specificity of the capsule is so great that even within a given species, immunologic subspecies or types may be distinguished as a result of even slight differences in the composition of the capsular material. For example, there are nearly 15 distinct immunologic types of the single species of *Streptococcus pneumoniae.* In addition to providing immunologic specificity, providing protection against phagocytosis, and functioning as virulence factors, capsules also serve as osmotic barriers since they themselves consist of almost 95 percent water, which prevents the too-rapid flux of water into or out of the cell.

Other Surface Appendages

Several groups of bacteria secrete discernible structures, which function physically to stick or hold these cells to surfaces. These structures are referred to as holdfasts, and usually occur on bacteria existing in the aquatic environment; these are prosthecate bacteria.

A variety of bacteria, also found free-living in the natural environment—especially in environments rich in organic compounds and reduced metallic salts—form sheaths or tubes that surround and enclose these cells. In comparison to the capsule, the sheath is a very complex chemical structure.

CELL WALL

It was clear from van Leeuwenhoek's initial observations of the various shapes of bacteria that a structure must be present on these bacteria to provide and maintain these various morphotypes. Since the internal cytoplasm does not mix freely with the external environment, the existence of a rigid limiting layer, or cell wall, is required (Fig. 3–9a, b). The cell wall, (specifically its peptidoglycan, (see page 68) gives the cell its shape and protects the cell cytoplasm from osmotic pressure differences that are exerted between the intracellular and extracellular environments. The cell wall is also the primary "sieve" in the transport of molecules into the cell. It also functions as an anchor for the capsule, as well as for pili, fimbriae, and flagella, and it is the primary receptor for the absorption of specific viruses or bacteriophages prior to their transport into the cytoplasm.

With the exception of the members of the taxonomic group, *Mollicutes* (i.e., *Mycoplasma, Acholeplasma, Spiroplasma,* PPLO, and the archebacteria, *Halobacterium, Methanobacterium*), the rigidity and strength of the bacterial cell wall is due to a network of fibers composed of heteropolymers of the chemical class of mucopolysaccharides commonly referred to as the mucopeptide, mucocomplex, or peptidoglycan. These fibers form a tough network or **sacculus** that completely surrounds the cell.

In the *Mollicutes,* the cytoplasm is enclosed by a single, thin cell membrane, approximately 7.5 nm thick (Fig. 3–10). This membrane functions as both the cell wall and the cytoplasmic membrane (see further on). Without a cell wall to provide rigidity these

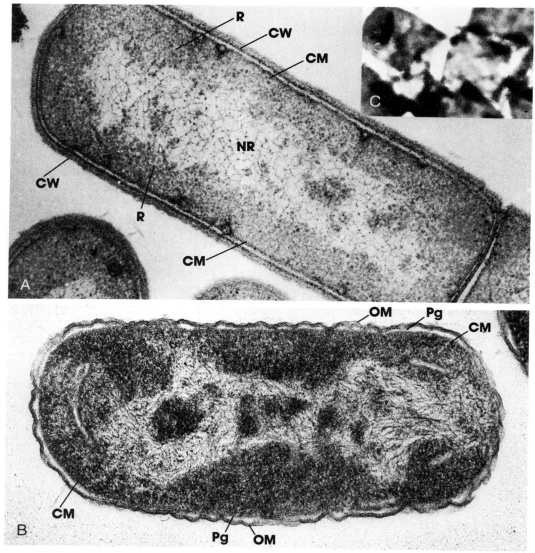

Figure 3–9 ■ Electron photomicrographs of *(A)* the gram-positive bacterium, *Bacillus macroides*, and *(B)* the gram-negative, *Escherichia coli*. In *A*, the thick cell wall (CW) surrounds the thin cytoplasmic membrane (CM), which encloses the cytoplasmic region containing electron-dense ribosomes (R) and a fibrillal nucleoid (NR). *B*, The outer membrane (OM) is external to the very thin peptidoglycan (Pg), which encloses the unit cytoplasmic membrane (CM). *C*, Isolated cell wall fragments from *B. macroides*. Note that the fragments maintain their rod-appearance, a result of the chemical construction of the peptidoglycan. NR = nuclear region; R = ribosomes.

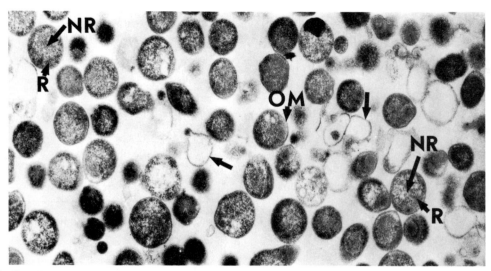

Figure 3–10 ■ Electron photomicrograph of the wall-less bacterium, *Mycoplasma capricolum*. Note the absence of the cell wall. The cell is surrounded by a thin cell membrane. The *arrows* indicate the thin outer membrane. NR = nuclear region; OM = outer membrane; R = ribosomes. (Courtesy of Dr. Schlomo Rottem.)

microorganisms must live in an environment where the osmotic pressure is such that it will not rupture the cells; hence, the very restricted ecologic environment in which these "wall-less" bacteria live. It is probably more useful to divide the *Mollicutes* into the wall-less *Mycoplasmas* and the peptidoglycan-less *Archebacteria*.

The ability of bacterial cells to retain or release specific dyes in the classic gram-staining technique has resulted in a clear separation of bacteria into two major groups: those that retain the blue dye crystal violet after treatment with iodine, alcohol, and counterstaining with the red dye safranin, and those that do not do so. Gram-positive cells retain the blue crystal violet and stain blue, while Gram-negative bacteria do not retain this dye and thus stain red with safranin after alcohol treatment. The characteristic morphology of gram-positive and gram-negative cell walls is seen in Figure 3–8c, d. Immediately apparent is that the cell walls of these two major groups of bacteria are visibly different. Cell walls of gram-positive bacteria are thicker (15 to 50 nm) than those of gram-negative bacteria (7.5 to 10 nm). Some cell walls of gram-positive bacteria have been observed to reach thicknesses of 80 nm, and, depending upon the growth conditions, stage of growth, as well as C- and N- sources, the gram-positive cell wall can constitute between 20 and 40 percent of the cellular dry weight. The cytoplasmic membrane (see further on) adheres very tightly to the internal aspect of the cell wall in gram-positive bacteria.

The cell wall of gram-negative bacteria is both morphologically and chemically more complex than that of gram-positive bacteria. It consists of several membranes (see page 72 for discussion of the concept of a membrane) that lay outside of the cytoplasmic membrane and that enclose the electron-dense cytoplasmic region. The multilayered arrangement of the gram-negative cell wall and the fact that it cannot be separated as a unit (as can the gram-positive cell wall) have resulted in this layer being referred to as the *cell envelope*. The outermost layer of the cell envelope then is referred to as the *outer membrane*. This layer is approximately 7.5 to 10 nm thick and encloses an electron transparent space, the *periplasmic space*. The periplasmic space contains a variety of hydrolytic enzymes and chemotactic stimulants involved in the hydrolysis of large macromolecules and chemical attraction, respectively. Within the periplasmic space is a very thin peptidoglycan layer, that is approximately 3 to 4 nm thick. The cell wall of gram-negative bacteria consists of two layers; the outer membrane and the peptidoglycan layer enclose a periplasmic space; together they form the gram-negative cell envelope. The gram-positive bacterial cell wall consists of one thick layer.

Chemistry of the Peptidoglycan

The peptidoglycan is unique to the cell wall of essentially all prokaryotes (with the exceptions noted earlier); it has not been found in eukaryotes. It is responsible for the maintenance of cell shape and rigidity. The chemical composition of the cell walls of gram-positive and gram-negative bacteria is seen in Table 3–2. Gram-positive cell walls contain relatively high amounts of amino sugars (i.e., 15 to 20 percent), no lipids, and only minor amounts of amino acids. In contrast, the cell walls of gram-negative bacteria (outer membrane and peptidoglycan) are rich in lipid (10 to 20 percent), have a low amino sugar content (2 to 5 percent), and contain the full complement of amino acids that are found routinely in proteins.

The chemical structure and molecular configuration of the peptidoglycan are seen in Figure 3–11a, b. Chemically, the peptidoglycan consists of two sugars, N-acetylglucosamine and N-acetylmuramic acid, at least four amino acids, usually glutamic acid, alanine, glycine, and lysine (Fig. 3–11b). Diaminopimelic acid can substitute for lysine (Fig. 3–12). The gram-positive cell wall consists almost entirely of peptidoglycan. The N-acetylglucosamine and N-acetylmuramic acid are chemically linked together into a linear polymer of approximately 40 to 50 disaccharides, or glycan units. The repeating N-acetylglucosaminyl-N-acetylmuramyl dimers that

Table 3–2 ■ Basic chemical composition of gram-positive and gram-negative cell walls

Cell Wall Component	Gram-positive	Gram-negative
Peptidoglycan	+	+
Teichoic acid and/or Teichuronic acid } =	+	–
Polysaccharide	+	+
Protein	±	+
Lipid	–	+
Lipopolysaccharide	–	+
Lipoprotein	–	+

+ = routinely present; – = routinely absent; ± = usually absent, but present in some genera.

form the glycan are covalently connected by random cross-links between short tetrapeptides that originate from the muramyl residues. Not all of the muramyl peptide chains are linked together through interpeptide bonding; the degree of cross-linking of the peptidoglycan will affect its rigidity as well as its strength. Therefore, the thick gram-positive cell wall has an extremely strong tensile structure, consisting of many (between 15 and 50) peptidoglycan layers,

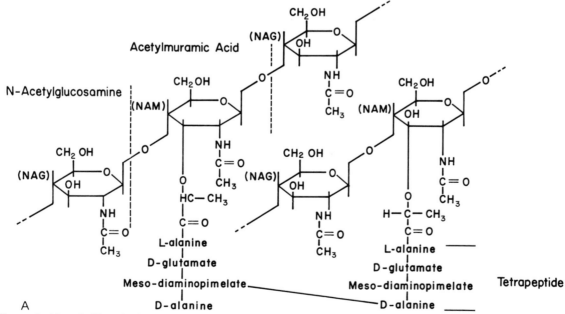

Figure 3–11 ■ A, Chemical structure of a classic peptidoglycan fragment. The branching structure consists of repeating units of an N-acetyl-glucosamine and an N-acetyl-muramic acid. This glycan chain is joined to other glycan chains by tetrapeptide links consisting of L-alanine, D-glutamic acid, lysine of meso-diaminopenalic acid, and D-alanine. The interpeptide bridge between meso-diaminopenalic acid and D-alanine can consist of several different amino acids. B, The chemical structure of the N-acetyl-glucosamine-N-acetyl-muramic acid tetrapeptide is seen.

Illustration continued on opposite page

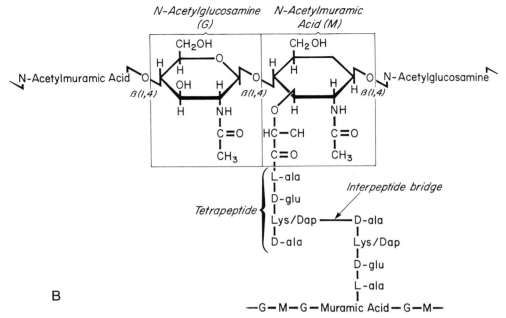

N-Acetylglucosamine (G) N-Acetylmuramic Acid (M)

Figure 3–11 ■ Continued.

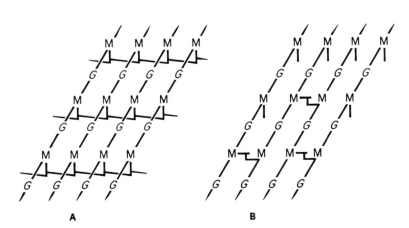

Figure 3–12 ■ Chemical structure of diaminopimelic acid and lysine.

Diaminopimelic Acid

Lysine

Figure 3–13 ■ Diagrammatic representation of a segment of the peptidoglycan showing the cross-bridging of the molecule. This cross-bridging provides the rigidity and strength to the peptidoglycan. N = N-acetylmuramic acid; G = N-acetyl-glucosamine.

A   B

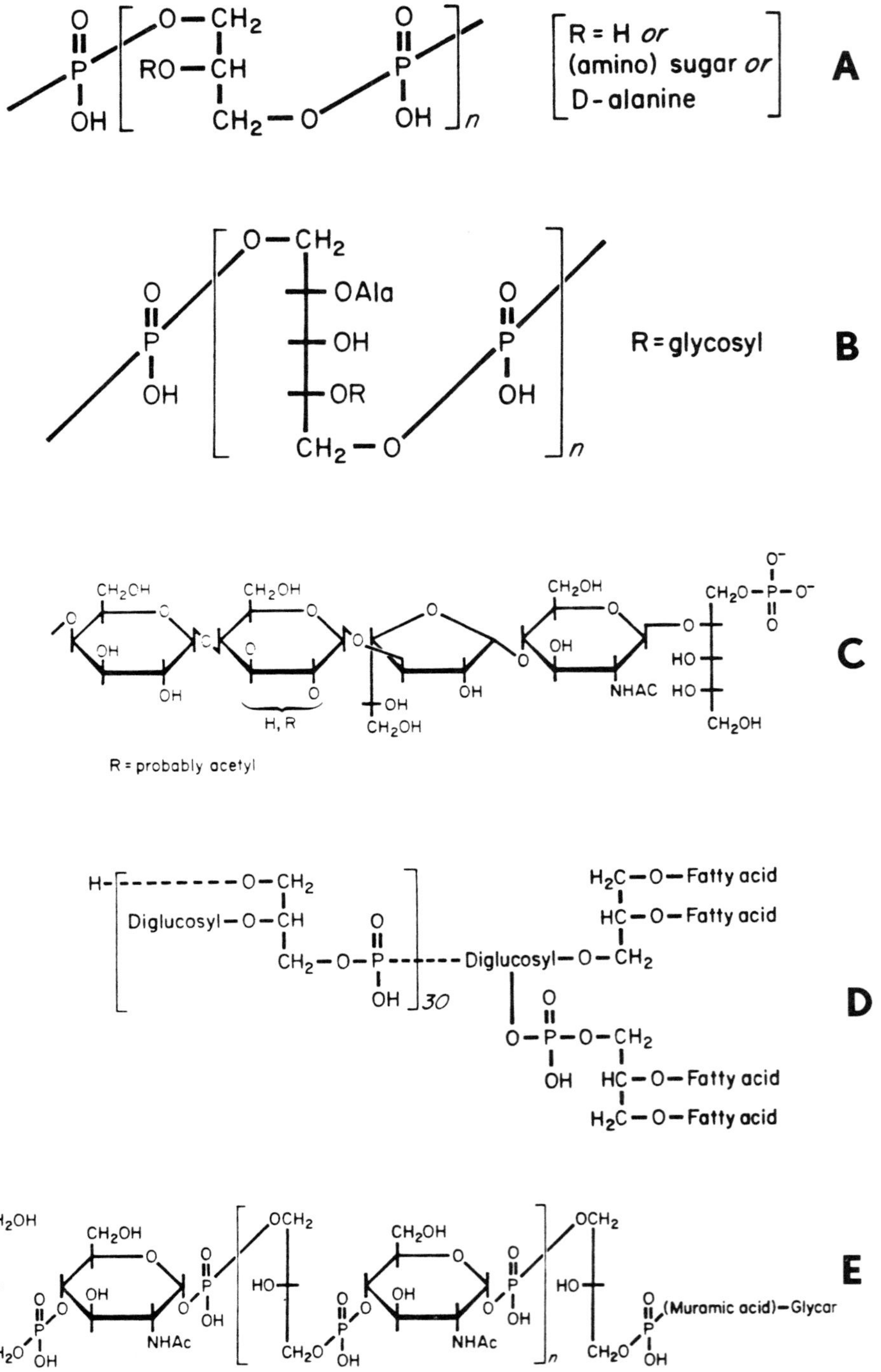

Figure 3–14 ■ Chemical structure of various teichoic acids that constitute a portion of the gram-positive cell wall. *A,* Glycerol teichoic acid. *B,* Ribitol teichoic acid. *C,* Teichoic acid of *Streptococcus pneumoniae* capsule. The structure consists of oligoglycosyl ribitol units. *D,* Lipoteichoic acid of *Streptococcus faecalis.* The diglycosyl units consist of glucose a,1–2 glucose molecules, or sometimes referred to as kojibiose. *E,* Repeating unit of *N*-acetyl-glucosamine-1-phosphate-glycosyl-phosphate. These sugar molecules are present in the backbone chain of selected peptidoglycans.

whereas the gram-negative peptidoglycan has been estimated to be only one layer thick, and consequently is a much more fragile cell wall (compare Figs. 3–9a, b, and 3–13). In order to add more vertical stability to the gram-negative cell envelope, two proteins bind the outer membrane to the peptidoglycan in this group. These proteins, the *matrix proteins* and the *Braun lipoproteins*, are inserted into the outer membrane, providing this vertical stability to the outer membrane–peptidoglycan complex by providing a chemical link between these two envelope layers (see Fig. 3–18). The peptidoglycan does, however, maintain the shape and rigidity of the cell.

Teichoic Acids

In addition to the peptidoglycan, the gram-positive cell wall also contains uronic acids (Fig. 3–14). Teichoic, teichuronic, and lipoteichoic acids are the major uronic acid constituents. These amphipathic linear polyalcohol phosphate molecules are linked together as glycerol-sugar-phosphate polymers. They have not been observed in gram-negative bacteria; their formation is dependent upon growth conditions, and not all species of gram-positive bacteria form them. The predominant uronic acids are either glycerol or ribitol, and these are linked via phosphodiester bonds to the *N*-acetylmuramic acid of the cell wall glycan strands. The polyalcohol phosphate molecules are inserted into the pre-existing cell wall as a teichoic acid–peptidoglycan complex. Not all of the teichoic acid termini originate from the cell wall itself. The fatty acid, or acylated teichoic acid (lipoteichoic acid, or LTA), penetrates through the cell wall, with the lipid moiety intercalating the phospholipids of the cytoplasmic membrane (Fig. 3–15).

Function of the teichoic acids ▪ While the exact function of these teichoic or uronic acids in the bacterial cell wall is still unclear, it has been postulated that since one end of the molecule probably emerges from the surface of the cell, they may contribute to the overall negative-charge density of the cell surface. This large negative charge on their surface makes them very effective molecules, and lipoteichoic acids are recognized as strong adhesins, especially in the attachment of streptococci to mammalian cells. In addition to attachment to mammalian tissues, these molecules may adhere to red blood cells, tooth surfaces, and the numerous other surfaces that routinely are positively charged. The teichoic acids are also the major antigenic components of the gram-positive cell surface.

The Gram-Negative Envelope: Its Chemistry and Function

Chemically, the outer membrane consists of approximately 20 to 25 percent phospholipid and 45 to 50 percent protein, with the remainder (about 30 percent) consisting of the unique glycolipid, the *lipopolysaccharide*, or LPS (Fig. 3–16). The LPS is found only in gram-negative bacteria.

Structurally, the outer membrane consists of two layers arranged in the characteristic bilayer common to all biologic membranes (see page 74). The outer layer—or outer leaflet—of the outer membrane contains, in addition to these phospholipids, the lipopolysaccharide. The inner leaflet of the outer membrane consists primarily of phospho-

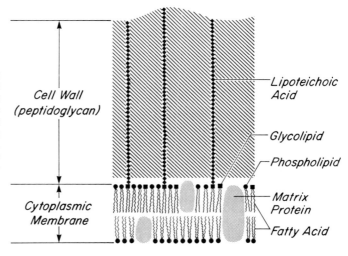

Figure 3–15 ▪ Diagrammatic representation of the insertion of the lipoteichoic acid into the gram-positive cell wall. The lipoteichoic acid inserts directly through the cell wall into glycolipid moieties. Teichoic acid molecules (not shown), devoid of their acyl groups, can insert directly into the matrix of the cell wall. (Redrawn from Stanier, R., et al. [eds.]: The Microbial World, ed. 5. Prentice-Hall, Englewood Cliffs, NJ, 1986.)

Cell Wall (peptidoglycan)

Cytoplasmic Membrane

Lipoteichoic Acid

Glycolipid

Phospholipid

Matrix Protein

Fatty Acid

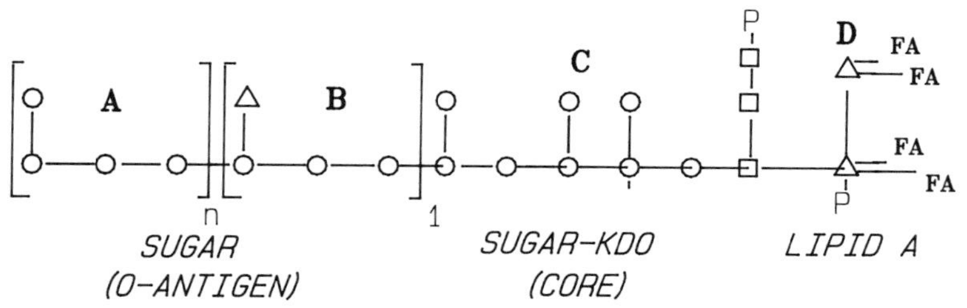

A=Various O-antigen sugars: i.e., rhamnose, mannose
  abequose, galactose

B=O-antigen sugar repeat
C= N-acetylglucosamine (△), glucose, galactose, heptose (○)
  2-Keto, 3-deoxy-octanoate, KDO (□)

D= b-1-6-linked N-acetylated glucosamine+
  at least 7 fatty acids (FA)

Figure 3–16 ■ Schematic representation of lipopolysaccharide from *Salmonella typhimurium*. The lipid backbone (lipid A) is composed of B 1-6-linked *N*-acetylated glucosamine monosaccharides (GlcNAc). The fatty acids (Fa) vary among C-12, C-14, C-16, OH-C-16, and OH-C-12 compounds. The number and type of lipid A fatty acids vary among bacterial species. In addition, phosphate esters (P), amino groups (not shown), or both are substituted at the 1 and 4′ positions of the nonreducing and reducing glucosamines, respectively (see Fig. 3–44). An eight-carbon keto sugar 2-keto,3-deoxy-octanoic acid, KDO, links the lipid A and polysaccharide portions of the molecule. The number of KDOs is variable among species. The remainder of the core sugars include heptose, glucose, galactose, and *N*-acetylglucosamine. The O-antigen sugars in *S. typhimurium* include galactose, rhamnose, mannose, and abequose. (Reproduced with permission of Hitchcock, P. J., et al.: J. Bacteriol. 166:699, 1986.)

lipids. The presence of the LPS in the outer leaflet and of the phospholipids in the inner leaflet produces the structural asymmetry characteristic of the gram-negative outer membrane; that is, the outer leaflet of the outer membrane is more electron-dense than the inner leaflet.

One of the primary functions of the outer membrane is to act as a molecular sieve, excluding the transfer, both into and out of the cell molecules, with molecular weights exceeding 700. Molecules with a molecular weight greater than 700 enter the cell via specific proteins, referred to as *porin proteins.* The outer membrane also functions as a bacterial virus (bacteriophage) receptor and as an antigenic determinant. The outer membrane prevents the penetration of antibiotics, detergents, and other harmful molecules into the cell.

The LPS consists of three regions: the O-specific polysaccharide, the core polysaccharide, and the lipid A (Fig. 3–16). The O-specific polysaccharide, or O-somatic antigen, provides the cell with its unique antigenic makeup. The core polysaccharide joins the lipid A to the O-specific polysaccharide and consists of the unique molecule, 2-keto-3-deoxy-octanoate (KDO), and a seven-carbon heptose sugar. The lipid A is highly hydrophobic and is embedded in the outer leaflet of the outer membrane. It consists of a phosphorylated glucosamine disaccharide that is esterified with long-chain fatty acids, usually C14, C16, and C18 carbon chain lengths. In addition to these fatty acids, the lipid A contains hydroxy fatty acids. These fatty acids have been postulated to function as the **endotoxin.**

Functionally, the LPS acts to protect the cell from the action of antibody and complement, is a bacteriophage receptor, and is one of the major endotoxic molecules of gram-negative bacteria; hence, it is considered an important virulence factor of these bacteria. Depending upon the lipid A type, dosage, and route of lipid A injection, it can cause hemorrhage, fever, tumor necrosis, fatal shock, septicemia, and even abortion.

CYTOPLASMIC MEMBRANE

In both animal and plant cells, the cytoplasm is not readily differentiated from the outer integument, or cytoplasmic membrane; however, in prokaryotic cells, the cytoplasmic membrane is a distinct and, in most cases, a readily separable component of the cell (see Figs. 3–1*a*, 3–8*d*, 3–9, and 3–17*a*). In gram-positive bacteria the cytoplasmic mem-

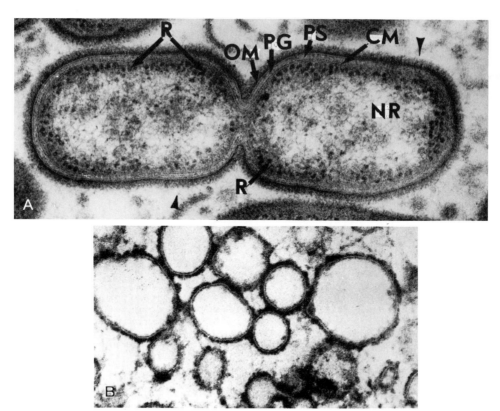

Figure 3–17 ■ Electron photomicrographs of whole cells *(A)* of the gram-negative bacterium *Bacteroides gingivalis,* and *(B)* isolated outer membrane. *Arrows* point to the thick capsule. R = ribosomes; OM = outer membrane; PG = peptidoglycan; PS = periplasmic space; CM = cytoplasmic membrane; NR = nuclear region.

brane is in close association with the cell wall (see Figs. 3–1a, 3–8e), while in gram-negative cells it lies just below the thin peptidoglycan layer (see Figs. 3–8d, 3–9b, and 3–17a). It consists of three distinct layers, or leaflets: the outer and inner layers, which are separated from each other by a middle layer (Figs. 3–17b, 3–18). The outer and inner layers are approximately 2 to 2.5 nm thick, while the middle layer is approximately 5 nm thick (Fig. 3–18). Therefore, the cytoplasmic membrane is approximately 10 nm in diameter, with an average diameter of 7.5 nm. This construction is referred to as a **"unit membrane."** Chemically, the outer and inner layers are composed of approximately 70 percent protein, with the middle layer 30 percent lipid. In addition to fatty acids in this central hydrophobic region of the membrane, phospholipids and transmembrane proteins (e.g., permeases) also exist. The polar or hydrophilic head groups of the phospholipids are located at the outer surface of the hydrophobic region of the membrane, with the hydrophobic fatty acid "tails" extending into the central region of the membrane. The structural and permease proteins traverse the hydrophobic region. The nature of these transmembrane proteins, as well as the fact that the individual lipids within the membrane leaflets are free to exchange with each other within the leaflets, has resulted in the concept of the fluid mosaic model for biologic membranes (Fig. 3–19). This model describes a membrane that is considered highly "plastic" and that is capable of adjusting to changes in both temperature and nutritional conditions. However, while the phospholipids of the cytoplasmic membrane provide for a two-dimensional fluid, the large amount of protein within the membrane provides for membrane stability, especially with respect to the individual membrane proteins.

In summary then, from a functional point of view, the cytoplasmic membrane is one of the most important components of the bacterial cell, in fact, of all cells. Without a functional cytoplasmic membrane the cell would not survive—it is the site of anabolic and catabolic metabolism and regulates the transport of molecules into and out of the cell.

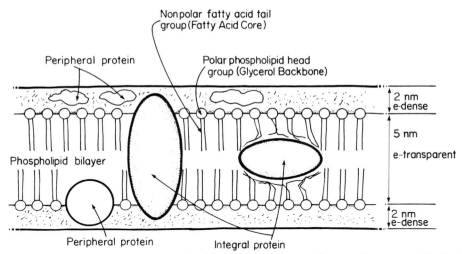

Figure 3–18 ■ Diagrammatic representation of a classic unit membrane. The membrane consists of a "sandwich" of hydrophilic protein, which encloses a hydrophobic lipid layer. Proteins exist in the peripheral region of the membrane as well as traversing the membrane. The integral proteins function to transport material from the outside to the inside of the cell as well as providing structural integrity. The phospholipid head groups are embedded in the protein layers, and the fatty acid tails extend into the central region of the membrane.

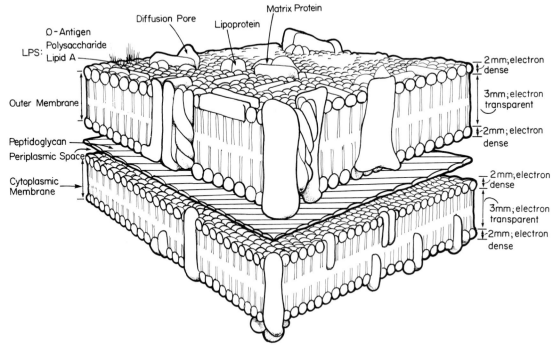

Figure 3–19 ■ Three-dimensional representation of the cell envelope of a gram-negative bacterium. The cell envelope consists of a thick outer membrane, an intermediate peptidoglycan layer, and the underlying cytoplasmic membrane. Both the cytoplasmic membrane and the outer membrane are of unit construction (see Fig. 3–18). Diffusion pores, lipoprotein, and matrix proteins emerge from the surface of the membrane. Also, the O-antigen of the lipopolysaccharide emerges from the outer membrane surface as thin hair-like structures. Lipid A of the lipopolysaccharide is embedded in the outer membrane.

THE CYTOPLASM AND ITS INCLUSIONS

The bacterial cytoplasm consists of all of the structures and substances enclosed by the cytoplasmic membrane (Figs. 3–1a; 3–8b through e; 3–9a, b; 3–10; and 3–17a). The cytoplasm itself, excluding the nuclear region, consists of a complex mixture of ions, amino acids, proteins, and lipid complexes. These materials serve as the building blocks for cellular biosynthesis and energy production. The cytoplasm also contains the various RNAs and the multitude of electron-opaque ribosomes that intertwine with and surround the nuclear region required for protein synthesis. The cytoplasm also contains the storage granules that are formed in response to the cells' chemical and physical environment. Basically then, the bacterial cytoplasm consists of a central nuclear region surrounded by ribosomes mixed in a "sea" of enzymes, cofactors, amino acids, and vitamins, as well as a multitude of other ions and molecules.

Ribosomes

The ribosome is the most abundant inclusion in the bacterial cytoplasm (see Figs. 3–1a; 3–8b through e; 3–9a, b; and 3–17a). It consists of approximately 40 percent protein and 60 percent RNA. Its exclusive function is protein synthesis. When ribosomes are centrifuged at high speed they move with a specific rate known as the sedimentation rate. The sedimentation rate, or Svedborg (S̈), of the bacterial ribosome is 70 S̈, while that of the eukaryotic ribosome is 80 S̈. The eukaryotic ribosome is larger than the bacterial ribosome. Three types of RNA exist: ribosomal RNA (r-RNA), amino acid transfer RNA (t-RNA), and messenger RNA (m-RNA). (The reader is referred to a recent textbook of biochemistry for a description of the role of these RNA molecules in protein synthesis, as well as to pages 100 to 106 of this chapter.)

Nuclear Region and Nuclear Elements

The development of specific staining techniques and improved methods of cell preservation combined with electron microscopy revealed that bacteria contained a non-membrane bound region that was equivalent to the eukaryotic nucleus. This fibrous region of the bacterial cell was determined to be the nucleus or nucleoid because of its non-membrane bound character (see Figs. 3–1a; 3–8b through e; 3–9a, b; 3–10; and 3–17a). Studies

of bacterial genetics described the bacterial genetic material, or genome, as individual genetic determinants (i.e., genes) arranged in a linear fashion along a long circular strand of DNA. This DNA strand, if laid open, would stretch almost 1400 μm (remember, the average bacterium is approximately 1 μm in diameter!). In terms of molecular weight, or mass, the bacterial genome varies over a wide range; for example, *Mycoplasma* species have a relatively small genome of from 0.45 to 1.1 $\times$ 10^9 daltons (1.2 $\times$ 10^6 bases, or 1000 genes), and the gram-positive cocci and rods, as well as gram-negative bacteria (i.e., *E. coli* and *Bacteroides*), have very large genomes on the order of 2.8 $\times$ 10^9 daltons (4.2 $\times$ 10^6 bases, or approximately 3000 genes).

While the nuclear region contains the genetic material of the cell, many bacteria also contain DNA molecules that are independent of the nuclear region. These small, extrachromosomal DNAs, which have molecular masses of between 1 and 113 $\times$ 10^6 daltons, are referred to as **plasmids.** The plasmids are self-replicating small circular molecules of DNA. Plasmids typically contain approximately 0.1 to 0.2 percent of the DNA of the cell's chromosome. While plasmids are not essential for the survival of the bacterial cell, they do carry a variety of important genetic functions.

Bacterial Storage Granules and Inclusions

During their growth and metabolism, bacteria accumulate a variety of storage products in their cytoplasm (Fig. 3–20; Table 3–3). These metabolic products are formed as a result of the environment, as well as the metabolism by the cell of the large number of carbohydrates, lipids, and proteins that they can utilize. These inclusions include both membrane-limited and non–membrane-limited structures (Table 3–3).

Growth and Division

In order for cells to perpetuate themselves, they must grow—that is, increase in mass and size in an orderly fashion—and reproduce or divide. Not only must the cell separate physically, but it must also separate all of its cellular components including RNA, DNA, membranes, and so forth, into equal parts to be shared among the daughter progeny. For a cell to be successful in growth, division and survival the individual cellular components must increase prior to cell divi-

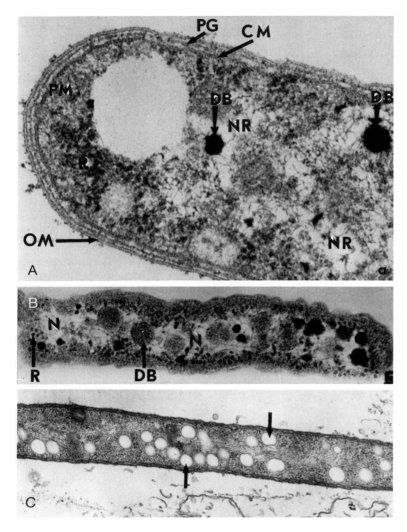

Figure 3–20 ■ Electron photomicrographs of various bacterial inclusions. *A* and *B,* The small, dense, spherical bodies or dense bodies (DB) are probably polyphosphate. Note their proximity to the fibrous nucleoid (N). In *B,* the cytoplasmic region also contains electron dense ribosomes (R), and storage granules of unknown chemistry and function. *C,* Electron transparent storage granules *(arrows)* traverse the cytoplasmic region. Note that these structures are surrounded by a thin layer. R = ribosomes; OM = outer membrane; PG = peptidoglycan; CM = cytoplasmic membrane.

sion. The cell's metabolic and biosynthetic constituents must also increase in an orderly series of events. All of these events are predetermined by the cells' genetic information. When all of these events have taken place and the cell reaches a genetically predetermined size and volume, it divides into two identical copies of itself. By definition then, *growth* is the orderly increase or synthesis of all cellular constituents from extracellular nutrients, the ultimate result of this increase being division.

TRANSVERSE OR BINARY CELL DIVISION

Growth of bacteria can be separated into two distinct stages: an increase in cell mass such as elongation of a bacillus, or an increase in size or volume such as in a coccus; and the division of these cells into two new daughter cells. While various modes of cell division occur in prokaryotic cells (Fig. 3–21), the most common mechanism of bacterial cell division then can be described as a binary or transverse division, or *binary fission* (Figs. 3–21 and 3–22). With only minor special differences, the majority of gram-positive and gram-negative bacteria divide in an identical fashion. Ideally, bacterial binary fission consists of at least three steps (Fig. 3–22):

1. During an initial growth or division period, bacilli will increase in both length and volume, while cocci will increase in volume. The nuclear material separates into two approximately equal halves, with one of the nuclear segments being attached to the cytoplasmic membrane.

2. Late in this initial division period, division septa or cross-walls develop. The septum is routinely formed at the approximate center of the dividing cell, and is the result of the ingrowth of the cell wall. Septum

Table 3–3 ■ Prokaryotic inclusions

Inclusion	Membrane-limited*	Shape	Formed in Presence of	Function
Polyglycoside	−	Sphere-rod	Excess C; limiting N, S, P; cell age	Carbohydrate storage
Polyphosphate	−	Sphere	Excess PO_4	Phosphate storage
Cyanopcin	−	Undulating flattened sac	Limiting essential nutrients. N-fixation	N-reserve during N-fixation
Phycobilisome	−	Sphere-rod	Light energy receptors	Receptors of light-energy chlorophyll
Poly B-hydroxybutyrate	+	Sphere	Excess glucose or acetate	Energy and C-storage
Sulfur	+	Sphere-globular subunits	Growth in presence of H_2S	Sulfur oxidation when H_2S becomes limiting
Gas vacuole	+	Stacks-hollow cylinders with conical ends		Movement of cells in vertical plane
Carboxysome	+	Spheres, polyhedral particles paracrystalline	Ribulose-1-5-diphosphate carboxylase	CO_2-fixation
Chlorosome	+	Oblong vesicles	Light—contains chlorophyll	Storage of chlorophyll for photosynthesis
Magnetosome	+	Linear array cuboidal particles	Contains Fe_3O_4 or magnetite (lodestone)	Orientation in magnetic field

*Membrane usually consists of one-half unit membrane, 3 to 4 nm thick.

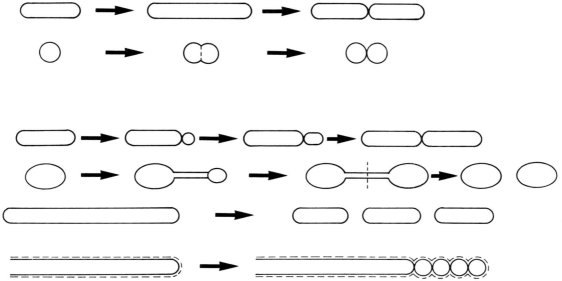

Figure 3–21 ■ Diagrammatic representation of various modes of bacterial cell division. The cells routinely divide by transverse binary fission. Several cells also form bud-like structures from the terminal portions of the cell.

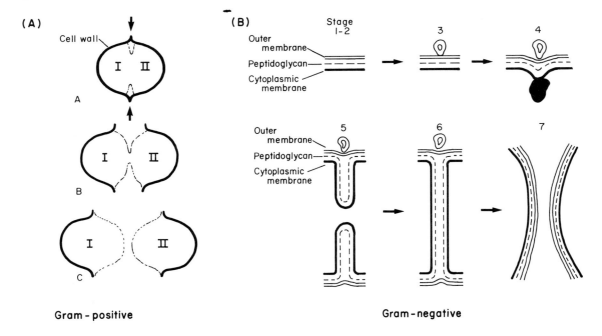

SEPTUM FORMATION

Figure 3–22 ■ Diagrammatic representation of septum formation and cell division in gram-positive and gram-negative bacteria. In gram-positive cell division *(A)* the cell wall is seen to grow into the cell as a septum until cell division is completed. In contrast, gram-negative septum formation *(B)*, involves the constriction of the outer membrane, peptidoglycan as well as cytoplasmic membrane. The septum ingrows forming a division plane, at which time it separates to form a new outer membrane and two daughter cells. (Adapted from Burdett, I. D., and Murray, R. G.: J. Bacteriol. 119:1029, 1974.)

formation at the approximate center of the cell is common among rods and bacilli. While there has been a large body of early descriptions of a "constrictive division" in gram-negative bacteria (a pinching of the central region of the cell to form two identical daughter cells), in fact the outer membrane is maintained as a rigid layer, with septum formation occurring as an ingrowth of the cytoplasmic membrane and peptidoglycan. Therefore, the completed septum consists of two "lamellae" of peptidoglycan that are separated by a gap.

3. In gram-positive bacteria, cell separation or binary fission occurs as the result of hydrolytic cleavage of the ingrowing peptidoglycan by specific hydrolytic enzymes, or amidases, while in gram-negative bacteria cell separation occurs by the ingrowth of the outer membrane after septum formation has been completed. This ingrowth of the outer membrane results in the physical separation of the cells into two identical daughter cells.

OTHER MECHANISMS OF BACTERIAL CELL DIVISION

Bacteria such as *Hyphomicrobium*, *Corynebacterium*, and *Mycobacterium* divide by *bud-*

ding, a process that is very similar to that seen in fungi and budding yeast cells. The budding cells originate as an outgrowth of the original, or mother, cell that eventually reaches a size equal to that of the mother cell. The bud then separates from its mother cell to undertake an independent existence. Several of the *Actinomycetes* form filamentous cells that reproduce by the formation of spores from a chain of cells, or by a simple fragmentation of the original filament into "new" cells.

GROWTH AND ENUMERATION OF BACTERIA

The basic events of bacterial growth, or multiplication, are measured by determining increases in cell numbers as a function of time. Since it is only theoretically possible to study the growth and multiplication of one bacterium, or even of one cell as it forms into a mass of cells (i.e., into a culture), one must study large populations of cells when studying growth. Therefore, the growth characteristics that one observes are the result of, and are subject to, statistical interpretation. There

Table 3–4 ■ Representative procedure for determining bacterial growth

Technique	Application	Resultant Determination
Microscopic count	Enumeration of total bacterial number	Number of cells
Electronic count	Same as for microscopic count	As for microscopic count
Plate count	Enumeration of viable bacteria in culture	Colony-forming units
Membrane filter count	As plate count	As plate count
Absorbance	Microbiologic assay. Estimation of cell increase in broth, cultures, or aqueous suspensions.	Optical density
Nitrogen determination	Measurement of cell mass	Units of nitrogen
Dry weight determination	Same as for nitrogen determination	Units of dry weight of cells
Measurements of specific biochemical parameter	Microbiologic assays	Milliequivalents of acid per ml or per culture

Modified from Pelczar, M. J., Jr., Chan, B. C. S., and Krirg, N. R.: Microbiology, 5th ed. McGraw-Hill Book Co., New York, 1986.

are several methods for the study of bacterial growth (Table 3–4), and the reader is referred to any standard microbiology textbook for a complete description of the techniques for the measurement of this growth.

MATHEMATICS OF BACTERIAL GROWTH

For this discussion, we will consider a bacterial culture that is growing under optimal conditions of nutrients, temperature, pH, and atmospheric conditions. We will also assume that all of the cells within this bacterial population are alive—that is, viable— and that they are dividing by transverse binary fission. Under these conditions, the cells in the culture are dividing at a constant and geometric rate; in other words, they are dividing in an exponential fashion. Thus, one cell in this culture will give rise to two cells, two to four, four to eight, and so forth. This binary series (1, 2, 4, 8, 16, 32, 64, . . .) defines exponential growth. Clearly, cells growing in this way will increase in number at a very rapid rate and will produce very large populations of cells (10^7 to 10^{11} cells per

ml being possible). This binary increase in the bacterial cell number is referred to as the doubling time, or generation time, and is defined as the time required for the cell or population of cells to divide, or to double itself.

It is possible to express the generation time mathematically. If we assume that the bacterial culture just described is inoculated with 100 cells (10^2), and if at specified times (i.e., 20-minute intervals) a sample is removed from the culture and the number of viable cells determined, one could determine the generation time. So if at zero time and at 20-minute intervals thereafter, the viability of the culture was determined to be 100, 200, 400, 800, 1600, and 3200 cells, the generation or doubling time would be 20 minutes. The bacterial population would also be increasing by one exponent, 2^n. In Figure 3–23, we have plotted the increase in cell number both arithmetically and in logarithmic notation. Note that by plotting the logarithms of the cell number one can plot on one piece of graph paper the results of a very large increase in the number of cells. Fortunately for us, cells do not grow exponentially for very long periods of time, but eventually fall prey to the vagaries of the environment (see further on). This fact becomes very important since, if one considers the enteric bacterium *Escherichia coli* growing with a generation time of approximately 20 minutes, in 48 hours a population of cells representing 2.2×10^{43} would be produced. Considering that one cell weighs 10^{-12} g, the total weight of this culture would be approximately 2.5×10^{25} tons, or almost 4000 times the mass of the earth!

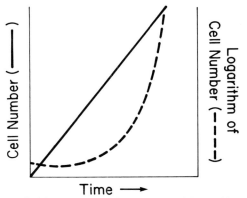

Figure 3–23 ■ Mathematical representation of bacterial growth. (---) = logarithm of number of bacteria versus time; (—) = arithmetic number of bacteria versus time. Generation time is determined from exponential curve and equals the time required for the culture to double.

THE BACTERIAL GROWTH CURVE

What are the events that occur when a culture of bacteria is inoculated into a suitable growth medium and provided with all appropriate requirements for maximum growth and division? If samples are taken from the culture as a function of time, as described earlier, and this is plotted as a function of either increase in optical density (turbidity) or any other cell component, then the result seen in Figure 3–24 occurs, which is typical of the growth of essentially all cell populations, both eukaryotic and prokaryotic, and is referred to as the *growth curve*. The growth of cells can be divided into at least four segments or growth phases: the *lag phase*, when there is no increase in cell number; the *logarithmic* or *exponential phase*, when the cells are dividing at a constant rate per unit time; the *stationary phase*, when maximum cell numbers are reached and the cell population stops active growth; and the *death* or *decline phase*, when the number of viable cells decreases, usually at an exponential rate.

Lag Phase

This phase of growth occurs when cells are transferred from one medium to another or from one environment to another. It is a phase of adjustment and represents the period required for the adaptation of the cells to the new environment. The cells in this phase often increase in total cell volume almost twofold or threefold, but they do not divide. These cells are rapidly synthesizing DNA, new protein, and new enzymes as a prerequisite to division.

Exponential Phase

It is in this phase that cells are dividing at both a constant and a geometric rate, as well as at a maximum rate. Not only are the cells dividing at a constant rate, but such cellular components as RNA, protein, dry weight, and cell wall polymers are all also increasing at a constant rate per unit time. Because the cells in the exponential phase are dividing at this maximum rate, they are much smaller in diameter than cells in the lag phase.

The exponential growth phase usually comes to an end owing to the depletion of essential nutrients, the depletion of oxygen in an aerobic culture, or the accumulation of toxic products.

Stationary Phase

During this portion of the growth phase there is a rapid decrease in the rate of cell division. Eventually a stage is reached where the total number of dividing cells will equal the number of dying cells, and a true stationary cell population occurs. The cells in this phase now turn all of their resources toward survival, and energy generation is harnessed to maintain osmotic barriers, motility, and the repair and resynthesis of essential macromolecules. The energy required to maintain cells in the stationary phase is called the *maintenance energy* and is obtained from the degradation of cellular storage products (i.e., glycogen, starch, lipids). After all of the storage products are exhausted, the cells turn next to the degradation of their own cellular components, which ultimately leads to the death phase.

Death Phase

As conditions become increasingly inimical, the cells reproduce more slowly, and death overtakes them in increasing numbers. The cells eventually enter the logarithmic death phase, during which the decrease in the number of cells occurs at a regular, unchanging rate, a rate that approximates that of the exponential growth phase but is of negative slope.

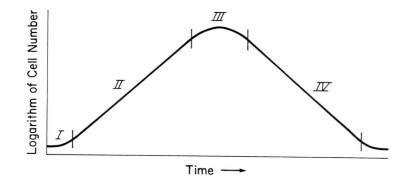

Figure 3–24 ■ Typical bacterial growth curve. The various growth phases are I, Lag phase; II, Log (logarithmic), or exponential phase; III, Stationary phase; IV, Death or decline phase.

Finally, conditions become such that an equilibrium is reached so that the rate of cell death and the increase in cell numbers tend to balance each other at a very low population level, and a phase of readjustment and final dormant phase are reached. The cells can exist in this condition for weeks or months, and complete sterility of the culture may not occur for a considerable length of time.

Physiology and Metabolism

Cell growth and division require that the cells obtain from their environment all of the necessary chemical constituents that are required for metabolism and the generation of energy (i.e., ATP; see page 83). The requirement for these chemical constituents for bacterial growth and metabolism is dependent upon the genetic make-up of the particular bacterial species. Some species have a very diverse nutritional flexibility (i.e., *Pseudomonas*), being capable of synthesizing many of their metabolites from simple precursors, whereas others have much more demanding nutritional requirements (i.e., *Bacteroides*) and require the input of more complex nutrients in order to grow and reproduce.

CARBOHYDRATE UTILIZATION

For purposes of our discussion of bacterial physiology, we will assume that the reader has some familiarity with the basic metabolic pathways for the utilization of sugars, amino acids, and lipids, as well as for the generation of energy by way of electron transport and anaerobic respiration. We will only present the basic information that is required for an understanding of the catabolism of these compounds by prokaryotic cells. The physiology of a cell can be considered under the general heading of *metabolism*, a process that denotes the chemical changes occurring in living cells. These metabolic changes can be divided into two basic groups, catabolism and anabolism.

Catabolism is the degradation (breakdown) of chemical compounds (substrates) into their constituent atoms, molecules, or molecular groups that will eventually be utilized for the synthesis of other carbon "skeletons," which will become part of larger molecules (macromolecules) of growing cells. Catabolism also includes the formation of the necessary energy for the cell to carry out its necessary macromolecular syntheses (i.e., cell wall formation, protein synthesis), as well as all of the other activities required of growing and metabolizing cells (motility, reproduction, taxis).

Anabolism refers to the conversion of the catabolically generated carbon skeletons into the macromolecules that constitute the physical and chemical make-up of the cell. It comprises all of the cell-building activities of the cell.

Clearly, catabolism and anabolism are interdependent processes; anabolic events occur to constantly replace cellular constituents that either have been used by the cell or need to be replaced, while catabolic events furnish the required materials and energy for these anabolic events to occur.

BASIC NUTRITIONAL REQUIREMENTS

The basic constituents of all cells are water, solids, and trace elements, with water accounting for between 80 and 90 percent of the total weight of a cell. In order for a cell to grow, it must obtain from the environment—or synthesize itself—all of its required basic cellular constituents. For example, the required oxygen and hydrogen are obtained from the hydrolysis of water, while essential carbon, nitrogen, phosphorus, and the other essential elements are provided to the cell from the environment (i.e., from the growth medium). Trace elements, such as magnesium (Mg), calcium (Ca), iron (Fe), manganese (Mn), and others, which are essential for the multitude of enzymatic reactions that occur in a cell, are usually supplied to the cell as *trace elements* in the water, from the growth vessels, and so on.

Carbon, the essential structural element of all cells, is provided to bacteria either by the dark reactions of photosynthesis through the Calvin cycle and the oxidation (loss of electrons or hydrogen) of inorganic carbon compounds, such as CO_2, or by the oxidation of organic compounds. Both mechanisms generate the needed carbon for the growth of the cell, as well as generating a large amount of the energy necessary for the cell. Nitrogen, which is required for protein synthesis, is usually supplied to the cell from amino acids as well as from the degradation of proteins in peptones, or from tryptones, which are constituents of many bacterial growth media. Several bacteria are capable of utilizing nitrogen in the form of NO_3^-, which is reduced (gain of electrons or hydrogen) to NH_3, which is then used in biosynthetic reactions. Some bacteria are capable of utilizing atmospheric dinitrogen (nitrogen fixation) from the atmosphere and of reducing it to NH_3.

Sulfur, another important element, especially of several amino acids, is usually supplied to bacteria by the direct metabolism of the sulfur-containing amino acids. For example, the sulfhydryl group ($-SH$) of methionine or cysteine is released by the oxidation of the amino acid with the formation of sulfate ($SO_4^=$), which like NO_3^- can be reduced to H_2S (or NH_3). The H_2S (NH_3) can then be used in further amino acid biosynthesis.

AUTOTROPHS AND HETEROTROPHS

Bacteria can be divided into two broad metabolic groups on the basis of their distinctive nutritional requirements: bacteria that use organic compounds as a source of electrons are referred to as heterotrophs, or organotrophs, and those that use an inorganic electron source are autotrophs, or lithotrophs. It is also possible to categorize bacteria in terms of the source of electrons in energy generation for ATP synthesis. Thus, photoautotrophs utilize light as an inorganic electron donor, while chemoautotrophs utilize inorganic molecules as sources of energy and electrons.

SOURCES OF ENERGY

In order to survive, all organisms must have some source of energy. We have described two of these sources: solar energy (phototrophs) and chemical energy (chemotrophs). We have already indicated that not only are bacteria capable of using both sources of energy but, among the large number of metabolic diverse bacteria, there is also a great diversity in chemotrophic energy metabolism. The three major mechanisms of energy generation in bacteria are respiration, fermentation, and anaerobic respiration. Accordingly, aerobic bacteria are able to use oxygen as a terminal electron acceptor, to reduce it to water, and, in this process of *aerobic respiration*, to form large amounts of energy as ATP (adenosine triphosphate). The oxidation of organic compounds (i.e., sugars) by respiratory means provides an enormous number and variety of bacteria with their

ATP. Some bacteria are capable of using organic compounds in the complete absence of oxygen, that is, under anaerobic conditions. This metabolic process is known as *fermentation*, and it produces not only ATP but also a variety of organic end products (i.e., alcohol from glucose in the yeast fermentation, or lactic acid in streptococci, depending upon the fermentative pathway used). Other bacteria are also capable of obtaining their energy while growing anaerobically; they do so if inorganic molecules such as NO_3^- or $SO_4^=$ are used as electron acceptors in the absence of oxygen. This anaerobic process of energy generation is referred to as *anaerobic respiration*.

Metabolism and Biosynthesis

From our brief introduction to the nutrition of bacteria, it should be clear that prokaryotic cells have a very diverse ability to metabolize an extraordinarily large number of organic and inorganic compounds. In fact, it is probably correct to assume that for essentially every natural compound that exists in our environment, as well as for many of the manufactured compounds, there is a microorganism in that environment that can metabolize it. The metabolism of all of these compounds serves one purpose—to provide the cell with the necessary carbon and energy for growth and reproduction. Even with this remarkable diversity in metabolism, there is a surprising degree of unity of the biochemical mechanisms for the overall metabolic processes. Therefore, no matter what the organism, the same building materials and essentially identical metabolic mechanisms exist—truly a "unity of biochemistry."

ENERGY REQUIREMENTS OF BACTERIA

Whether it be the formation of a simple compound or of a complex macromolecule, all biosynthetic processes require the input of energy; that is, they are endergonic reactions. The energy required to chemically "drive" these biosynthetic processes is routinely provided to the cell as ATP. ATP is the major energy currency of cells and is formed by a variety of catabolic reactions that are capable not only of producing this unique molecule but also, importantly, of transferring it to other energy-yielding exergonic reactions. It is the coupling of endergonic reactions with exergonic ones that permits the multitude of chemical reactions to proceed and the cell to grow and synthesize its numerous macromolecular components.

ATP Formation

The production of ATP is a function of the degree to which any organic compound is degraded; in fact, all energy-yielding reactions are the result of oxidation reactions. We have already discussed the fact that these oxidations can occur either in the presence of molecular oxygen with molecular oxygen serving as the terminal electron acceptor in aerobic respiration ($2H^+ + 2e^- + O_2 \rightarrow H_2O$), or under anaerobic conditions with inorganic molecules such as NO_3^- or $SO_4^=$ serving as electron acceptors in these energy-generating reactions ($2H^+ + 2e^- + NO_3^- \rightarrow NH_3$). *In all cases, however, it is the production of ATP in exergonic reactions and its transfer and use in endergonic reactions that link metabolism into a unified process.*

How is ATP produced in biologic reactions? For the most part, the oxidation reactions required for the generation of ATP in biologic systems (i.e., a bacterial cell) are the result of a series of interdependent reactions in which electrons are reversibly oxidized and reduced through a series of electron transfer reactions. These reactions, in which molecules are reversibly oxidized and reduced as electrons flow from a more negative electrical potential to a more positive one, constitute the electron transfer chain (see page 87 for an in-depth discussion of electron transport). At specific points along this electron transfer chain, energy as ATP is produced (Fig. 3–25a). The aerobic generation of ATP through this electron transport chain is referred to as *oxidative phosphorylation* (see further on for more discussion). Note in Figure 3–25a that simple examination of the electron transport chain does not provide any useful information as to how the passage of electrons through this series of electron carriers is capable of producing energy as ATP. Peter Mitchell in 1961 provided the most plausible hypothesis for how ATP generation could occur when electrons flow through the electron transport system (Fig. 3–25b). He proposed the *chemiosmotic hypothesis (proton motive force potential)*, in which ATP was formed by a change in electrical potential between the outside and inside of a membrane-bound organelle such as the eukaryotic mitochondrion or chloroplast or the prokaryotic cytoplasmic membrane. The flow of electrons through the electron transport system functions to release energy in such a way as to push positively charged hydrogen ions (i.e., H^+, protons) across the boundaries of the membrane. In the process of this proton flow there is the production of both a pH gradient and an electrical potential gradient because of the positive charge carried by the proton. The flow of hydrogen ions back across the membrane results in the production of ATP through this *proton motive force potential*. The flow of these electrons at specific sites within the membrane, known as the ATPase enzyme complex, results in the production of ATP.

EMBDEN-MEYERHOF-PARNAS PATHWAY—GLYCOLYSIS

Bacteria, as well as many animals and some plants, are able to metabolize or degrade carbohydrates such as starch, cellulose, dextrans, levans, glycogen, sucrose, lactose, and so forth, to a common intermediate, pyruvic acid (pyruvate). This degradation is routinely carried out by the Embden-Meyerhof-Parnas (EMP) glycolysis, or glycolytic, pathway (Fig. 3–26). In both humans and bacteria, the glycolytic pathway has common intermediates to pyruvic acid, and it is at pyruvate that metabolic specialization occurs. In humans, for example, pyruvate is metabolized to lactic acid in muscle glycolysis, while in yeasts, the pyruvate is converted to CO_2 and acetaldehyde, with the latter being converted to ethanol in the yeast fermentation. These latter reactions constitute the **alcoholic fermentation.** Note in Figure 3–26 that while ATP is required for the carbohydrate (i.e., glucose) to enter the pathway (the carbohydrate must first be "activated" by being phosphorylated), there is a net gain of two ATPs per mole of glucose degraded. Notice that the electron transfer molecule, pyridine nucleotide in its oxidized form (nicotinic acid adenine dinucleotide, NAD^+), which is reduced ($NADH_2$) in the upper portion of the EMP pathway, is reoxidized ($NADH + H^+ \rightarrow NAD^+$) in the conversion of pyruvate to reduced end products. It is essential that reduced pyridine nucleotide be regenerated so that the EMP pathway continues to function in the utilization of carbohydrates.

Basically, then, in the EMP pathway, glucose is first phosphorylated to produce an activated glucose-6-phosphate, which is ultimately split into two trioses, glyceraldehyde-3-phosphate (three-carbon units), which are

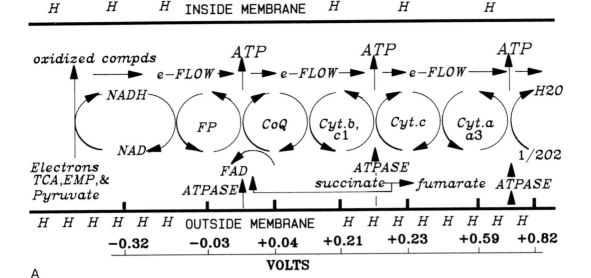

A

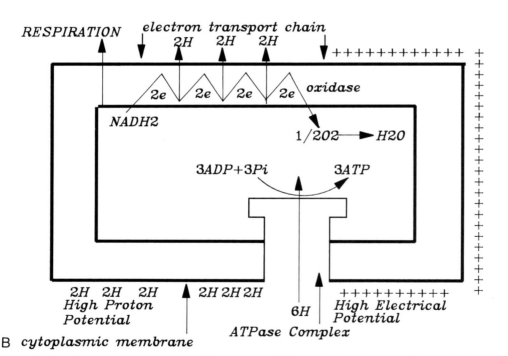

B cytoplasmic membrane

Figure 3–25 ■ *A,* Electron transport system (ETS) produces ATP by oxidative phosphorylation. Electrons from various electron generating cycles (TCA, EMP, pyruvate), are passed to NAD$^+$ and then to the electron acceptors such as flavoprotein (FP), coenzyme Q (CoQ), cytochromes b and c$_1$, cytochrome c, and cytochromes a and a$_3$. Each electron acceptor is reduced and reoxidized when it passes the electrons on to the next acceptor. Oxygen is ultimately reduced to form water in aerobic respiration; NO$_3^-$, and SO$_4^=$ are reduced to NH$_3$, and H$_2$S, respectively, in anaerobic respiration. Flow of electrons through ETS results in high H-ion concentration outside cytoplasmic membrane, and low concentration inside. The resultant pH and electrochemical gradient results in H ions being drawn back into the cell at ATPase sites in the membrane. The electrons that are transported down this voltage gradient liberate their energy, with the resultant formation of ATP at ATPase sites (see also Fig. 3–28b). *B,* Diagrammatic representation of the Mitchell or chemiosmotic hypothesis of energy generation. Electrons and protons (a hydrogen atom), which are generated by fatty acid and carbohydrate oxidation (i.e., respiration; see Fig. 3–28), are carried by electron carriers to an electron acceptor (i.e., O$_2$, NO$_3^-$, SO$_4^=$), which is reduced. The transport of electrons across the membrane results in the transport of protons to the outside of the membrane. This electron flow produces both a proton gradient and a gradient in electric potential, which functions to push protons back across the membrane at specific sites (ATPase complex) where ATP is generated by the process of oxidative phosphorylation.

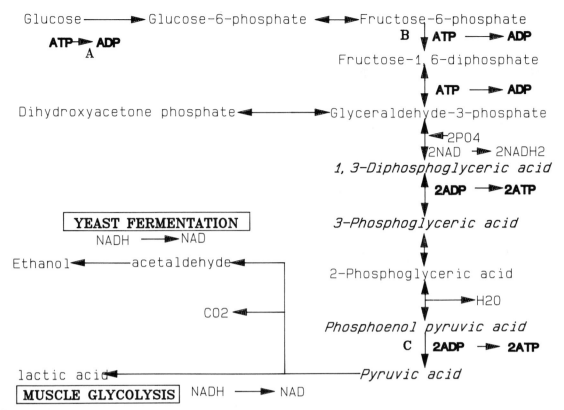

Figure 3–26 ■ The Embden-Meyerhof-Parnas (glycolytic) pathway of glucose catabolism. Enzymes (A, B, C) are for those steps which are not freely reversible. In the absence of oxygen, there is the formation of lactic acid (muscle) or CO_2 plus ethanol in the yeast (alcoholic) fermentation. Pyruvic acid is also the central compound in the formation of a large number of dissimilatory end-products of carbohydrates (see p. 90). The reactions of substrate-level phosphorylation are described in boldface italics. A = Hexokinase (glucose-6-phosphatase). B = Phosphofructokinase (fructose-1,6-diphosphatase). C = Pyruvate kinase (phosphoenol pyruvate synthase).

subsequently oxidized to pyruvate. The oxidation of glyceraldehyde-3-phosphate results in the release of a pair of electrons (two H atoms), which under anaerobic conditions are used to reduce the pyruvate to lactic acid or ethanol (Fig. 3–26). Under aerobic conditions, the electrons enter the respiratory chain (see Fig. 3–25a and below).

RESPIRATION

While the EMP pathway is the central pathway for carbohydrate metabolism, the conversion of glucose to pyruvic acid can be considered in reality to be an anaerobic process in that it can occur either in the presence or in the absence of oxygen. However, the majority of eukaryotes and prokaryotes (as well as humans) do not live in an anaerobic environment, and the carbohydrate that is metabolized to pyruvate in glycolysis is usually metabolized further under aerobic mechanisms involving oxygen. Thus, in humans

and in higher animals, although lactic acid is produced from the reduction of pyruvate by NADH (for the regeneration of NAD for further glycolysis), it is not the final end product of this metabolism. Instead, lactic acid is partly converted to the storage product, glycogen, and a portion of it is completely oxidized to CO_2 and water. This latter oxidation is the result of the process of *aerobic respiration* and is accomplished by the further oxidation of pyruvate through the *tricarboxylic acid cycle* (Krebs cycle, TCA cycle, citric acid cycle).

TRICARBOXYLIC ACID CYCLE—CITRIC ACID CYCLE

The TCA cycle (Fig. 3–27) is a true cycle (compared with the EMP pathway), in that the end product of the cycle, oxalacetic acid, is regenerated so as to react continuously with the acetyl-CoA that is supplied from glycolysis. (Citric acid, the result of the con-

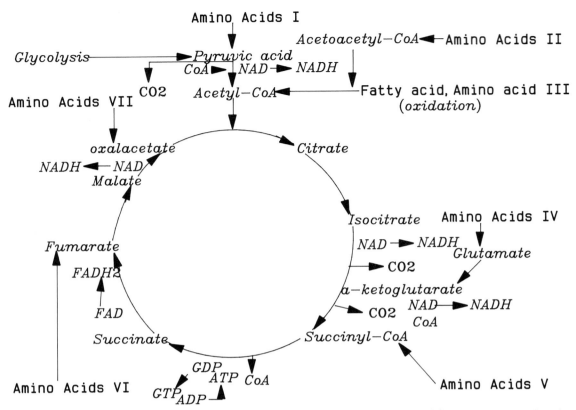

Figure 3–27 ■ The Krebs (tricarboxylic acid) cycle oxidizes pyruvic acid to three CO_2 molecules and transfers electrons to NAD^+ or FAD. The GTP formed is the only high-energy triphosphate formed directly. The four-carbon oxaloacetic acid is regenerated and can start another cycle by picking up another molecule of acetyl-CoA. The nucleotide reactions function to transfer electrons to the electron transport chain. Amino acids and fatty acids are oxidized at various points in the cycle. The CO_2 generated is utilized in CO_2-fixation via the Calvin cycle (see Fig. 3–36). Amino acids I, ala, cyst, gly, ser, threo; II, ala, tyros, leu, lys, trypt; III, isoleu, leu, trypt; IV, arg, hist, gluNH$_2$, prol; V, isoleu, Met, val; VI, tyr, ala; VII, asp.ac, aspNH$_2$.

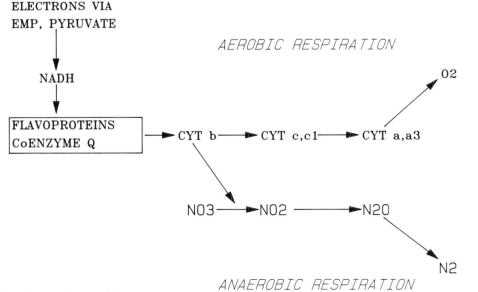

Figure 3–28 ■ Electron transport through aerobic and anaerobic respiration. Electrons generated from glycolysis pyruvate, TCA, are transferred to nucleotides and flavoproteins to the electron transport cytochromes. In aerobic respiration (see also Fig. 3–25), the electrons are passed to oxygen to form water, or are passed via anaerobic respiration to NO_3^- or $SO_4^=$ to generate N_2, NH_3, or H_2S.

densation of oxalacetic acid and acetyl-CoA, can be considered to be the start of the cycle.) The energy-rich acetyl-coenzyme-A (acetyl-CoA) is formed from pyruvate by an activation with coenzyme A. The citric acid is converted in a true cyclic fashion to a series of important intermediates, which can be used in a variety of other essential biosynthetic reactions. Therefore, the TCA cycle can be considered to be an *amphibolic cycle,* in that it functions in both catabolic as well as anabolic reactions. Basically, then, the TCA cycle has two major functions: to supply carbon skeletons for cell structure and to generate large numbers of electrons. It is these electrons that enter the aerobic or anaerobic *electron transport system* (Figs. 3–25a, 3–28) and are used for the generation of ATP.

ELECTRON TRANSPORT CHAIN— CYTOCHROME PATHWAY

The electron transport system exists in the eukaryotic mitochondrion and in the cytoplasmic membrane of prokaryotes. Its primary function is the transfer of the electrons generated in the TCA cycle by a reversible series of oxidation-reduction reactions involving specific enzymes and cofactors.

These enzymes and cofactors function as an internal oxidation/reduction system, transferring the electrons in stepwise fashion through the electron transport chain to an ultimate electron acceptor: oxygen in aerobic respiration (Fig. 3–25a) and an inorganic molecule (NO_3^- or $SO_4^=$) in anaerobic respiration (Fig. 3–28). Several important enzymes are involved in the initial steps of electron transport. These enzymes are the dehydrogenases, which have NAD or NADP (a phosphorylated pyridine nucleotide) as their coenzyme. A second dehydrogenase, the flavoproteins, is linked to NAD in the respiratory chain. These flavoproteins contain either flavin adenine dinucleotide (FAD) or its mononucleotide (FMN) as their prosthetic group. The vitamin riboflavin is the major part of the coenzyme, and it functions in the reversible transfer of electron pairs through the chain. The third enzyme in the electron transport system is the coenzyme, coenzyme Q, or ubiquinone, so named because of its ubiquitous nature in all cells. The other major class of oxidation/reduction compounds in the electron transport chain is the cytochromes (Fig. 3–29). The cytochromes are heme or iron (Fe) derivatives, which contain a single Fe atom. It is the Fe atom that is reversibly oxidized and reduced by the pas-

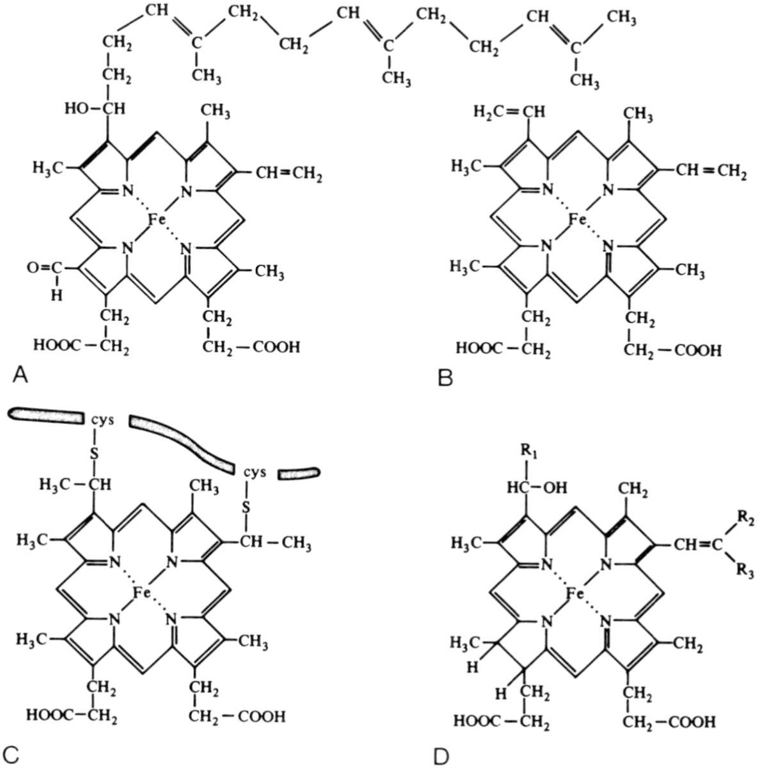

Figure 3–29 ■ The basic structure of various types of cytochromes showing their specific prosthetic groups. In the a-type cytochrome *(A)* the cytochromes contain a formyl group as the side chain. In *B,* the b-type cytochrome, the prosthetic group is a heme. The c-type cytochrome *(C)* the prosthetic group is linked to a protein by way of cysteine (cys) bridges. In *D,* the D-type cytochrome has as its prosthetic group a derivative of dihydroporphyrin. (From Gottschalk: Bacterial Metabolism, ed. 2, Springer Verlag, New York, 1986, with permission.)

sage of an electron through the chain. Interestingly, the initial electron transfer compounds, NAD, FAD, and coenzyme Q of the electron transport chain, all function in the transfer of two hydrogen atoms (i.e., $2H^+ + 2e^-$), while the cytochromes transfer only electrons. The proton portion of the hydrogen atom is associated with $-NH_2$ groups or $-COOH$ groups; however, they are also transferred to oxygen. The terminal cytochrome, cytochrome oxidase (cytochrome a/a3), contains copper; however, it is only cytochrome a3 that reacts with oxygen to produce water in aerobic respiration; NO_3^- or $SO_4^=$ produces NH_3 or H_2S, respectively, in anaerobic respiration (Fig. 3–28). Thus, the electron transport chain permits the flow of electrons (a pair of electrons or hydrogen atoms), so as to result in a stepwise release of energy, a portion of which is conserved as ATP. Remember, ATP is formed by way of proton motive force (see page 83), in which proton and electrical gradients are established so that there is a flow of electrons across a membrane with the generation of ATP (Fig. 3–25b). The remainder of the energy is released as heat.

GENERATION OF ENERGY AS ATP: A SUMMARY

Energy as ATP is generated at several places in the metabolism of a carbohydrate such as glucose to water, or other inorganic end products. ATP is formed in the EMP pathway from the transition between the EMP pathway and the TCA cycle, from the electrons that are released from the TCA cycle, and through the electron transport chain. The ATP yields from each of these metabolic pathways are seen in Figures 3–30 and 3–31. For each mole of glucose that enters the EMP pathway, eight ATPs are produced; the electrons that enter the electron transport chain from the TCA cycle function to oxidize 12 coenzymes, two FADH2 (1 from each turn of the TCA cycle), and 10 NADH2 (two from glycolysis, two from the transition between glycolysis and TCA, and six from the required two turns of the TCA cycle for each mole of glucose). Three ATPs are produced from each NADH2, two ATPs from each FADH2, and 34 ATPs from oxidative phosphorylation through the cytochrome system. The total yield of energy from the complete oxidation of one mole of glucose to $CO_2 + H_2O$ is therefore 38 ATPs; 34 ATPs are produced from oxidative phosphorylation, two ATPs from glycolysis, and two additional ATPs are produced from a guanosine triphosphate (GTP) reaction in the TCA cycle. Note that in glycolysis alone (that is, in the anaerobic oxidation of glucose to lactate or ethanol) only two ATPs per mole of glucose are produced. Clearly then, aerobic oxidation of glucose is a far more efficient

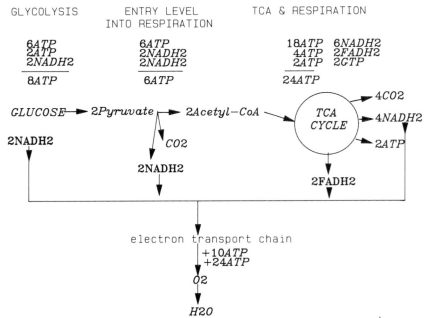

Figure 3–30 ■ Summary of energy yields of ATP in glycolysis, entry into respiration, and TCA and respiration. Note the dramatic differences in energy yield between aerobic respiration and glycolysis.

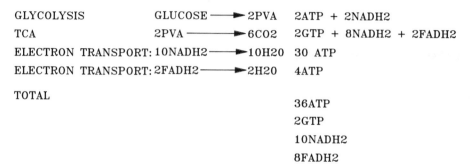

GLYCOLYSIS	GLUCOSE $\longrightarrow$ 2PVA	2ATP + 2NADH2
TCA	2PVA $\longrightarrow$ 6CO2	2GTP + 8NADH2 + 2FADH2
ELECTRON TRANSPORT:	10NADH2 $\longrightarrow$ 10H20	30 ATP
ELECTRON TRANSPORT:	2FADH2 $\longrightarrow$ 2H20	4ATP
TOTAL		36ATP
		2GTP
		10NADH2
		8FADH2

Figure 3–31 ■ Summary of maximum energy yield per mole of glucose metabolized by glycolysis and respiration.

energy-generating process than anaerobic metabolism.

FERMENTATION

Since anaerobic bacteria, as well as some facultative anaerobes, do not possess the cytochromes of the aerobic electron transport system, they cannot obtain energy via aerobic electron transport, that is, through oxidative phosphorylation. Bacteria growing in an anaerobic environment obtain their energy directly from glycolysis and from the process of substrate level phosphorylation (Fig. 3–26), or from anaerobic respiration (Fig. 3–28). Since substrate level phosphorylation is essentially the only mechanism of energy generation available to anaerobic bacteria, the energy obtained in these anaerobic processes is far below that obtained from aerobic respiration. Rather than pyruvate being converted to acetyl-CoA, and eventually metab-

olized through the TCA cycle, the pyruvate that is formed is reduced to a large number of end products characteristic of the specific bacterial species (Table 3–5 and Fig. 3–32). These specific anaerobic reactions are referred to as fermentation chemical reactions in which organic compounds serve as ultimate electron acceptors.

Several groups of bacteria including oral *Bacteroides* are even capable of fermenting amino acids; however, they do so in very complicated and specific ways and will not be considered here.

PENTOSE-PHOSPHATE PATHWAY— HEXOSE MONOPHOSPHATE SHUNT

This pathway for the catabolism of carbohydrates is similar to that of EMP. The pentose-phosphate pathway (Fig. 3–33), or hexose monophosphate shunt, possesses several of the reactions of glycolysis and therefore

Table 3–5 ■ Major end products of glucose dissimilation by representative prokaryotes*

Genera	Representative Products	Representative Genera*
Lactic acid bacteria		
Streptococcus	Lactic acid, acetic acid, formic acid, and ethyl	A, C
Lactobacillus	alcohol; only lactic acid homofermentative;	
Leuconostoc	lactic acid plus other compounds homofermentative	
Propionic acid bacteria		
Propionibacterium	Propionic acid, acetic acid, carbon dioxide	H
Veillonella		
Enterobacter group		
Escherichia	Formic acid, acetic acid, lactic acid, succinic	B, G
Enterobacter	acid, ethyl alcohol, carbon dioxide,	
Salmonella	hydrogen, 2,3-butylene glycol	
Acetone, butyl alcohol group		
Clostridium	Butyric acid, butyl alcohol, acetone, isopropyl	C, D, E, F
Eubacterium	alcohol, acetic acid, formic acid, ethyl	
Bacillus	alcohol, hydrogen, and carbon dioxide	
Acetic acid bacteria		
Acetobacter	Acetic acid, gluconic acid, kojic acid	

*See Figure 3–32.

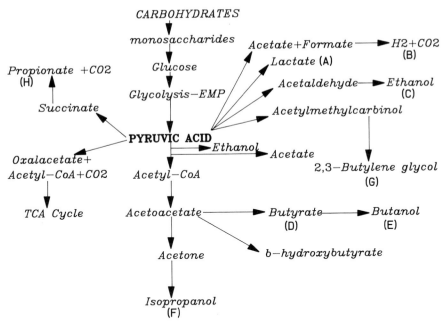

Figure 3–32 ■ Role of pyruvic acid in the formation of a variety of reduced end products from the dissimilation of glucose. The letters indicate representative groups of bacteria that dissimilate glucose to the end product in Table 3–5. (Adapted from Pelczar, M-J, Chan, ECS, Krieg, NR (eds): Microbiology, 5th Ed. McGraw Hill, New York, 1986.)

can be considered as a "shunt" pathway of glycolysis. In this catabolic pathway, notice that while electrons are generated from the oxidation of glucose, not much energy is produced as ATP; in fact, the major function of this pathway is to provide reducing power (NADPH) for the multitude of biosynthetic reactions of the cell that require this pyridine nucleotide, as well as pentose phosphates required for nucleotide biosynthesis.

ENTNER-DOUDOROFF PATHWAY

The Entner-Doudoroff pathway (Fig. 3–34) is confined to aerobic and anaerobic bacteria;

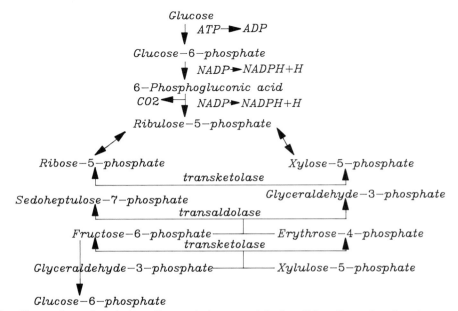

Figure 3–33 ■ The pentose phosphate pathway of glucose catabolism. This pathway functions to produce ribose-5-phosphate and NADPH + H⁺. The pyridine nucleotide serves as an important source of reducing power for fatty acid biosynthesis, while the ribose-5-phosphate functions in nucleotide biosynthesis.

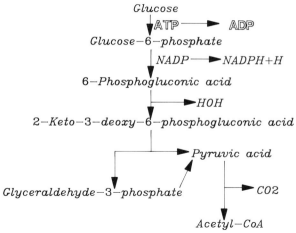

Figure 3–34 ■ The Entner-Doudoroff pathway of glucose catabolism. This metabolic pathway, for the dissimilation of glucose, occurs in selected gram-negative bacteria, especially *Pseudomonas* and *Azotobacter*.

it is absent from all eukaryotic cells so far examined. Identical to glycolysis and the hexose monophosphate shunt, glucose is phosphorylated by ATP. The glucose-6-phosphate formed in the Entner-Doudoroff pathway is converted to a gluconic acid, which is dehydrated, and then cleaved to the two trioses, pyruvic acid and glyceraldehyde-3-phosphate. These trioses are activated by coenzyme A, and the acetyl-CoA produced is catabolized via the TCA cycle. Energy and carbon skeletons are then produced as described for the TCA cycle and electron transport.

GLYOXYLATE CYCLE

Several bacteria, notably the members of the genus *Pseudomonas*, are capable of metabolizing acetic acid, as well as other higher fatty acids. Since eukaryotic cells are not required to metabolize acetate alone, the glyoxylic acid (or glyoxylate) cycle is limited to bacteria. In the glyoxylate cycle (Fig. 3–35), acetate is activated with coenzyme A to acetyl-CoA; however, there is no formation of pyruvate as an intermediate. The acetyl-CoA enters the glyoxylate cycle at two places by condensation reactions; the first is with oxalacetate to produce citrate identical to that found in the TCA cycle, and the second involves a condensation of the acetyl-CoA molecule with glyoxylate to produce malate. Both malate and citrate enter the TCA cycle. The two critical enzymes responsible for the functioning of the glyoxylate cycle are isocitrate lyase and malate synthase. Both enzymes function to replenish the pool of carbon for the TCA cycle, and are therefore known as anaplerotic enzymes, in that they maintain the necessary levels (pool) of intermediates for biosynthesis.

PHOTOSYNTHESIS

Plants, algae, and selected microorganisms in our environment are capable of utilizing light as a source of energy; that is, they are able to carry out the process of *photosynthesis*.

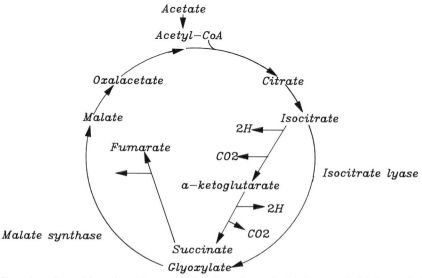

Figure 3–35 ■ The glyoxylic acid cycle or bypass. It functions to replenish the pool of intermediates of the TCA cycle. Isocitrate lyase and malate synthase are enzymes specific to the cycle. Note the reactions common to the TCA cycle. (Adapted from Pelczar et al. See Fig. 3–32. Ed. 5; and from J. Mandelstam, K. McQuillen, and I. Dawes (eds.): Biochemistry of Bacterial Growth. 3rd Ed. John Wiley & Sons, New York, 1982.)

Plants, blue-green bacteria (cyanobacteria), and algae carry out an aerobic, or *oxygenic*, *photosynthesis* in which the CO_2 generated in other metabolic reactions (i.e., TCA) is reduced to carbohydrate or cell material (CH_2O) in the presence of the chemical reductant, water:

$$2H_2O + CO_2 \xrightarrow{light} (CH_2O) + O_2 + H_2O$$

In contrast to plants, algae, and cyanobacteria, selected photosynthetic bacteria, while being able to use light as an energy source, cannot do so in the presence of oxygen. Further, they cannot use water as a reductant, and consequently do not produce oxygen as one of the end products of metabolism. They carry out an *anoxygenic photosynthesis* in which compounds other than water function as the chemical reductant. Hence,

$$2H_2A + CO_2 \xrightarrow{light} (CH_2O) + 2A + H_2O$$

Since the chemical reductant in the anoxygenic photosynthetic bacteria can be a variety of compounds, it is designated as H_2A. Inorganic compounds such as H_2, H_2S, and even S_2O_3, as well as organic compounds such as acetate, lactate, or succinate, can function as chemical reductants. The cell mass (CH_2O), which was formed from the CO_2 generated as a product of the TCA cycle (see Fig. 3–27), is "fixed" from the "dark reactions" of photosynthesis, or the Calvin cycle (Fig. 3–36). We refer the reader to any textbook of general microbiology or biochemistry for a discussion of photosynthesis.

SYNTHESIS OF MAJOR CELLULAR MACROMOLECULES

It should now be very clear that the generation of energy as ATP, and reducing power as pyridine nucleotide through the various catabolic cycles, functions to provide the cell with the ATP and pyridine nucleotides to drive the biosynthetic reactions necessary for the growth and anabolic reactions of the cell. Approximately 150 different small organic molecules are used for the biosynthesis of the basic cellular macromolecules (i.e., polysaccharides, lipids, proteins, and nucleic acids). In fact, these small organic molecules are synthesized from only 12 key precursor metabolites.

The biosynthesis of several selected macromolecules and their organization into functional units are common to most bacteria. We will assume that the reader is familiar with the synthesis of the amino acids and lipids. Both are synthesized from the end

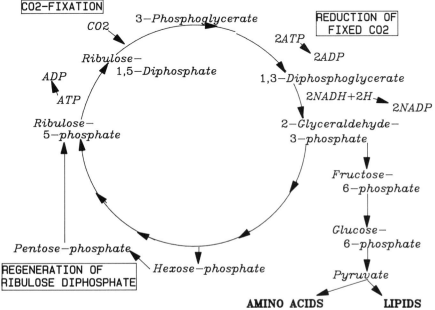

Figure 3–36 ■ Simplified version of the Calvin cycle. CO_2 is fixed autotrophically into organic molecules. These are the "dark reactions" of photosynthesis because no light is directly required for the reactions to proceed. However, light energy is required for the production of ATP and NADPH.

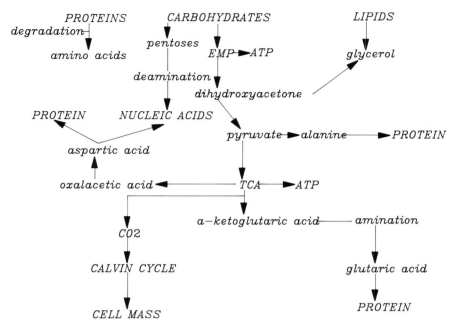

Figure 3-37 ■ Interrelationships among carbohydrates, lipids, and proteins leading to the synthesis of macromolecules.

products of the metabolic pathways that have already been discussed; the reader should familiarize him- or herself with these biosynthetic reactions by consulting a textbook of biochemistry. Figure 3–37 provides a basic summary of the interrelationships among carbohydrates, lipids, and proteins, which lead to the synthesis of macromolecules.

Purine and Pyrimidine Biosynthesis

The purines and pyrimidines (Fig. 3–38) are nucleic acid (DNA, RNA) precursors and are synthesized from several amino acids and CO_2 in a stepwise process that involves at least 12 different enzymes and at least five different compounds (Fig. 3–39a, b). The reader is referred to a textbook of biochemistry for a discussion of purine biosynthesis.

The purine and pyrimidine nucleotides (base-sugar-phosphate) are essential to a large number of critical biosynthetic functions of the cell. They are, for example, central components of several vitamins and coenzymes, and are essential compounds in cell wall molecules (peptidoglycan, lipopolysaccharide), as well as being involved in the formation of amino acids and complex lipids. Figure 3–40 describes in simplified fashion the basic biosynthetic pathways for the formation of the purine and pyrimidine ribonucleotide triphosphates.

The ribonucleotides (ribose-containing nu-

cleotides) are used as precursors for the synthesis of RNA (ribose nucleic acid), while the deoxyribonucleotides (deoxyribose-containing nucleotides) function in the synthesis of DNA (deoxyribose nucleic acid). The ribonucleotides are synthesized by the action of the phosphorylated pyridine nucleotide, NADP, and the enzyme thioredoxin reductase (Fig. 3–41). The nucleotides are reduced to the triphosphates, while the cofactor is reduced to the deoxyribose of the DNA. Energy is supplied as ATP.

POLYSACCHARIDE BIOSYNTHESIS

Activation may be required for some simple sugars to be able to pass through, or be transported across, bacterial membranes and cell walls. This activation usually entails a phosphorylation, in which a nucleotide phosphate in the presence of a specific enzyme (kinase) produces a sugar-phosphate. This sugar-phosphate is easily transported into the cell, as well as functioning as a precursor of polysaccharide formation. The nucleotide, uridine triphosphate (UTP), for example, activates glucose to UDP-glucose. This activated glucose (the glucose phosphate is a high-energy molecule) now has sufficient energy for the subsequent linkages of additional glucose molecules to form a glucose polymer, that is, a polysaccharide.

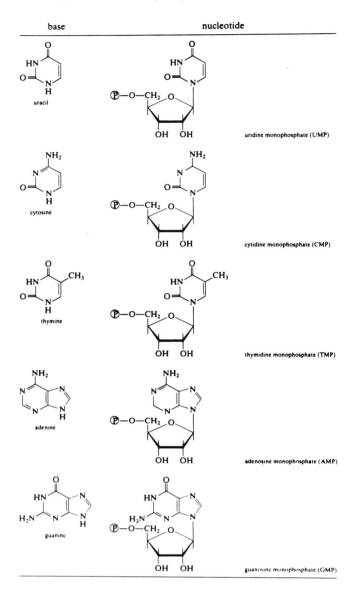

base   nucleotide

uracil

uridine monophosphate (UMP)

cytosine

cytidine monophosphate (CMP)

thymine

thymidine monophosphate (TMP)

adenine

adenosine monophosphate (AMP)

guanine

guanosine monophosphate (GMP)

Figure 3–38 ■ Important pyrimidines, purines, and corresponding nucleotides.

The type of sugar polymer formed, as well as its manner of linkage, is also determined by the monosaccharide composition and by the chemical interactions required for linkage. The homopolysaccharide (one sugar type) glycogen, for example, consists of poly-1,4-glucose units, and the glucose-glucose bonding occurs under the control of UDPG →UDP. The heteropolysaccharides (several different sugars) are composed of more than one sugar, and separate enzymes are required. These enzymes function to catalyze the addition of each sugar to the developing chain. Interestingly, in the formation of the important polysaccharides dextran, levan, and fructan, the nucleotide sugars (sugar + UTP sugar − PO_4 + UDP) are not involved in polymer formation, but these polymers are synthesized under the control of specific enzymes (i.e., dextransucrase):

sucrose + dextransucrase ⟶ dextran + fructose

The energy required for the synthesis of the polymer is obtained by the hydrolysis of the glycosydic bond of the sugar molecules.

PEPTIDOGLYCAN BIOSYNTHESIS

We have already indicated that the peptidoglycan maintains the shape and structural integrity of bacteria. It consists of repeating

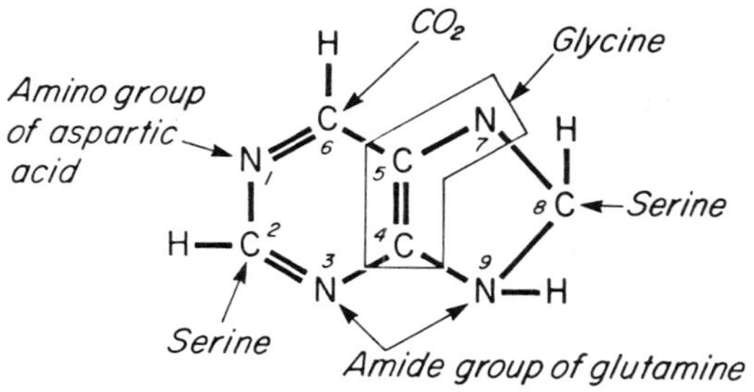

A

Purine Molecule

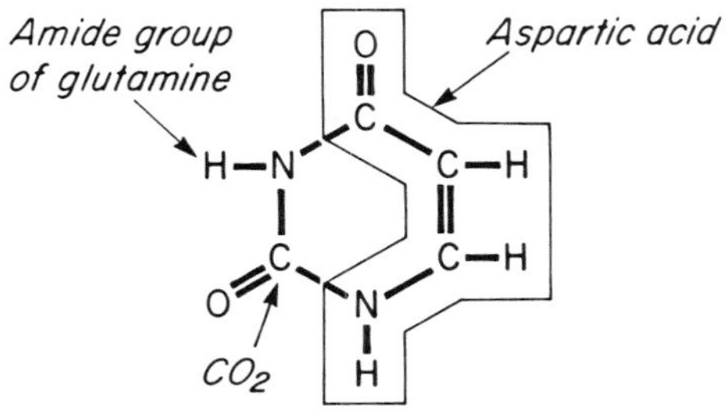

Figure 3–39 ■ Representation of the precursor molecules that are involved in the formation of purine (A) and pyrimidine (B) molecules. Each of the fragments of these two molecules are formed from the indicated amino acids or carbon dioxide.

B

Pyrimidine Molecule

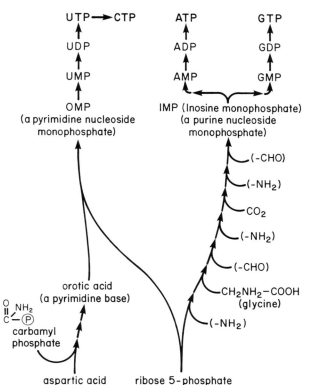

Figure 3–40 ■ Simplified generalized scheme for the formation of the various nucleotide phosphates. Aspartic acid ribose-5-phosphate undergoes a series of addition and deletion reactions to eventually form the purine and pyrimidine nucleotide monophosphates. These in turn are converted to the four purine and pyrimidine bases: uridine triphosphate, cytidine triphosphate, adenosine triphosphate, and guanosine triphosphate, respectively.

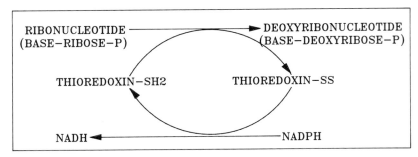

Figure 3–41 ■ Formation of deoxyribonucleotides from ribonucleotides. Pyridine nucleotide and the enzyme thioredoxin reductase function in the reduction of the ribonucleotide to the deoxyribonucleotide.

glycan polymer of *N*-acetylglucosamine and *N*-acetylmuramic acid to which peptide subunits are attached (see Fig. 3–11). The biosynthesis of the peptidoglycan takes place in four distinct stages and at distinct locations within the bacterial cell (Fig. 3–42):

Stages 1 and 2 ■ Both stage 1 and stage 2 are carried out in the cell cytoplasm and involve the formation of UDP-sugars. UDP-*N*-acetylglucosamine and UDP-*N*-acetylmu-

ramic acid are formed as a result of ATP-requiring reactions. The specific amino acids are then sequentially added to form the UDP-sugar-pentapeptide, and after elimination of one terminal amino acid the tetrapeptide is attached to a lactylcarboxyl group of *N*-acetylmuramic acid. An amino acid bridge connects the terminal carboxyl group of each side chain with the free amino group of lysine or diaminopimelic acid.

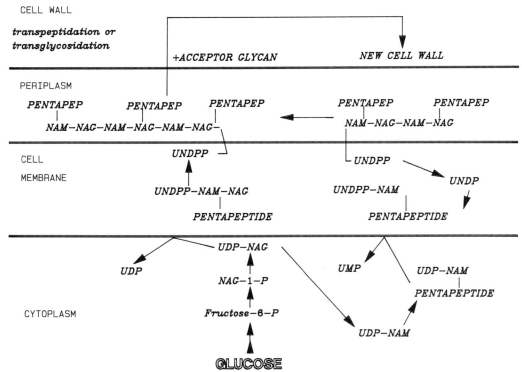

Figure 3–42 ■ Diagrammatic representation of the formation of a new cell wall. New cell wall synthesis occurs in three regions of the cell: in the cytoplasm, in the periplasm and cell membrane, and on the cell wall. Glucose is utilized in the cytoplasmic region to form uridine dinucleotide phosphates (see Fig. 3–40), which "carry" muramic acid pentapeptides to the cell membrane. The UDP-pentapeptide is covalently linked to an *N*-acetylglucosamine. This unit, formed in the cell membrane is then carried by an undecaprenol C55 lipid carrier (UND) through the cell membrane, where it is further linked to additional *N*-acetylmuramic acid and *N*-acetylglucosamine repeating units. This entire unit then is transferred from the periplasm to the growing cell wall. The peptide-linked and sugar-linked cell wall is formed at the outer surface by transpeptidation and transglycosidation reactions.

Stage 3 ■ The nucleotide-sugar pentapeptide formed in the cytoplasm is then transported to the cell surface by a specific carrier molecule, an isoprenoid c_{55}-carrier lipid, *bactoprenol* or *undecaprenol*. After linkage of this carrier to the UDP-sugar-pentapeptide, *N*-acetylglucosamine molecules are added to it in the periplasma, and the entire repeating unit is then transported across the cytoplasmic membrane where it is chemically linked to an "acceptor" of partially completed polymer in the developing cell wall. The isoprenoid carrier is regenerated by the removal of an inorganic phosphate by the action of a phosphatase enzyme.

Stage 4 ■ The final stage in the formation of the peptidoglycan is the cross-linking of the polypeptide chains in the cell wall matrix itself. Cross-linking occurs either directly, as an amide bond between diaminopimelic acid

or lysine and the penultimate D-alanine of an adjacent peptidoglycan chain, or indirectly, by the addition of a pentaglycine bridge between the penultimate D-alanine. In both cases the D-alanine is released into the bacterial cytoplasm to be utilized in other chemical reactions.

LIPOPOLYSACCHARIDE BIOSYNTHESIS

The basic structure of the lipopolysaccharide is seen in Figure 3–16, and its mechanism of synthesis and transport in Figure 3–43. The lipid A is the endotoxic portion of the LPS and is covalently linked to the polysaccharide core. The O-antigen contains a variety of sugar residues, which provide it with the immunologic specificity characteristic of the large number of gram-negative bacteria.

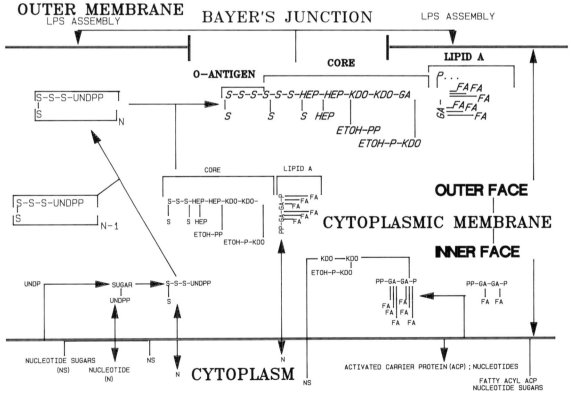

Figure 3–43 ■ Diagrammatic representation of the formation of lipopolysaccharide. Synthesis of the lipopolysaccharide occurs in the cell cytoplasm, on the membrane surfaces of the cytoplasmic membrane, and on the surface of the outer membrane. The lipopolysaccharide is formed from nucleotide sugars (NS) and fatty acyl nucleotide sugars, which are formed in the cytoplasm. These two units are transported to the interface of the cytoplasmic membrane by C55-undecaprenol lipid carriers (UND), as well as by activated carrier proteins (ACP). These two units, the sugars and fatty acyl units, are elongated on the inner face of the cytoplasmic membrane. The three components of the lipopolysaccharide molecule—the core, lipid A, and O-antigen—are then transferred to the outer face of the outer membrane where they are linked by covalent linkage into small O-antigen, core, and lipid A complexes. These complexes are then transferred through the Bayer's junction in the outer membrane, where they are assembled along the outer membrane surface into the completed lipopolysaccharide structure.

Core Polysaccharide

The core polysaccharides are routinely heptose phosphate residues, which are linked to a unique 8-carbon sugar acid, 2-keto-3-deoxyoctanoate, or KDO. It is the KDO that links the O-antigen and core polysaccharide to the lipid A. Initial synthesis of the LPS occurs in the bacterial cytoplasm where the O-antigenic sugars are attached to the polysaccharide backbone. The UDP-activated sugar precursors are then transferred from the cytoplasm to a lipid carrier, undecaprenyl phosphate similar to that involved in peptidoglycan synthesis. In LPS synthesis, the undecaprenyl phosphate exists in the cytoplasmic membrane. The soluble sugar precursors are first polymerized into the O-antigen subunits, which are then attached to the lipid A core polysaccharide to form the complete LPS molecule. The entire completed LPS molecule is then translocated to the outer membrane by an as yet unknown mechanism.

O-Antigen

We have already indicated that the O-antigen is covalently linked to the core polysaccharide through heptose and KDO. Two important characteristics of the linkage of the O-antigen to the inner core should be noted: (1) the disaccharides are linked together by pyrophosphate (P-P) bridges rather than by glycosidic ones, and (2) the free (open) positions of the disaccharides are esterified with fatty acyl residues. These fatty acyl residues are exceedingly important in the stabilization of the LPS in the outer membrane, as they are able to penetrate into the hydrophobic portion of the membrane where they are held securely.

Lipid A

Mild acetic acid hydrolysis of the entire molecule easily removes the lipid A from the O-polysaccharide and KDO-heptose. Chemically, the lipid A consists of D-glucosamine-4-phosphate, which is linked to several long-chain fatty acids and to the phospholipid ethanolamine (Fig. 3–44). Its synthesis is basically identical to that of the synthesis of the phospholipids. However, one major difference between the lipid A and the membrane phospholipids is that in the lipid A hydroxy fatty acids predominate. The hydroxy fatty acids are linked to the glucosamine disac-

Figure 3–44 ■ Chemical structure of the lipid A from *Salmonella* species. The structure consists of a central backbone of B-1, 6-linked, d-glycosamine disaccharide units which have at positions 4' and 1 phosphomonoester residues. Long-chain fatty acids of 10, 12, 14, and 16 carbons are linked to the amino and hydroxyl groups of the glucosamine disaccharides. The molar ratios of the various fatty acids are indicated in the lower portion of the figure. (From Lüderitz, O., et al.: Naturwissenschaften 65:578, 1978, with permission.)

charides through either ether or amide linkages. The disaccharide also carries a phosphate group as well as a pyrophosphorylethanolamine residue. Intramuscular or intravenous injection of small amounts of the isolated lipid A into animals (such as mice, hamsters, and guinea pigs) results in endotoxemia; the *lipid A is therefore considered to be the endotoxic portion of the LPS.* Injection of large amounts of lipid A into animals can result in fetal shock.

NUCLEIC ACID BIOSYNTHESIS

Replication of DNA

Structure of DNA ■ From the reader's understanding of basic genetics, the genetics discussed in this chapter, and the previous discussion of growth and reproduction, it should be clear that in order for a cell to perpetuate itself unchanged, it must be able to provide its "daughters" with a complete and accurate copy of its genetic material. In order to do this correctly, the cell's genetic material, DNA (deoxyribose nucleic acid), must be faithfully duplicated without errors (mutation). In Figure 3–45 a portion of the long (molecular weight, 10^6 daltons) DNA is shown. Chemically, the DNA molecule consists of a repeating nucleic acid monomer or nucleotide of the four bases—adenine, cytosine, guanine, and thymine—and the five-carbon sugar (pentose) deoxyribose arranged in a double helix. The bases are chemically linked together as base pairs of adeninethymine and guanine-cytosine, which are themselves linked together through a backbone of covalently linked sugars that alternate with phosphate groups. The process of DNA duplication (replication) begins by the breaking of the H-bonds between the adenine-thymine (A-T) and guanine-cytosine (G-

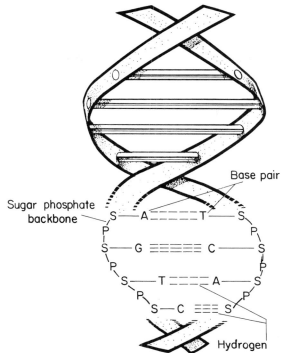

Figure 3–45 ■ Diagrammatic representation of a portion of the helical DNA molecule. The alpha-helix consists of repeating units of a sugar phosphate backbone. The two helices are connected by complementary base pairs consisting of adenine (A)–thymine (T), and guanine (G)–cytosine (C). The base pairs are connected by hydrogen bonding.

C) base pairs at specific points in the double helix. This results in the separation of the two individual helices at those points. Each of the separate strands is then used as a template for the synthesis from the 5' end of the molecule to the 3' end of a new strand of DNA that is *complementary* to the original strand (Fig. 3–46). This results in the formation of two new DNA strands that are identical to that of the parent molecule. Note that the nucleotide pairs in the new strand are in

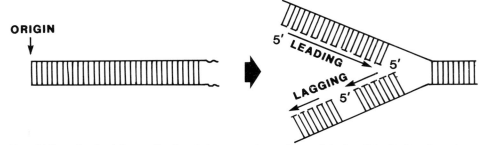

Figure 3–46 ■ DNA synthesis at the replication fork proceeds *continuously* in the 5' to 3' direction along only one strand of DNA, called the leading strand. Because DNA polymerases can synthesize from d NMPs only in the 5' to 3' direction, as portions of the lagging strand are exposed, complementary DNA is synthesized *discontinuously* as fragments of DNA. As a final step the fragments are linked together by the enzyme DNA ligase.

the same order and arrangement as they were in the original strand. This occurs because the order and arrangement of the nucleotides in the "old half" of the newly formed double helix was conserved in its original form. Thus, the original double helix has now produced two complete double helices, each of which is an exact replica of the original. Since each of the two new double helices consists of one chain of the old double helix, plus a new complementary chain, this mode of replication is referred to as *semiconservative replication*.

How does a bacterial chromosome replicate? How does it "know" where to begin the replication of the DNA molecule? When the bacterial chromosome duplicates itself during cell division, there is a unique point, or "point of origin," at which replication is initiated. Although there are many points of origin in the eukaryotic chromosome, there is only one such point in the bacterial chromosome. During this replication from the point of origin, the bacterial chromosome replicates in a bidirectional fashion, with replication beginning at the point of origin and then proceeding in both directions at an equal rate (Fig. 3–47). Replication is completed 180 degrees from its origin. The entire process of replication is very complex both genetically and biochemically, with a number of replication proteins being associated in a multienzyme complex, or replication apparatus. We will not discuss them in this chapter; however, any textbook of genetics or microbiology will suffice to describe the replication process in detail.

Replication of RNA

Structure of RNA ■ The RNA molecule consists of the sugar ribose and the bases adenine, guanine, cytosine, and uracil, which is substituted for thymine. In contrast to the double stranded–helix DNA molecule, RNA is usually single stranded. There are three unique forms of RNA: messenger-RNA (m-RNA), transfer-RNA (t-RNA), and ribosomal-RNA (r-RNA). m-RNA is considered to be the "messenger" of the genes of the DNA molecule and is in fact a true linear copy of that molecule. As such, it consists of nucleotide triplets, or *triplet codons*, which carry the genetic information for the synthesis of the 20 naturally occurring amino acids within a developing polypeptide chain (Table 3–6). The t-RNA carries the specific amino acids to the ribosomes for their incorporation into the growing polypeptide chain, which

will eventually make the specific protein that was dictated by the DNA by m-RNA. The r-RNAs also carry triplet codons; however, these codons function to indicate the starting and stopping points of the polypeptide in the protein synthetic process. Genetically, they carry the requisite information to signal chemically for a stop in protein synthesis; the "stop" codons are sometimes referred to as "nonsense codons," in that they do not carry information for the production of an amino acid. The t-RNAs also function with the ribosomal protein in the physical structure of the ribosome, the site of protein synthesis.

RNA Synthesis (Transcription)

The synthesis of the RNA molecule is very similar to that which we have described for DNA synthesis; however, new RNA strands are synthesized on a *DNA template*, and specific base pairing occurs by complementary bonding (Fig. 3–48). The major difference between DNA synthesis and RNA synthesis is that in the latter the phosphodiester bonds between adjacent bases are formed by the enzyme DNA-dependent RNA polymerase. RNA synthesis also differs from DNA synthesis in that newly formed RNAs are synthesized from short segments of DNA, and therefore require a much finer degree of control. This control is effected by genetic "signals" being built into the DNA molecule that indicate to the DNA-dependent RNA polymerase exactly which portions of it are to be copied. Importantly, since only one DNA strand is used in the synthesis of an RNA molecule, and since the two DNA strands are complementary, there must be a mechanism for choosing the correct strand for RNA synthesis—that is, the strand that carries the appropriate genetic information. The mechanism has developed so that the correct strand is distinguished from its complementary strand, and this information-bearing strand is referred to as the *sense strand*. It is only this sense strand that is copied (Fig. 3–48).

Finally, in order for RNA synthesis to occur, the RNA polymerase must bind to a segment of the DNA molecule, the *promoter region*. This promoter region consists of a sequence of bases (recognized by the RNA polymerase) that precedes the gene(s) that are to be transcribed. The RNA polymerase then travels down the sense strands of DNA, transcribing a series of genes until it recognizes a "stop" codon (also known as a ter-

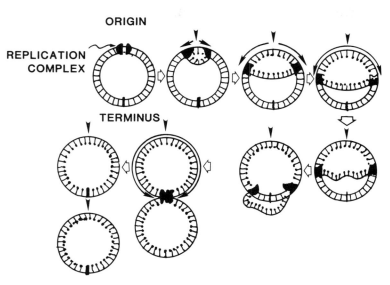

Figure 3–47 ■ Replications of the bacterial chromosome occurs in a bidirectional manner. Replication is initiated by binding of the replication complex at the origin, designated *ori*, and terminated at a point opposite *ori* on the circular chromosome. The replication rate is 800 nucleotides per second per replication fork and is independent of the growth rate. Since there are two replication forks per chromosome, a bacterial chromosome of 3.8×10^6 base pairs will be replicated in 40 minutes.

Table 3–6 ■ The genetic code*

5'-OH Terminal Base		Middle Base				3'-OH Terminal Base
		U	*C*	*A*	*G*	
U	UUU	Phe(F)	UCU Ser(S)	UAU Tyr(Y)	UGU Cys(C)	U
	UUC	Phe(F)	UCC Ser(S)	UAC Tyr(Y)	UGC Cys(C)	C
	UUA	Leu(L)	UCA Ser(S)	UAA Termination	UGA Termination	A
	UUG	Leu(L)	UCG Ser(S)	UAG Termination	UGG Trp	G
C	CUU	Leu(L)	CCU Pro(P)	CAU His(H)	CGU Arg(R)	U
	CUC	Leu(L)	CCC Pro(P)	CAC His(H)	CGC Arg(R)	C
	CUA	Leu(L)	CGA Pro(P)	CAA Gln(O)	CGA Arg(R)	A
	CUG	Leu(L)	CCG Pro(P)	CAG Gln(O)	CGG Arg(R)	G
A	AUU	Ile(I)	ACU Thr(T)	AAU Asn(N)	AGU Ser(S)	U
	AUC	Ile(I)	ACC Thr(T)	AAC Asn(N)	AGC Ser(S)	C
	AUA	Ile(I)	ACA Thr(T)	AAA Lys(K)	AGA Arg(R)	A
	AUG	Met(M)	ACG Thr(T)	AAG Lys(K)	AGG Arg(R)	G
	AUG	IMet				
G	GUU	Val(V)	GCU Ala(A)	GAU Asp(D)	GGU Gly(G)	U
	GUC	Val(V)	GCC Ala(A)	GAC Asp(D)	GGC Gly(G)	C
	GUA	Val(V)	GCA Ala(A)	GAA Glu(E)	GGA Gly(G)	A
	GUG	Val(V)	GCG Ala(A)	GAG Glu(E)	GGG Gly(G)	G

*All but four of the triplets of nucleotides are allocated to specific amino acids. UUA, UAG, and UGA indicate chain termination, while AUG represents the chain-initiating *N*-formyl-methionine. Both three-letter and one-letter abbreviations are shown for the amino acids; e.g., phenylalanine, PHE(F).

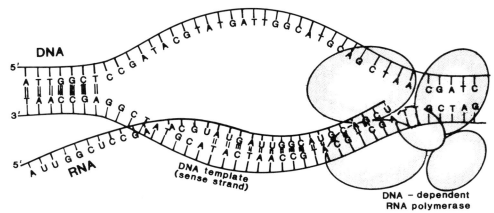

Figure 3–48 ■ Transcription is the synthesis of RNA on a DNA template. The strands of the DNA molecule are unwound for a short distance. Then the enzyme complex, DNA-dependent RNA polymerase, uses ribonucleotide triphosphates (ATP, CTP, GTP, or UTP) and the sense strand of the unwound DNA as a template for the synthesis of a single strand of RNA complementary to the DNA. Note the complementary pairing G to C and A to U (rather than A to T as in DNA).

mination codon, or terminator) and falls off the DNA, releasing a strand of m-RNA into the cytoplasm (Fig. 3–49). This m-RNA molecule is a *polycistronic message* (or transcript) of RNA since it contains the sequence of more than one gene.

PROTEIN SYNTHESIS (Translation)

From our discussion here, as well as from the reader's own knowledge of chemistry and biology, it should be clear that all of the essential biochemical reactions that occur in

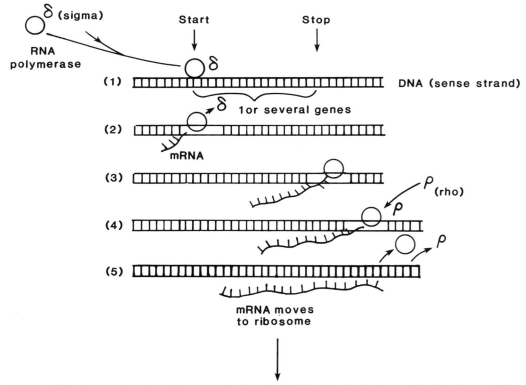

Figure 3–49 ■ DNA transcription. A gene or group of sequentially transcribed genes (operon) has a start signal (promotor) sequence where the DNA-dependent RNA polymerase binds with the help of the sigma factor. The helix unwinds and the RNA polymerase begins the synthesis of complementary RNA to one strand, the sense strand (see also Fig. 3–48) of DNA *(2 and 3)*. One or several genes may be encoded for on a single mRNA molecule, or RNA transcript. Once the RNA polymerase reaches the stop signal, which may or may not require the binding of an additional protein called *rho (4)*, it falls off the DNA strand, releasing the mRNA *(5)*, which then moves onto ribosomal complex formation for protein synthesis.

a cell are catalyzed by specific enzymes (proteins), and that the structure of all proteins is determined by the nucleotide sequence in the DNA molecule (see Table 3–1). The specific piece of DNA that designates a specific protein is the *structural gene*. How does it do so? From our brief descriptions earlier, it is clear that the information in the DNA molecule is transferred to the various RNAs and that these in turn function to arrange the amino acids in their unique order on the ribosome to produce a polypeptide, which eventually forms a functional protein (Figs. 3–50 and 3–51). The sequence of events from the conversion of the information in the DNA molecule to a functional protein comprises the events of *transcription* and *translation*. All three classes of RNA participate in the protein-forming reactions of translation (see earlier). In one sense, translation (protein synthesis) involves a different alphabet from replication and transcription. In translation, the alphabet consists of amino acids instead of nucleotides. A sequence of nucleotides results in DNA or RNA molecules, whereas an orderly sequence of amino acids results in a protein, just as sequences of letters result in a sentence.

The process of protein synthesis involves the *activation* of a specific amino acid and its attachment to the t-RNA molecule that contains the codon for that particular amino acid (Fig. 3–52). This t-RNA molecule then functions to "pass on" the amino acid to a specific site on another molecule of RNA, the m-RNA, which is recognized by the complementarity of the triplet codons on the RNA molecules. The genetic information for the production of the specific t-RNA–amino acid complex is carried by the m-RNA. Subse-

quent to the attachment of the first amino acid on the RNA molecule, a second amino acid, again designated by a specific m-RNA, is transferred to the ribosome (by t-RNA), with the formation of a peptide bond and the initiation of a large polypeptide and eventually a functional protein. When the polypeptide is of a specific length (as designated by the DNA molecule and molecular information for the formation of that protein), the polypeptide synthesis is terminated and the protein is liberated from the m-RNA–ribosome complex by a termination signal, again from a specific codon. Remember, these codons constitute the "start" and "stop" codons.

The events of protein synthesis can be summarized in the following way (Fig. 3–52):

1. The amino acids to be used in the synthesis of a specific protein are activated by an amino acyl-tRNA synthetase plus ATP.

2. The activated amino acid next binds to a t-RNA molecule, a reaction catalyzed by the enzyme that was originally bound to the amino acid. The amino acid to be carried to the ribosome for polypeptide formation is linked to the terminal nucleotide of the t-RNA molecule.

3. The t-RNA–amino acid complex is carried to the surface of the ribosome, where it (the amino acid) is added to the growing polypeptide chain (initiation).

4. On the surface of the ribosome one end of an m-RNA molecule binds at a specific site, such that the reading or translation of the m-RNA codon occurs in the correct sequence.

5. The first t-RNA–amino acid complex attaches to the chain-initiating codon of the m-RNA molecule.

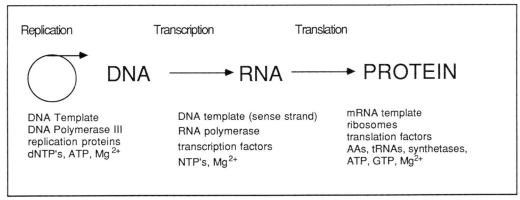

Replication	Transcription	Translation
DNA	⟶ RNA	⟶ PROTEIN
DNA Template DNA Polymerase III replication proteins dNTP's, ATP, Mg^{2+}	DNA template (sense strand) RNA polymerase transcription factors NTP's, Mg^{2+}	mRNA template ribosomes translation factors AAs, tRNAs, synthetases, ATP, GTP, Mg^{2+}

Figure 3–50 ■ The flow of genetic information in prokaryotes is unidirectional: from DNA to RNA to protein. Reverse transcription, the production of DNA on RNA templates, occurs in eukaryotic cells. (Adapted from Glass, R. E.: Gene Function.)

DNA

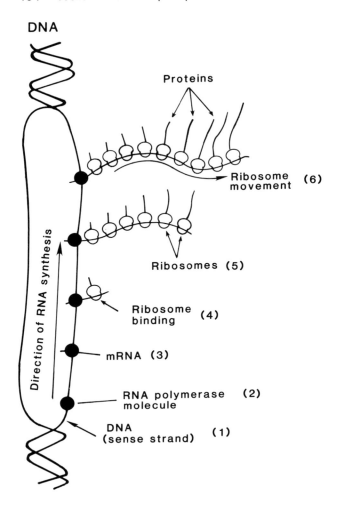

Figure 3–51 ■ mRNA is transcribed into protein in a continuous manner in which mRNA synthesis (transcription) and protein synthesis (translation) can actually occur simultaneously. As the mRNA is elongated *(3)* ribosomes can bind *(4* and *5)* and begin translation. Several ribosomes translate one mRNA molecule at a time, forming a complex known as a polyribosome *(6)*.

6. A second t-RNA–amino acid complex is transported to the ribosome and binds at the first codon site (step 1, elongation).

7. A dipeptide bond is formed between the carboxyl group of t-RNA–amino acid complex 2 and the amino group of t-RNA–amino acid complex 1. The formation of this initial dipeptide bond results in the release of t-RNA1. The m-RNA is then moved along the ribosome to a position adjacent to the next codon, so as to be ready for the next t-RNA–amino acid complex (step 2, elongation).

8. Peptide formation continues in this fashion until the peptide chain is of the appropriate length. The termination of the amino acid addition process results from interaction of a nonsense or termination codon.

9. The completed polypeptide chain dissociates from the terminal t-RNA molecule and is organized into a functional protein by the appropriate folding and bending of the polypeptide.

REGULATION OF CELLULAR ACTIVITIES

Bacteria need to be extremely economical with their energy supply; they must synthesize only those cellular materials that they require. The control of protein synthesis—that is, regulation of gene expression—can be accomplished at two stages: either by regulating DNA transcription (mRNA synthesis) or by regulating RNA translation (protein synthesis). Although regulating translation is an effective means of regulating enzyme levels, it is also wasteful. Regulation at the level of transcription is not only more energy efficient, but it also allows the *coordinate regulation* of linked as well as unlinked genes. For example, several enzymes are necessary for the metabolism of lactose by bacteria. If lactose is not present or available to the bacterial cell, then it would be wasteful for the cell to synthesize the lactose-utilizing enzymes. If the synthesis of each of the

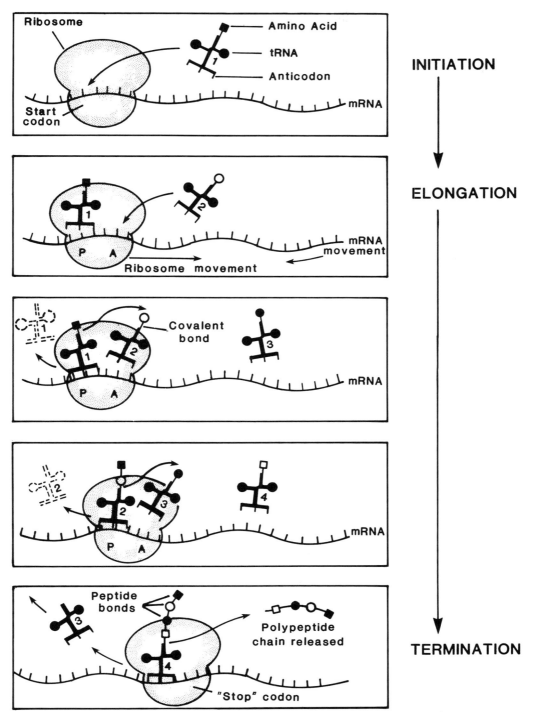

INITIATION

ELONGATION

TERMINATION

Figure 3–52 ▪ Stages of protein synthesis (translation). See text for description.

enzymes required for lactose utilization is regulated by the same promoter sequence on the DNA, then either all the enzymes are synthesized or none of them are synthesized (i.e., they are under *coordinate regulation*). Consequently, most gene regulation in prokaryotes occurs via transcription, by controlling initiation and termination rates of the synthesis of m-RNA. This regulation requires the interaction of certain regulatory molecules and specific DNA sequences in the promotor region of the DNA.

The *regulatory molecules* are small diffusible proteins or organic molecules that can interact with the regulatory regions (see further on). The activity of regulatory molecules (proteins) is often modified by *effector* molecules such as sugars or RNA. The regulatory proteins are multimeric, allosteric proteins with recognition sites for both DNA and the particular effector molecule. These effector proteins are *constitutive* (i.e., synthesized at a constant rate independent of the genes they control) and may either prevent or promote transcription. Regulatory proteins that prevent transcription are called *repressors* and function by *negative control,* whereas those that promote transcription are called *activators* and function by *positive control.*

The DNA regulatory region at which these molecules function contains three main elements: a *promoter* (P), in which transcription is initiated (where the RNA polymerase binds); a repressor binding region, or *operator* (O); and a promoter-potentiation site where the activator interacts. These sites are not necessarily physically distinct and, although a promoter is necessary, only one of the other two sites may be present in any regulatory region.

The lac operon (Fig. 3–53) is an example of an operon regulated by *negative control* or *negative repression*. Regulation of this *operon* (a series of structural genes under control of the same promoter and regulatory region) is mediated by the protein encoded by the lac I regulatory gene, a gene not contained in the lac operon itself. The regulatory protein is produced constitutively and binds to the operator site of the lac operon, preventing passage of RNA polymerase, and thus, transcription. When lactose or an analogue of lactose enters the cell, it will bind to the allosteric regulatory protein, change its conformation, and inhibit its binding to the operator. Thus, the RNA polymerase is free to move down the DNA and transcribe the rest of the operon (which contains gene-encoding enzymes needed for the utilization of lactose).

Some operons are regulated in an opposite manner from the lac operon. Examples of these are the operons encoding enzymes involved in the catabolism of maltose and arabinose (Fig. 3–54). The regulatory proteins for these operons form a complex with each specific sugar and this complex then binds near the promoter, allowing RNA polymerase binding and transcription of the operon. These operons are under *positive control* or regulation.

Extrachromosomal DNA

Some bacteria contain extrachromosomal DNA molecules that are distinct *replicons,* that is, they are not covalently linked to the chromosome. These covalently closed circular molecules of DNA, called *plasmids* (Fig. 3–55), range in size from less than 1 kb (1000 bases) to well over 100 kb, exist in the cytoplasm, and reproduce independently of the chromosome. Many, but not all, bacteria contain plasmids, and some bacteria contain more than one type of plasmid. Because plasmids replicate independently of the bacterial chromosome, there are often several identical copies of a plasmid per cell; these are called *multicopy plasmids.* Plasmids code for genes not essential for growth of the cell but for properties that might be advantageous in certain environments. For example, plasmids called *R factors* carry genes that confer resistance to antibiotics. Other plas-

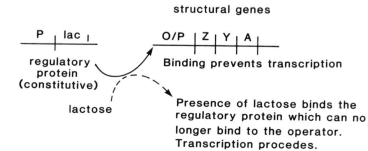

structural genes

Binding prevents transcription

Presence of lactose binds the regulatory protein which can no longer bind to the operator. Transcription procedes.

Figure 3–53 ■ The lactose operon of *E. coli* is under negative control.

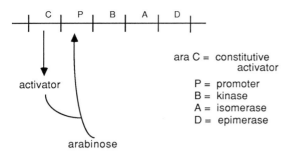

ara C = constitutive activator

P = promoter
B = kinase
A = isomerase
D = epimerase

Figure 3–54 ■ The arabinose operon of *E. coli* is under positive control. Unless the activator is coupled to arabinose, it cannot bind to the regulatory sequence and RNA polymerase cannot bind to the promoter. When arabinose is present, it combines with the activator, and this complex binds to the regulatory region, thereby promoting the binding of RNA polymerase, and transcription occurs.

mids may encode genes for surface structures, resistance to heavy metals, toxins, and a variety of other proteins and virulence factors. Plasmids have been found in oral gram-positive organisms such as *Streptococcus* spp., but evidence indicates that they occur less frequently in oral gram-negative species such as *Bacteroides*.

Conjugation

Certain plasmids may be transferred from cell to cell in a process called conjugation (explained later). One of these *conjugative plasmids* is the F plasmid of *E. coli*. This plasmid is 94.5 kb in size (2 percent the size of the *E. coli* chromosome) and approximately one third of the plasmid DNA encodes for genes involved in the transfer of DNA. Cells that carry an F plasmid, *F⁺ bacteria* (also called male cells), produce long, thin pili (F or sex pili) that are hollow, protein appendages several microns in length and 8 nm in diameter. When F⁺ cells and F⁻ cells (those lacking an F plasmid, or female cells) are mixed, *conjugal pairs* (or *mating pairs*) form by the attachment of a male sex F pilus to the surface of a female cell (Fig. 3–56). By an as yet unknown mechanism, a single linear strand of the F plasmid is transferred to the recipient cell (Fig. 3–56), probably through the hollow pilus, or *mating tube*. This transfer is always initiated at a unique site on the plasmid called *ori T* (origin of transfer) and occurs at a rate of 10^4 nucleotides (bases) per minute. At 37°C the transfer of the entire F plasmid is thus complete in 2 minutes. After the transfer of the F plasmid is complete, the recipient (female) cell is then an F⁺ (male) cell, since the F plasmid contains the genes that encode for pilus expression.

F plasmids may at times *integrate* (insert themselves) into the bacterial chromosome. This occurs at frequencies of 10^{-5} (1 in 100,000) to 10^{-7} (1 in 10,000,000) per generation of bacteria. Bacteria that contain an F plasmid integrated into their chromosome are called *Hfr* cells since they give a *h*igh(H) *fr*equency(fr) of transfer and *r*ecombination of their genes into a recipient (F⁻) cell. This high rate of recombination occurs when the

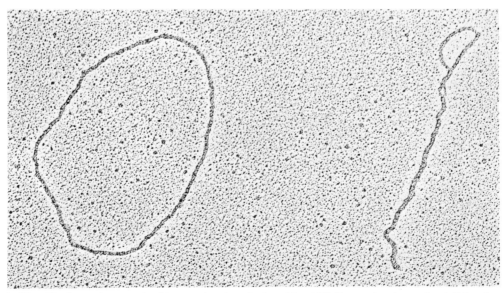

Figure 3–55 ■ Electron micrograph of two molecules of plasmid col E1. The molecule on the left is relaxed and the one on the right, supertwisted. (Courtesy of Dr. D. Lang.)

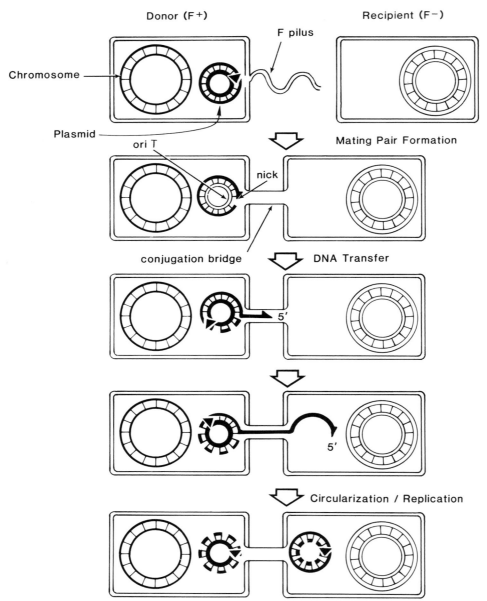

Figure 3–56 ■ The first step in the transfer of an F plasmid is donor cell–to–recipient cell contact, mediated by the F pilus of the donor cell, resulting in mating pair formation. Once the conjugation bridge has been formed, possibly utilizing the hollow F pilus itself, a nick at the origin of transfer site (*ori* T) generates a 5′ end of single-stranded DNA, which is transferred to the recipient cell. In order for the transferred DNA to become an autonomously replicating DNA element, a complementary strand of DNA must be produced in the recipient cell to form a double-stranded DNA molecule and this double-stranded molecule must circularize. This is, thus, a rolling-circle mode of replication.

F plasmid is transferred as described earlier for F⁺ cells, but because the leading edge of the F⁺ factor is now attached to the chromosome, transfer of the chromosome also occurs. The transfer of the *cointegrate* DNA (F factor and chromosomal DNA) occurs at the same rate as that of the F plasmid alone, and thus requires approximately 100 minutes for transfer of the entire chromosome. However, transfer of the entire chromosome

rarely occurs, since any minute disruption of mating pairs breaks the cell-to-cell contact and shears the donor DNA, terminating DNA transfer. The transfer of chromosomal genes during Hfr-mediated pairing occurs in a highly reproducible order since the transfer always begins at the point of origin and proceeds in one direction. The time of entry of donor genes (the time required for each particular gene to be transferred) is a measure of relative (molecular) distances on the chromosome. This is why distances between genes on genetic maps of bacterial chromosomes are expressed in minutes.

In addition to F plasmids, R plasmids (plasmids that confer resistance to antibiotics) are also conjugative plasmids. Many R plasmids carry genes that confer resistances to several classes of antibiotics. The presence of transmissible plasmids that carry multiple genes encoding resistance factors for several antibiotics explains the occurrence and rapid spread of multiply resistant microorganisms. Some of these multiply resistant plasmids may even be transferred from one bacterial species to another. To make matters worse, plasmid-mediated drug resistance can be somewhat nonspecific, conferring resistance not only to a certain antibiotic but also to its synthetic derivatives. Since conjugation commonly occurs in nature, it is probably the most frequent mechanism of transfer of antibiotic resistance in vivo.

Some bacteria are able to transfer their genetic material in the absence of pili (see further on). In gram-positive bacteria such as *Streptococcus faecalis*, it has been postulated that a "sex phenome" may be present on the bacterial cell surface, which induces the cells to mate. However, it is not clear whether such a substance actually exists in bacteria.

Transformation

Conjugative as well as nonconjugative plasmids and pieces of bacterial chromosomes can be transferred from cell to cell by a process called *transformation*. During transformation naked DNA is taken up by "competent" cells. A state of *competency* is induced when certain bacterial species are treated with calcium and magnesium chloride. This treatment induces some unknown state in the bacterial cell that allows the transport of a DNA molecule through the cell membrane(s) and peptidoglycan and into the cytoplasm. Transformation of gram-negative bacteria usually requires closed circular DNA, whereas *Bacillus* spp. are transformed more efficiently by linear (cut) DNA.

As soon as a plasmid has been introduced into a cell via transformation, it can replicate and its genes will be expressed by the recipient cell. However, pieces of a chromosome that are introduced into a recipient cell by transformation must first *recombine* with (insert into) the recipient chromosome before the genes are expressed. This process of inserting into the chromosome, *homologous recombination* (Fig. 3–57), occurs when two sequences of DNA that are identical or nearly identical to one another align and form complementary base-pairing between strands of

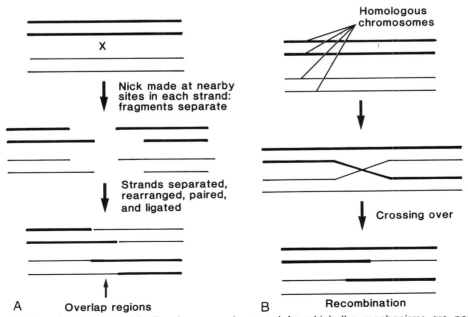

Figure 3–57 ■ Homologous recombination is a complex event for which the mechanisms are not yet fully understood. The recombination process can be simplistically diagrammed as in *A* or *B*, in which two double-stranded DNA molecules are broken and rejoined. Experiments have determined that the joining requires homologous base-pairing and that overlap regions are present at many stages in the recombination process. DNA replication does not appear to be required for recombination to occur.

DNA unwound from two different DNA molecules. This puts the identical (or *homologous*) sequences in exact register. Subsequent to this, the two internal strands of homologous DNA break and are religated (recombined), but the ligation occurs between the broken ends of the two opposing strands, which results in a cross-over product. This crossing over must occur at two sites in order for a new sequence to be inserted into the chromosome during transformation. Transformation is commonly used in the laboratory for purposes of genetic analysis and for DNA cloning (see later discussion of cloning) and may occur in nature.

BACTERIAL VIRUSES

Viruses that infect and grow in bacteria are called *bacteriophages* (Fig. 3–58) and may be considered as specialized extrachromosomal DNA elements that have the added capabilities to encode a (viral) protein coat and kill the host cell. Bacteriophages have no metabolic or synthetic capabilities of their own and must rely entirely on the host for these functions, so they are unable to multiply in the absence of a sensitive host. Bacteriophages consist of a replicon of genetic material (DNA or RNA) encapsulated by a protein coat (head *capsid*) (Table 3–7), which acts as a vehicle for transfer of the replicon. In addition, some bacteriophages have a protein tail through which the phage particles attach to the host cell surface as an initial step of infecting the host. There are two types of phages: (1) *virulent* phages, which multiply within a susceptible host cell, giving rise to progeny phage and resulting in host cell lysis and death (Fig. 3–59); and (2) *temperate* phages, which have the ability to either enter the lytic cycle as virulent phages or *lysogenize* the host cell (Fig. 3–60). While in the lysogenic state, the phage nucleic acid integrates into the chromosome and thus undergoes controlled replication within the cell without causing host cell lysis.

Phage genomes (DNA) vary from a few kilobases (encoding three proteins) to well over 100 kilobases, encoding 135 genes (see Table 3–7), or 4 percent of the size of a bacterial chromosome.

Bacteriophages can mediate the transfer of small segments of chromosomal (or even plasmid) DNA between cells, by a process called *transduction*. This phage-mediated gene transfer results in either movement of random regions of DNA (*generalized transduction*) or transfer of certain limited portions of the bacterial chromosome (*specialized transduction*). Some phages can facilitate either type of transduction while others are limited to one type or the other.

Generalized Transduction

During maturation of phage particles in the cytoplasm of the bacterial cell, occasionally a small amount of the bacterial DNA will

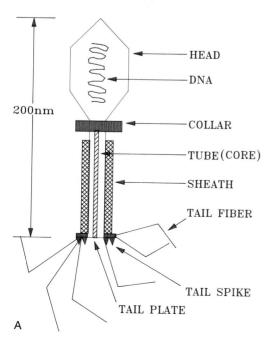

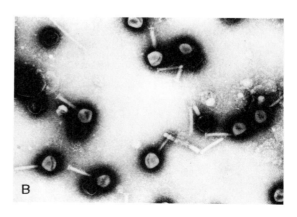

Figure 3–58 ▪ Schematic representation *(A)* and electron photomicrograph *(B)* of T-2 bacteriophage of the bacterial virus T-2. This bacteriophage consists of a large diamond-shaped head, which encloses doubled-stranded DNA. The head is attached to a long thin tail by a collar. The tail fibers attach to the tail plate.

HEAD

DNA

200nm

COLLAR

TUBE (CORE)

SHEATH

TAIL FIBER

TAIL SPIKE

TAIL PLATE

A

Table 3–7 ■ Comparison of bacteriophage characteristics[a]

Phage	Class[b]	Infective Cycle[c]	Virion Characteristics		Viral Genome	
			Head Size (nm)	Tail (nm)	Size[c] (kb)	Form
	lambdoid	temperate[d]	60	135 × 15	48.6	ds, linear
P1	—	temperate[e]	65	150 × 12	91.5	ds, linear
P2	—	temperate	60	135 × 10	33	ds, linear
Mu	—	temperate	54	135 × 18	38	ds, linear
T4	T-even	virulent	80 × 110	98 × 20	166	ds, linear
T7	T-odd	virulent	58	20 × 19	40	ds, linear
O × 174	isometric	virulent[e]	25	—	5.4	ss, circular
M13	filamentous	virulent	—	900 × 9	6.4	ss, circular
MS2	RNA phage	virulent	26	—	3.6	ss, linear, RNA

[a]Adapted from Bukhari et al. (1977), Luria et al. (1978), and *Gene Function*, R. Glass (1982).
[b]Abbreviations: kb, 10^3 nucleotides: female (F −)- or male (F +)-specific.
[c]In the lysogenic mode, phages lambda and P2 integrate at specific chromosomal sites, designated att B, att[P2]H and att[P2]H (at 17, 43, and 86 minutes, respectively): MU integrates at random. Phage P1 can either exist autonomously or inserted in the chromosome in the prophage state.
[e]P1 has a broad host range, O × 174 infects *E. coli* strain C but is unable to adsorb to wild-type K12.

be erroneously packaged by the phage capsid. This erroneous packaging occurs randomly and thus can include any part of the bacterial DNA. The phage particle containing bacterial host DNA then continues the maturation cycle as normal and is able to infect another cell, eventually injecting the bacterial DNA along with the rest of the viral DNA. In order for this transferred (injected) donor chromosomal DNA fragment to be expressed and maintained stably by the recipient cell, it must be recombined (via homologous recombination) into the recipient host cell genome.

Specialized Transduction

Upon phage infection with specialized transducing phages, the viral DNA inserts into the host cell's chromosome at a specific site. For the temperate bacteriophage *lambda*, the site is designated *att B* and lies between the bacterial *gal* and *bio* genes. Integration of the circular phage genome occurs through homologous recombination (analogous to insertion of the F plasmid at specific sites on the bacterial chromosome to form an Hfr). Upon excision of the phage DNA, some adjacent chromosomal DNA may be accidentally excised and packaged in the viral capsid along with the viral DNA. (When this happens with lambda phage, *gal* or *bio* genes are excised along with the phage DNA.) This bacterial DNA is then injected into the next bacterial host. This type of transduction is "specialized" since only specific regions of the chromosomal DNA (that which is directly adjacent to the integrated viral DNA) are

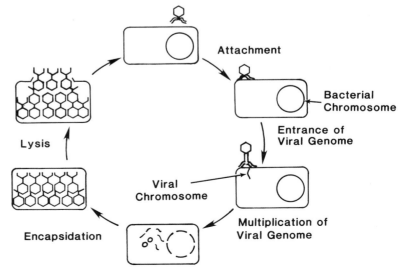

Figure 3–59 ■ The lytic life cycle of a bacteriophage begins when the phage attaches to the surface of the bacterial host. After injection of the phage genome into the host, the host's metabolism is controlled by the phage genome, which encodes and directs the synthesis of phage progeny and finally lysis of the host cell. (Typically, 50 to 200 bacteriophages are produced per infected cell.) The released progeny phage are then able to attach and infect other susceptible bacterial hosts.

Attachment

Bacterial Chromosome

Entrance of Viral Genome

Multiplication of Viral Genome

Viral Chromosome

Encapsidation

Lysis

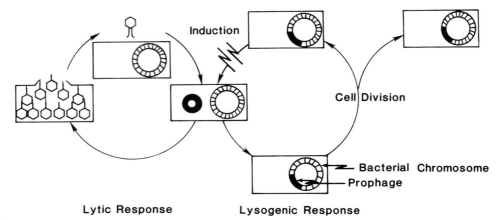

Lytic Response · Lysogenic Response

Figure 3–60 ■ A temperate bacteriophage can enter into one of two life cycles. Upon infection of the bacterial host, it can continue through the lytic cycle, resulting in the production of numerous infective viral particles and lysis of the host (see Fig. 3–13). Alternatively, it may enter the lysogenic cycle, in which the bacteriophage genome is integrated into the bacterial chromosome as a prophage or the genome may be present as a stably inherited autonomous genetic element, identical to a plasmid. The lysogenic cycle may continue through numerous cell divisions until interference with the host's cell metabolism or DNA synthesis induces a change from the lysogenic cycle to the lytic cycle.

transduced. Both types of transduction occur in nature and have been used for many years by scientists studying gene expression and for genetic mapping.

We have now discussed three different modes of gene transfer in bacteria. The properties of transformation, conjugation, and transduction are summarized in Table 3–8.

MUTATION

The DNA of an organism may be damaged or changed during cell growth by factors in either its internal or external environment. If the change is permanent (i.e., one that is heritable), the change is called a *mutation* and the organism whose DNA is mutated is called a *mutant* organism. Mutations may inactivate a gene product, modify its activity, or, very infrequently, create a new property of the gene product. Mutations that inactivate es-

sential genes are, of course, lethal to the cell. Nonlethal mutations affecting dispensible gene products may result in such things as a change in growth requirements, the ability to survive in the presence of cidal (lethal) agents, resistance to bacteriophages, or no phenotypic change at all.

Mutation Classification

A mutation that affects just one nucleotide is referred to as a *point mutation*. Examples of this type of mutation include *base pair substitutions* (the replacement of one base by another) and *frameshift mutations* (the addition or deletion of one or more base pairs), which alter the translational reading frame. Base pair substitutions may result in a *missense mutation*, which results in the encoding of a different amino acid from the wild type protein, or a *nonsense mutation*, which results in a codon (UAG, UAA, or UGA) that codes for

Table 3–8 ■ Characteristics of gene transfer in bacteria

Characteristic	Transformation	Conjugation	Transduction
Mode of DNA transfer	Across the cell membrane of the recipient	Through pill after cell-to-cell contact	Within the protein coat of a bacteriophage
Bacteria involved	Both gram + and gram −	Almost only gram −	Both gram + and gram −
Amount of donor DNA transferred	About 20 genes	From 20 genes to entire chromosome	About 20 genes
Plasmid transfer	Yes	Yes	Yes
Resistance to deoxyribonuclease (degrades DNA)	No	Yes	Yes
Unidirectional transfer	No	Yes	No
Important as exchange mechanism in nature	Probably	Yes	Yes

termination of polypeptide synthesis. In this case termination occurs too soon, resulting in a *truncated* (or shortened) protein that is inactive.

Spontaneous mutations occur naturally at a rate of 10^{-8} per generation and are the result of DNA replication errors from within the bacterium. *Induced mutations* are caused by external factors such as irradiation, chemical substances, or heat. Induced mutations occur at a variable but greater frequency than spontaneous mutations.

Chemical Mutagens (Table 3–9)

Several chemical compounds originally thought to be safe are now known to be mutagenic agents, causing chromosomal damage in a wide range of organisms including prokaryotes and humans. These chemical mutagens can be divided into three main groups according to their mode of action: *base analogues,* compounds that alter the structure of nucleic acids (*base modifiers*), and DNA-binding or *intercalating agents.* The base analogues such as 5-bromouracil and 2-amino-

purine have structures similar to thymine and adenine, respectively. Introduction of these base analogues instead of the normal base into the DNA during DNA synthesis results in mispairing at the site of the modified base during replication.

Some chemical mutagens directly modify template DNA in situ. Nitrous acid and hydroxylamine behave in this manner, resulting in incorrect base pairing in daughter cells. Alkylating agents (the largest class of mutagens) alkylate several components of DNA and induce mutations both directly through mispairing and indirectly by error-prone repair (as described for thymine-thymine dimers further on).

Compounds that intercalate (insert) between stacked nucleotide bases, such as acridine orange and ethidium bromide, cause frameshift mutations by an as yet unknown mechanism.

Exposure of bacteria to ultraviolet irradiation (254 nm) generates pyrimidine dimers (usually thymine-thymine) in the DNA. Thymine dimers are unable to form hydrogen bonds (base pair) so bacterial repair mechanisms are called upon to excise and repair the affected bases. During this repair, mistakes may be made in the insertion of bases, resulting in a mutated gene.

Table 3–9 ■ Mutagenic Agents and Their Specificities

Mutagenic Agent	Specificity	Mechanism[a]
Spontaneous	Substitution	Mispairing
	Frameshift	Slipping
	Multisite	Recombination
	All types	Misrepair
UV radiation	All types	Misrepair
Base analogue		
5'-bromouracil	A·T↔G·C[b]	Mispairing
2'-aminopurine	G·C↔A·T	Mispairing
Base modifiers		
nitrous acid	A·T↔G·C	Mispairing
hydrozylamine	G·C↔A·T	Mispairing
alkylating agents	Mainly transitions[d]	Mispairing
	All types	Mispairing
Intercalators	Frameshift	Slipping
	All types[e]	Misrepair

[a]Mispairing (nonstandard base pairing) may arise spontaneously or through the presence of nucleotide derivatives. Slipping refers to imperfect pairing between complementary strands due to base sequence redundancy. All types of mutations may be induced indirectly by faulty repair mechanisms (misrepair).

[b]G·C↔A·T is most common.

[c]A·T↔G·C transitions occur 10- to 20-fold more frequently.

[d]EMS and MNNG are highly specific for G·C↔A·T transitions (though other mutations are induced by error-prone repair).

[e]The wide range of lesions induced by international chemical reference (ICR) compounds may stem from their alkylating side chain.

TRANSPOSONS

Transposons (TN) (Table 3–10) are *genetic elements* (short sequences of DNA) that translocate between DNA sequences of no apparent homology; that is, they "jump" from one site to another in no apparent pattern. There appear to be no specific sequences that transposons recognize; they can even transpose between a plasmid and a chromosome.

Transposons vary in size from 4 to 21 kb and contain coding regions that confer resistance to one or more antibiotics or even to toxin genes. One striking characteristic of transposons is that they have terminal inverted or direct repeats (see Table 3–10), which are required for transposition activity.

Transposons are ubiquitous in prokaryotic cells. For example, the antibiotic resistance genes of several R plasmids are transposon-like structures. The frequency of transposon transposition varies from 10^{-3} to 10^{-6}, depending on the particular transposon. Transposition is relatively nonspecific, yet is not entirely random because insertion can occur in any gene; however, there are certain "hot spots" on the chromosome where insertions

Table 3–10 ■ Properties of transposable genetic elements[a]

Genetic Elements	Size (bp)[b]	Terminal Repetition Element[c]	Drug Resistance[d]
Tn1 (Tn2, Tn3)[e]	4,957	38 bp inverted	Ampicillin
Tn5	5,400	1,450 bp inverted	Kanamycin
Tn9	2,638	ISI direct	Chloramphenicol
Tn10	9,300	1,400 inverted	Tetracycline
Bacteriophages			
Mu	38,000	11 bp inverted	—
	48,600	—	—

[a] After Calos and Miller (1980) and *Gene Function*, R. E. Glass (1982).
[b] bp = base pairs.
[c] Refers to direct repetitions flanking inserting element. The 15 bp terminal repeat associated with prophage lambda represents the common core 0 present in both att B and att P.
[d] Refers to antibiotic resistance encoded by transposon.
[e] Tn1, Tn2, and Tn3 are very similar (the complete DNA sequence of Tn3 is known).

occur more frequently than other sites. The location of these "hot spots" depends on the particular transposon.

The insertion of a transposon in a gene interrupts that gene, resulting in gene inactivation, or mutation. This type of *insertional inactivation* has frequently been used to generate mutations in specific genes for genetic studies. Just as a transposon jumps into a gene, it can as easily jump out.

This "jumping out," or *excision*, may reactivate the mutated (target) gene if the excision is precise, or may result in a deletion of adjoining chromosomal or plasmid DNA when excision is not precise (i.e., some of the adjoining DNA is removed with the transposon excision). Regardless of whether or not the excision is precise, the transposon remains intact and can subsequently insert into another gene and begin the process once again.

GENETIC ENGINEERING

The discovery and isolation of (bacterial) enzymes that cut and paste (*restrict* and *ligate*, respectively) pieces of DNA in a test tube has allowed the combining of fragments of DNA from different organisms in order to produce new combinations or sequences of DNA, or *recombinant DNA*. The application of this technology has already resulted in the production of quantities of highly purified vital proteins such as human insulin, interferon, interleukin II, and human growth hormones. A multitude of bacterial genes have also been cloned. Figure 3–61 outlines a general procedure for cloning antigens of any bacterial cell, in this case genes of *Bacteroides* spp. Initially, chromosomal DNA is isolated from the donor bacterium and is restricted by an *endonuclease* (an enzyme that cuts

DNA), which recognizes a certain DNA sequence (usually 4 to 6 bases in length) and makes a staggered cut in that particular sequence (see Fig. 3–18), wherever that sequence occurs in the chromosome. The *vector* DNA, which is either a plasmid or bacteriophage genome (in this case the multicopy plasmid, pUC9), is also restricted with the same enzyme and thus has staggered (*sticky*) ends complementary to those of the chromosomal DNA pieces. Upon mixing these two DNA species in the presence of the enzyme ligase (a DNA pasting-together enzyme), the complementary ends recombine in a random fashion. When both ends of the plasmid vector are ligated to the opposite ends of a piece of the chromosomal DNA (Fig. 3–62), a covalently closed circular (CCC) piece of recombinant DNA is formed. Under appropriate laboratory-induced conditions (salt washes and heat shock, see *transformation*), E. coli bacteria will take up CCC DNA into their cytoplasm. Like a naturally occurring plasmid, this recombinant plasmid will then be replicated and its genes transcribed into protein by the host cell. Since the plasmid encodes (in this case) for ampicillin resistance, cells that have taken up a plasmid can be selected on medium containing ampicillin. Because each gene on the recombinant plasmid may be expressed, the donor bacterial DNA that is ligated into the plasmid vector will also be transcribed into RNA, and the RNA will be translated into the appropriate protein(s) by the E. coli host. Suppose, for instance, that a piece of *Bacteroides* DNA that encodes a *Bacteroides* surface protein (or antigen) is ligated into the plasmid vector, and the resulting recombinant plasmid is used to transform an E. coli cell. This E. coli cell will then synthesize the *Bacteroides* surface antigen. The transformed E. coli cell is thus a kind of hybrid cell that can be identi-

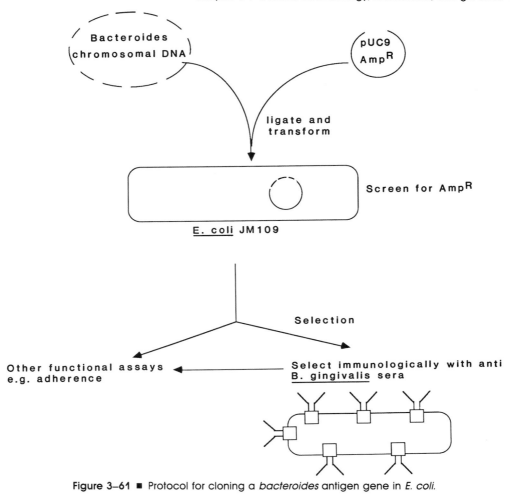

Figure 3–61 ■ Protocol for cloning a *bacteroides* antigen gene in *E. coli.*

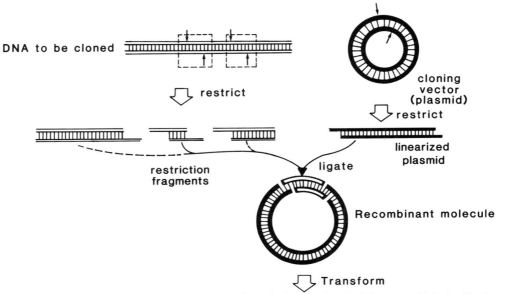

Figure 3–62 ■ The DNA to be cloned *(white)* and the cloning vector *(solid)* are restricted with the same endonuclease to generate fragments of DNA with "sticky" or complementary ends. The recombinant molecule is formed in vitro when the "sticky" ends from one source of DNA anneal (in the presence of the enzyme ligase) with the complementary ends of the vector DNA. The recombinant DNA molecule is then used to transform a suitable host, often an *E. coli* strain.

fied in the midst of thousands of other *E. coli* transformants (which contain other pieces of the *Bacteroides* chromosome) by the fact that this particular transformant, or clone, will react with anti-*Bacteroides* antisera. In this way, one gene and its product (the antigen) can be isolated and studied independently of other *Bacteroides* genes. In addition, once a gene is cloned into *E. coli,* it may be producd in large quantities by the *E. coli* cell.

Because of the universal genetic code, virtually any DNA can be used as donor DNA, and bacteriophages, in addition to certain plasmids, can be used as cloning vectors. Genes can be cloned into several gram-positive species of bacteria as well as other gram-negative species besides *E. coli.* Depending on the gene to be cloned, a variety of clone selection techniques can also be used.

Several genes of dentally important bacteria have been cloned. These include virulence genes of *Streptococcus mutans* (including glucosyl-transferase) and *S. sanguis*; a gene encoding *B. gingivalis* pili; a fimbrial gene of *Actinomyces vicosus*; a gene encoding a protease of *B. gingivalis*; and surface antigen genes of *A. actinomycetemcomitans, B. gingi-*

valis, B. intermedius, and *Eikenella corrodens.* Several of these cloned proteins are likely candidates for vaccines.

DNA PROBES

Recognizing the principle that a single-stranded piece of DNA will voraciously bind to a complementary single strand of DNA, researchers have created DNA probes. The probes are used to detect the presence of a particular gene or sequence of DNA in a particular DNA preparation (Fig. 3–63). These probes are selected fragments of DNA that contain specific gene sequences. Almost any DNA segment can be selected as a probe. If a desired DNA sequence is known, the probe can even be synthesized. To make it possible to visualize the probe, either radioactive or enzymatic labels are attached.

Several DNA probes are already used in clinical diagnostic laboratories to rapidly detect the presence of specific viruses and bacteria, as well as a variety of human genes and mutations. The great advantages of DNA-probe diagnostic tests are their specific-

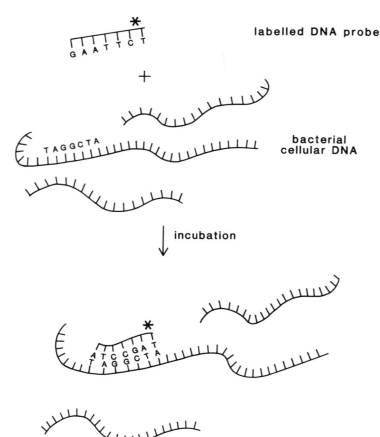

labelled DNA probe

bacterial cellular DNA

Figure 3–63 ■ DNA probes allow the detection of specific genes or DNA sequences. In the hypothetical case depicted here, the probe DNA contains a sequence specific for a certain species of bacteria. The target (bacterial cellular DNA) could be from a plaque sample. If the particular species for which the DNA probe is specific is present in the plaque, then that complementary DNA sequence will be present in the bacterial cellular DNA and the probe will bind to the target DNA. This type of assay only works with single-stranded DNA, so that prior to incubation of the target DNA with the probe, the DNA is denatured by heat to generate single strands of the DNA.

ity and speed. Among the DNA probes currently in use are those for (1) the screening for presence of the AIDS virus in donated blood; (2) testing for bacterial meningitis, yielding results in 10 minutes; (3) testing for streptococcal throat infection requiring 1 hour; and (4) testing for the presence of *Neisseria gonorrhoeae*, genital herpes, or *chlamydia*.

Several DNA probes have recently been developed for the detection of various periodontopathic species of bacteria. These are now being tested in clinical trials. Since these tests are relatively simple and specific, coupled with the development of nonradioactive techniques for labeling probes, it may be possible in the near future to detect the presence of these bacteria during a routine dental examination. This information would undoubtedly be helpful in identifying potential disease sites before tissue breakdown occurs.

THE NATURE OF BACTERIAL VIRULENCE

A *pathogenic microorganism* is one that is capable of producing disease in a susceptible host. Some bacteria are extremely pathogenic. For example, *Treponema pallidum*, the infectious agent of syphilis, has a minimal infectious dose estimated at 1 to 3 microorganisms. Other bacteria, such as *Vibrio cholerae*, which have a minimal infectious dose of 1×10^8 bacteria, are much less pathogenic. Bacteria that cause disease are *virulent* microorganisms—that is, they have the capacity to overcome host defense mechanisms. Virulence is actually the product of many interacting variables, involving both the microorganism and the host. A *virulence factor* is one property or characteristic of a pathogenic microorganism that allows the organism to cause disease. The sum total of virulence factors of a pathogenic bacterium is the mechanisms by which the bacterium evades the host's defensive mechanisms, establishes an infection, and damages host cells. *Infection,* as defined for this textbook, is an invasion of the host by a pathogenic microorganism or its products, resulting in disease in the host. Bacteria may establish an infection by two mechanisms: (1) colonization and invasion of tissues of the host, and (2) the production of toxins that may disseminate and produce cytotoxic effects on tissues distant from the initial site of infection. Therefore, in order for an infection to occur in a host,

the infecting organism (*etiologic agent*) must be able to (1) gain access to host tissue, (2) multiply in host tissue, (3) resist host defense mechanisms, and (4) damage host tissues. The last part of this chapter will discuss the microbial (virulence) factors involved in the establishment of an infection.

BACTERIAL ADHERENCE

For the most part, in order for bacteria to cause disease, they must first enter and establish themselves in the host tissue. The primary mechanism by which bacteria establish themselves is by adherence to host tissue. In a vast majority of diseases, an individual becomes infected by colonization of mucosal surfaces of the upper respiratory tract, the intestinal tract, and/or the genitourinary tract. Because secretions (including saliva), ciliary action, peristalsis, desquamation, excretion, coughing, sneezing, swallowing, and blood flow wash away or remove unattached bacteria from these mucosal surfaces, attachment of the invading microorganism to host cells is a requirement of all pathogens of mucosal surfaces, including the oral cavity. It has been estimated that each one of us swallows approximately 1 liter of saliva a day! It is thus not surprising that unattached bacteria are washed away faster than they multiply (divide).

The requirement for the attachment of bacteria to host tissues prior to infection is founded on the following evidence:

1. In vitro experiments have indicated that the propensity of certain bacteria to infect specific tissues is comparable to the ability of these bacteria to adhere to the tissue (Table 3–11). In no case has it been demonstrated that a high incidence of infection by a specific pathogen is associated with poor adherence of that pathogen to the isolated tissue in vivo. For example, several streptococcal species colonize the oral cavity but with differing predilections. *S. salivaris* is primarily found on the dorsum of the tongue and on the buccal mucosa, while *S. mutans* and *S. mitis* are found abundantly in dental plaque (*S. mutans* is recovered in high numbers from supragingival plaque), but in low numbers on mucosal surfaces. In vitro, these species are found to adhere to tissue cells of the tissue type that they colonize but not to other cells or other dental surfaces.

2. Bacterial variants that are found to have a reduced capacity to adhere in vitro have

Table 3–11 ■ Relationship between site of infection and in vitro adherence

Site of Infection	Source of Target Cell	Organism	Relative Adherence to Target Cell (in vitro)	Relative Incidence of Infection
Endocarditis	Heart-valve endothelium	Streptococci (viridans group), staphylococci	Good	High
		E. coli	Poor	Low
		Pseudomonas	Good	High (in heroin-using adults)
Mucosal colonization	Buccal mucosa	S. mitis	Poor	Low
		S. salivarius	Good	High
		E. coli	Good	Low
Pyoderma	Skin epithelium	S. pyogenes		
		Skin strain	Good	High
		Pharyngeal strain	Low	Moderate
Pharyngitis	Buccal cells	S. pyogenes		
		Skin strain	Moderate	Low
		Pharyngeal strains	Good	High
Cervicitis	Vaginal cells	Anaerobic bacteria	Poor	Low
		N. gonorrhoeae	Good	High
		S. agalactiae (group B)	Moderate	None
		C. vaginale	Moderate	Intermediate
Pyelonephritis	Uroepithelial cells	E. coli		
		Pyelonephritis strains	Good	High
		Nonpyelonephritis strains		

decreased infectivity in vivo (see Table 3–12). For instance, certain colony types of *Neisseria gonorrhoeae* that have a very limited ability to adhere to genital epithelial cells are unable to cause human infection in vivo, whereas colony types that adhere well in vitro have a high infectivity rate in vivo. The same is true of variants of several other pathogens including *Salmonella, E. coli, Proteus mirabilis,* streptococci, and *Actinomyces viscosus.*

3. The bacterial binding capacity of epithelial cells from individuals prone to certain bacterial infections is sometimes higher than those tissues from uninfected individuals (Table 3–13). For example, greater numbers of uropathogenic *E. coli* bind to urinary tract epithelial cells of women who have recurrent urinary tract infections than to urinary tract epithelial cells of normal women; cells of individuals with virus infections bind more *Streptococcus sanguis* than cells from uninfected individuals; and certain strains of piglets that are susceptible to diarrhea caused by *E. coli* (which have the k88 adhesin) bind more *E. coli* than do other piglets.

Bacterial adherence is mediated by bacterial cell surface structures called *adhesins,* which recognize specific receptors on the particular host cell surface (Fig. 3–64). The occurrence and distribution of host cell recep-

Table 3–12 ■ Relationship between epithelial cell adherence in vitro and bacterial infectivity in vivo

Bacteria	Bacterial Variants	Relative Adherence In Vitro	Relative Infectivity In Vivo
A. viscosus	Fimbriate	Good	High
	Nonfimbriate	Poor	Low
Gonococci	T₁ (fimbriate)	Good	High
	T₄ (nonfimbriate)	Poor	Low
E. coli (enterotoxigenic)	CF +	Good	High
	CF −	Poor	Low
Streptococci	Dextran +	Good	High
	Dextran −	Poor	Low
Salmonella	Fimbriate	Good	High
	Nonfimbriate	Poor	Moderate
E. coli	K88 +	Good	High
	K88 −	Poor	Low
P. mirabilis	Fimbriate	Good	High
	Nonfimbriate	Poor	Low
B. pertussis	Fimbriate	Good	High
	Nonfimbriate	Poor	Low

Table 3–13 ■ Correlation between in vitro adherence to target host cells and predisposition to acquire infection

Subjects	Bacteria	Target Cells	Target Cells from	Relative in vitro Adherence
Females with recurrent urinary tract infections	E. coli	Vaginal periurethral epithelial cells	Subject	High
			Normal	Low
Individuals with damaged heart valves (i.e., rheumatic heart disease)	Streptococci	Endothelium of heart valves	Damaged	High
			Normal	Low
Individuals with viral infections	S. sanguis, S. agalactiae	Tissue culture cells	Virus-infected culture	High
			Uninfected culture	Low
Staphylococcal carriers	S. aureus	Nasal epithelium	Carrier	High
			Noncarrier	Low
Genetic variants of pigs	E. coli K88	Intestinal epithelium	K88-resistant phenotype	Low
			K88-susceptible phenotype	High
Primates	N. gonorrhoeae	Organ cultures of oviducts	Human	High
			Nonprimate	Low

tors for particular (bacterial) adhesins determines the tissue and species *tropisms* (specificities) of bacteria.

Because both bacterial and tissue cell surfaces are net negatively charged, bacteria must overcome this repulsion by charge and hydrophobicity localization. To this end, bacterial adhesins are commonly located on surface appendages such as fimbriae (Table 3–14).

There are several pathogens for which adherence mechanisms are known in detail (Table 3–14). *Actinomyces viscosus* strain T14V, an etiologic agent of root caries in rats, mice, and probably humans, synthesizes at least two antigenically distinct types of fimbriae, designated type 1 and type 2. Type 2 fimbriae mediate lactose-sensitive adherence of *A. viscosus* to several species of streptococci and to neuraminidase-treated erythrocytes. Type 1 fimbriae, on the other hand, mediate the adsorption of strain T14V to saliva-treated hydroxyapatite (SHA), a surface that mimics the saliva-coated tooth surface. This adsorption is not inhibited by lactose. The receptors on the SHA surface for the actinomyces type 1 fimbriae are a specific class of salivary proteins, proline-rich-proteins (PRPs). Since these proteins are a component of saliva that preferentially adsorb to the tooth surface, it

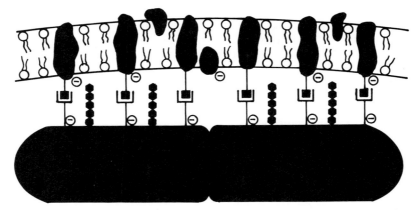

Figure 3–64 ■ Attachment of a bacterial cell to a host cell membrane or surface usually occurs by *specific* binding of bacterial cell structures (adhesins ५) to target host cell receptors (↓). Because there is a net negative charge on both cell surfaces, the bacterial cell may contain hydrophobic molecules (⊖), which are attracted toward phospholipid molecules (hydrophobic) in the host cell membrane. Several different types of bacterial cell surface structures may act as adhesins, see Table 3–14. (From Beachey, Bacterial Adherence. Chapman and Hall, London, 1980, pp 1–29, with permission.)

	Table 3–14 ■ Specific adhesins and receptors of various bacteria	
Bacteria	**Adhesin**	**Receptor**
S. pyogenes	LTA-M protein fibrillae	Fibronectin
E. coli	Type 1 fimbriae	D-mannose
Klebsiella aerogenes		
K. pneumoniae		
Serratia marcescens		
Shigella flexneri		
Enterobacter cloacae		
Salmonella typhi		
S. paratyphi A		
S. paratyphi B		
S. typhimurium		
Citrobacter freundii		
E. coli (uropathogenic)	MR fimbriae	GalNacoal-3GalNacbl-3-Galal-4Galbl-4GlcCer (Globotetraosylceramide and Globotriosylceramide)
	MR and type 1 fimbriae	Same as above plus D-mannose
E. coli CFA 1 CFA 11	MR fimbriae	?Gal Nacbl-4-Galal-4GlcCer (GM$_2$ ganglioside)
E. coli K88	MR fimbriae	?b-D-Gal or GalNac and GlcNac
A. viscosus	Type 1 fibrillae	Proline-rich protein or glycoprotein
Vibrio cholera	Fimbriae	Fucose and mannose
Mycoplasma	Membrane protein	Sialic acid, glycophorin
Neisseria gonorrhoeae	Fimbriae	Galbl-3GalNac-bl-4Gal
Proteus species	Fimbriae (type 4)	?
Bordetella pertussis	Fimbriae	? Sterol
Pseudomonas aeruginosa	Fimbriae	?
Chlamydia	?	N-acetylglucosamine

is thought that the type 1 fimbriae are the principal adhesins involved in the adherence of *A. viscosus* to tooth surfaces in vivo.

Group A streptococci (i.e., *S. pyogenes,* the etiologic agent of pharyngitis, rheumatic fever, and glomerulonephritis) binds to epithelial cells by M-protein lipoteichoic acid (LTA) complexes present on the surface of the streptococci. The LTA molecules, which consist entirely of glycerol-PO$_4$, are anchored to the cytoplasmic membrane by covalent binding to the membrane glycolipids. The host epithelial receptor for the LTA adhesin is probably the membrane protein, fibronectin. Both purified LTA and antibodies to LTA (but not those to other surface antigens) block adherence of streptococci to cell membranes.

Type 1 fimbriae are one of several adhesins that mediate the binding of *E. coli* to host epithelial cells. Since the binding of type 1 fimbriae to epithelial cells can be inhibited by the presence of mannose, it appears that the epithelial cell receptor contains mannose since cells treated with concanavalin A, a plant lectin that binds to mannose residues, also prevents adherence of *E. coli* to the epithelial cells.

Once bacteria have colonized a target tissue, fimbriae may be detrimental to the bacterial cells since their presence may increase the chance of phagocytosis. Consequently,

after the initial colonization bacteria may undergo phenotypic changes and no longer synthesize fimbriae. This appears to be the case with pyelonephritic *E. coli*. While the *E. coli* are infecting the lower urinary tract and bladder, they contain high numbers of type 1 fimbriae. However, once the infection progresses to the kidneys, the cells contain very few, if any, fimbriae.

It should now be obvious that the adherence of bacteria to host tissues promotes colonization and facilitates penetration of target tissues by virulent bacteria. This adherence of bacteria to host tissue cells, may, in certain cases, permit a close association between the toxigenic bacteria and their target tissues. This close association may enhance the activity of the toxins by delivering the toxin directly to the target tissue. For example, *Vibrio cholerae* (the causative agent of cholera) adherence to the intestinal mucosa facilitates the local delivery of the cholera toxin (choleragen) to the intestinal cells. In a similar fashion, attachment of enteropathogenic *E. coli* to intestinal epithelial cells allows local delivery of the enterotoxin to the intestinal mucosal cells, resulting in traveler's diarrhea. *S. mutans* cells use sucrose to produce extracellular capsular polysaccharides, or *glucans,* which allow the cells to adhere to the tooth surface, primarily in protected fissures and indentations. As a byproduct of their metabolism, *S. mutans* cells produce lactic acid, a toxic end product, since a sufficient buildup of this acid causes demineralization of the tooth surface and, thus, ultimately caries. If the streptococci were not closely attached to the tooth surface, the acid would be quickly diluted and neutralized by saliva.

VIRULENCE FACTORS

During the infection process, not only must microbial components or products adhere to host tissues and resists host defense mechanisms, but also they must damage tissue, either directly, by production of toxins, or indirectly, by induction of an immunopathologic response. In the following section, we will discuss in more detail bacterial components that are determinants of disease.

Surface Appendages

As discussed previously in this chapter, bacterial pili (fimbriae) commonly function as adhesins (see Table 3–14). Several pathogenic bacteria contain more than one type of fimbriae and thus more than one type of adhesin. As discussed earlier the F pili of gram-negative bacteria attach to neighboring cells and facilitate the transfer of DNA from cell to cell. This DNA exchange mechanism mediates the transfer of antibiotic resistance genes as well as virulence genes (including genes encoding various types of fimbriae) between cells.

Extracellular Capsules and Slime

As we mentioned previously in this chapter, the capsule of *S. mutans* is required for adherence and virulence, but a capsule that functions as an adhesin is relatively unusual for pathogenic bacteria, and recent evidence suggests that capsules of some pathogens such as *A. viscosus*, *Neisseria meningitidis*, and *S. pneumoniae* may actually result in reduced adherence. However, the overall effect of the presence of extracellular polysaccharides is a substantial increase in virulence. This is due primarily to the antiphagocytic properties of capsules. Several pathogens for which capsules have been shown to decrease *opsonization* and have antiphagocytic properties are listed in Table 3–15. In mixed infections, the presence of a capsule of one bacterial species may protect neighboring unrelated bacteria from phagocytosis. Polysaccharide capsules may also hinder the effects of antibiotics in vivo by preventing the antibiotic from coming into direct contact with the bacterial outer membrane or cell wall.

A detailed series of studies of *Bacteroides fragilis* has shown that strains that produce a capsule are virulent (able to cause abscess formation), whereas strains without a capsule are avirulent. The virulent property of the capsule was proved further when implantation of the purified capsular polysaccharide into rats produced abscesses in all rats tested.

Lipopolysaccharides

Lipopolysaccharides (endotoxin; LPS) elicit a broad spectrum of pathophysiologic prop-

Table 3–15 ■ Invasive factors of microbial species pathogenic to mankind

Invasive Factor	Bacterial Source	Activity
Capsule	Streptococcus pneumoniae Klebsiella pneumoniae Hemophilus influenzae Bacillus anthracis Yersinia pestis	Inhibits phagocytosis
M protein of cell wall	Group A streptococci	Inhibits phagocytosis
Extracellular enzymes	Clostridium perfringens	
Collagenase	Bacteroides gingivalis	Hydrolyzes collagen
Hyaluronidase	Staphylococci, streptococci, Clostridia	Hydrolyzes hyaluronic acid
Lecithinase	Clostridium perfringens	Hydrolyzes lecithin
Coagulase	Staphylococcus aureus	Clots fibrin
Fibrinolysin (kinase)	Staphylococci, streptococci	Lysis of fibrin clots
Proteases, nucleases and lipases	Staphylococci, streptococci, Bacteroides species	Depolymerization of proteins, nucleic acids, and fats
Leukocidin	Staphylococci, streptococci	Lysis of red blood cells
Hemolysin	Actinobacillus actinomycetemcomitans	Lysis of PMNs
IgA protease	B. gingivalis B. intermedius Oral streptococci Neisseria gonorrhoeae	Cleavage/inactivation of IgA

erties (Table 3–16), and depending upon the amount the host encounters, can result in cardiovascular collapse and even death within an hour or two. Experimental findings indicate that irreversible hemorrhagic shock is due primarily to adsorption of LPS from the bowel. Most of the endotoxic biologic properties are directly attributable to the lipid A portion of the molecule; however, the polysaccharide moiety confers resistance to neutrophils, is a major antigen for many bacterial species, and also functions to neutralize serum components.

The direct role of LPS in many chronic human diseases is ill defined, but several characteristics of typhoid fever and meningococcal septicemia are compatible with the known effects of LPS. Endotoxins are incompletely neutralized by antibodies (against the O-antigen component) and are stable to heat and even autoclaving. It should be noted that medical apparatus, especially that used for intravenous administrations, which may become contaminated by gram-negative organisms, is not detoxified by autoclaving and should not be used.

There is evidence that LPS may contribute to much of the tissue damage, especially bone resorption, in periodontal diseases. Several LPSs from putative periodontopath-ogenic species have been purified and the biologic effects studied. The chemical composition of the LPSs of *Bacteroides* species, *Eikenella corrodens*, and *Capnocytophaga* differs from that of the classic or enteric (*E. coli* and *S. typhimurium*) LPS, while that of *A. actinomycetemcomitans* appears to be quite similar to *Salmonella typhimurium* LPS. The LPSs of *Eikenella* and *A. actinomycetemcomitans* are stimulatory to bone resorption when tested in in vitro assays, and purified *E. corrodens* LPS by itself causes loss of periapical bone in vivo. The mechanisms by which these LPSs cause bone resorption are not known, but it is known that the uptake of Ca^{++} is inhibited; therefore, the resorption is probably not via stimulation of osteoclastic activity. In addition to their effects on bone, these same LPSs are also mitogenic to B cells (independent of T cells) and *A. actinomycetemcomitans* LPS aggregates platelets and is toxic to macrophages.

Several pathogenic bacteria, including suspected periodontal pathogens (i.e., *Bacteroides* species and *A. actinomycetemcomitans*), produce copious amounts of membrane blebs, which may be a mechanism for delivery of membrane-bound LPS to distant sites in the absence of lysis of the bacteria. This blebbing may have important implications in periodontal diseases, especially since it has been demonstrated that LPS can be found in periodontal tissues in the absence of penetration by bacteria.

CELL WALL COMPONENTS

In addition to maintaining the shape of bacterial cells and serving as a protective barrier, peptidoglycan (see earlier discussion) may also have virulence-associated properties. For instance, it can activate complement, has pyrogenic activity, has been shown to interfere with phagocytosis, and may contribute to damage of fallopian tubes during gonococcal infections. Streptococcal peptidoglycan contributes to the development of a chronic inflammatory response in a rheumatoid arthritis model system. The peptidoglycans of oral species of bacteria have been shown to be mitogenic and to stimulate bone loss in an in vitro assay. Purified preparations of peptidoglycans from oral isolates of *Bacteroides*, *Eikenella*, and *Actinomyces* are toxic to macrophages at high concentrations (greater than 50 µg/ml), and at lower concentrations significantly inhibit lysozyme activity.

Table 3–16 ■ Biologic properties of lipopolysaccharides

Activity	Effect/Mechanism
Pyrogenicity	Causes fever by release of pyrogen from phagocytic cells
Mitogenic for T-cells	Stimulates T-cells, independent of B cells
Irreversible shock	Death
Cardiovascular collapse	Death
Necrosis of tumors	Stimulates macrophages
Cytotoxic to fibroblasts	Kills fibroblast in vitro
Chemotactic to PMNs	
Activates complement	Altered resistance to bacterial infections alternate pathway, independent of Ab
Platelet aggregation	Thrombosis in vitro?
Bone resorption	Loss of periodontal bone
Hemorrhage	
Intravascular coagulation	Activation of clotting factors
Leukopenia and leukocytosis	Decrease in number of circulating lymphocytes, granulocytes
Interferes with gluconeogenesis and glycogenesis	Loss of hepatic glycogen

EXOTOXINS

Both gram-negative and gram-positive bacteria have been shown to produce diffusible protein molecules, or exotoxins, that injure tissue directly. These toxins are usually heat labile, have been shown to have a direct necrotic effect on tissues with which they come in contact and are among the most powerful poisons known to humans (Table 3–17). For example, 1 mg of tetanus toxin is enough to kill 1 million guinea pigs. The potency of these toxins is often expressed as the LD_{50}, which is the amount required to kill 50 percent of a test population of individuals. Most exotoxins can be inactivated by

chemical treatment, which results in retention of the antigenic properties of the active toxin molecule. These chemically detoxified proteins, or *toxoids*, are used in many instances to stimulate a protective immune response (i.e., diphtheria and pertussis toxoids). The pharmacologic actions of most exotoxins are known and are generally quite slow, often requiring several days for full activity (Table 3–17). Many exotoxins are plasmid-encoded, and several have been cloned. Few exotoxins from oral isolates have been identified. However, *A. actinomycetemcomitans* isolates produce a leukotoxin that is released in blebs from the bacterial cell surface. This heat-labile, soluble toxin destroys

Table 3–17 ■ Exotoxins produced by various toxigenic bacteria

Microbial Species	Disease	Toxin Designation	Activity or Effect of Toxin
Bacillus anthracis	Anthrax	Factors 1, 2, and 3	Pulmonary edema, capillary thrombosis
Yersinia pestis (Pasteurella pestis)	Plague	Plague toxin	Lethality in mice related to anti-cAMP effects and shift in hormone balance
Corynebacterium diphtheriae	Diphtheria	Diphtheria toxin	An inhibitor of protein synthesis; causes necrosis of tissue
Streptococcus pyogenes	Pyogenic infections	Streptolysin 0	Hemolysin
		Streptolysin S	Hemolysin; cytotoxic for many subcelluar organelles
	Scarlet fever	Erythrogenic toxin	Rash
Staphylococcus aureus	Pyogenic infections	Alpha toxin	Hemolytic, dermonecrotic; paralysis of smooth muscle
		Delta toxin	Hemolytic and dermonecrotic
		Leukocidin	Leukolytic
	Food poisoning	Enterotoxin	Vomiting and diarrhea
	Scalded skin syndrome	Exfoliatin	Exfoliation
Vibrio cholerae	Cholera	Enterotoxin (choleragen)	Activates adenyl cyclase with increased hypersecretion of Cl^-, HCO_3^-, and H_2O
Escherichia coli	Infant diarrhea	Enterotoxin	Activates adenyl cyclase (?)
	Traveler's diarrhea		
Pseudomonas aeruginosa	Opportunistic pathogen in burn patients, the immunosuppressed, and those with cystic fibrosis	Exotoxin	Possible effects on liver (?)
Clostridium tetani	Tetanus	Tetanospasmin	Blocks nerve transmission in CNS, resulting in spastic paralysis
Clostridium botulinum	Botulism	Types A, B, E, and F principal cause of botulism in humans	Acts on peripheral nervous system: blocks release of acteylcholine, resulting in flaccid paralysis
Clostridium perfringens	Gas gangrene	Alpha toxin	A lecithinase: lyses RBCs and leukocytes
		Kappa toxin	A collagenase: attacks connective tissue
		Theta toxin	Hemolysin
	Food poisoning	Enterotoxin	Vomiting, diarrhea
Clostridium novyi, C. septicum, and *C. sporogenes*	Gas gangrene	Alpha toxin	Lecithinase: lyses RBCs and leukocytes
Shigella dysenteriae	Bacillary dysentery	Enterotoxin	May be involved in diarrhea
Actinobacillus actinomycetemcomitans	Juvenile periodontosis	Leukotoxin	Leukolytic

human and monkey blood PMNs and gingival crevice PMNs but not other human cells or PMNs from a variety of other species. The leukotoxic activity does not require phagocytosis of the bacteria, but binding of the leukotoxin to the target cell membrane is an initial and prerequisite step in the cytotoxic reaction. Leukotoxic activity can be inhibited by sera from patients with juvenile periodontitis.

HYDROLYTIC ENZYMES

Most pathogenic species of bacteria synthesize a variety of enzymes that are useful to them in the host-parasite confrontation. Many gram-negative bacteria contain proteolytic and hydrolytic enzymes in their periplasmic space. In addition, both gram-negative and gram-positive organisms may produce extracellular lytic enzymes that increase the virulence of certain pathogenic species (see Table 3–15). These enzymes, for the most part, function to provide nutrients for growth and contribute to the invasiveness of the organism. For instance, *B. gingivalis* produces a collagenase as well as high levels of peptidases. These peptidases are active on glycine-proline peptides, peptides that are major components of collagen of the periodontal ligament. *Capnocytophaga* species possess peptidase as well as acid and alkaline phosphatases, which may degrade bone proteins.

Several pathogenic bacteria produce proteolytic enzymes that degrade human serum proteins. IgG, IgM, C_3, and C_5 are degraded by *B. gingivalis* isolates, whereas strains of *B. intermedius* degrade IgG and C_3. The degradation of serum components may cause reduced phagocytosis and a subsequent reduction of bactericidal activity by PMNs. This may explain why *B. gingivalis* promotes the survival of avirulent bacteria in polymicrobial infections in guinea pigs and inhibits phagocytosis of other bacteria present in in vitro assays.

IgA protease is an important virulence factor in some bacterial infections of the mucous membranes, particularly gonorrhea. Since IgA is the primary antibody present in mucous membrane secretions and is a potent host defensive mechanism that can prevent bacterial adherence to the host cells, it is not surprising that the ability to produce an IgA protease would be clearly advantageous to a mucosal surface pathogen. Of 21 bacterial species found to produce an IgA-cleaving enzyme (out of 800 tested), more than half are oral streptococci or species associated with destructive periodontal disease. The remaining positive isolates include respiratory tract pathogens and *Neisseria gonorrhoeae*. The periodontal disease–associated isolates that were found to produce an IgA protease included several species of *Bacteroides* and *Capnocytophaga*. Interestingly, nonoral *Bacteroides* species were unable to cause degradation of IgA. The *Bacteroides* IgA protease is different from all other IgA proteases in that it results in total destruction of the IgA molecule, whereas the others cleave the immunoglobulin at only one site.

REFERENCES*

Structure

Bayer, M. E.: Areas of adhesion between wall and membrane of *Escherichia coli*. J. Gen. Microbiol. 53:345, 1968.

Costerton, J. W.: How bacteria stick. Sci. Am., 238:86, 1978.

Costerton, J. W.: The role of electron microscopy in the elucidation of bacterial structure and function. Ann. Rev. Microbiol. 33:459, 1979.

Leive, L. (ed.): Bacterial Membranes and Walls. Marcel Dekker, New York, 1973.

Nikaido, H., and Nakae, T.: The outer membrane of gram-negative bacteria. Adv. Microbiol. Physiol. 20:163, 1979.

Nikaido, H., and Varra, M.: Molecular basis of the permeability of bacterial outer membrane. Microbiol. Rev. 49:1, 1985.

Osborn, M. J., and Wu, H. C. P.: Proteins of the outer membrane of gram-negative bacteria. Ann. Rev. Microbiol. 34:369, 1980.

Pettijohn, D. E.: Prokaryotic DNA in nucleoid structure. CRC Crit. Rev. Biochem. 4:175, 1976.

Salton, M. R. J., and Owen, P.: Bacterial membrane structure. Ann. Rev. Microbiol. 30:451, 1976.

Schleifer, K. H., and Kandler, O.: Peptidoglycan types of bacterial cell walls and their taxonomic implications. Bacteriol. Rev. 36:407, 1972.

Shiveley, J. M.: Inclusion bodies of procaryotes. Ann. Rev. Microbiol. 28:167, 1974.

Shockman, G. D., and Barrett, J. F.: Structure, function and assembly of cell walls of gram-positive bacteria. Ann. Rev. Microbiol. 37:501, 1983.

Silverman, M., and Simon, M. I.: Bacterial flagella. Ann. Rev. Microbiol. 31:397, 1977.

Ward, J. B.: Teichoic and teichuronic acids: Biosynthesis, assembly, and location. Microbiol. Rev. 45:211, 1981.

Wittman, H. G.: Components of bacterial ribosomes. Ann. Rev. Biochem. 51:155, 1982.

Wittmann, H. G.: Architecture of prokaryotic ribosomes. Ann. Rev. Biochem. 52:35, 1983.

*The references listed here represent an assortment of articles and books that will be useful to the reader in extending and interpreting this chapter. We have listed the titles under major subject headings for ease of locating useful information.

Metabolism

Dagley, S., and Nicholson, D. E.: An Introduction to Metabolic Pathways. Blackwell Scientific, Oxford and Edinburgh, 1970.

Gottschalk, G.: Bacterial Metabolism. Springer-Verlag, New York, 1979.

Gottschalk, G., and Andreesen, J. R.: Energy metabolism in anaerobes. In Quayle, J. R. (ed.): International Review of Biochemistry, Vol. 21. Springer-Verlag, New York, 1979, pp. 5–115.

Haddock, B. A., and Jones, C. W.: Bacterial respiration. Bacteriol. Rev. 41:47, 1977.

Ingeledew, W. J., and Poole, R. K.: The respiratory chains of *Escherichia coli*. Microbiol. Rev. 48:181, 1984.

Jones, C. W.: Bacterial respiration and photosynthesis. Thomas Nelson and Sons, Walton-on-Thames, Surrey, England, 1982.

Moat, A. G.: Microbial Physiology. John Wiley and Sons, New York, 1979.

Racker, E.: From Pasteur to Mitchell; a hundred years of bioenergetics. Fed. Proc. 39:210, 1980.

Rose, A. H.: Chemical Microbiology, ed. 3. Plenum, New York, 1976.

Zeikus, I. G.: Chemical and fuel production by anaerobic bacteria. Ann. Rev. Microbiol., 34:423, 1980.

Biosynthesis

Caskey, C. T.: Peptide chain termination. Trends Biochem. Sci. 5:234, 1980.

Clark, B.: The elongation step of protein biosynthesis. Trends Biochem. Sci. 5:207, 1980.

Hunt, T.: The initiation of protein synthesis. Trends Biochem. Sci. 5:178, 1980.

Kozak, M.: Comparison of initiation of protein synthesis in prokaryotes, eukaryotes and organelles. Microbiol. Rev. 47:1, 1983.

Preiss, J.: Bacterial glycogen synthesis and its regulation. Ann. Rev. Microbiol. 38:419, 1984.

Troy, F. A., II: The chemistry and biosynthesis of selected bacterial capsular polymers. Ann. Rev. Microbiol. 33:519, 1979.

Growth

Bauchop, T., and Elsden, S. R.: The growth of microorganisms in relation to their energy supply. J. Gen. Microbiol. 23:457, 1960.

Cole, R. M., and Hahn, J. J.: Cell wall replication in *Streptococcus pyogenes*. Science 135:722, 1962.

Ingraham, J. L., Maaloe, O., and Neidhardt, F. C.: Growth of the Bacterial Cell. Sinauer Assoc., Sunderland, MA, 1983.

Pooley, H. M.: Localized insertion of new cell wall in *Bacillus subtilis*. Nature 274:264, 1978.

Genetics

Alberts, B., Bray, D., Lewis, J., Raff, M., Roberts, K., and Watson, J. D.: Molecular Biology of the Cell. Garland Publishing, New York, 1983.

Clewell, D. B.: Plasmids, drug resistance and gene transfer in the genus *Streptococcus*. Microbiol. Rev. 45:409, 1981.

Lewin, B.: Genes III, ed. 3. John Wiley and Sons, New York, 1987.

Nossal, N. G.: Prokaryotic DNA replication systems. Ann. Rev. Biochem. 52:581, 1983.

Smith, H. O., and Danner, D. B.: Genetic transformation. Ann. Rev. Biochem. 50:41, 1981.

chapter 4

Bacterial classification

Joseph J. Zambon, D.D.S., Ph.D.

Since 1743 when Antonie van Leeuwenhoek first used light microscopy to examine scrapings from human teeth, microbiologists have been confronted with the problem of making comparisons between microorganisms. They needed to make these comparisons for a number of reasons. First, they sought to provide an orderly framework to the catalogue of microbial life forms that can assume an almost limitless variety of shapes and growth requirements. Second, a system of bacterial classification was needed in order for scientists to communicate with one another and to answer the question: Is the microorganism isolated by scientist A the same as the microorganism isolated by scientist B? Finally, and most important for the health-related professions, a system of bacterial classification was necessary for the diagnosis of infectious diseases and to answer the question: What is the microorganism responsible for causing a patient's illness?

For all of these reasons, bacterial classification is an essential component of modern microbiology. It is also an ever-changing process much to the dismay of the casual observer. As more is learned of certain microorganisms, and as better techniques are used to examine bacteria, old groupings are dissolved and new taxonomies are formulated. A classic example is that of the black-pigmented *Bacteroides* species (Fig. 4–1). Originally, these microorganisms were classified as *Bacterium melaninogenicum*. As these microorganisms were more intensively studied, it became clear that there were significant differences among strains of *Bacteroides melaninogenicus* in their ability to ferment sug-

ars. Based on these sugar fermentations and other biochemical characteristics, the species *Bacteroides melaninogenicus* was divided into three subspecies. The strongly fermentative strains were categorized as *Bacteroides melaninogenicus*, subspecies *melaninogenicus*, while the nonfermentative strains were categorized as *Bacteroides melaninogenicus*, subspecies *asaccharolyticus*. Strains that were intermediate in their ability to ferment sugars were categorized as *Bacteroides melaninogenicus*, subspecies *intermedius*. Subsequent examination of these same species using newly developed molecular biology techniques revealed significant differences in the sequence of deoxyribonucleic acid bases. Based on these data, each of the subspecies was elevated to species status as *Bacteroides melaninogenicus*, *Bacteroides asaccharolyticus*, and *Bacteroides intermedius*, respectively. Each of these changes may appear trivial or even deliberately confusing to those unfamiliar with bacterial taxonomy, but each change is made only after consideration of appropriate data.

Dating back to the work *Species Plantarum* by the Swedish taxonomist Linnaeus, published in 1753, bacteria have been categorized into a taxonomic hierarchy (Table 4–1), and in this hierarchy, they have been named using a two-part **epithet**. This is the same convention used to name animal or plant species. In zoology and botany, however, a species can be defined in more precise terms than is possible in microbiology. In these disciplines, species are the smallest group that can sexually interact to produce fertile offspring. This definition is inappropriate for bacterial species, which most often reproduce

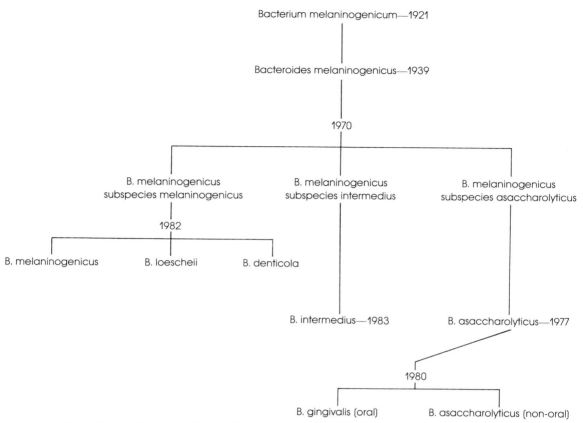

Figure 4–1 ■ Changes in the classification of the oral black-pigmented *Bacteroides* species.

asexually and which are not so clearly delineated as plant and animal species. Bacterial species are considered to represent a group of strains that share a number of common features. A bacterial strain is defined as the descendant of a single pure (**axenic)** culture.

The first part of a bacterial name is the *genus* name which is, by convention, a latinized, usually descriptive word, spelled with a capital letter. The second part of this binomial name, or *binonem,* is the *specific* epithet, which is, by convention, spelled with a lower case letter. Some species, as in the example of *Bacteroides melaninogenicus* described earlier, may also make use of a *subspecies epithet,* for example, *Bacteroides melaninogenicus,* subsp. *intermedius.* Many species names are descriptive. *Actinobacillus actinomycetemcomitans* is such a descriptive species name. "Ac-

tinobacillus" refers to the fact that microorganisms in this genus exhibit a star-shaped formation (hence, "actino" for star) in the center of the colonies on agar surfaces and the bacterial cells are short rods ("bacillus"). The specific epithet "actinomycetemcomitans" refers to the fact that this microorganism was first isolated together with *Actinomyces israelii* from lesions of cervicofocial actinomycosis. Hence, "actinomycetemcomitans" means "together with *Actinomyces.*"

Since bacterial species are not defined in relation to reproductive ability as are species of whales, for example, microbiologists use other features of the microorganism to make groupings or **taxa.** The earliest groupings, and those which are still commonly used today, are based on relatively easy to define properties (Table 4–2). These include the size and shape of the bacterial cells seen under the light microscope, the ability to hold certain stains such as the Giemsa and Gram stains, evidence of cellular motility as seen using phase contrast or darkfield microscopy, ability to grow at different temperatures and in different gaseous environments, the size and shape of the bacterial colony on certain

Table 4–1 ■ Hierarchy of bacteria taxa	
Rank	
Kingdom	Family
Division	Genus
Class	Species
Order	

Table 4–2 ■ Typical features for the phenotypic classification of bacteria

1. Cellular characteristics
   a. Gram stain
   b. Size
   c. Shape
   d. Presence of flagella, fimbria
   e. Motility
2. Colony characteristics
   a. Size
   b. Shape
   c. Color
   d. Consistency
   e. Edge
3. Physiologic characteristics
   a. Temperature for optimum growth
   b. Growth environment
      1. Aerobic
      2. CO_2 enriched air
      3. Anaerobic
      4. Facultative
   c. Biochemical reactions
      1. Indole
      2. Nitrate/nitrite reduction
      3. H_2S production
      4. Gas production
   d. Fermentation of specific sugars
   e. Pattern of metabolic acids as determined by gas-liquid chromatography

types of media—there are literally hundreds of properties that can characterize a bacterium and that can be used in categorization. As our knowledge and methods have improved, additional properties have been examined and incorporated into these schemes. The analysis of metabolic acid end products by gas-liquid chromatography is one such development that is now standard practice in the identification and taxonomy of bacteria.

The most basic analysis in taxonomy is an examination of the bacterial genome, which generally range from 1 to 8×10^9 daltons (Table 4–3). All other phenotypic properties such as bacterial size, shape, and metabolism

Table 4–3 ■ Methods for the classification of bacteria

I. Phenotypic
II. Genetic—Based on DNA analysis
   1. Per cent guanine plus cytosine
      a. Thermal denaturation
      b. Buoyant density centrifugation
   2. DNA base sequence
      DNA-DNA hybridization
III. Chemotaxonomy
   1. Lipids
   2. Cell wall polymers
   3. Isoprenoid quinones
   4. Cytochromes
   5. Bacterial enzymes
IV. Serology

are based on the kind and arrangement of nucleotides in the bacterial DNA. Several techniques have been developed for use in bacterial taxonomy, based on characterization of the bacterial genome. First is the determination of deoxyribonucleic acid base composition or the mole percent guanine plus cytosine content (**mol% G + C**). As the name implies, this method gives information on the amount of the specific nucleotide bases, guanine and cytosine, in bacterial DNA. In eukaryotic cells this percentage varies within a very small range, but in prokaryotic cells it can vary from 25 to 75 percent. The calculation of mol% G+ C is commonly performed in one of two ways, either by a thermal denaturation or by buoyant density (isopyknic) centrifugation. In the former method, DNA is purified from the bacterial cell and the absorbance in the ultraviolet region is measured as the preparation is slowly heated. Increasing temperature will disrupt the hydrogens bonds linking the paired DNA strands and resulting in increased absorbance. This absorbance can then be plotted, and the midpoint of the curve, known as the melting temperature, or T_m, is then used to calculate the mol% G + C. The buoyant density method involves centrifugation of purified bacterial DNA in a cesium chloride gradient. At equilibrium, the density of the bacterial DNA can be calculated from its position in the cesium chloride gradient, and from this the mol% G + C can be determined. By either thermal denaturation or the buoyant density method, the mol% G + C gives information only on the composition of the bacterial genome, and even distantly related bacterial species can have the same mol% G + C. Neither technique provides information on the sequence of base pairs. This information is much more valuable since microorganisms possessing bacterial genomes with identical sequences are likely to be members of the same bacterial species. Sequence homology can also be used to infer evolutionary relationships between microorganisms. In zoology and botany, evolutionary relationships between species can be derived by examination of fossil records. However, there is very little available in the way of microbial fossil data and the evolution of bacterial species has been very difficult to examine. Analysis of the DNA sequence in the entire bacterial genome, and especially in particular "target" genes, can be useful for these types of studies.

Several methods have been developed to examine DNA base sequence homology, including DNA-DNA hybridization. These same techniques are also being used in the diagnosis of bacterial infections by means of species-specific "DNA probes." DNA-DNA hybridization techniques involve the purification of bacterial DNA from one species and breaking the double-stranded DNA helix into single strands using either thermal denaturation or alkali treatment. These single DNA strands are immobilized onto a substrate such as a nitrocellulose filter and are then reacted with radiolabeled, single-stranded DNA from another bacterial strain. At points on the DNA strands where there are complementary bases, a heteroduplex will form. For identical microorganisms, there should be 100 percent hybridization (see Chapter 2). Between less closely related microorganisms, there is less heteroduplex formation and more areas of single-strandedness. Following the hybridization reaction between strands, the mixture is treated with an enzyme, DNAase, which cleaves the unpaired, single-strand DNA but leaves the heteroduplexes untouched. The degree of DNA hybridization is then measured by determining the amount of radioactivity bound to the substrate.

Since DNA base content and base sequence reflect the entire basis for other phenotypic properties expressed by the microorganism, these assays are thought to reflect bacterial relationships, and hence bacterial taxonomy, more accurately than other tests. However, even the bacterial genome within a single species can change. It can vary over time, for example, as genetic elements are transferred between microorganisms by means of transduction and conjugation (see Chapter 2). Bacterial taxonomy, whether based on phen-

otypic traits or on the bacterial genome, can also be expected to change.

One specialized area of research in bacterial taxonomy is known as **numeric (phenetic)** taxonomy. Using this approach, a large number of traits (usually 100 to 200) such as Gram stain characteristics, motility, sugar fermentations, and biochemical reactions are determined in a group of microorganisms. Each trait or character is assigned a value of 1; that is, no more weight is assigned to one feature as compared with any other feature. Thus, in numeric taxonomy, gram-positivity or negativity, which is generally considered to be an "important" trait, is weighted the same as fermentation of individual sugars. By compiling the number of similar features among different strains, referred to as "operational taxonomic units," the degree of relatedness can be calculated and expressed as a simple matching coefficient or percent similarity. By means of statistical calculations including "cluster analysis" or "ordination" which are often derived through the use of computers, similar strains can be grouped together. The relationships among strains can be plotted as a **dendogram** (Fig. 4–2) for data derived by cluster analysis or as a **taxonomic map** for data derived from ordination.

Prior to January 1, 1980, the complete list of bacterial names contained microorganisms for which **type strains**—the standard reference bacteria strain which is used to define a bacterial species—did not exist. Some of these strains dated back to the 1800s and had undergone numerous reclassifications. Starting on January 1, 1980, however, all accepted bacterial names were listed in a publication, "Approved Lists of Bacterial Names." In or-

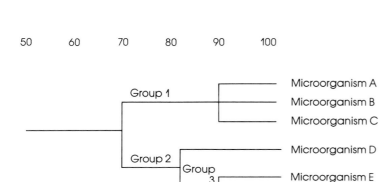

Figure 4–2 ■ Dendogram of a hypothetical microorganism.

der for a bacterial name to be accepted, that is, to have scientific standing, it must appear on this list. New species or reclassifications of existing species must be published in the *International Journal of Systematic Bacteriology*. Subsequent questions on the validity of a bacterial species are reviewed by the Judicial Commission of the International Union of Microbiological Societies.

In addition to the methods described earlier for the classification of bacteria, there are two other methods that have been useful. These are chemotaxonomy and serology. **Chemotaxonomy** makes use of physical and chemical characteristics for the classification of bacteria. There are a number of factors that can be measured, including lipids, cell wall polymers, isoprenoid quinones (which are a special class of cell membrane lipids), cytochromes, and bacterial enzymes. In addition, the pattern of soluble proteins extracted from bacterial cells can be ''fingerprinted'' by the use of two-dimensional electrophoresis.

Serotaxonomy involves the use of antigen-antibody reactions for bacterial classification. Special serodiagnostic reagents are developed to detect the presence of particular antigens. A group of bacterial strains can then be distinguished based on the presence of these antigens. For example, the causative microorganism of dental caries, *Streptococcus mutans*, has been divided into a number of serologic groups, or serogroups.

REFERENCES

Johnson, J. L.: Use of nucleic acid homologies in the taxonomy of anaerobic bacteria. Int. J. Syst. Bacteriol. 28:308, 1973.

Skerman, V. B. D., McGowan, V., and Sneath, P. H. A. (eds.): Approved lists of bacterial names. Int. J. Syst. Bacteriol. 30:225, 1980.

Sneath, P. H. A.: Classification of microorganisms. *In* Norris, J. R., and Richmond, M.H. (eds.): Essays in Microbiology. John Wiley, Chichester, UK, 1978.

Willcox, W. R., Lapage, S. P., and Holmes, B.: A review of numerical methods in bacterial identification. Antonie van Leeuwenhoek Journal of Microbiology and Serology 46:233, 1980.

section II

General bacteriology

chapter 5

Normal microbial flora of the human body

William F. Liljemark, D.D.S., Ph.D. □ Cynthia G. Bloomquist, B.A.

CHAPTER OUTLINE

- THE NORMAL ORAL FLORA: IS IT COMPULSORY?
- THE NORMAL FLORA OF THE HUMAN ORGANISM
- CONCEPTS AND TERMS FOR THE STUDY OF NORMAL MICROBIAL FLORA
- THE NORMAL FLORA'S SIGNIFICANCE IN THE HUMAN HOST
- THE NORMAL MICROBIAL FLORA OF THE BODY BY ANATOMIC REGION

The Normal Oral Flora: Is It Compulsory?

Pasteur hypothesized that the normal bacterial flora was essential to life. This has been disproved by the living experiment that occurs when animals are aseptically delivered from their mothers and raised in a sterile environment with sterilized water and food. These *germ-free* animals have been extensively studied in contrast to their conventional counterparts. Their anatomic development differs in that they have an enormously enlarged cecum, greatly diminished peristalsis, a thinner alimentary lamina propria, shallower crypts of Lieberkuhn, a more regular epithelium, and shorter-lived enterocytes. Further, the intestinal epithelium renewal rate is half that of conventional animals. The immune system of the germ-free animal is also markedly underdeveloped. The reticuloendothelial system, lymph nodes, and immunoglobulin levels are greatly decreased. Germ-free animals have a weak, delayed hypersensitivity, which probably results from a lack of stimulation of their immune systems. Germ-free animals live almost twice as long as conventional animals, and they eventually die of intestinal atonia, whereas conventional animals frequently die of infections.

Thus, although the indigenous flora is not essential for life and, indeed, may even shorten it, the normal flora profoundly affects the host in many ways.

The Normal Flora of the Human Organism

Human beings have diverse microbial flora associated with their skin and mucous membranes from shortly after birth until death.

The normal adult is composed of over 10^{14} cells, of which about 10 percent or (10^{13}) are human cells. The various body surfaces and the gastrointestinal tract of humans contain about 10^{14} prokaryotic and eukaryotic microbial cells, including one arthropod, numerous protozoans, several dozen fungi, and over 700 distinct species of bacteria. These high cell numbers are due to the great density of microbes found on or in the various body surfaces (Table 5–1). There are from 10^3 cells per cm^2 of skin to greater than 10^{11} cells per gram of dental plaque or feces. Considering that a gram of water occupies 10^{12} cubic microns, that same gram could contain, at most, 10^{12} bacteria, supposing the organisms were 1 micron in diameter. In reality, for example, packed cells of streptococci contain about 2.3×10^{11} cells per gram.

Concepts and Terms for the Study of Normal Microbial Flora

The fields of medical microbiology, microbial ecology, and epidemiology have evolved as separate disciplines. Because of this, many synonyms are used to describe the normal flora.

The term "normal flora" collectively describes the various microbial types frequently found by culture or microscopy on the skin or mucous membranes, and in certain body cavities in normal, healthy individuals. The species and numbers of the flora vary in different areas of the body, and sometimes at different ages. Normal flora is used as a synonym for *indigenous microflora* and *endogenous flora*. Indigenous species are *amphibiotic* in humans and are defined as (1) frequently encountered in one or more typical human anatomic regions, (2) found at least as often in the absence of disease as in its presence, and (3) having as their primary habitat the human species.

The term "amphibiotic" also describes the relationship between two organisms. Thus the amphibiont, in relation to its host, can be assigned a space between *symbiosis* (that is, the living together of two dissimilar organisms, with both organisms benefiting, which is not the case for the normal flora and the human host) and pathogenicity (see definition further on). The typical amphibiont that constitutes the normal flora is obligately parasitic (nonsaprophytic) and not overtly, actively, or obligately pathogenic in

a particular host. The amphibionts that compose the normal flora would, when disturbed, promptly re-establish themselves in a stable ecosystem.

Some members of the normal flora are found at a low frequency in the human population and are not pathogenic for their particular host, but are potentially pathogenic for other members of the population. These hosts are commonly called *carriers*. The *pathogenicity* of any microorganism denotes the ability to cause disease. *Virulence* introduces the concept of degree—that is, virulent organisms exhibit pathogenicity when introduced into the host in very small numbers. It is frequently measured by the number of microorganisms necessary to kill 50 per cent of a given host and is termed the **LD**$_{50}$ (*median lethal dose*). Different strains of a bacterial species vary in their ability to cause disease. For example, type 3 *Streptococcus pneumoniae* strains are more virulent than other polysaccharide types. Similarly, one strain of *Salmonella typhimurium* may have an LD$_{50}$ for mice of 100 cells, and another strain an LD$_{50}$ of 1000 cells. The median lethal dose is bacterial strain–specific, as well as the host animal species–specific. The virulence of members of the normal flora is usually low in an uncompromised host.

Infection refers to the presence and multiplication of a microorganism in body tissues. *Infectious disease* is the clinical expression of an infection that disrupts the host while producing a characteristic group of symptoms. Infections caused by the normal flora are sometimes called *endogenous infections*. Specifically, these occur from traumatic disruptions to skin or mucous membrane by outside forces (broken bones, cuts, burns, bullets, and so forth) or by health personnel (e.g., nasogastric and endotracheal tubes, IVs, catheters, scalpels). Endogenous infections usually result when an indigenous microbe is thrust into an unusual anatomic region (e.g., a human bite). Infections caused by endogenous microbes, called *opportunistic infections*, also occur at a microbe's usual anatomic habitat following a disease or other predisposing factor (such as debilitating chronic conditions such as diabetes mellitus or alcoholism, stomach ulcers, colon and other invasive cancers, antibiotics, immune and nutritional deficiencies, stresses), which compromise the host. Both endogenous and opportunistic infections can be *iatrogenic* or "healer induced." When infections arise in a hospital they are called *nosocomial* or "hospital acquired."

Table 5–1 ■ Distribution of flora in the healthy human body

Body Site	Flora	Number of Organisms
Blood	Sterile, occasional transient low-level bacteremia from trauma	—
Cerebrospinal fluid, tissues, uterus and fallopian tubes, middle ear, paranasal sinuses	Sterile	—
Skin, external ear	*Staphylococcus epidermidis*, *Corynebacterium* sp., *Propionibacterium acnes*, *Lactobacillus* sp., *Micrococcus* sp., fungi	$10^3–10^4/cm^2$ (10^6 axilla and groin)
Conjunctiva	*Staphylococcus epidermidis*, *Corynebacterium* and *Propionibacterium* sp.	Few (17–46% sterile)
Nose and nasopharynx	*Staphylococcus epidermidis*, *Corynebacterium* sp., *Staphylococcus aureus*, *Propionibacterium acnes* (nares), *Hemophilus parainfluenzae*	$10^5/ml$
Oropharynx	Alpha and nonhemolytic *Streptococcus* sp., *Neisseria* and *Branhamella* sp., enterococci, *Corynebacterium* sp., *Bacteroides* and *Fusobacterium* sp., *Staphylococcus* sp.	$10^7/ml$
Oral cavity	See Chapter 25	$10^8/ml$ saliva and $10^{11}/g$ plaque
Esophagus	Transient oral flora	—
Stomach	Transient oral flora and organisms from food	$0–10^3/ml$ normal fasting individual, dependent on pH
Small intestine		$0–10^4/ml$
upper	*Streptococcus* sp., *Lactobacillus* sp., *Staphylococcus* sp., yeasts	
distal	*Bacteriodes* sp., coliforms, enterococci, *Streptococcus* sp.	~ $10^4/ml$
Colon		
Breastfed infant	*Bifidobacterium* sp., *Lactobacillus* sp., enterococci	?
After weaning	*Bacteroides* sp., *Bifidobacterium* sp., *Eubacterium* sp., *Lactobacillus* sp., *Peptostreptococcus* sp., *Ruminococcus* sp., *Streptococcus* sp., coliforms	$10^{11}/g$ feces
Kidneys and urinary bladder	Usually sterile except for anterior urethra	—
Anterior urethra	*Staphylococcus epidermidis*, *Corynebacterium* sp., *Streptococcus faecalis*	—
Urine, midstream	Same as anterior urethra	$0–10^3/ml$
Vagina		
prepubertal and postmenopausal	Skin and colonic species	?
childbearing years	*Peptococcus* sp., anaerobic and facultative *Lactobacillus* sp., *Staphylococcus epidermidis*, *Neisseria* sp., *Bacteroides* sp.	$10^9/g$ secretions

Many of today's serious nosocomial infections are caused by *Escherichia coli*, *Klebsiella pneumoniae*, *Staphylococcus aureus*, and *Proteus mirabilis*. These organisms are frequently members of the normal human flora. Inasmuch as these bacteria are not considered to be highly virulent in their usual habitat in a human, they are considered "nonpathogens." However, when the health of a host is compromised, or a microbe is inserted into a new environment, a relatively less virulent "nonpathogen" may quickly become a pathogen.

Prevalence describes the percent of a particular site of the population sampled that contains a certain organism, at a certain time or age. For example, approximately 40 percent of the anterior nares of adults contain *S. aureus*. A synonym is *frequency*, as it also refers to a percent at a given time. These terms should *not* be confused with *incidence*, which refers to the rate at which a certain event occurs, as in the number of new cases of a specific disease occurring during a certain period.

The Normal Flora's Significance to the Human Host

Knowledge of the specific habitats and diverse roles of the normal flora is necessary for the dentist. The normal flora serves both as a defense mechanism against infection from exogenous microbes and as a source of potentially virulent organisms. The study of the normal flora is important for a number of reasons:

1. In countries with active public health programs, infections are more often a result of indigenous bacteria rather than of exogenous pathogenic microorganisms. For example, one in 20 people admitted to hospitals develops a nosocomial infection. In 1984, 40 percent of such infections were urinary tract infections, usually caused by indigenous bacteria introduced through catheterization. This represents 600,000 infections per year in the United States. Similarly, *Candida albicans* is a normal, albeit not ubiquitous, microbial member of the mouth, pharynx, small intestine, and colon. An opportunistic infection by *C. albicans* in the oral cavity or vagina (thrush or candidiasis) is often seen in conjunction with broad-spectrum antimicrobial therapy; overgrowth can also occur in the colon in conjunction with neomycin therapy, which causes a diarrhea consisting of almost a pure growth of *C. albicans*.

2. The normal microbial flora may provide protection from similar but more pathogenic species. For example, bacteriocidal antibodies to *Neisseria meningitidis*, a common causative agent of spinal meningitis, have been found in children colonized with a normal resident, *N. lactamicus*. These provide at least partial protection against all capsular types of *N. meningitidis*.

This example suggests the significant contribution made by the indigenous microflora to the general immunity of the host. It is apparent, teleologically, that many of the indigenous microbes are closely related to their more virulent relatives and often possess common antigens. Humans have frequent transient bacteremias from chewing and from breaks in the skin and mucous membranes. We have thus acquired low-level circulating antibody titers against most of our indigenous flora which may cross-react, thus elevating the host's immunity to exogenous pathogens.

3. The normal microflora provides a barrier to *colonization* (see definition later) by exogenous bacteria via the spatial inhibition of potential adhesion sites, by physiologic competition for limited nutrients, or by inhibitory substances produced by the normal species. A widely studied bovine and porcine example is the exquisite sensitivity of newborn calves or piglets to colonization by the piliated enterotoxigenic strains of *Escherichia coli*, which causes a potentially fatal diarrhea. This susceptibility to enteropathic *E. coli* decreases sharply with age, and disappears 4 to 6 days after birth, as the intestinal epithelia of these animals are then sufficiently colonized with bacteria. This protection is termed *bacterial interference*.

Alternately, in certain cases, the indigenous microflora actually assists exogenous pathogens. A prime example is that of *Entamoeba histolytica*, the causative agent of amebic dysentery, which colonizes a germ-free animal, but will not cause disease unless the animal is subsequently conventionalized with one or more of the normal gastrointestinal microorganisms.

4. Lastly, the normal flora has been suggested to have an effect on the nutrition of the host. It is well established in rodents, via coprophagy, that quantities of vitamins are absorbed from the feces. The dependence of the microbial intestinal flora to aid digestion in ruminants is also essential. Similarly the production of vitamin B_{12} by certain intestinal bacteria has been suggested as a nutritional source for humans. However, the human colon has little absorptive capacity, and any significant contribution to host nutrition or aid in digestion is unlikely.

FACTORS INFLUENCING THE COMPOSITION OF NORMAL FLORA

Acquisition of the Normal Flora

The healthy term neonate has a fairly gentle introduction to the microbial world. Cultures of the nose, nasopharynx, oropharynx, umbilicus, rectum, and feces are often negative on the first day of life. The skin is colonized during vaginal births and contains a sparse population of cocci and corynebacteria. The nasopharynx of the newborn is sterile, but within 2 or 3 days the infant acquires the normal flora of the mother or caretaker. The newborn's mouth is sometimes sterile or contains the same organisms as the mother's vagina. These organisms diminish in number, and a few days after birth are replaced largely by the caretaker's flora. Within 4 to 12 hours after birth, alpha and nonhemolytic streptococci become established as the prominent members of the mucous membranes of the mouth and oropharynx, and remain so for life.

The gastrointestinal tract of the newborn is usually sterile. Under normal conditions, intestinal flora are established during the first 24 hours. The stool of the breastfed infant is soft, light yellow-brown, with a faint, acidic odor. *Lactobacillus bifidus* is prominent, as are enterococci, coliforms, and streptococci. In contrast, artificially fed infants have hard, dark, foul-smelling stools that contain *Lactobacillus acidophilus,* coliforms, enterococci, and anaerobic species. *L. bifidus* may again predominate following the addition of 12 percent lactose to formula. Remarkably, by 5 to 7 days, the intestinal flora of the formula-fed infant contains the same complexity of anaerobes as the adult.

The vulva of the newborn is also sterile. After 24 hours it gradually acquires a rich and varied flora of corynebacteria, micrococci, and nonhemolytic streptococci. Two or 3 days after birth, estrogen from the maternal circulation induces the deposition of glycogen in the vaginal epithelium, which facilitates the growth of lactobacilli. These organisms produce acid from glycogen, and a flora like that of the adult female develops. After the passively transferred estrogen is gone, the glycogen, lactobacilli, and acid disappear, and the pH again becomes alkaline. At puberty the glycogen again appears and an adult flora with lactobacilli reappears.

SPECIFICITY OF MICROBIAL ADHERENCE MECHANISMS AND FACTORS AFFECTING COLONIZATION

In vitro and *in vivo* studies of the interactions between bacteria and the human host have led to an understanding of the role of colonization in the ecologic development and maintenance of a characteristic flora. The relative ability to adhere (**avidity**) of a number of bacterial species and their natural distribution despite the moving streams that bathe the different epithelial surfaces have been found to correlate positively with their in vitro adherence to different epithelial cell lines. An example of this tissue tropism is the difference between the adherence of *Streptococcus pyogenes* (group A streptococci) and *Escherichia coli.* Both of these bacteria adhere avidly to human epithelial cells; however, *S. pyogenes* is virtually limited to the pharynges and skin epithelial cells, whereas *E. coli* are rarely found at these sites but adheres avidly to periurethral epithelial cells.

Bacterial adherence is thus remarkably cell- and surface-specific, which appears to be mediated by the attraction of species-specific microbial *adhesins* (some of which are *lectins*) to complementary host cell–specific receptors. The bacterial adhesins are sometimes, but not always, found on the surface appendages of bacteria, termed *pili* in gram-negative species and *fimbrae* in gram-positive species (see Chapter 3). Clearly, the extent to which an organism can attach to a particular surface will influence the extent to which it can colonize. Adherence is not the only prerequisite for colonization. The ability to survive the local environmental conditions (that is, the amount of oxygen, pH, nutritional sources, bacterial antagonists and symbionts, the unidirectional flow of fluids over epithelial surfaces, mucociliary clearing systems, epithelial cell turnover, local immune systems, and nonspecific host antimicrobial agents) is necessary for colonization. Obviously, the ability to grow under these environmental conditions is also essential.

The Normal Microbial Flora of the Body by Anatomic Region

SKIN

The composition of the skin's microbial flora (Table 5–2) varies according to age and the environment due to different levels of moisture, body temperature, and concentration of skin surface lipids. For example, the perineum and toe webs are higher in moisture and are more frequently colonized by gram-negative bacilli than are drier areas of skin.

Staphylococcus epidermidis (biotype I) constitutes a major proportion of the flora, constituting more than 90 percent of the resident flora in some areas. *S. epidermidis* frequently causes an endogenous infection following the insertion of a ventriculoatrial shunt in the treatment of hydrocephalus. *S. aureus* is found on the skin of the arms and trunk of

Table 5–2 ■ Cultivable microflora of the human skin

Species	Prevalence
Staphylococcus epidermidis	85–100
Staphylococcus aureus	5–25
Propionibacterium acnes	100
Corynebacterium sp.	55
Lactobacillus sp.	55
Micrococcus luteus	20–40
Acinetobacter calcoaceticus	20–30
Fungi* (especially lipophilic yeasts but not C. albicans)	40–80
Candida parapsilosis	1–15
Pityosporum sp.*	Common
Dermatophytic fungi† (Epidermophyton floccosum, Microsporum sp., Trichophyton sp.)	Common

*Especially in areas rich in sebaceous glands.
†Found on nonliving surfaces (hair, nails, keratinized skin).

5 to 25 percent of the population and reflects the density of colonization in the nose. The perianal skin is more frequently colonized and can be considered the major habitat of this species. The nonlipophilic Corynebacterium species are frequently found on glabrous skin, while Propionibacterium acnes is ubiquitous and more common in areas rich in sebaceous glands, such as the axilla and face. Consequently, children younger than age 10 are rarely colonized with P. acnes, due to the lack of sebum secretion before puberty. Gram-negative bacteria are usually found only in the moist intertrigenous areas and include Acinetobacter species and occasionally others such as Klebsiella pneumoniae (as well as enterococci, E. coli, and Proteus species). Two lipophilic yeasts, Pityosporum ovale and P. obiculare, are present on the scalp or chest and back. Nonlipophilic yeasts, such as Torulopsis glabrata, are variably present. Candida albicans is not considered a normal resident of the skin. Other fungi and yeasts are sometimes present in skin folds. Dermatophytic fungi, which only grow on nonliving body structures (hair, keratinized skin, and nails), are often found. Demodex folliculorum, or the follicle mite, resides in and around the eyelashes and the hair follicles of the outer nose folds and chin.

Although the skin is constantly contaminated with organisms from exogenous and endogenous sources, it normally supports the growth of only three major types of bacteria. This is remarkably apparent, especially in the perianal area, which is in regular contact with the concentrated and varied fecal flora, but which, within an hour or so

of defecation, retains only the resident staphylococci and corynebacteria. The external skin is highly acidic and dry and is constantly shedding, making it unfavorable for colonization by exogenous species. The metabolic activity of the normal gram-positive flora also contributes to the stable ecosystem of the skin by breaking down the complex lipids in sebum, produced by the sebaceous glands, producing a fatty acid coating that inhibits the growth of many pathogenic bacteria and fungi. Further, sweat glands secrete lysozyme, which interferes with cell wall synthesis and keeps the numbers of the resident gram-positive species in check.

The microbial flora of the external ear is similar to the flora on skin rich in sebaceous glands. S. epidermidis and Propionibacterium species predominate. Acid-fast nonpathogenic Mycobacterium species are also found.

CONJUNCTIVA (EYE)

The flora of the conjunctival sac is sparse (Table 5–3). Approximately 17 to 49 percent of culture samples are negative. The predominant microorganisms are Corynebacterium species, Propionibacterium species, and S. epidermidis. These species presumably arise from the skin-like flora of the eyelids. A gram-negative species resembling hemophilus, called Moraxella, is also found here. Conjunctival flora is held in check by the mechanical flow of tears, the presence of the antibacterial enzyme lysozyme, and the production of other inhibitors by the normal eye flora (see subsequent section on the oropharynx).

NOSE AND NASOPHARYNX

The anterior nares have a flora somewhat similar to that of the skin (Table 5–4). The

Table 5–3 ■ Cultivable microflora of the conjunctiva

Species	Prevalence (%)
Staphylococcus epidermidis	32–68
Staphylococcus aureus	6–28
Corynebacterium and Propionibacterium sp.	27–58
Moraxella sp.	Frequent
Hemophilus parainfluenzae	25
Fungi (often airborne Aspergillus sp)	6–24
Pseudomonas aeruginosa	1–7

Table 5–4 ■ Cultivable microflora of the nose and nasopharynx	
Species	**Prevalence**
Staphylococcus epidermidis*	90
Staphylococcus aureus*	30–40
Corynebacterium sp.	55
Propionibacterium acnes*	30–40
Hemophilus parainfluenzae	35–65
Hemophilus influenzae	12
Branhamella catarrhalis	12
Streptococcus pneumoniae	0–17
Streptococcus pyogenes (Group A)	1–5
Alpha hemolytic or nonhemolytic streptococci	Uncommon
Moraxella nonliquefaciens	5–10
Neisseria meningitidis	0–10

*Especially anterior nares.

posterior nares, nasopharynx, and sinuses are more difficult to culture, and studies of the flora in these areas are limited. In health the sinuses are considered to be sterile. The anterior nares and nasopharynx share many similar species with the oropharynx, but there are notable exceptions. Especially apparent is the presence of staphylococci, and the absence of alpha or nonhemolytic streptococci, in the nose and nasopharynx. The opposite occurs in the oropharynx. The anterior nares are especially associated with staphylococci; either *S. epidermidis* or *S. aureus* predominate. *Corynebacterium* species, *Propionibacterium* species, and *H. parainfluenzae* are also frequently found in the nose and nasopharynx. *Streptococcus pneumoniae, H. influenzae, C. diphtheriae* and *Bordetella pertussis* are also found in some individuals.

Some species of the normal nasal flora are not ubiquitous but are commonly found in a small fixed percentage of the healthy population. These "carriers" provide a reservoir of potentially virulent species for other members of the population, especially those in a compromised state. Although the perineum could be considered its major residence, *S. aureus* is estimated to be found in 20 to 85 percent of the anterior nares in a healthy population, with a figure of 30 to 40 percent probably being most accurate, half being permanent carriers and half transient carriers of several weeks or less. Although the nose and nasopharynx flora is the most probable source of the microbes associated with sinusitis and otitis media, a diagnosis based on its flora correlates poorly with these diseases and does not aid diagnosis. The adult nasopharyngeal carrier is also important in the transmission of spinal meningitidis by *Neisseria meningitidis* and provides a reservoir for

infection of individuals living in close quarters. An interepidemic carriage rate of 5 to 30 percent can be compared with meningococcal disease in military populations, which is associated with carriage rates as high as 90 percent.

OROPHARYNX

The most important group of microorganisms native to the oropharyx, uniquely different than the nasopharynx, is the predominant alpha and nonhemolytic streptococci (Table 5–5). Often erroneously called "viridans streptococci," this group contains a wide variety of species with unique colonization patterns. These species are frequent members of the oral cavity (see Chapter 25). It is more than possible that the species present on the buccal mucosa are also present on the oropharyngeal mucosa, especially those species shed from the various oral surfaces present in high numbers in saliva. However, the oropharyngeal flora is not identical to the salivary flora. For example,

Table 5–5 ■ Cultivable microflora of the oropharynx	
Species	**Prevalence**
Alpha and nonhemolytic Streptococcus, sp.	93–99
S. salivarius	50–75
S. sanguis	25–75
S. mitis	25–75
S. milleri	25–75
S. mutans	25–75
Streptococcus sp. (Group D)	90–100
Streptococcus pneumoniae	1–50
Streptococcus pyogenes (group A)	1–6
Neisseria sp. and Branhamella catarrhalis	81–97
Neisseria meningitidis	5–15
Corynebacterium sp.	15–90
Propionibacterium acnes	11–12
Staphylococcus epidermidis	3–70
Staphylococcus aureus	35–40
Hemophilus parainfluenzae	20–35
Hemophilus influenzae	5–20
Lactobacillus sp.	1–37
Bacteroides sp.	Common
Fusobacterium necrophorum	Common
Anaerobic Micrococcus sp.	11–12
Acinetobacter calcoaceticus	5–30
Peptostreptococcus sp.	10
Klebsiella pneumoniae	5
Pseudomonas aeruginosa	5
Candida albicans	3–6
Actinomyces sp.	Common
Mycoplasma sp.	Common

S. mutans has been suggested to be a member of the normal oropharyngeal flora. It is not known to adhere with any degree of avidity to epithelial cells; rather, it colonizes the hard surfaces of teeth. Consequently, *S. mutans* may be just a transitory member of the salivary flora, not a resident of the oropharynx.

Other than the predominant alpha and nonhaemolytic streptococci, *Neisseria* species and *Branhamella catarrhalis*, are frequently found. *B. catarrhalis* is an occasional serious causative agent of pneumonia, suppurative sinusitis, and otitis media. *Corynebacterium* species, *Propionibacterium* species, *Hemophilus parainfluenzae*, and *H. influenzae* are also present, as are staphylococci, lactobacilli, *Acinetobacter* species, *Mycoplasma* species and spirochetes.

The oropharynx also contains a number of anaerobes, but studies of the anaerobic species have been limited. *Bacteroides* species, *Fusobacterium necrophorum*, and certain anaerobic cocci have been cited. Similar to the nasopharynx, the oropharynx is also the site of carriage of a number of potentially virulent organisms, such as the only pathogenic member of the corynebacteria, *C. diphtheriae*. Although asymptomatic carriage of this microbe is not found in an adequately immunized population, depressed urban areas and the native population of Alaska constitute a current reservoir of this disease. In tropical areas, the skin is also a reservoir. Other potential pathogens carried in the normal oropharyngeal flora are *Klebsiella pneumoniae, Pseudomonas aeruginosa, Streptococcus pneumoniae, N. meningitidis,* and *Proteus mirabilis.*

One of the best examples of the normal flora's positive role in host defense can be seen in seriously ill patients. There is a markedly increased susceptibility of the respiratory tract of seriously ill patients to colonization by gram-negative bacilli. Gram-negative colonization has been positively correlated with the loss of fibronectin, a high molecular weight protein, present on the surface of normal oropharyngeal epithelial cells. Fibronectin is thought to promote the attachment of the indigenous gram-positive species, which normally interfere with the attachment of gram-negative bacterial pathogens such as *Pseudomonas aeruginosa.* The sequelae following the eradication of the predominant streptococci with high doses of penicillin can cause a similar gram-negative overgrowth.

The healthy climax community of the oropharynx is maintained by several species.

Alpha hemolytic streptococci and nonpathogenic *Neisseria* species (and *S. epidermidis*, found most often in the nose) are known to inhibit the colonization of *S. aureus, N. meningitidis,* and *Streptococcus pyogenes* (group A streptococci). Children with high numbers of alpha-hemolytic streptococci are not colonized following exposure to Group A streptococci. Further, strains of *S. salivarius* and *S. mitis* have been shown to produce a cell-free filtrate called enocin capable of inhibiting *S. pyogenes* by interference with pantothenate utilization.

GASTROINTESTINAL TRACT

The intraluminal environment of the stomach is usually sterile. Studies have shown low counts of alpha-hemolytic streptococci, anaerobic cocci, lactobacilli, *S. epidermidis,* and *Candida albicans* that tend toward zero several hours after meals. These are transitory species from saliva and ingested materials. Gastric pH is the major factor controlling microbial growth in the stomach.

The flora of the small intestine is highly dependent on the location of sampling. The upper small intestine is usually sterile or has similar species and counts as the stomach. Coliforms and *Bacteroides* species are rarely present. The lower small intestine contains a flora that closely approximates the colon but with much lower counts (10^5 versus 10^{11}). The nature of the streptococci change from primarily alpha-hemolytic in the upper small intestine to enterococci (or group D streptococci) in the lower small intestine. The lower intestine also has some coliforms and the beginning of an anaerobic flora.

The normal colonic microbial flora is the same as the feces because of the difficulties associated with sampling the intestinal epithelium. Microbial counts in the transverse colon are two to three logarithmic values lower than fecal samples. The "holding" function of the colon allows certain organisms to multiply. Although there are substantial quantitative differences at various locations of the colon versus fecal flora, there are no marked qualitative differences in the major groups of bacteria.

Bacteroides thetaiotaomicron is the most prevalent and numerically predominant fecal species (Table 5–6). Other *Bacteroides* species are common, especially *B. vulgatus, B. distonis,* and *B. fragilis* (these species were formerly classified as subspecies of *B. fragilis*). *Eubac-*

Table 5–6 ■ Cultivable microflora of the colon (feces)	
Species	Prevalence
Bacteroides sp.*	99
B. thetaiotaomicron	87
B. vulgatus	70
B. distasonis	53
B. fragilis	49
Eubacterium sp.*	94
E. aerofaciens	49
E. lentum	43
Bifidobacterium sp.*	74
B. adolescentis	55
Lactobacillus sp*	78
L. acidophilus	45
Peptostreptococcus sp.*	45
P. productus	30
Ruminococcus sp.*	45
Anaerobic Streptococcus sp.*	34
S. intermedius	28
Facultative Streptococcus sp.	99
S. faecalis	80
S. faecium group	31
S. mitis	31
S. lactis	28
S. bovis	18
Escherichia coli	93
Fusobacterium sp.*	18
Bacillus sp.*	82
Clostridium sp.*	100
Propionibacterium acnes	9
Actinomyces naeslundii	6
Veillonella sp.	34
Klebsiella pneumoniae	20
Staphylococcus epidermidis	31
Staphylococcus aureus	11
Pseudomonas aeruginosa	11
Candida albicans	14
Other yeasts	36
Spirochetes	Common
Various protozoa	?
Mycoplasma sp.	Common

*Numerous other species in the genera occur as well.

terium species and anaerobic cocci are found in high numbers (*Peptostreptococcus* species, *Veillonella* species, *Acidaminococcus* species, and anaerobic streptococci, especially *Streptococcus intermedius*). *Lactobacillus* species, especially *L. acidophilus,* are also prevalent. The facultative streptococci, *Bacillus* species, and *Clostridium* species are prevalent, and probably represent species arising from oral secretions and ingested materials, respectively. More than 450 bacterial species are found, including those associated with the skin (staphylococci) and pharynges (gram-negative species). Some fungi and yeasts, such as *Candida albicans,* also occur. Various protozoa, *Mycoplasma* species and spirochetes, are often found. Spirochetes, fusiform bacilli, and cocci have been seen attached to the epithelial surfaces of the colon when examined by electron microscopy.

GENITOURINARY TRACT

Secretions around the female urethra and uncircumsized male contain a flora similar to that of the skin, as well as *Mycobacterium smegmatis,* a harmless microbe sometimes confused with *Mycobacterium tuberculosis.* The skin flora frequently present in the distal urethra of both sexes contains *Corynebacterium* species, nonhemolytic streptococci, and *S. epidermis,* as well as *Streptococcus faecalis.* The internal urethra, bladder, urine, and kidneys are usually sterile.

The adult female genitourinary tract has a microbial flora constantly changing with the variation of the menstrual cycle. Although complex, fewer species are present than in the oral or colonic flora. The major aerobic and facultative strains are *Streptococcus epidermidis,* staphylococci, lactobacilli, and corynebacteria. Lactobacilli, combining both facultative and aerobic species, are the species most commonly associated with vaginal flora, and constitute a large portion of the bacteria present (Table 5–7). They are so named because they produce lactic acid and help maintain the pH of the vagina and external cervical os at approximately 4.4 to 4.6.

Anaerobic bacteria predominate over aerobic bacteria 10-fold. Peptococci are the most frequently found and are numerically predominant. Peptostreptococci, anaerobic lactobacilli, eubacteria, anaerobic gram-negative bacteria, *Mycoplasma* species and spirochetes

Table 5–7 ■ Cultivable microflora of the vagina	
Species	Prevalence
Peptococcus sp.	64
Anaerobic Lactobacillus sp., L. fermentum	45
Facultative Lactobacillus sp.	50
Staphylococcus epidermidis	28–94
Staphylococcus aureus	5–15
Branhamella catarrhalis and Neisseria sp.	60–80
Bacteroides sp.	60–80
Corynebacterium sp.	38–76
Peptostreptococcus sp.	30–40
Eubacterium sp.	5–23
Enterobacteriaceae sp.	18–40
Candida albicans	30–50
Streptococcus sp.	
Alpha hemolytic	14
Group B (S. agalactiae)	20–40
Enterococci (group D)	30–80
Nonhemolytic (not B or D)	36
Torulopsis glabrata	Common
Escherichia coli	9–27
Trichomonas vaginalis	10–25
Mycoplasma sp.	Common

are also found. *Staphylococcus aureus* has been found in 15 percent of healthy women, and is correlated positively with nasal carriage. Further, 60 percent of the women with vaginal *S. aureus* also had nasal *S. auresus*, versus 23 percent of women without vaginal *S. aureus*.

REFERENCES

Beachey, E. H.: Bacterial adherence: Adhesin-receptor interactions mediating the attachment of bacteria to mucosal surfaces. J. Infect. Dis. 143:325, 1981.

Gibbons, R. J.: Adherence of bacteria to host tissue. In Schlessinger, D. (ed.): Microbiology 1977. American Society for Microbiology, Washington, DC, p. 395, 1977.

Goldmann, D. A., Leclair, J., and Macone, A.: Bacterial colonization of neonates admitted to an intensive care environment. J Pediatrics 93:288, 1978.

Hentges, D. J.: *Human Intestinal Microflora in Health and Disease*. Academic Press, New York, 1983.

Johnston, D. A., and Bodey, G. P.: Semiquantitative oropharyngeal culture technique. Appl. Microbiol 20:218, 1970.

Mackowiak, P. A.: The normal microbial flora. N. Eng. J. Med. 307:83, 1982.

Marples, M. J.: Life on the human skin. Sci. Am. 220:108, 1969.

Martin, R. R., Buttram, V., Besch, P., Kirkland, J. J., and Petty, G. P.: Nasal and vaginal *Staphylococcus aureus* in young women: Quantitative studies. Ann. Int. Med. 96:951, 1982.

Onderdonk, A. B., Zamardhi, G. R., Walsh, J. A., Mellor, R. D., Munoz, A., and Kass, E. H.: Methods for quantitative and qualitative evaluation of vaginal microflora during menstruation. Appl. Environ. Microbiol. 51:333, 1986.

Rosebury, T.: Microorganisms Indigenous to Man. McGraw-Hill, New York, 1962.

Savage, D. C.: Microbial ecology of the gastrointestinal tract. Ann. Rev. Microbiol. 31:1781, 1977.

Savage, D. C., and Fletcher, M. (eds.): Bacterial Adhesion: Mechanisms and Physiological Significance. Plenum Press, New York, 1985.

Woods, D. E., Straus, D. C., Johanson, W. G., and Bass, J. A.: Role of fibronectin in the prevention of adherence of *Pseudomonas aeruginosa* to buccal cells. J. Infect. Dis. 143:784, 1981.

chapter 6

The streptococci

Burton Rosan, D.D.S., M.Sc.

The Pyogenic Streptococci (Streptococcus pyogenes, the "Lancefield Group Streptococci")

The streptococci are gram-positive coccal bacteria that divide in one plane. Since they do not separate easily after division, they tend to form small or long chains and thus can be distinguished from staphylococci which usually divide in different planes leading to bunches, or grape-like clusters, of cocci (Fig. 6–1). The streptococci also differ from the staphylococci because they are catalase negative, whereas all the staphylococci are catalase positive. The streptococci constitute a major population in the oral cavity. Several different species are found associated with the different ecologic niches in the mouth. Thus, *Streptococcus sanguis* and *S. mutans* are found in dental plaque, whereas *S. salivarius* is found primarily on the tongue and *S. mitis* on other mucosal tissues. It is also clear that these species are associated with different diseases (e.g., *S. mutans* causes dental caries, whereas *S. sanguis* is frequently involved in subacute bacterial endocarditis). Therefore,

an understanding of the taxonomy of these bacteria provides information about the factors involved in the virulence of these organisms. This is not an easy task because taxonomic schemes were developed long before bacterial genetics was understood, at a time when the relationship between structure and function among bacteria was generally based on speculation rather than fact. Much of the knowledge of these relationships in streptococci stems from studies of *S. pyogenes*, an organism involved in systemic diseases (e.g., streptococcal pharyngitis, scarlet fever, rheumatic fever, and various types of skin infections). Since patients with a history of rheumatic fever often pose special problems in dental therapy, it is important to study the pyogenic cocci as an etiologic agent in these diseases and to establish the appropriate background for the study of the oral streptococci.

HEMOLYSIS AND THE STREPTOCOCCI

Blood and blood products have been used as a constituent of bacterial media from the earliest days of bacteriology when it was

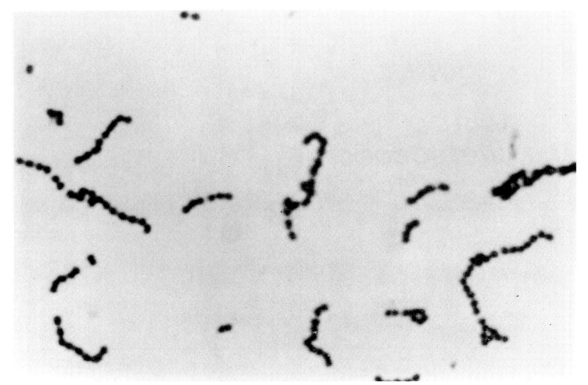

Figure 6–1 ■ Gram stain of group A streptococci. (From Schneierson, S. S.: Atlas of Diagnostic Microbiology. North Chicago, IL, Abbot Laboratories, 1965, with permission.)

observed that the streptococci isolated from purulent throat and skin infections often caused complete lysis of red blood cells ("*hemo*-lysis"). This was easily recognized in a blood agar medium as a zone of complete clearing around the colonies. Other streptococci also found in the oropharynx that did not appear associated with local disease caused a type of "incomplete lysis," in which the red blood cells shrink and take on a greenish tinge. The latter phenomenon occurs only in the presence of oxygen and is due to the reduction of hemoglobin. This incomplete hemolysis was called alpha hemolysis (α-hemolysis) and the streptococci that produced it were designated *Streptococcus viridans*, whereas the complete lysis of the red blood cells was called beta hemolysis (β-hemolysis) and the organisms causing it were called *Streptococcus hemolyticus*. We now know that both names are misnomers and that there are many species that cause α hemolysis, many others that cause β hemolysis, and some species that produce both types of hemolysis, depending on strain and growth conditions. There are also many streptococci that are anhemolytic; the latter are often referred to as the gamma (γ) streptococci. The story of the hemolysis and the

α-streptococci will unfold in discussing the oral streptococci but for the moment let us concentrate on unraveling the tale of the β hemolytic streptococci and the diseases associated with these organisms.

THE LANCEFIELD SEROLOGIC GROUPING SCHEME

It soon became clear that the simple definition of hemolysis was not sufficient to distinguish among the streptococci causing disease. Particularly difficult was a group of β hemolytic streptococci that caused a mammary gland infection in cattle (bovine mastitis). The organism appeared almost identical to the organisms causing streptococcal pharyngitis in humans. If the organisms were the same, the bovine source could be important in the transmission of the infection. Attempts to distinguish the organisms by the usual biochemical methods—that is, fermentation of sugars—were not very fruitful. Thus, attention was focused on developing a serologic method of distinguishing among the β hemolytic streptococci. Rebecca Lancefield, a student of Landsteiner, the discoverer of the ABO blood groups, found that heating the streptococci at 100°C for 10 minutes at pH 2 extracted components from the streptococci. Extracts from the human β hemolytic streptococci reacted with rabbit antisera prepared against the human isolates but not against the bovine isolates. These isolates were called the Lancefield serologic group A and were given the species designation of *S. pyogenes*. In contrast, extracts from the bovine strains reacted with homologous antisera (antisera prepared against the bovine strain) but not with antisera prepared against the human strains. These strains were called the Lancefield group C and actually were found to contain several different species based on biochemical differences (*S. equisimalis, S. zooepidemicus*, and *S. dysgalactiae*). Because of its simplicity and accuracy, the Lancefield extraction procedure became the basis for establishing the Lancefield serologic grouping scheme, which is still employed to identify many streptococci (Table 6–1). There are now about 19 groups (A through S) recognized. In addition to its importance in differentiating among the streptococci, the Lancefield extraction was an important milestone in developing methods to determine the composition and structure of the bacterial cell wall.

The Group Antigens ("C" Carbohydrate)

Although earlier studies suggested that the antigen in the Lancefield extract responsible for the reaction was protein, or "nucleoprotein," subsequent studies proved conclusively that the antigens responsible for distinguishing between the Lancefield groups A

and C were carbohydrates (polysaccharides). The localization of these polysaccharides and other wall polymers is shown diagrammatically in Figure 6–2. The cell wall is composed of the peptidoglycan to which is linked the polysaccharide and the outer surface proteins. An early generic term for the streptococcal polysaccharides, regardless of source, was *C carbohydrate*. As shown in Figure 6–3B, the backbone of the C carbohydrate from both groups A and C streptococci is composed of rhamnose and *N*-acetyl-glucosamine. Branches of *N*-acetyl-glucosamine are responsible for the serologic specificity of the group A polysaccharide (Fig. 6–2A), whereas the group C polysaccharide contains *N*-acetyl-galactosamine branches (Fig. 6–2C). Thus, it appears that subtle differences in composition determine the serologic specificity of some of the Lancefield groups and may be related to the normal habitat of the streptococci. (These concepts will appear again in discussing the exquisite specificity in the ecology of the oral streptococci.) As more C carbohydrates from other serologic groups were examined, it was found that not all were true carbohydrates. Some (e.g., Groups D, H, and N) were composed of teichoic acids (see page 154), components also associated with the cell surface. One of the functions of teichoic acid may be the attachment of streptococci to tissue cells.

The Type Antigens: The M Proteins

It soon became clear that not all group A streptococci were equally virulent. In an attempt to define the basis of virulence Lance-

Table 6–1 ■ Diseases caused by streptococci

Serologic Group	Species	Diseases
Group A	*Streptococcus pyogenes*	**Acute** Pharyngitis, pyoderma (impetigo), erysipelas, scarlet fever, pneumonia, otitis media, sinusitis, puerperal fever, septicemia
		Post-streptococal Rheumatic fever, glomerulonephritis
Group B	*S. agalactiae*	Neonatal sepsis, meninigitis, puerpual sepsis
Group C	*S. equisimilis, S. equi, S. dysgalactiae, S. zooepidemicus*	Bovine mastitis, mild pharyngitis in humans
Group D	*S. faecalis, S. faecium, S. durans*	Genitourinary infections, wound infections, root canal infections, endocarditis
Group H	*S. sanguis*	Dental plaque, endocarditis

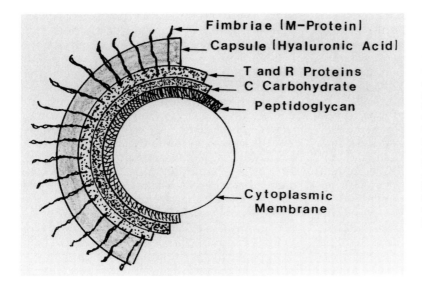

Fimbriae (M-Protein)
Capsule (Hyaluronic Acid)
T and R Proteins
C Carbohydrate
Peptidoglycan
Cytoplasmic Membrane

Figure 6–2 ■ Diagrammatic representation of the cell wall of a streptococcus. The fimbriae are shown as if they are separated from the T and R proteins; however, these proteins may also be fimbrial. The separation between the proteins and carbohydrate is for illustrative purposes, and there is no clear evidence to support a distinctly layered appearance for these surface components. The teichoic acids are not shown but would be found attached to cell membrane (see Fig. 6–11).

field and her coworkers found that only cells containing a trypsin-sensitive protein, called the "M" protein, were virulent. This name was chosen because the protein was present only in cells from "matt"-like rough colonies, which characterized the more virulent strains. Subsequent studies showed that these rough colonies resulted from the digestion of the capsular hyaluronic acid present on the group A streptococci by the organism's own hyaluronidase (see further on). To date, some 53 different M types have been identified; some (such as M type 3) are more closely associated with throat infections and rheumatic fever, whereas others (such as M type 12) are more closely associated with skin infections and nephritis. Antibodies against M proteins are opsonic (i.e., they stimulate phagocytosis) and protect the animals and humans against infection by the same M type strain. The antibody can also be used diagnostically to characterize the M type of an isolated strain; this is very important epidemiologically for identifying the source of the organism in an epidemic. The fact that the antibody against the M protein completely

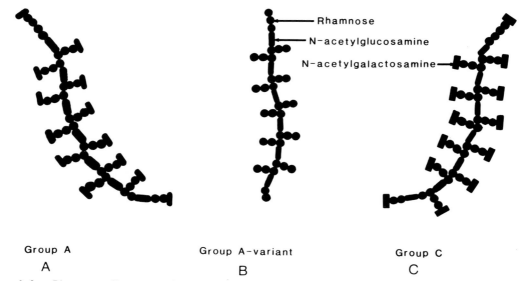

Rhamnose
N-acetylglucosamine
N-acetylgalactosamine

Group A
A

Group A-variant
B

Group C
C

Figure 6–3 ■ Diagrammatic representation of the C-carbohydrate of the β-hemolytic streptococci. The center diagram (B) represents the backbone structure composed of rhamnose and N-acetylglucosamine. This structure has actually been found in a mutant of the group A streptococcus called "A-variant." This polysaccharide is devoid of side chains. On the left (A), the polysaccharide of the group A streptococci is shown with its N-acetylglucosamine residues. On the right (C) is the structure of the polysaccharide of the group C streptococci.

protects against the infection indicates this protein is a major virulence factor of the group A streptococci. Subsequent studies showed that the group A streptococci contained other proteins in their cell wall (e.g., T and R), which were also useful in their classification.

THE VIRULENCE FACTORS

Somatic

Although the M protein is the principal virulence factor in the group A streptococci, these organisms contain a number of other components associated with virulence. These may be divided into three categories: (1) the **somatic** virulence factors, which are associated with structural components of the cell surfaces; (2) **spreading factors**; and (3) **erythrogenic toxin**, which causes scarlet fever. Table 6–2 lists these factors, their pathogenic activity, and whether they are immunogenic. At the top of the list is, of course, the M protein, which, as indicated previously is both antiphagocytic and immunogenic (induces an antibody response). The hyaluronic acid capsule, which also appears to be antiphagocytic, does not induce antibody, because its composition is the same as the hyaluronic acid found in human connective tissues. An extract containing the group A polysaccharide and fragments of peptidoglycan (group A polysaccharide complex) produces recurrent inflammatory lesions in rabbits resembling the joint and skin lesions seen in patients with rheumatic disease. Although no direct etiologic connection has been made between these diseases and the group A polysaccharide complex, there is a direct connection between infection with group A streptococci and rheumatic fever. The virulence factor involved in this relationship seems to be a component of the protoplast membrane of the streptococcus. It appears that this component, possibly an actin-like protein in the streptococcal cell membrane, induces an antibody that cross-reacts with an antigen in the heart tissue. This *autoimmune* reaction results in an inflammatory lesion closely associated with rheumatic heart disease.

Spreading Factors (Extracellular Enzymes)

In addition to the somatic components that appear to be involved in the virulence of the group A streptococci, these bacteria produce a number of extracellular enzymes—some that lyse host cells and others that can hydrolyze a number of macromolecules found in host tissues. These properties enable these streptococci to cause infections characterized by suppurative exudates, which spread along fascial planes. These spreading infections sharply contrast with the localized suppurative swellings associated with staphylococcal infections (see Chapter 7). Although the actual degree to which these spreading factors contribute to the virulence of the group A streptococci has never been established, these enzymes have become important both diagnostically and, paradoxically, in the treatment of postoperative swellings, and recently for dissolving clots in coronary arteries.

Streptolysin O ■ This oxygen-labile hemolysin is a potent immunogen, and antibodies against this component are produced

Table 6–2 ■ Virulence factors of the group A streptococci

Structural Components	Biologic Activity	Antigenicity
Hyaluronic acid capsule	Antiphagocytic	No
M protein	Antiphagocytic attachment to cells	Yes
Peptidoglycan–C polysaccharide complex	Recurrent inflammation of joints and skin	Yes
Lipoteichoic acid	Attachment to cells	Yes
Protoplast membranes	Antigenically similar to heart tissues	Yes
Extracellular enzymes (spreading factors)		
Streptolysin O (O_2 sensitive)	Hemolysin, cardiotoxic	Yes
Streptolysin S (O_2 stable)	Hemolysin, leukotoxic	No
Hyaluronidase	Hyaluronic acid depolymerase	Yes
Streptokinase	Digests fibrin	Yes
DNAse	Hydrolyzes DNA	Yes
NADase	Hydrolyzes nicotinamide adenine dinucleotide	Yes
Proteases	Hydrolyzes protein	Yes

during active streptococcal infection. These antibodies form the basis for the *antistreptolysin O* (ASO titer) assay for streptococcal infection. This hemolysin has been reported to have cardiotoxic properties. The importance of such observations is based on there still being some conjecture about the etiology of rheumatic carditis, although most investigators now consider it to be an autoimmune disease. However, despite its cardiotoxicity, no one has satisfactorily explained how this hemolysin affects heart tissue in the presence of high ASO titers generally present in patients with rheumatic fever.

Streptolysin S ■ This is the oxygen-stable hemolysin responsible for the hemolysis seen on blood agar plates. It also appears to have leukotoxic effects, although its relationship to disease is not understood; unlike most proteins, it is a poor antigen.

Hyaluronidase ■ As indicated previously, the group A streptococci produce both hyaluronic acid and the enzyme hyaluronidase, which removes the capsule. Presumably, the hyaluronidase functions in disease by breaking down the ground substance (hyaluronic acid) of connective tissue and allowing the organisms to spread. Although the streptococcal strains possessing this enzyme appear to be more virulent, the contribution of hyaluronidase and other spreading factors has not been quantitated. However, it is clear that these enzymes are produced during infection because increased antibody titers to them occur in patients with group A streptococcal disease. Thus, even if these enzymes do not play a crucial role in the disease process, they are diagnostically important since there are several clinical tests for streptococcal infection based on combinations of these antigens.

Streptokinase ■ This enzyme converts serum plasminogen to plasmin, an enzyme that digests fibrin. Presumably, dissolving fibrin clots can aid in the spread of the streptococci and thus intensify an infection. However, the major importance of this fibrinolysin as well as several other streptococcal enzymes is their use in chemotherapeutic preparations that dissolve the blood clots and emboli found in many thrombocytic diseases.

Streptodornase ■ This enzyme hydrolyzes DNA which is found in large amounts in purulent exudates as a result of lysis of the phagocytic cells. The lysis leads to decreased viscosity of the exudate and enhanced spread of organisms. However, many other inflammatory diseases, including those which result in thrombi, have exudates containing DNA. The viscosity of these exudates reduces the effectiveness of the phagocytic mechanisms necessary to "clean up" these exudates. In some types of infections, the combination of the fibrin clot and the viscosity prevents antibiotics from efficiently reaching the bacteria. Again, combinations of the streptococcal enzymes have been developed for therapeutic use to reduce the viscosity of exudates. Perhaps it is the ultimate paradox that the bacterial virulence factors become the agents used to reduce the severity of certain infections.

Other Spreading Factors ■ There are many other streptococcal enzymes that hydrolyze host components. Among them are nicotinamide adenine diphosphorylase (NADase) and various proteases.

Erythrogenic toxin ■ Some strains of *S. pyogenes* carry a lysogenic phage; when the phage DNA is incorporated into the streptococcal chromosome, the organism produces a toxin responsible for the scarlet fever rash. Before the antibiotic era, scarlet fever was feared because it often preceded symptoms of rheumatic fever and a prolonged illness. It is now considered a symptom in some cases of streptococcal pharyngitis and not essential for development of rheumatic fever. Indeed, the rash may have the beneficial effect of alerting both the patient and the physician to the seriousness of the "sore throat."

Because scarlet fever resulted in so many untoward reactions and its rash mimicked other skin infections, tests for both susceptibility and diagnosis were developed.

Dick test ■ This is a test for susceptibility to scarlet fever and consists of injecting a small amount of bacterial culture filtrate containing the erythrogenic toxin intradermally. In the absence of circulating antibody against the toxin, an area of redness is seen on the skin in 8 to 24 hours. The test is rarely used today.

The Schultz-Charlton test ■ This is a diagnostic test for scarlet fever. It consists of injecting a small amount of antitoxin into the rash; if the erythema disappears (i.e., the skin blanches) for a few minutes, it can be deduced that the rash was due to the erythrogenic toxin.

PATHOGENESIS OF STREPTOCOCCAL PHARYNGITIS

The local streptococcal lesion can be divided into three stages: attachment, spreading, and recovery.

Attachment

It has been estimated that approximately 2 $\times$ 10^6 organisms are necessary to initiate a lesion. A number of studies suggest bacterial attachment is mediated by lipoteichoic acid, which binds to the epithelial cell surface via their lipid ends. There is also some evidence that M protein and perhaps also the C polysaccharide take part in attachment. Regardless of the exact molecular mechanism of attachment, the bacteria proliferate and probably gain access to the underlying connective tissues via microscopic breaks in the epithelium. As in most infectious diseases, there is a prompt and vigorous inflammatory response mounted by the host to eliminate the bacteria. This response is characterized by a fluid exudate (edema) and primarily a polymorphonuclear (PMN) cellular infiltrate.

Spreading

The PMNs cannot phagocytize the organisms efficiently, allowing the streptococci to multiply rapidly in the connective tissue. The PMNs die, releasing their intracellular components (proteins, nucleic acids, and so on). The viscosity of this suppurative exudate might ordinarily confine this infection locally, but S. pyogenes produces the DNAses, proteases, and streptokinases that hydrolyze these components and allow the organisms to spread. In addition, they produce hyaluronidase, which breaks down the ground substance, allowing even further spread of the bacteria. If unchecked by the administration of appropriate antibiotics or the production of sufficient M protein antibodies, the organisms may gain entrance to the cervical lymph nodes or the sinuses, draining the ear and nasal pharynx to cause septicemia, that is, circulation of virulent bacteria in the blood, or blood poisoning.

Recovery

Even if untreated, most patients with streptococcal sore throat eventually recover because of the production of antibodies to M protein. These antibodies are opsonic and enhance phagocytosis but are specific for the M type antigen that induced them. However, recovery from the local disease does not necessarily mean that all is well. Approximately 3 per cent of the patients will develop a poststreptococcal disease called rheumatic fever, which can be more life-threatening than the local infection. It is the danger of rheumatic fever that necessitates the rapid and accurate diagnosis of all pharyngitis.

CLINICAL SIGNS AND SYMPTOMS OF STREPTOCOCCAL PHARYNGITIS

Streptococcal pharyngitis is characterized by a short incubation period (2 to 3 days), a high fever (103 to 104°F), pain, chills, headache, and often stomach cramps. The throat, particularly the tonsils or the tonsillar fauces, may appear "beefy red," a suppurative exudate may be present, and the cervical lymph nodes are enlarged and painful. A comparison of the incidence of antibodies to streptococcal products with the number of known cases of streptococcal disease suggests that perhaps as many as 20 per cent may be asymptomatic (subclinical). In addition to pharyngitis, the group A streptococci cause a number of other serious diseases; for example, puerperal fever (a septicemia originating from an infected uterus following delivery or abortion), skin infections, and occasionally acute endocarditis.

DIAGNOSIS

Because of the seriousness of poststreptococcal diseases and the similarity of symptoms of streptococcal sore throat and other upper respiratory diseases—for example, mononucleosis, adenovirus infection, influenza, diphtheria, and fusospirochetal infection (this is just an abbreviated list)—a differential diagnosis is essential. As in most infectious diseases, diagnosis is based first on the clinical signs and symptoms and then on the appropriate laboratory tests.

Throat Culture

The throat swab is plated on blood agar and also placed in an enrichment broth, in case the numbers of group A streptococci in the sample might be low. The sample from the broth is also plated on blood agar. The presence of β-hemolytic, bacitracin-sensitive streptococci is diagnostic for streptococcal pharyngitis. Bacitracin discs are often used because group A streptococci are particularly sensitive to this antibiotic. A catalase test should also be performed but cannot be done on blood agar plates because the erythrocytes are rich in this enzyme. Once the organism has been isolated, it should be screened for antibiotic sensitivity and it may be serotyped if necessary.

Serologic Tests

Although these tests are not necessary for the diagnosis of the local infection, it is often prudent to take a sample of the so-called acute phase serum from the patient with a diagnosed group A streptococcal infection. If complications develop, an increased titer of the "convalescent phase serum" compared with the "acute phase serum" is important in the diagnosis of poststreptococcal disease.

Antistreptolysin O (ASO) titer ■ This test has already been described briefly in connection with the virulence of streptolysin O. In this test, the patient's sera, usually both acute and convalescent samples, are mixed with streptolysin prior to adding the erythrocytes. The reduction of hemolysis in the sample compared with a normal serum control, which allows complete hemolysis to occur, is used as a measure of the amount of antibody present. Patients who have had a streptococcal infection show significantly less hemolysis in the convalescent serum compared with the acute serum. This indicates that more antibody (i.e., an increase in ASO titer) is present.

Antihyaluronidase titer ■ This test measures the antibody to streptococcal hyaluronidase. This test, as well as the anti-DNAse titer, is used primarily when the infection is suspected but the ASO test is inconclusive.

Streptozyme Test ■ This is a patented test kit in which the erythrocytes have been coated with several streptococcal enzymes (e.g., streptolysin, hyaluronidase, DNAse, and protease). Addition of patient's serum containing antibody against any one of these enzymes will cause hemagglutination.

EPIDEMIOLOGY

Streptococcal sore throat is usually spread by aerosol droplets from carriers, often asymptomatic children. As in many other infectious diseases, "lowered resistance" of the patient—because of an antecedent respiratory infection, crowded housing (socioeconomic factors), or seasonal factors—appears to be an important factor in the individual's susceptibility to infection. Indeed, during periods of rapid army mobilization, the barracks were often sources of streptococcal epidemics, and it was common practice to give

recruits prophylactic antibiotic therapy. The mortality rate prior to antibiotic therapy was 1 to 3 per cent. Although antibiotics seem to have diminished the severity of poststreptococcal complications such as rheumatic fever and glomerulonephritis, the actual incidence of these diseases is about the same.

TREATMENT

Penicillin is still the antibiotic of choice, since few of the group A streptococci have developed resistance to it. In patients allergic to penicillin, erythromycin is used. The physician will usually maintain therapy for at least 10 days in cases of proven group A infection. Sulphonamides are not used, because they do not prevent the poststreptococcal complications. Tetracyclines are also not used, because many streptococci are resistant to these drugs.

PREVENTION

Although type-specific immunity to M protein has been demonstrated, there are too many M types to make a vaccine feasible. Moreover, purification of the proteins is difficult. There are also some antigenic substances in purified M proteins that may immunologically cross-react with heart tissues. Techniques of gene cloning may provide a highly purified M protein or active fractions of M protein suitable for vaccines in the future.

RHEUMATIC FEVER

As indicated previously, rheumatic fever is not an active infection but usually results from a previous group A streptococcal pharyngitis. Indeed, the diagnosis is based on a set of signs and symptoms known as the Ducket-Jones criteria, shown in Table 6–3. A combination of major and minor criteria is necessary to establish the diagnosis of rheumatic fever. Some understanding of the pathogenesis of this disease is necessary for the dentist because patients with histories of rheumatic carditis have a predilection for endocarditis following dental therapy.

It is generally agreed that no streptococcal toxin is responsible for the scarring and subsequent stenosis of the coronary valves associated with rheumatic fever. Rather it ap-

Table 6–3 ■ Criteria for diagnosis of rheumatic fever (Duckett-Jones)

Major Signs or Symptoms	Minor Signs or Symptoms
Carditis	Fever
Murmurs	Arthralgia (joint pain)
Pericarditis	Previous rheumatic
Congestive heart failure	fever or rheumatic
Polyarthritis	heart disease
Chorea (uncoordinated	Increase in
movements)	erythrocyte
Erythema marginatum	sedimentation rate
Subcutaneous nodules	Positive C-reactive
	protein
	Leukocytosis
Evidence of previous streptococcal infection	
Scarlet fever	
Positive group A streptococcal culture	
Rise in ASO titer or titer against other sreptococcal protein	

pears that some component of the plasma membrane of the streptococci has antigenic determinants similar to the proteins in the coronary valves. These proteins are different enough to be recognized as foreign by the immune system and thus antibodies are produced against them. The antibodies cross-react with the proteins in the valves, which results in complement-fixation and initiates an Arthus-like reaction in the valves. The inflammatory reaction in the valves may result in scarring, subsequent stenosis, and the inability of the valves to function properly. Because of the mechanics of blood flow, the mitral valve seems to be more frequently affected than other cardiac valves. It is also, at least partially, the fluid mechanics that concentrate the bacteria resulting from bacteremia at the site of the damaged value. These bacteria, commonly oral streptococci, appear to attach readily to damaged valves and initiate infective endocarditis, which is a potentially fatal disease. This infection is described in more detail in the section on oral streptococci.

Streptococcus Pneumoniae

Pneumococcal pneumonia is still among the most frequent causes of death associated with infectious disease, particularly in people with lowered resistance (i.e., geriatric populations, patients receiving cancer chemotherapy or immunosuppressive therapy, and patients with diabetes or influenza). The epithet "Captain of the Men of Death" is still appropriately applied to this disease. In addition to its importance clinically, much of our knowledge of the molecular basis of virulence and microbial genetics stems from studies of *Streptococcus pneumoniae*. Thus, the organism and the diseases it causes provides an excellent model for studying the molecular basis of infectious disease.

Physiology

As with all streptococci, the organism is gram-positive and catalase-negative. It is α hemolytic under aerobic conditions but does produce an oxygen-labile hemolysin, which results in β hemolysis under anaerobic conditions and thus causes it to differ from most of the α hemolytic streptococci found in the oral pharynx, in which no hemolysis is observed under anaerobic conditions. Another useful property that distinguishes *S. pneumoniae* from other viridans streptococci is its sensitivity to a chemical called Optochin (ethyl cuprin hydrochloride). Thus, a simple diagnostic test for pneumococcal pneumonia is to plate a sputum sample on blood agar and place an Optochin disk over the streak. After incubation, the presence of α hemolytic colonies containing ovoid pairs of gram-positive cocci (diplococci, Fig. 6–4A), which are sensitive to Optochin, is diagnostic for this disease.

SEROLOGY

Capsular Polysaccharides

The most distinctive feature of *S. pneumoniae* is a capsule composed of a polysaccharide that can be visualized by several special staining techniques (Fig. 6–4B). The polysaccharide is not only shed from the surface, but because the organism tends to lyse spontaneously as it ages (autolyze), relatively large quantities of the polysaccharide are found in the spent medium. The lysis is due to a specific enzyme that cleaves the peptidoglycan of the pneumococcus. This *pneumococcal autolysin* is activated by bile salts such as desoxycholate. Indeed, a bile solubility test was once used to diagnose pneumococcal infections. The polysaccharide can be easily recovered from the spent medium and autolyzed cell cultures by relatively simple procedures. Figure 6–5 is a diagrammatic representation of the structure of the serotype III polysaccharide. This polysaccharide is composed of alternating units of glucose and

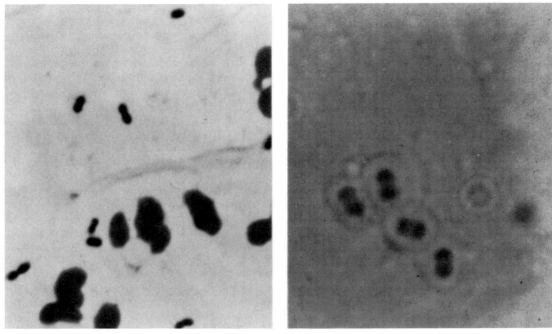

Figure 6–4 ■ *A,* Gram stain of *Streptococcus pneumoniae* in suppurative exudate. *B,* Quellung reaction (capsular swelling test). (From Schneierson, S. S.: Atlas of Diagnostic Microbiology. Abbot Laboratories, North Chicago, IL, 1965, with permission.)

glucuronic acid. There are some 80 different serologically distinct types of pneumococcal polysaccharides, many with markedly different compositions. As suggested by their name, these polysaccharides are strongly immunogenic and form the basis for a serologic classification scheme used to distinguish the various strains. Fortunately, only about 14 of these serotypes are responsible for over 90 per cent of the infectious disease caused by this species.

Transformation of Serotypes

You may recall from Chapter 3 that the molecular biology revolution originated with the observation that the capsular type of pneumococcus could be transformed by adding an extract of smooth cells of one type to rough cells derived from another type (rough cells are those that have lost their capsular polysaccharide, generally as a result of being cultured in vitro). The discovery by Avery and his colleagues that the transforming agent was DNA is responsible for this revolution.

Species-Specific Antigen

A component of the cell wall originally called the "C" substance (not to be confused with the "C" carbohydrate of the β hemolytic streptococci), but now known to be a specific type of ribitol teichoic acid containing choline, appears to be common to most strains of *S. pneumoniae*. Thus, this is one of the rare

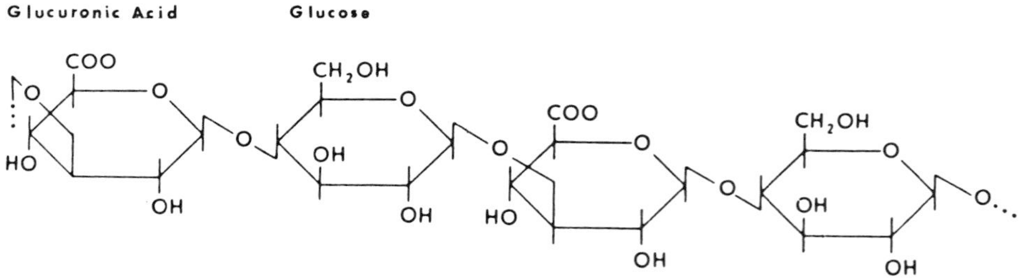

Glucuronic Acid   **Glucose**

Figure 6–5 ■ Structure of pneumococcal serotype 3 capsular polysaccharide.

bacterial antigens that are species specific. However, it is the type-specific polysaccharide antigens that are clinically important. (The "C" substance is used clinically for testing for the presence of a blood component with which it reacts. This is called the **C-reactive protein** [CRP] test).

The Capsular Swelling Test

Antisera against the specific pneumococcal polysaccharide will precipitate the molecule from solutions, agglutinate cells containing the polysaccharide capsule, or cause the capsule to "swell." The **Quellung** (German for swelling) **reaction**, or capsular swelling test, is most frequently used for diagnosis because of its simplicity and specificity. It consists of incubating a wet mount containing pneumococcal cells with antisera. The antibodies react with the polysaccharide in the capsule, perhaps changing its refractive index. When viewed in a microscope it appears that the capsule has swollen (see Fig. 6–4B). This test can often be carried out directly on fresh sputum samples of patients with suspected pneumococcal pneumonia, thereby speeding the diagnosis significantly. This test was especially important in the pre-antibiotic era when the only specific treatment for pneumococcal pneumonia was administration of antisera produced in horses. It was obviously important to choose the right horse (sic). Since death from pneumococcal pneumonia can occur within 6 days, rapid diagnosis was and still is essential. The antibodies against the capsular polysaccharide are both diagnostic and therapeutic, indicating that the capsule functions as the major virulence component of this species.

Virulence Factors

Capsular Polysaccharides ■ The capsular polysaccharides are not only the major antigens of *S. pneumoniae* but also the most important virulence factors. It has been suggested that the hydrophilic nature of the capsule prevents their phagocytosis by polymorphonuclear leukocytes. Thus, the capsules of the pneumococci are said to be *antiphagocytic* and, despite their completely different nature, to perform the same function as the M protein of the group A streptococci. When coated with specific antibody, the bacteria are readily phagocytized. (As mentioned previously, the process of anti-body-enhanced phagocytosis is called opsonization.) Indeed, the resolution of pneumococcal pneumonia occurs by a process called "crisis," which is associated with the production of opsonizing antibody by the patient (see further on).

Toxins ■ The beta (β) hemolysin has already been described; this component is said to have leukocidin properties (i.e., it can destroy human leukocytes). In addition, in many cases of pneumococcal pneumonia, in which the bacterial infection appears to be eliminated with effective antibiotic therapy, the patients still die with symptoms resembling a true toxemia (circulating toxin). An intensive search for such a toxin, however, has still not been completely successful.

Pathogenesis of Lobar Pneumonia

The disease is generally divided into four stages: (1) proliferation, (2) early consolidation, (3) advanced consolidation, and (4) resolution by crisis or death by complication. The beginning of the disease is often associated with an upper respiratory infection such as influenza. This results in reduced ciliary and epiglottal reflexes and a thick, copious mucous secretion. The pneumococci, which become trapped in this viscous mucous, are aspirated into the alveoli where they resist phagocytosis and multiply (proliferation). The bacteria induce an inflammatory reaction initially characterized by increased fluid (edema—early consolidation). This is followed by the cellular portion of the inflammatory response—the polymorphonuclear leukocytes attempt to phagocytose the bacteria, die, and lyse. Death of phagocytes results in a thick, purulent exudate, or pus (advanced consolidation). All this occurs in the relatively short time of 2 to 6 days and is characterized by sudden high fever, coughing, pain on breathing, and hypoxia (lack of oxygen). Resolution is associated with a sudden, copious perspiration ("sweats") and a drop in fever. It is due to the production of opsonizing antibodies. However, in many cases, particularly in older patients ("old man's friend") or in those with lowered resistance, the organisms enter the bloodstream (bacteremia) and are distributed to other vital organs such as the meninges, where their multiplication often leads to rapid death (death by complication). Indeed, prior to the antibiotic era 36 per cent of patients died of this disease.

Diagnosis

In addition to the clinical signs and symptoms, radiographs, sputum cultures, and blood cultures are taken. As indicated previously, before the advent of antibiotics it was routine to perform a Quellung test on the sputum sample. The presence of α hemolytic, Optochin-sensitive, gram-positive diplococci is diagnostic for infection with *S. pneumoniae*. A positive blood culture portends very serious consequences.

Treatment

Penicillin is still the antibiotic of choice, with erythromycin being used in patients allergic to penicillin. In recent years there have been strains reported that are resistant to multiple antibiotics, suggesting a plasmid mediated transfer. Because of the appearance of such strains and the inability to control the disease in some patients, a vaccine has been developed.

Prevention

Since this is a disease with lowered resistance, maintenance of good health is clearly one preventive method. However, a vaccine has been developed which contains 14 capsular polysaccharides representing the most common disease-producing strains. The vaccine seems to be particularly valuable for compromised patients such as those with Hodgkin's disease or sickle cell anemia, splenectomized patients, and miners exposed to various dusts. It also has been effective in reducing the frequency of middle ear infection in children particularly subject to this infection.

The Oral Streptococci

The oral streptococci constitute one of the most populous groups of bacteria in the mouth. Recent studies have divided these organisms into ever more numerous species; that is, *Streptococcus mutans* has now been split into several species—*S. mutans*, *S. sobrinus* (the latter two species are mostly human strains), *S. rattus*, *S. cricetus*, and *S. ferus*. However, in this chapter we will take the point of view of the "lumper" rather than the "splitter" in order to provide the student with a basic grasp of the major properties of the streptococcal groups in the mouth: all these species will be considered under the rubric of *S. mutans*. Similar taxonomic changes have occurred among other streptococcal groups in the mouth. However, our discussion will center on the *four* major streptococcal physiologic groups recognized in the mouth: *S. salivarius*, *S. mitis* (*S. mitior*), *S. sanguis*, and *S. mutans*. With the exception of *S. salivarius*, most of the strains of these species produce a greenish zone of alpha (α) hemolysis around colonies on blood agar. Because of this, they have previously been referred to as *S. viridans*, and indeed even today one sees this term used in some articles. However, this is the ultimate in "lumping" and truly is a misnomer. Its use makes it difficult to understand the relationship of each of the major streptococcal groups to its ecologic niche within the oral cavity and to disease. Thus, although *S. salivarius* is often considered a member of this group, it rarely if ever produces alpha hemolysis. Its normal habitat is the tongue, from which large numbers are shed, and it is the predominant organism in saliva. For this reason, the detection of *S. salivarius* is an indication of salivary contamination, just as *Escherichia coli* is an indicator of fecal contamination. Although all the data are not yet in, it appears that *S. mitis* is more commonly found on the buccal mucous membranes (nonkeratinized), whereas *S. sanguis* and *S. mutans* are the quintessential tooth organisms; moreover, the latter species appears to be the most cariogenic of the oral streptococci. Obviously, such differences in ecologic distribution and disease potential suggest not only specific attachment of the bacteria to the tissues but also metabolic differences which provide selective advantages for each species to exist in its distinct ecologic niche. The remainder of this section will deal with exploring the structure-function relationships that might account for the differences in ecology and particularly the enhanced cariogenicity of *S. mutans*.

STREPTOCOCCUS SALIVARIUS

Physiology

This species is the most easily identified oral streptococcus because it forms "gumdrop" colonies on agar medium containing sucrose. Typical colonies of this organism grown on mitis-salivarius agar (MSA) are highly convex in shape and look like gumdrop candies. The component responsible for this type of colony is an extracellular levan

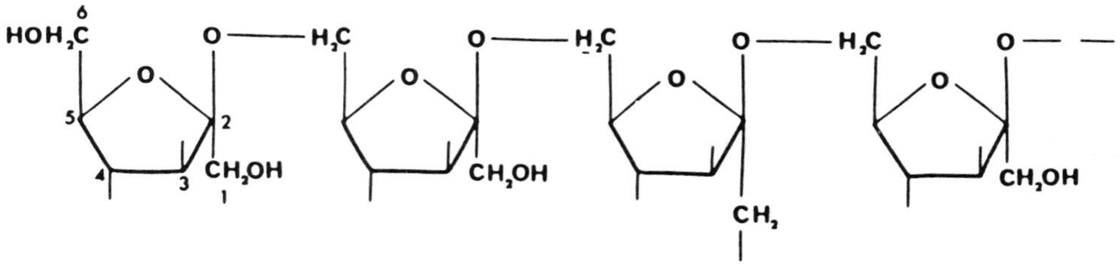

Figure 6–6 ■ Structure of levan from *Streptococcus salivarius.* (From Newbrun, E.: Cardiology. Williams & Wilkins, Baltimore, 1983, with permission.)

produced from sucrose in the medium. As shown in Figure 6–6, a levan is a linear polymer of fructose, which is synthesized by an enzyme on the surface of *S. salivarius* called a fructosyltransferase or a levan-sucrase. This enzyme cleaves the high energy glycosidic bond between glucose and fructose in sucrose and uses part of the energy released during hydrolysis to link the fructose units together to form the levan. The residual glucose that results from this hydrolysis is converted to lactate via the Embden-Meyerhof pathway. It is important to remember that only a small part of the sucrose is used to form the levan. Most of this substrate is converted to fructose and glucose by the enzyme invertase (see further on); these monosaccharides are then metabolized by the usual glycolytic pathways. It should also be noted that the disaccharide sucrose is unusual in possessing the high-energy glycosidic bond between glucose and fructose, thus making it the only dietary substrate usually available for this type of polymer formation. Similar kinds of reactions take place among the other oral streptococci, but they result in the formation of dextrans, polymers of glucose. Table 6–4 lists the biochemical reactions of the oral streptococci

commonly employed to identify them; however, adequate identification for most clinical purposes can often be achieved using just a few of these tests. Thus, the minimum properties that would identify the majority of *S. salivarius* are gram-positive cocci in chains that are catalase-negative, show no hemolysis, and form gumdrop colonies on MSA. However, commercial testing is now available that uses as many as 20 different tests to identify the streptococci precisely. The simplicity and accuracy of these tests have led to the replacement of the more cumbersome tube fermentation tests.

Serology

Although serology is probably less important in the taxonomy of *S. salivarius* than in the beta (β) hemolytic streptococci, it has great potential as a tool for probing the relationship of bacterial surface to the ecology of these organisms. Most strains of *S. salivarius* belong to Lancefield group K, although some strains contain the group F antigen and others the group O antigen. The antigens defining these groups are either cell wall or capsular polysaccharides distinct from the levans produced by this species. It appears that

Table 6–4 ■ Biochemical identification of oral streptococci				
Tests	S. salivarius	S. sanguis	S. mitis	S. mutans
Hemolysis	Nonhemolytic	Alpha	Alpha	Alpha
Catalase	Neg.	Neg.	Neg.	Neg.
Arginine hydrolysis	Neg.	Pos.	Neg.	Neg.*
Esculin hydrolysis	Neg.	Pos.	Neg./pos.	Pos.
Levan ("gumdrop" colonies)	Pos.	Neg.	Neg.	Neg.
Dextran	Neg.	Pos.†	Pos.†	Pos.†
Mannitol	Neg.	Neg.	Neg.	Pos.
Sorbitol	Neg.	Neg.	Neg.	Pos.
Inulin	Pos.	Pos.	Neg.	Pos.
Peroxide production	Neg.	Pos.	Pos.	Var.‡

*The serotype b strains *(S. rattus)* do hydrolyze arginine.
†Some strains do produce small amounts of levan but do not form "gumdrop" colonies.
‡Var. = variable.

those strains containing the K antigen adhere more strongly to human buccal epithelial cells in vitro than the K-negative strains. However, many strains, regardless of antigenic composition, aggregate with strains of *Veillonella* species, which are gram-negative anaerobic cocci that are major residents of the human tongue. *S. salivarius* is rarely found in dental plaque and, correspondingly, generally does not adhere well to saliva-coated hydroxyapatite, an in vitro model for dental plaque formation. Thus, the surface of this species seems to contain one or more components that favor its attachment to the tongue or bacteria associated with the tongue, and perhaps it is not surprising that this organ is its major habitat in the human oral cavity.

Fimbriae

The components responsible for bacterial attachment to tissues are called *adhesins* and appear to be associated with structures on the bacterial surfaces called *fimbriae* (these may be analogous to structures called pili found in gram-negative bacteria). A comparison of the fimbriae of various oral streptococci is shown in the transmission electron micrograph in Figure 6–7. Although the fimbriae appear to be delicate in these thin sections from which the water has been removed following fixation, negative staining of the whole organism, as seen in Figure 6–8, suggests they may be more substantial and firmly bound into the cell wall. It is evident, however, that both the quantity and quality of the fimbriae differ among the oral streptococci. *S. salivarius* contains numerous long fimbriae, whereas the fimbriae in some strains of *S. sanguis* are shorter and appear to be less dense. Other strains of *S. sanguis* have large, dense fimbriae, but these are localized to one area of the cell wall. Strains possessing these polarized fimbriae are often found adhering to strains of *Bacterionema matruchotii* or *Fusobacterium nucleatum* in aggregates known as "corncobs," found on the

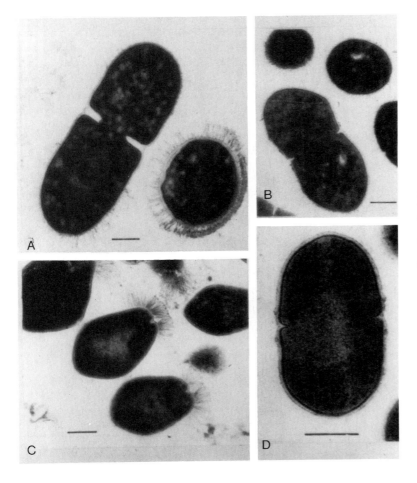

Figure 6–7 ■ Transmission electron micrographs of oral streptococci. *A, Streptococcus salivarius. B, Streptococcus sanguis* (typical plaque isolate). *C, Streptococcus sanguis* (corncob-forming strain with localized fimbriae) *D, Streptococcus mutans.*

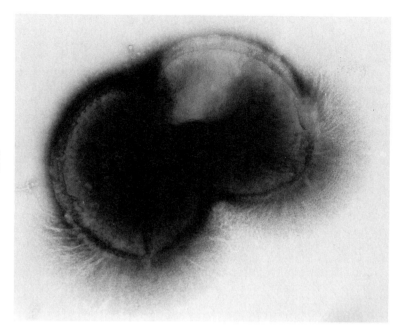

Figure 6–8. ■ Negative stain of corncob-forming strain. (Courtesy of Dr. Pauline Handley.)

surface of supragingival plaque (see Fig. 26–11, Chapter 26). *S. mutans* does not appear to have a significant amount of fimbriae compared with the other oral streptococci. The fimbriae of *S. mitis* appear similar to those of *S. sanguis,* but the antigenic composition of the surface as well as the chemical composition of cell walls of *S. mitis* and *S. sanguis* differ. In the final analysis, it is the molecular composition of the fimbriae, not their appearance, that governs where the bacterium will reside. Efforts directed at plaque prevention are attempting to identify these molecules and to develop specific biologic or chemotherapeutic reagents that will inhibit their activity.

STREPTOCOCCUS SANGUIS

The name of this organism is descriptive of its isolation from blood cultures of patients with subacute bacterial endocarditis ("sanguine" is Latin for blood). It is still among the most frequent species isolated from the patients with this disease and is also among the most frequent organisms isolated from dental plaque. Since endocarditis often results from a bacteremia following dental treatment, a simple deduction leads to the conclusion that these plaque bacteria may enter the circulation during dental treatment to cause this very serious and often fatal disease. Thus, an appreciation of the struc-

ture-function relationships of this organism is essential for understanding plaque formation and maturation as well as the pathogenesis of endocarditis.

Physiology

It has only been within the last 20 years that an acceptable physiologic classification of the "viridans streptococci" has been developed (note that the latter descriptive terminology is acceptable, whereas *S. viridans* is not). In any event a comparison of some of the physiologic characteristics of these organisms is provided in Table 6–4. Examination of this table suggests that *S. sanguis* may be reasonably identified by its failure to ferment either mannitol or sorbitol and its ability to produce ammonia and carbon dioxide from arginine. (Since *S. milleri* resembles *S. sanguis* in many respects, no separate discussion of this species will be included here.)

Arginine hydrolase ■ The arginine hydrolase pathway results in the breakdown of arginine into urea and finally into ammonia and carbon dioxide. This reaction can provide energy for growth of the bacteria in the absence of fermentable carbohydrate and enables *S. sanguis* to exist in plaque in the absence of fermentable carbohydrates. Moreover, the production of ammonia may neutralize acids produced by bacterial fermentation, providing an environment more suitable for bacterial growth. It has been suggested that this pathway may be the reason *S. sanguis* is less cariogenic than most strains of *S. mutans*, which do not possess this pathway. Indeed, the possibility that one could reduce the acidity of plaque by the formation of ammonia from metabolizable urea was the basis of an earlier anticariogenic toothpaste. More recently a group of investigators developed a tetrapeptide called Sialin, containing arginine and other basic amino acids; this peptide was metabolized by dental plaque and salivary sediments to yield ammonia. Measurements of plaque pH using *Stephan Curves* (see Chapter 27) indicated that plaque or salivary sediment (an in vitro model for plaque) treated with Sialin did not show the usual dramatic fall in pH after a sugar rinse compared with untreated plaque. It is clear that this clinical approach to caries prevention was based on the idea that organisms like *S. sanguis* can cause an increase in plaque pH if given the appropriate substrate. Unfortunately, clinical trials indicate that this approach to plaque prevention is not cost effective.

Dextran formation ■ Another property of ecologic interest in *S. sanguis* is the production of dextrans. These glucose polymers, like the polymers of fructose, are produced enzymatically from sucrose by dextransucrase or glucosyltransferase. These enzymes are associated with the surface of this organism, although their exact mode of attachment to the cell wall is still unknown. Most dextran produced by *S. sanguis* is of the "soluble" variety, which means it is predominantly a linear polymer of α-1,6 glucosyl pyranose (Fig. 6–9). The dextran accumulates in the

spent medium and can be readily precipitated from the medium by the addition of an equal volume of ethanol. The aqueous solubility of the α-1,6 dextrans makes their contribution to the attachment process questionable; however, the *S. sanguis* enzymes may bind the more insoluble dextrans produced by *S. mutans*, providing a mechanism of attachment of this more cariogenic organism to dental plaque. Although more cariogenic, this latter species generally has a much lower ability to adhere to tooth surface than does *S. sanguis*.

Glycogen storage ■ Many oral streptococci are capable of producing internal stores of glycogen (intracellular polysaccharide, or IPS), which can be metabolized and used as energy source during periods when external sugars are not available.

Peroxide production ■ Although classically it has been stated that streptococci possess no direct pathway to oxygen, it is clear that several species do produce small amounts of H_2O_2. Presumably this is due to the direct transfer of hydrogen from reduced flavoprotein to molecular oxygen; however, the exact pathway is still unknown. Since these organisms do not possess a catalase or peroxidase, the peroxide accumulates and may become toxic. This is one reason anaerobic incubation is often used to grow these bacteria. Indeed, even small amounts of dissolved oxygen in the medium can result in quite marked cytotoxic effects, as shown in Figure 6–10. *S. sanguis* cells formed large pleomorphic rods when grown in flasks that permit a large surface area of the medium to be exposed to the air and absorb oxygen.

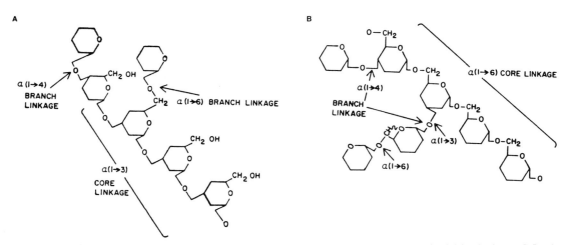

Figure 6–9 ■ *A,* Dextran containing α(1,6)-glucose backbone and side chain typical of soluble dextrans. *B,* Dextran with α(1,3)-glucose side chains. The extent of these α(1,3) linkages determines the solubility of the dextran. (From Loesche, J. W.: Dental Caries, A Treatable Infection. Charles C Thomas, Springfield, IL, 1982, with permission.)

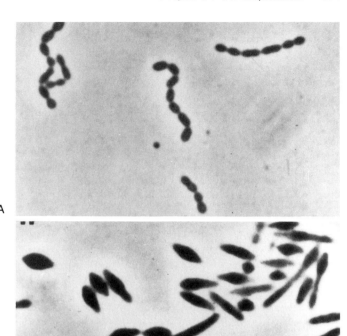

Figure 6–10 ■ Effects of oxygen on the shape of *S. sanguis* cells. *A*, Normal cells grown under anaerobic or microaerophilic conditions. *B*, Cells grown in cultures that have been shaken to increase concentration of dissolved oxygen.

The viability of these rod-shaped forms is low compared with the usual coccal forms of the organism (Fig. 6–10*A*). The peroxide not only is autotoxic, but also can inhibit other bacteria. This may explain why the presence of *S. sanguis* in plaque has been suggested to be beneficial. (In addition, a bacteriocin produced by *S. sanguis* has also been found to inhibit certain gram-negative plaque bacteria.) An additional role for streptococcal H_2O_2 may be as a substrate for the lactoperoxidase in saliva. This enzyme catalized the oxidation of thiocyanate (SCN^-) ion to hypothiocyanate ($OSCN^-$) in the presence of H_2O_2. The hypothiocyanate is also toxic to many streptococci and lactobacilli, although an exact role for this reaction in vivo has not yet been described. In any case, it is clear that *S. sanguis*, by both its numbers in plaque and its range of metabolic activities, can play an important role in oral ecology.

Serology

Group H antigen ■ If confusion were said to exist in the physiologic classification of the oral streptococci, then "chaos" would be a mild description for the serologic classification. Indeed, the two problems were interrelated because the inadequate physiologic classification led to using strains that were not properly speciated for immunization. Even today, one of the largest commercial suppliers still uses an antiserum that probably does not detect the true group H antigen (the most common antigen in *S. sanguis*) for its serologic identification. Thus, many strains being used for oral ecologic studies are often actually a different streptococcal species than the one the author thought he or she was investigating. This has led to confusion in deciding which organisms live in which place.

Recent studies have shown that the group H antigen is a membrane lipoteichoic acid (LTA) containing a small number of α-glucosyl units, which form the antigenic determinant. Thus, it is homologous with the group D and group N antigens, which are also membrane LTAs but of different serologic specificity. Since some teichoic acid is present on the surface of the organism, it has been speculated that this component is responsible for the adherence of *S. sanguis* to salivary pellicle. These speculations were stimulated by the observation that LTA is believed to play an important role in the adhesion of group A streptococci to epithelial cells presumably via the lipid end of the molecule. As shown in Figure 6–11, LTA is an amphipathic molecule, of which one end is a hydrophobic lipid and the other end a hydrophilic lipid. Several studies suggested that attachment to salivary pellicle is mediated by hydrophobic interactions, which could involve LTA. Others have suggested the hydrophilic portion of the molecule interacts with the phosphate or calcium ion in the hydroxyapatite or sulfate groups in the salivary pellicle. However, the evidence to support any of these hypotheses is not yet convincing. Indeed, the major biologic function of LTA is still unknown, possibly because no LTA-negative mutant has been isolated. However, *S. mitis* strains do not contain LTA yet appear to adhere well, particularly to buccal epithelial cells.

Type antigens ■ In contrast to the group A streptococci, the antigen that separates the group H streptococci into two serotypes is a polysaccharide that is similar in some respects to the polysaccharide that forms the group-specific antigen in the β hemolytic

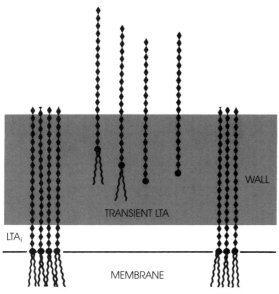

Figure 6–11 ■ Diagrammatic representation of attachment and secretion of teichoic acids. The LTA$_i$ is the lipoteichoic attached to the cell membrane via the lipid *(wavy line)* end. Some of the lipid may be lost during passage through the wall (deacylation); the deacylated teichoic acid accumulates in the wall and is also found in the spent medium. Note that the proposed orientation of the LTA in the cell wall would make it difficult for the molecule's lipid end to function in attachment. (From Wilken and Knox: Prog Immunol *3*:135–143, 1977, with permission.)

WALL

TRANSIENT LTA

LTA$_i$

MEMBRANE

streptococci. These paradoxes serve to illustrate that in discussing serologic groups and types, operational definitions are used (i.e., a group contains the largest number of strains, whereas a serotype is a smaller part of the group). There is no theoretic significance in the concept of serologic group or type; it is merely a convenient means allowing us to categorize bacteria. Group antigens may be polysaccharides, teichoic acids, or proteins. The same spectrum of molecules can be associated with type specificity. (The group A streptococci are defined by a polysaccharide and typed by protein; the pneumococci are typed by polysaccharides.) The importance of type specificity among strains of *S. sanguis* is that the type 1 strains appear to adhere better to salivary pellicles than the type 2 strains. However, it is not clear whether differences in the type-specific polysaccharides or other surface components are responsible for differences in adhesion.

Other surface antigens ■ The importance of microbial adhesion as a virulence factor was first pointed out by dental researchers who have been studying the molecular basis for the specificity bacterial attachment to various surfaces. The oral streptococci have been important models because of the clear ecologic differences among the various species. Although these investigations are still ongoing, they have shown that the picture of a simple surface composed of only a few different antigenic polymers is inaccurate (see Fig. 6–2). Indeed, it appears that in addition to the peptidoglycan, *S. sanguis* contains one or more polysaccharides, several forms of teichoic acids, and perhaps nine or more different proteins or glycoproteins. A major goal of current investigations is to determine which components function as adhesins.

STREPTOCOCCUS MITIS (S. MITIOR, MITEOR, S. SANGUIS—BIOTYPE II, NUTRITIONALLY VARIANT STREPTOCOCCI [NVS], S. ORALIS)

Although placed in parentheses, the other names listed have been used to describe similar organisms. Indeed, it is now being proposed that only *S. oralis* is correct for some of these species, although very few investigators prefer it. However, this surfeit of names for what are at the very least similar organisms illustrates one of the major problems in trying to study the relationship between structure and biologic activity among oral streptococci. The difficulty in defining this species is that they do little physiologically and are antigenically heterogeneous. Thus, there are few positive characteristics for defining them. Indeed, they are classically defined by exclusion (i.e., if an oral streptococcus is not *S. salivarius*, *S. sanguis*, or *S. mutans*, then it must be *S. mitis*).

Physiology

Table 6–4 illustrates the difficulty in identifying *S. mitis*; very few characteristics are positive and these do not differentiate this species from other oral streptococci. Until recently, there was not a single characteristic distinctly associated with *S. mitis*. However, a group of α hemolytic streptococci requiring cysteine and vitamin B_6 for growth was isolated from patients with endocarditis. These organisms, called nutritionally variant strains (NVS), produced a red chromophore when heated at pH 2 to extract the Lancefield antigens. These strains appear to be similar to *S. mitis*, except the latter do not require cysteine or vitamin B_6 for growth. However, they also produce the chromophore when treated with acid. Although the nature of this chromophore has not been established, it could prove of great value in identifying *S. mitis* species.

Serology

The difficulties in identifying *S. mitis* are not eased by using serology. Antisera prepared against an individual strain are often strain specific—that is, they only react with antigens from the strain that induced them. When cross-reactions are present, they do not appear to define any large groups, but react rather haphazardly with various strains. Although *S. mitis* is often called *S. sanguis II*, not only does it lack the group H antigen, but also no LTA has been found in any of the strains tested. Thus, it appears to be the only group of streptococci and indeed perhaps the only species among the *Lactobacillaceae* that does not contain LTA. Indeed, *S. mitis* is one of the few gram-positive bacteria that do not contain LTA. It is interesting to speculate that the absence of this molecule may be related to the minimal metabolic capabilities of this species. Many strains of this species react with Lancefield group K antiserum, but the exact nature of this reaction is not known, nor has the relationship of this reaction to the group K–positive

strains of *S. salivarius* been investigated. Thus, for the most part *S. mitis* is still identified after all the other possibilities have been eliminated.

STREPTOCOCCUS MUTANS

As indicated previously, there is now good genetic evidence that the species previously called *S. mutans* really consists of several different species. The latter epithet has been reserved primarily for strains of serotypes c, e, and f that reside in human hosts. Other species that are physiologically very similar to *S. mutans* are found in rodents (e.g., *S. rattus*, *S. cricetus*, and *S. ferrus*). The physiology of these organisms, particularly their carbohydrate metabolism, is so similar that it is logical to consider them as the "mutans" group. Moreover, these metabolic properties are intimately related to their ability to cause dental caries.

Physiology

Fermentation ∎ In contrast to many of the other oral streptococci, which ferment only a small variety of carbohydrates, *S. mutans* group ferments many sugars. In particular, their ability to ferment *mannitol* and *sorbitol*, sugar alcohols derived from mannose and glucose, respectively, distinguishes them from other oral streptococci. Indeed, so consistent are these properties that attempts have been made to use them as rapid screening methods for the identification of these organisms. With the exception of some strains of *S. rattus*, the mutans group does not hydrolyze arginine. Thus, a working definition of *S. mutans* would be α hemolytic streptococci, which ferment mannitol and sorbitol but do not hydrolyze arginine. In addition to fermenting a wider variety of sugars, these organisms show quantitative differences in the amount of acid produced from glucose. *S. mutans* accumulates more acid and causes a larger drop in pH on solid media than do *S. sanguis* strains.

Sucrose metabolism

Dextran ∎ As indicated previously, many oral streptococci can synthesize carbohydrate polymers from sucrose utilizing the cleavage of the high-energy glycosidic bond in sucrose as an energy source. In the *S. mutans* group of organisms the glucosyltransferase predominates and the major carbohydrate produced is a dextran (glucan). In contrast to the linear α-1,6 dextran produced by *S. sanguis,* the polymer produced by *S. mutans* contains up to 40 per cent α(1,3)-branches, as shown in Figure 6–10. This renders the polymer much less soluble and so distinctly different in properties from the usual dextran that it has been called a *mutan.* The mutan is relatively insoluble and its presence on the bacterial surface causes it to become "sticky" so that the bacteria do not separate easily. At one time, this property was believed important in bacterial adherence to tooth surfaces but now it is believed to be more important in holding plaque together (cohesion) rather than initiating attachment via the salivary pellicle. The importance of mutan production in dental caries has been established by examining mutants which have a reduced capacity or have lost the ability to produce insoluble dextrans and are no longer as cariogenic as the parent strains. The importance of glucosyltransferase in relationship to dental caries has resulted in attempts to develop vaccines or other chemotherapeutic agents which would interfere with its activity and thereby possibly reduce dental caries (see Chapter 27). Although the fructose released during the formation of the mutan is utilized to produce acid and potentiates the cariogenic capacity of these organisms, only a small part of the total dietary sucrose is needed to produce even relatively large amounts of the mutan associated with these organisms. Most sucrose is metabolized via another pathway.

Invertase ■ The hydrolysis of sucrose to glucose and fructose by the enzyme invertase represents the dominant pathway of sucrose metabolism in *S. mutans* and other oral streptococci. These monosaccharides are transported into the cell via a proton motor force (PMF) or through the phosphotransferase system (PTS). The latter involves the phosphorylation of the monosaccharide prior to transport across the cell membrane. The phosphate donor is phosphoenolpyruvate (PEP), a product of the Embden-Meyerhof pathway. The contribution of each of these transport systems is dependent upon the growth rate of the bacteria and the concentration of the sucrose in the medium. In the presence of sugar limitation, PTS is favored, whereas the PMF transport system is favored when there is excess carbohydrate. Perhaps more important, these factors also determine the amounts and types of end products produced. Thus, sugar excess also favors lactate formation, as opposed to sugar limitation in

which larger quantities of acetate, formate, and ethanol are produced. These findings explain the special relationship between sucrose metabolism and dental caries.

Selectivity of sucrose for **S. mutans** ■ The special relationship between sucrose and *S. mutans* has been used to formulate media containing high concentrations of the sugar (20 per cent), which inhibit other streptococci but permit *S. mutans* to grow. Further selectivity is provided by adding bacitracin to the medium (MSB), since *S. mutans* is more resistant to this antibiotic than are other oral streptococci.

Serology

Serotypes ■ The differentiation of *S. mutans* into serotypes antedates the division of the group into different species. Indeed, as indicated at the beginning of this section, there is a close association between the serotype and the species. The serotype antigens are cell wall polysaccharides composed of rhamnose, glucose, and, in some serotypes, galactose. The serologic specificity resides in terminal sugar linkages, which are sometimes similar enough to result in cross-reactions among some types. These can often be removed by absorbing the antibody with cells of the cross-reacting species, resulting in a type-specific antiserum. However, in some instances—that is, in serotypes a and d—the polysaccharides do carry two distinct antigenic determinants. The presence of these type-specific antigens has provided a means of rapid identification of the species and has also been used in studies localizing these organisms in human dental plaque. The exact biologic role for these polymers is still not completely understood nor is it known if they play some role in virulence. Table 6–5

Table 6–5 ■ Species and serotypes and the mutans streptococci

Species	Serotypes	Antigenic Determinants*
S. mutans	c	Glucose-α(1,4)-glucose
S. ferus	c	
S. mutans		Glucose-β(1,6)-glucose and Glucose-β(1,4)-glucose
S. mutans	f	Glucose-α(1,6)-glucose
S. rattus	b	Galactose
S. cricetus	a	Glucose-β(1,6)-glucose
S. sobrinus	d	Galactose-β(1,6)-glucose
S. sobrinus	g	β-galactose

*The backbones of these polysaccharides are composed predominantly of Rhamnose.

lists the relationship between species, serotypes, and specific antigenic determinants of the cell wall polysaccharides among the *S. mutans* group.

Protein antigens ■ In addition to the polysaccharide type-specific antigens, an important protein antigen has been identified in *S. mutans*. This antigen—variously identified as antigen I/II, B, P1, and SPaA—is important because antibodies that react with this protein appear to be protective against dental caries. The antigen has been purified to homogeneity from culture supernatants of *S. mutans*, where it accumulates in relatively large amounts in certain strains. The exact biologic role for this protein remains unknown, although it has been suggested to act as an adhesin for the initial attachment of these organisms to the salivary pedicle. Attempts are being made to prepare large quantities of this antigen by gene-cloning methods so that its exact role in the carious process can be assessed. The availability of this protein will also enable studies of its usefulness as a caries vaccine. Unfortunately, some investigators have found that antibodies against this protein appear to cross-react with human heart tissues. Since it has been suggested that cross-reactions between streptococcal antibodies and heart tissues could be a factor in rheumatic heart disease, it is hardly likely that such a vaccine will be permitted to be used until its cross-reactive properties can be eliminated. In this case, the skills of the microbial geneticist are called upon to dissect and clone the portion of the gene that produces proteins for protective vaccines and to eliminate those portions responsible for cardiac cross-reactions.

chapter 7

The staphylococci

Burton Rosan D.D.S., M.Sc.

Although similar to the streptococci in shape, smears of staphylococci reveal bunches of gram-positive cocci similar to clusters of grapes. Indeed, the name derives from the Greek "staphyle," a bunch of grapes. These bunches result from the division of this species in different planes rather than in a single plane, as streptococci divide (Table 7–1). However, the novice often confuses the two genera in Gram stains. This confusion can easily be eliminated by placing a couple of drops of 3 percent H_2O_2 on a colony (as long as it is not on blood agar). If bubbles of O_2 are detected, catalase is present and the organism must be a *Staphylococcus*; no bubbles indicates the organism is probably a *Streptococcus*. The two species of staphylococci most commonly found in humans are *S. aureus* and *S. epidermidis*. As the latter name indicates, this species is found primarily residing on the skin and is generally considered to be nonpathogenic. In contrast, *S. aureus* is a potential pathogen and may be carried asymptomatically in the nasopharynx of up to 40 percent of individuals. It is probably from this site that it finds its way to the oral cavity where it is occasionally found in low numbers (i.e., 350 organisms per milliliter saliva). Thus, it does not usually play a significant role in intraoral infections but may cause serious infections associated with accidental or surgically induced wounds, including those around the head and neck. In addition there are strains that produce an enterotoxin that causes a type of food poisoning.

Physiology

The staphylococci prefer aerobic conditions, although they will grow anaerobically. They produce much larger colonies than the streptococci (1 to 4 mm in diameter), and *S. aureus* may be golden yellow owing to carotenoid pigments. However, pigment production is variable and cannot be used as a valid guide to speciation. The two most important characteristics distinguishing the nonpathogenic *S. epidermidis* from the pathogenic *S. aureus* are coagulase production and mannitol fermentation (Table 7–2). Coagulase is an extracellular enzyme produced by pathogenic strains of staphylococci, which activates either prothrombin or a similar substance that induces the conversion of fibrinogen to

Table 7–1 ■ Comparison of staphylococci and streptococci

Staphylococci	Streptococci
Cocci arranged in bunches	Cocci arranged in chains
Catalase-positive	Catalase negative
Salt tolerant	Sensitive to high salt*
Facultative aerobe	Facultative anaerobe
Localized-type infection	Spreading-type infection
Coagulase-positive	Coagulase-negative (usually)
Antibiotic resistance	Most sensitive to penicillin†

*Except *S. faecalis*, which is tolerant of salt at concentrations up to 6.5%.
†Except *S. faecalis*, which tends to be resistant to high concentrations of penicillin and other antibiotics.

fibrin. In addition, most pathogenic strains produce DNAse. The staphylococci are among the hardiest of all non–spore-forming bacteria and are resistant to heating at 60°C for 30 minutes and may be stored at 4°C for long periods without affecting viability. They are also resistant to high concentrations of NaCl. These properties have been utilized to prepare a selective and differential medium called mannitol salt agar, which contains 7.5 percent NaCl, 1 percent mannitol, and phenol red, an acid-base indicator. The presence of *S. aureus* in a clinical sample is assumed if growth occurs and mannitol is fermented.

Antibiotic Resistance

Perhaps no other species symbolizes the success—as well as the major weakness—of the "antibiotic revolution." Thus, the initial success in the treatment of staphylococcal infections with penicillin was followed very shortly by the realization that these organisms become resistant to this antibiotic. It soon became apparent that as rapidly as new

Table 7–2 ■ Comparison of the human staphylococci

Staphylococcus aureus	Staphylococcus epidermidis
Coagulase-positive	Coagulase-negative
Ferments mannitol	Does not ferment mannitol
DNAse-positive	DNAse-negative
Found in upper nasal pharynx	Found on skin
Pathogenic	Nonpathogenic

antibiotics that inhibited *S. aureus* were put into use, resistant organisms appeared to develop. It is now known that penicillin resistance is often associated with an enzyme, penicillinase, which is coded for by a gene on a plasmid. Studies have established that these plasmids may carry several antibiotic resistant genes and thus have been called resistance transfer factors (RTFs). In staphylococci, these factors may be transferred rapidly among strains by a bacteriophage vector through the process of transduction (see Chapter 3). Thus, although the development of staphylococcal resistance to penicillin was disappointing, it has helped our understanding of microbial genetics, which may aid in controlling bacterial infections, cancer, and other diseases in which genetic changes or anomalies occur.

Bacteriophage Typing

The patterns of lytic specificity between the phage and host have been used as a means of typing the staphylococci. It is generally not necessary to phage type an infection due to *S. aureus*, but every so often there is an outbreak of staphylococcal infection following surgery or in a hospital nursery. These outbreaks can have tragic consequences, and it is essential to determine if the same phage type is causing all the infections. Once this is determined, the carrier is sought by matching the phage types carried by patients or hospital personnel with the types isolated from the infections. (It is usually the hospital personnel who become carriers.) In this way, the carrier can be identified and appropriate isolation procedures taken.

Somatic Antigens

CAPSULES

Polysaccharide capsules that appear to be antiphagocytic have been identified. This slime layer may be associated with the ability of some pathogenic strains to adhere to catheters and other materials and thus to provide a nidus for infection.

TEICHOIC ACIDS

Ribitol Teichoic Acid

Staphylococci have ribitol teichoic acid in their cell walls. The antigenic determinant of these teichoic acids is usually a hexosamine residue. Such hexosamine residues are widely distributed among other bacteria and in eukaryotic cells and thus they may be responsible for the large number of serologic cross-reactions often observed with staphylococcal antisera.

Glycerol Teichoic Acid

The glycerol teichoic acids have the same structure and cytoplasmic membrane association as those found in streptococci. The antigenic determinant is often the same hexosamine that determines the specificity of the cell wall ribitol teichoic acid and this results in some confusion between the two. In strains of *S. epidermidis,* the antigenic determinant of the teichoic acid is glucose.

PROTEIN A

The surface of many staphylococcal strains contains a protein that binds to the Fc region of most IgG subclasses of mammalian species. In humans, all IgG subclasses except IgG3 bind. Most IgM and IgA subclasses except IgG3 are not bound. In addition to these immunochemical interactions, protein A–Fc interactions associated with cell surface can lead to a variety of biologic effects. These include both systemic and local anaphylactic reactions; the latter show the typical wheal and erythema reaction associated with histamine release. Arthus reactions associated with complement activation by both the classic and alternate pathways are also produced by protein A–Fc interactions. Opsonic antibody may be blocked because of competition of protein A for the Fc receptors on phagocytes. It has also been observed that protein A activates B lymphocytes but not T lymphocytes.

BOUND COAGULASE (CLUMPING FACTOR)

If plasma is mixed with staphylococci on a slide, the organisms will agglutinate. This is due to a component similar or identical to coagulase, which in the process of inducing the cross-linking of the fibrinogen chains results in clumping of the bacteria. This can be used as a rapid screening test for the presence of coagulase. However, other or-

ganisms, such as *Streptococcus faecalis,* can also clump in the presence of plasma and therefore the test must be interpreted with caution.

Virulence Factors

COAGULASE

As indicated previously, this enzyme is found in most pathogenic strains of *S. aureus* and causes plasma to clot.

OTHER ENZYMES

These organisms produce hyaluronidase and a fibrinolysin called staphylokinase, which, like its streptococcal counterpart, causes dissolution of fibrin clots. It also produces DNAses and RNAses.

HEMOLYSINS

The staphylococci produce at least four distinct hemolysins, which unfortunately have been labeled with Greek letters and are often confused with the types of hemolysis found in the streptococci. All the hemolysins in the staphylococci cause complete lysis of erythrocytes. The major differences among them involve the kind of erythrocytes they lyse and the conditions under which lysis occurs.

α-Hemolysin

This is the major hemolysin in this organism. It does not lyse human red blood cells but will lyse rabbit erythrocytes; it does affect human platelets.

β-Hemolysin

This is the so-called hot-cold hemolysin and is more commonly found in *S. aureus* strains isolated from animals. It is best observed by placing sheep blood agar plates at 4°C after growth has occurred. After overnight incubation in the cold, the plates are transferred to 37°C for several hours. Zones of hemolysis will often be seen surrounding the golden colonies of staphylococci. In addition to sheep blood, human and guinea pig blood also show this same phenomenon, but these red blood cells are less efficient, apparently owing to the lower content of sphingomyelin in their membranes.

Other Hemolysins

Two other hemolysins, the δ and γ, have been described. In addition, a leukocidin is found in most *S. aureus* strains.

EPIDERMOLYTIC TOXIN

This toxin causes a number of skin lesions. Its activity is associated with cleavage of desmosomes, which connect cells in the lower layers of the epidermis.

ENTEROTOXINS

These are relatively heat-stable and trypsin-resistant toxins produced by 50 percent of *S. aureus* strains. They are one of the major causes of food poisonings associated with the "church picnic" type of syndrome in which pre-prepared foods, such as salads, whipped creams, and so forth, become contaminated with staphylococci which grow and produce toxins if the foods are not kept cold. Within 4 to 6 hours following ingestion of these preformed toxins, the patient exhibit symptoms of diarrhea and nausea, which may last up to 24 hours. In a famous episode at a meeting of the American Society for Microbiology in Chicago in the 1950s, the members were served a Cherries Jubilee dessert at the annual banquet. Despite the fact that this was a flaming dessert, the whipped cream had sat at room temperature for too long. Some time in the early dawn the sudden flushing of hundreds of toilets resulted in a temporary water shortage. In fact, such episodes are not uncommon with this toxin. Fortunately, these types of food poisonings are transient and generally self-limiting with little permanent damage to the individual.

TOXIC SHOCK SYNDROME TOXIN 1 (TSST-1)

Toxic shock syndrome was first reported in 1978 in menstruating women using a particular kind of extra-absorbent tampon. In rather short order, the etiology was determined to be *S. aureus* strains producing a toxin eventually named toxic shock syndrome toxin 1 (TSST-1). In many respects, the toxin resembled one of the types of enterotoxin produced by this species and indeed had originally been named staphylococcal enterotoxin F. Although the exact pathogenesis of the disease is still not clear, it appears that the tampons allowed a more aerobic environment than the less absorbent older variety tampons. This favored the overgrowth of the staphylococci. If TSST-1 is produced, it gives rise to a toxemia that may enhance the activity of endotoxin several thousand times. Since small amounts of endotoxin are nearly always available from the large number of indigenous gram-negative organisms, it is possible that this enhancement may lead to the profound shock and death associated with this disease.

Pathogenesis of Staphylococcal Disease

Although much remains to be known about diseases associated with the staphylococcal toxins, many common staphylococcal diseases appear to be associated with the multiplication and spread of the organism at local sites. Occasionally, if the local infection is particularly severe or if the patient is in poor health, the organism may invade other tissues or enter the bloodstream, leading to a septicemia. The most common local infection is the boil or furuncle, which is associated with the blockage of a sebaceous gland and the overgrowth of the staphylococci in this location. In this small lesion many of the characteristics of the more serious staphylococcal lesions are observed. First and more characteristic of staphylococcal infection is the suppuration which often localizes to form an abscess. The pus consists of necrotic cells that have released their cytoplasmic proteins and of nucleic acids, which cause a viscous consistency and give the exudate its yellowish green color. The wall of fibrin that surrounds the abscess may be due to the release of coagulase from the bacteria. It is noteworthy that in streptococcal infections, in which spreading factors are dominant extracellular products, the infections spread rather than remaining localized. In general, these small boils heal without consequence, but occasionally several boils may coalesce to form a carbuncle, which can be more serious. Sometimes the bacteria spread to bone where they may set up an osteomyelitis (a "furuncle of the osseous medulla"). However, osteomyelitis usually occurs following traumatic wounds—for example, fractures, particularly those of the compound type in which bone is exposed. Staphylococcal wound infections have signs and symptoms similar to those of the local abscess, except that the initiating factor may be a traumatic or a surgically created wound.

The exact role of the various virulence factors (i.e., hemolysins, enzymes, coagulase, and toxins) in these infections is not clear, so that it has not been possible to develop a specific vaccine against this disease. Indeed, it appears that most of us have relatively high antibody titers against many of the components found in staphylococci, yet few of us appear immune to the various diseases caused by this organism. Herein lies the danger and the challenge, since it is most discouraging to observe patients developing a staphylococcal infection following what appears to be successful surgery.

Treatment

As indicated previously, laboratory diagnosis is relatively easy, since the presence of gram-positive, catalase-positive cocci, in bunches, that ferment mannitol and produce coagulase, establishes the diagnosis of an *S. aureus* wound infection. It is obviously essential to establish antibiotic susceptibility of the strain, as this may be the key aspect of successful therapy. Antibiotic resistant strains are ubiquitous, particularly in hospital populations. In general until the exact antibiotic sensitivities are established, the synthetic penicillins (i.e., methicillin or oxacillin), which are not hydrolyzed by penicillinase, may be used. Alternatively, many clinicians start with the cephalosporin type of antibiotic. Whatever the final choice, the therapy must be intensive. Drainage should be established as soon as the suppuration is evident, since these lesions do not respond to antibiotic therapy alone.

chapter 8

Genus Actinomyces *and other* filamentous bacteria

Richard P. Ellen, D.D.S.

Members of the genus *Actinomyces* and other gram-positive filamentous bacteria in the family *Actinomycetaceae* are common within the indigenous microflora colonizing the mouths of humans and various other animals. Interest in these bacteria derives from their amphipathic relationship with the host. They are commensals that usually co-exist peacefully with their hosts, but, under some conditions, they emerge as opportunistic pathogens involved in infections of both soft tissues and teeth. Of the oral *Actinomycetaceae*, the genus *Actinomyces* has been studied the most thoroughly in terms of taxonomy, pathogenicity, natural ecology, and interbacterial relationships within the oral microbial community.

Taxonomy

The oral gram-positive filamentous bacteria have an entangled history in all three interrelated areas of taxonomy: classification, nomenclature, and identification. The inclusion in the family *Actinomycetaceae* of major genera and species has changed considerably over the years, depending on the criteria used for clustering or separating clinical isolates. Confusion with fungi by pathologists and use of the name "Actinomyces" as an erroneous descriptor for aerobic *Streptomyces* in some countries persists even today. Freshly isolated gram-positive filaments are often difficult to assign beyond genus level, especially when trying to keep the number of laboratory tests to a minimum. Attempts will be made in this chapter to present a simplified taxonomy, citing historic references only to clarify points of interest. Emphasis will be placed on the genus *Actinomyces* when examples and illustrations are presented.

CLASSIFICATION AND NOMENCLATURE

Members of the family *Actinomycetaceae* have many features in common. They are all gram-positive, nonmotile, non–acid-fast, non–spore-forming bacilli with a tendency to grow as branched filaments in tissues and under some laboratory conditions. They often demonstrate polymorphism; one gram-stained smear may contain cells of different shapes—filaments mixed with diphtheroids, short rods, or even coccobacilli. This can be very confusing to novice microbiologists who should follow the recommendation to sub-culture single colonies of a new isolate several times prior to confirming it as a pure culture. *Actinomycetaceae* genera all ferment carbohydrates. A rather obvious comon trait is that all members of *Actinomycetaceae* are true bacteria with the following characteristics distinguishing them from fungi:

1. They are prokaryotic.
2. They have typical bacterial cell wall composition, lacking chitin.
3. Although they may branch, branching cells have a similar diameter; they do not produce aerial hyphae.
4. They are sensitive to antibiotics that are active against bacteria.

Why, then, the name "Actinomyces," which means "ray fungus"? The name was chosen more than 100 years ago as a metaphor describing the histopathologic appearance of debris from soft tissue lesions caused by these infectious agents. Regulations governing microbial nomenclature honor precedent; thus, the name "Actinomyces" remains, even though it is literally inaccurate.

Clustering members of this family into species by overall similarity or separating them by their degree of difference has been an ever-changing exercise influenced a great deal by available technology. The current classification scheme reflects a composite that evolved mostly from a dizzying array of microbiologic tests of physiologic traits, serology, and acid end-product analysis. Recently, analysis of cell wall chemistry, total protein profiles, DNA homology, and the use of computer-assisted numerical taxonomy to cluster the findings for isolates into a managable expression of degree of similarity has greatly influenced classification. Currently, *Actinomycetaceae* is composed of the five genera listed in Table 8–1: *Actinomyces, Arachnia, Bifidobacterium, Bacterionema,* and *Rothia*. Only two of these genera, *Actinomyces* and *Bifidobacterium*, currently contain more than one species (Table 8–2).

Genus *Actinomyces* contains six species (see Table 8–1). *Actinomyces bovis, A. israelii,* and *A. meyeri* are considered strictly anaerobic; *A. naeslundii, A. viscosus,* and *A. odontolyticus* are facultatively anaerobic but often grow better on primary isolation under anaerobic conditions or in an environment with high levels of CO_2. *A. israelii* can be further divided into two serotypes. *A. naeslundii* and human isolates of *A. viscosus* are so similar by standard microbiologic tests (except for catalase activity, for which *A. viscosus* is positive) and by virtue of their similar cell wall structure and

Table 8–1 ■ Classification and identification of genera in *Actinomycetaceae*

Genus	Species	Growth Environment	Acid End Products
Actinomyces*	bovis israelii meyeri	Anaerobic	Acetic Lactic Succinic
	naeslundii viscosus odontolyticus	Facultatively anaerobic	
Arachnia†	propionica	Anaerobic	Acetic Propionic Succinic
Bifidobacterium†	24 species	Anaerobic	Acetic Lactic
Bacterionema†	matruchotii	Facultatively anaerobic	Acetic Propionic Lactic Formic
Rothia	dentocariosa	Aerobic	Acetic Lactic Succinic

*Recent proposals would add three species: *A. howellii* and *A. hordeovulneris*, which, like *A. bovis*, are indigenous to nonhuman animal species, and *A. pyogenes*, a reclassification of *Corynebacterium pyogenes*.

†These genera are classified in *Actinomycetaceae* because they demonstrate branching during laboratory cultivation. Proposals have been raised to move them to other families:

Arachnia → *Propionibacteriaceae*
Bifidobacterium → *Lactobacillaceae*
Bacterionema → *Corynebacteriaceae* or *Mycobacteriaceae*

Table 8–2 ■ Filament facts

Actinomyces bovis—Not isolated from human mouth
    —Associated with "lumpy jaw" (actinomycosis) in cattle
A. israelii—Isolated from human plaque, calculus, tonsillar crypts
    —Associated with most cases of human actinomycosis
    —Increased proportions in plaque under nonhygienic conditions
    —Recently shown to coaggregate with *Cytophaga*, gram-negative gliding bacteria
A. odontolyticus—Despite name, role in caries etiology has not been established
    —Requires serum for growth; forms reddish colonies on blood agar
    —Found in dental plaque, but no specific relationship to disease established
A. naeslundii—Preferentially colonizes tongue and other mucosal surfaces
    —Can colonize oral cavity prior to tooth eruption
    —Induces periodontal disease and root caries in animals
    —Adheres to mucosal cells and oral streptococci via type 2 fibril-borne lectin specific for β-galactosides
    —Associated with some cases of actinomycosis
A. viscosus—Only catalase-positive member of genus *Actinomyces*
    —Preferentially colonizes teeth
    —Does not often colonize predentate infants
    —Induces periodontal lesions and root caries in animals
    —Numerical association with human gingivitis
    —Influences gingival inflammatory response via several pathways
    —Prevalent in established human root caries, but also on noncarious surfaces
    —Adheres to pellicle via type 1 fibrils and to epithelial cells and oral streptococci by type 2 fibril-associated lectin
A. meyeri—Previously classified in genus *Actinobacterium*
    —Isolated from plaque, but association with disease not established
Arachnia propionica—Produces propionic acid; cell wall has diaminopimelic acid
    —Some taxonomists have proposed moving *Arachnia* to family *Propionibacteriaceae*
    —Associated with some cases of human actinomycosis
Bifidobacterium spp.—Isolated from dental plaque and from deep dentinal carious lesions
    —Not known to be associated with etiology of any oral diseases
    —"Bifid" morphology helps to differentiate from anaerobic lactobacilli
Bacterionema matruchotii—Isolated from dental plaque
    —Not known to be associated with etiology of dental diseases
    —Long filaments with short, thick terminal bacillus yields characteristic "whip handle" morphology
    —Composes central filament of "corn-cob" formations (*S. sanguis* cells bound to *B. matruchotii*) at salivary interface of supragingival plaque
    —Has been used to study bacterial calcification and calculus formation
Rothia dentocariosa—Despite name, role in caries etiology doubtful
    —Commonly isolated from dental plaque and root caries
    —Aerobic
    —Highly pleomorphic; often cocci mixed with filaments
    —Has been shown to induce gingival inflammation in laboratory rodents

serologic cross-reactivity that merger into one species has been suggested. However, on the basis of some distinct surface antigens, incomplete DNA homology, separation into distinct clusters by numerical taxonomy, and a recently demonstrated difference in total protein profiles, the maintenance of two separate species containing subgroups reflecting serotype specificity seems warranted (Fig. 8–1). It is interesting to note that by the criteria of serology, DNA homology, and numerical taxonomy, *Actinomyces viscosus* strains isolated from the mouths of rodents bear little relation to isolates from humans. However, rodent isolates have priority for the designation *A. viscosus* ("viscosus" because they grow as a cohesive slime) by being the first to be described under this name. They had originally been described in a new but now defunct genus *Odontomyces* ("odonto" meaning tooth; "myces" from "Actinomyces").

IDENTIFICATION

Appropriate classification finds its clinical significance in identification of new isolates and determination of their association with health status. Optimally, identification is the use of a minimum number of rapid tests, which allows assignment to a given species in the classification scheme. A combination of acid end-product analysis, serology, and a few biochemical tests is usually sufficient to identify these bacteria to genus level. However, at species level, fresh isolates of

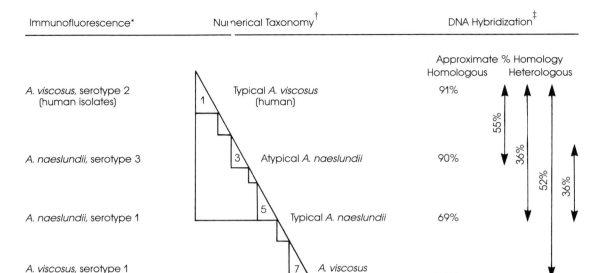

Figure 8–1 ■ Comparison of three *Actinomyces viscosus* and *A. naeslundii* classification schemes based on serology,* numerical taxonomy,† and DNA homology.‡
*Adapted from Slack, J. M., and Gerencser, M. A.: Actinomyces, Filamentous Bacteria. Biology and Pathogenicity. Burgess Publishing, Minneapolis, 1975.
†Adapted from Fillery, E. D., et al.: A comparison of strains of bacteria designated *Actinomyces viscosus* and *Actinomyces naeslundii*. Caries Res 12:299, 1978.
‡Adapted from Coykendall, A. L., and Munzenmaier, A. J.: Deoxyribonucleic acid hybridization among strains of *Actinomyces viscosus* and *Actinomyces naeslundii*. Int J Syst Bacteriol 29:234, 1979.

oral gram-positive rods frequently challenge the concept of easy identification because their response in microbiologic tests is so wide-ranging, and the classification defining species relies on a combination of "chemotaxonomic" methods. Gas chromatography of acid end products of glucose metabolism is often essential (see Table 8–1). For example, it is difficult to differentiate *Actinomyces israelii* from *Arachnia propionica* by typical bench microbiology tests, although they are classified in separate genera. They are best differentiated by acid end-product analysis. Both produce acetic and succinic acids, but *A. propionica* also produces propionic acid (hence its name), while *A. israelii*, like all *Actinomyces* species, produces lactic acid. Chemical analysis of cell wall sugars is also useful; diaminopimelic acid is found in *A. propionica* but not in *A. israelii* walls. Members of *Actinomycetaceae* must also be differentiated from other gram-positive bacilli, which are not members of this family, including some genera that are morphologically and metabolically rather similar ((*Propionibacterium, Corynebacterium, Eubacterium*).

One of the fastest and surest identification methods for this group is the use of serology, especially by fluorescence microscopy. Immunofluorescence reagents can discriminate among genera and among serotypes within the genus *Actinomyces*. Figure 8–2 is an example of a positive test result, which also demonstrates typical *Actinomyces* cell morphology. The identification scheme of Slack and Gerencser, which uses specific antisera prepared by absorbing out problematic cross-reacting antibodies, has received wide acceptance. Antibody-mediated bacterial agglutination tests are also accurate for intergeneric identification and identification of major *A. viscosus* and *A. naeslundii* subgroups based on more laborious numerical taxonomy and DNA homology. It is interesting to note the degree of agreement among different approaches for grouping *A. viscosus* and *A. naeslundii* (Fig. 8–1).

Pathogenicity

ACTINOMYCOSIS

Of the *Actinomyces* species described, all but *A. bovis* are prevalent in the human oral cavity. They are often isolated in significant levels from dental plaque and calculus, as well as from the tongue, tonsils, and other soft tissues. Opportunistic infections may arise following traumatic injury and the in-

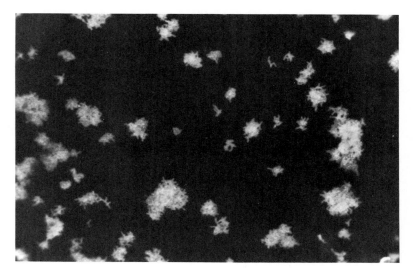

Figure 8–2 ■ Example of typical *Actinomyces* morphology in a positive immunofluorescence test.

troduction of contaminated debris into the tissues. Actinomycosis is a chronic, granulomatous, soft tissue infection with foci of abscesses and suppuration through draining sinuses. It is most common in the cervicofacial region (Fig. 8–3), draining intraorally or through the skin of the face or neck. Actinomycosis can also affect the lower respiratory tract via aspiration or inhalation of contaminated material from the mouth and may occasionally affect the abdomen following surgical or accidental trauma. Actinomycetes have also been isolated from persistent infections of the urogenital tract of some women who use intrauterine birth control devices. Actinomycosis is not a common disease, but it can be fatal.

In addition to the clinical appearance and case history, examination of draining pus for so-called sulfur granules helps to establish a tentative diagnosis of actinomycosis. The gross appearance of these granules, as seen under low-power magnification, is an irregularly shaped, yellowish mass of radiating filaments. Under high-power magnification, filaments and club-shaped extensions are clearly evident (Fig. 8–4). Infected tissues should be biopsied, sectioned, and stained for histopathologic assessment. Such preparations usually contain the granules, digested cellular debris, and mixed populations of polymorphonuclear leukocytes and lymphocytes, surrounded by fibrous connective tissue. Diagnosis of actinomycosis should be confirmed by cultivation or by immunofluorescence. For the sake of clarity, "sulfur gran-

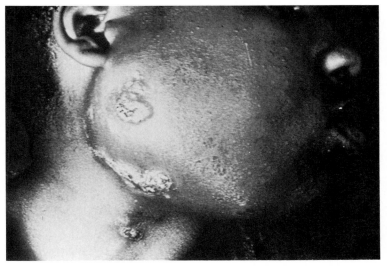

Figure 8–3 ■ Human cervicofacial actinomycosis.

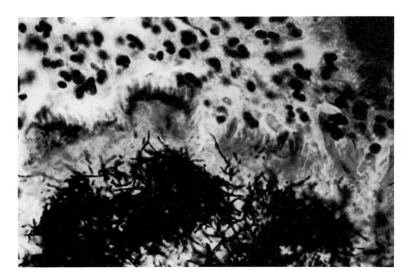

Figure 8–4 ■ Microscopic appearance of a sulfur granule obtained from a human actinomycotic lesion.

ules,'' despite their yellow color, are likely devoid of significant sulfur and their ''ray fungus''–appearing filaments are bacteria.

Actinomycosis lesions often contain a mixed microflora. By far, the most common species is *Actinomyces israelii*, but some lesions yield *A. naeslundii*, *A. viscosus*, or *Arachnia propionica*. *Actinomyces bovis* causes similar infections in cattle. Along with anaerobic streptococci, gram-negative bacteria have been isolated from mixed actinomycotic lesions; the most common are pigmented *Bacteroides* and *Actinobacillus actinomycetemcomitans*—this significant periodontal pathogen was named for its actinomycosis connection! The relative contribution of the individual species to pathogenicity of mixed actinomycosis infections has not been clearly established, but their common colonization of teeth and periodontal pockets suggests an intraoral reservoir for infecting other tissues. It should not be surprising that trauma to the teeth or jaws and bite wounds are often the opportunistic events predisposing to actinomycosis. Treatment of actinomycosis is often difficult and protracted because the mixed flora massed in the center of the ''sulfur granules'' is relatively ''protected'' from host defenses. Surgical excision and drainage is usually required, as well as extended antibiotic therapy, usually with drugs in the penicillin family.

Very little is known of the pathogenesis of actinomycosis, but it has been suggested that *A. israelii* may suppress some immunity functions which, in turn, may favor chronicity. Likewise, little is known of the intraoral ecology of *A. israelii* other than its enrichment in anaerobic environments such as periodontal pockets and thick supragingival plaques associated with gingivitis. Aside from recent reports that strains of *A. israelii* adhere to enamel and cementum, and that they coaggregate with oral *Cytophaga* strains, there has been no concerted effort to study factors favoring its establishment in the mouth or its mode of transmission among humans.

PERIODONTAL DISEASES

As a group, the gram-positive filamentous rods increase in proportion relative to other bacteria in the microflora soon after cessation of oral hygiene practices. Thus, they have the opportunity, along with other bacteria in early plaque, to stimulate inflammatory responses in the gingiva. Yet, because fluctuations in their subgingival populations (along with other gram-positive bacteria) are usually inversely related to the severity of destructive periodontal lesions in the adjacent tissues, they are not considered among the highly pathogenic species involved in progressive periodonitis in humans.

Actinomyces viscosus is the only member of this group to be studied in depth for its periodontal pathogenic potential, probably because it was originally isolated from, and shown to be responsible for, naturally occurring transmissible periodontitis in laboratory rodents (Fig. 8–5). However, very few potential virulence traits that might account for direct tissue damage have been documented for this species. It produces few potent proteolytic or other hydrolytic enzymes; its acid

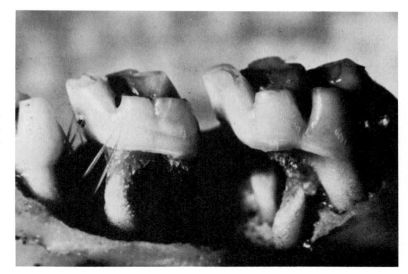

Figure 8–5 ■ Periodontitis and root surface caries induced experimentally by *A. viscosus* infection.

end products are not significantly more toxic than those of other bacteria; and it does not produce volatile sulfur-containing compounds like hydrogen sulfide or methyl mercaptan. In contrast, the evidence is very strong that *A. viscosus* can stimulate an inflammatory response, leading to tissue damage indirectly (Table 8–3). The fact that humans demonstrate elevated levels of *A. viscosus* and simultaneously elevated hypersensitivity reactions specific for *A. viscosus* antigens during the onset of experimental gingivitis probably means that it is involved in the etiology of gingivitis and, possibly, of mild cases of periodontitis.

Gram-positive bacteria, like *A. viscosus*, may also be involved in the sequence of events leading to more rapidly destructive periodontitis by creating an environment suitable for outgrowth of more virulent gram-negative species. The cartoon in Figure 8–6 illustrates this point. It is well known that the environment in dental plaque becomes more anaerobic with time because of utilization of oxygen by bacteria. *Actinomyces viscosus* is also known to promote adhesion of the periodontal pathogen *Bacteroides gingivalis* to dental plaque and to produce succinate, a growth-stimulating factor for *B. gingivalis*. Moreover, the increased bleeding and pocket depth occurring via the inflammatory response also encourages the emergence of fastidious, gram-negative anaerobes.

DENTAL ROOT SURFACE CARIES

Filamentous bacteria are very numerous in supragingival root surface plaques and plaques overlying established carious lesions on roots. While these bacteria have little coronal cariogenic activity in experimental animals, *A. viscosus* and *A. naeslundii* strains isolated from human root decay have been shown repeatedly to induce root surface caries in laboratory rodents (see Fig. 8–5). *A. viscosus* ferments sugars, yielding acid end products, and isolates from root lesions store intracellular polysaccharides, which may contribute to prolonged acid release. However, *A. viscosus* is not as rapidly acidogenic as *Streptococcus mutans*, a known cariogenic species, when grown on a variety of dietary carbohydrates (Fig. 8–7). Although *A. viscosus* is considered to be a principal root caries pathogen, its frequent isolation from caries-

---

Table 8–3 ■ Mechanisms by which *Actinomyces viscosus* affects periodontal health

Elaborates factors chemotactic for polymorphonuclear leukocytes.
Causes release of hydrolytic enzymes from leukocytes and
  macrophages.
Alters fibroblast function.
Mitogenically stimulates lymphocytes (polyclonal activator).
Antigenically stimulates host hypersensitivity.
Stimulates osteoclastic bone resorption.

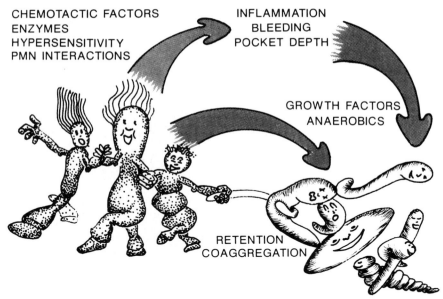

Figure 8–6 ■ Direct and indirect ways by which *A. viscosus* and other gram-positive bacteria promote the emergence of virulent gram-negative bacteria in the periodontal microflora.

free root surfaces renders it a poor choice as a microbiologic marker for assessing patients' root caries risk or for monitoring success of preventive or therapeutic measures.

Ecology of Actinomyces viscosus *and* A. naeslundii

ESTABLISHMENT AND DISTRIBUTION

In contrast to the paucity of information on the oral ecology of *A. israelii* and *A.*

odontolyticus, much is known about *A. viscosus* and *A. naeslundii* owing to the interest generated by their frequent isolation from humans and demonstrated periodontal pathogenicity in laboratory animals. Figure 8–8 illustrates the host age at which these species establish in the human mouth, relative to some of the oral streptococci. Although almost identical in their physiologic traits and nutrient requirements, *A. viscosus* and *A. naeslundii* differ in the host age at which they appear in the mouth and in the surfaces that they preferentially colonize. *A. naeslundii* col-

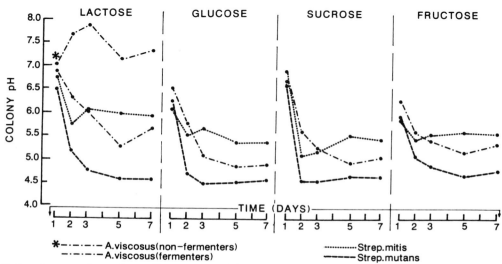

Figure 8–7 ■ Comparative colony pH responses of *A. viscosus* and oral streptococci to dietary carbohydrates. (From Ellen, R. P., and Onose, H.: Arch Oral Biol 23:105, 1978.)

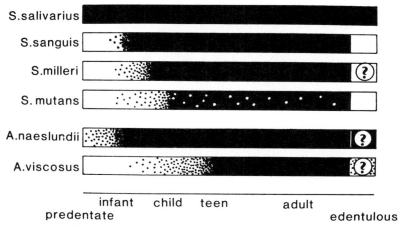

Figure 8–8 ■ Comparative oral isolation frequencies for *A. viscosus, A. naeslundii,* and oral streptococci during the human lifespan. Solid black bars represent virtually 100 per cent carrier state in the population. (From Ellen, R. P.: Oral colonization by Gram-positive bacteria significant to periodontal disease. In Genco, R. J., and Mergenhagen, S. E. [eds.]: Host-Parasite Interactions in Periodontal Diseases. ASM Publications, Washington, DC, 1982, pp 98–111, with permission.)

onizes the tongue more readily and usually accounts for a greater proportion of the salivary microflora than *A. viscosus.* Therefore, conditions favor its intraoral establishment prior to tooth eruption. In contrast, *A. viscosus* colonizes teeth more efficiently than mucosal surfaces. Thus, establishment is often delayed until after teeth erupt and even longer, depending on the effective dose transmitted by saliva of individuals with whom the child has contact. These colonization differences are relative in that, in adults, *A. naeslundii* does colonize teeth and *A. viscosus* colonizes mucosal surfaces, but not to the same extent. Differences in their colonization patterns probably reflect their relative abilities to attach to differing receptors on the various surfaces of the mouth.

SURFACE PROPERTIES AND ADHERENCE

Although *A. viscosus* strains have been found to synthesize capsules of both fructan and heteropolysaccharide types, such extracellular polymers do not appear to function in adhesion. Both *A. viscosus* and *A. naeslundii* elaborate long surface appendages termed *fibrils,* or *fimbriae* (Fig. 8–9). These are composed almost entirely of proteins, and they carry some of the antigens that differentiate the two species. The fibrils help foster the attachment of *A. viscosus* and *A. naeslundii* to host surfaces and to other bacteria in dental plaque. Although morphologically similar, two types of distinct populations of fibrils have been described immunochemically and functionally. Type 1 is likely involved in

Figure 8–9 ■ Electron photomicrograph of shadow cast *A. viscosus* cell. The long fibrils are clearly evident. (From Masuda, N., Ellen, R. P., and Grove, D. A.: J Bacteriol 147:1095, 1981.)

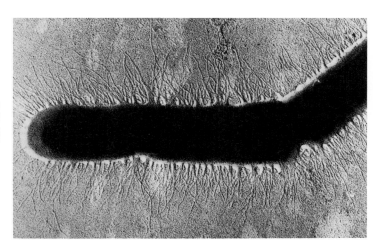

adherence to salivary pellicle coating the teeth. Recent work suggests that proline-rich proteins with affinity for hydroxyapatite may serve as its pellicle receptor. Type 2 functions in *Actinomyces* interactions with host epithelial and red blood cell membranes as well as with other bacteria such as various streptococci. Type 2 fibrils carry a protein that functions as a lectin with specific binding recognition for oligosaccharides terminating in beta-linked galactose. Target galactosides in membrane glycoproteins or glycolipids are often in a position penultimate to sialic acids; *A. viscosus* and *A. naeslundii* can actually promote their own adherence by producing sialidases to cleave the sialic acid, thereby exposing the beta-linked galactosides. Relative abilities to bind to oral surfaces may reflect differences in the distribution of type 1 and type 2 fibrils on *A. viscosus* and *A. naeslundii* cell surfaces. There is some evidence that typical *A. naeslundii* strains are less well fimbriated and are devoid of type 1 fibrils, rendering them inefficient in binding to salivary pellicle. The fibril composition on atypical *A. naeslundii* (serotype 3, see Fig. 8–1) is more closely related to *A. viscosus*, and both of these adhere efficiently to salivary pellicle.

ADDITIONAL READING

Bowden, G. H., and Hardie, J. M.: Commensal and pathogenic *Actinomyces* species in man. In Sykes, G., and Skinner, F. A. (eds): *Actinomycetales*: Characteristics and Practical Importance. Academic Press, New York, 1973.

Bowden, G. H., Hardie, J. M., and Fillery, E. D.: Antigens from *Actinomyces* species and their value in identification. J. Dent. Res. 55(special issue A): 192, 1976.

Cisar, J. O., Sandberg, A. L., and Mergenhagen, S. E.: The function and distribution of different fimbriae on strains of *Actinomyces viscosus* and *Actinomyces naeslundii*. J. Dent. Res. 63:393, 1984.

Clark, W. B.: *Actinomyces* fimbriae and adherence to hydroxyapatite. In Mergenhagen, S. E., and Rosan, B. (eds): Molecular Basis of Oral Microbial Adhesion. American Society of Microbiologists, Washington, DC, 1985.

Coykendall, A. L., and Munzenmaier, A. J.: Deoxyribonucleic acid hybridization among strains of *Actinomyces viscosus* and *Actinomyces naeslundii*. Int. J. Syst. Bacteriol. 29:234, 1979.

Ellen, R. P.: Oral colonization by Gram-positive bacteria significant to periodontal disease. In Genco, R. J., and Mergenhagen, S. E. (eds.): Host-Parasite Interactions in Periodontal Diseases. American Society of Microbiologists, Washington, DC, 1982.

Fillery, E. D., Bowden, G. H., and Hardie, J. M.: A comparison of strains of bacteria designated *Actinomyces viscosus* and *Actinomyces naeslundii*. Caries Res. 12:299, 1978.

Goodfellow, M., Mordarski, M., and Williams, S. T.: The Biology of the Actinomycetes. Academic Press, London, 1984.

Holmberg, K., and Nord, C.-E.: Numerical taxonomy and laboratory identification of *Actinomyces* and *Arachnia* and some related bacteria. J. Gen. Microbiol. 91:17, 1975.

Howell, A., Jordan, H. V., George, L. K., and Pine, L.: *Odontomyces viscosus*, gen. nov., spec. nov.: A filamentous microorganism isolated from periodontal plaque in hamsters. Sabouraudia 4:65, 1965.

Jordan, H. V., and Keyes, P. H.: Studies on the bacteriology of hamster periodontal diseases. Am. J. Pathol. 46:843, 1965.

Pine, L., and George, L. K.: Classification and phylogenetic relationship of microaerophilic actinomycetes. Int. J. Syst. Bacteriol. 20:445, 1970.

Rǎsić, J. L., and Kurman, J. A.: Bifidobacteria and Their Role. Experientia Supplementum, Vol. 39, Birkhäuser Verlag, Basel, 1983.

Schofield, G. M., and Schaal, K. P.: A numerical taxonomy study of members of the *Actinomycetaceae* and related taxa. J. Gen. Microbiol. 127:237, 1981.

Slack, J. M., and Gerencser, M. A.: *Actinomyces*, Filamentous Bacteria. Biology and Pathogenicity. Burgess Publishing, Minneapolis, 1975.

van der Hoeven, J. S.: The role of *Actinomyces viscosus* in dental plaque. Ecological and biochemical aspects. Thesis. University of Nijmegen, Nijmegen, The Netherlands, 1974.

chapter 9

Haemophilus and Pasteurella

Thomas V. Potts, D.D.S., Ph.D.

CHAPTER OUTLINE

- THE GENUS HAEMOPHILUS
- THE GENUS PASTEURELLA

The Genus Haemophilus

The name "haemophilus" is Greek for "blood-lover" and is derived from the observation that most organisms in this genus require one or two growth factors which are present in blood (Table 9–1). The factors supplied by blood were originally termed X factor and V factor, and have subsequently been identified—X factor is protoporphyrin IX or protoheme, and V factor is nicotinamide adenine dinucleotide (NAD). The only *Haemophilus* species that can grow in the absence of X and V factors are *Haemophilus aphrophilus* and *Haemophilus actinomycetemcomitans* (previously *Actinobacillus actinomycetemcomitans* [see Chapter 17]).

Bacteria from the genus *Haemophilus* are gram-negative, nonmotile, short rods or coccobacilli, which may become pleomorphic and form long filaments, especially under poor growth conditions. All *Haemophilus* species can reduce nitrates and ferment carbohydrates. The ecologic niche of these organisms is primarily the mucous membranes of a variety of animal species where they occur as obligate parasites. The proportion of guanine plus cytosine in the DNA of these organisms has been measured in the range of 35 to 44 percent (Table 9–2).

Virtually all saliva samples and over 95 per cent of supragingival and subgingival dental plaque samples harbor some haemophili. The five species of haemophili commonly found in the human oral cavity include *Haemophilus parainfluenzae, Haemophilus aphrophilus, Haemophilus paraphrophilus,* "*Haemophilus actinomycetemcomitans,*" and *Haemophilus segnis. Haemophilus influenzae* is occasionally also isolated from oral specimens; however, it is primarily a resident of the nasopharynx (Table 9–2).

H. actinomycetemcomitans, H. aphrophilus, H. paraphrophilus, and *H. segnis* are significantly interrelated as measured by DNA-DNA homology (Table 9–3) and occupy the same ecologic site in dental plaque.

The presence of haemophili in dental plaque is inversely related to the presence of dark-pigmented bacteroides and spirochetes. Plaque containing a high proportion of either dark-pigmented *Bacteroides* species or spirochetes virtually never contains a high proportion of haemophili. While this observation has not been completely explained, the *Haemophilus* species are facultative anaerobes in contrast to the spirochetes and *Bacteroides* species, which are obligate anaerobes. As a result, the facultative and obligate anaerobes might be expected to occupy somewhat different ecologic niches.

Table 9–1 ■ Haemophili growth requirements and enzymatic activity

Species	X Factor Requirement	V Factor Requirement	Catalase	Oxidase
H. actinomycetemcomitans	−	−	+	−
H. aphrophilus	−	−	−	−
H. paraphrophilus	−	+	−	−
H. influenzae	+	+	+	
H. aegyptius	+	+	+	
H. parainfluenzae	−	+	+	+
H. segnis	−	+	+	−
H. ducreyi	+	−	−	+

HAEMOPHILUS APHROPHILUS AND H. PARAPHROPHILUS

H. aphrophilus and *H. paraphrophilus* are very closely related organisms, as evidenced by DNA-DNA homologies in excess of 70 percent (Table 9–3). The differentiating characteristic is the requirement for V factor by *H. paraphrophilus* (see Table 9–1). *H. aphrophilus* and *H. paraphrophilus* are isolated infrequently from smooth surface plaques and saliva. Plaque formation by these organisms occurs readily in vitro and is not dependent on the presence of sucrose or the production of extracellular polysaccharides. The causes of adhesion and aggregation of these organisms are not known.

H. aphrophilus infections of medical importance are relatively rare, with the vast majority of these diagnosed as either endocarditis or brain abscess. In patients with endocarditis, a significant number were reported to have undergone dental treatment prior to the onset of symptoms. The most common predisposing conditions were rheumatic heart disease and valvular lesions. Many of these infections are fatal, with a 27 per cent mortality rate.

HAEMOPHILUS SEGNIS

Haemophilus segnis is very similar to *H. parainfluenzae* on the basis of morphologic and biochemical criteria (see Table 9–1). However, DNA-DNA hybridization has shown that these organisms are not closely related (Table 9–3). *H. segnis* isolates make up a substantial fraction of the haemophili found in mature dental plaque but are infrequently isolated from either saliva or early dental plaque (Table 9–4). This organism fails to form plaque in vitro, and the factors determining its association with mature smooth surface plaques are unknown.

H. segnis has recently been described and differentiated from *H. parainfluenzae*. Consequently, there are little data regarding its involvement in human disease. It is not known to be associated with any dental diseases.

HAEMOPHILUS ACTINOMYCETEMCOMITANS (PREVIOUSLY ACTINOBACILLUS ACTINOMYCETEMCOMITANS)

H. actinomycetemcomitans is found as part of the normal flora of the oral cavity in up to 36 percent of the population. It is routinely isolated from supragingival plaque and from subgingival plaque, and may be found attached to the buccal mucosa. *H. actinomycetemcomitans* does not require X or V factors and, unlike *H. aphrophilus*, is catalase-positive (see Table 9–1).

Table 9–2 ■ Primary site of isolation and DNA comparisons

Species	Site	DNA % Guanine + Cytosine
H. actinomycetemcomitans	Dental plaque	45–47
H. aphrophilus	Dental plaque	43–44
H. paraphrophilus	Dental plaque	43–44
H. segnis	Saliva and dental plaque	39–40
H. influenzae	Nasopharynx	39–40
H. aegyptius	Conjunctiva	39–40
H. parainfluenzae	Saliva and dental plaque	35–38
H. ducreyi	Genitalia	38

Table 9–3 ■ Homology of Haemophilus species

Species	% Homology Determined With DNA Probes to		
	Parainfluenzae	Actinomycetemcomitans	Aphrophilus
H. parainfluenzae	70–100	12–16	15
H. actinomycetemcomitans	5–9	69–100	30–39
H. aphrophilus	10–16	30–35	90–100
H. paraphrophilus	11–12	32–37	73–77
H. segnis	9–14	31	34
H. influenzae	7–17	6–9	6

H. actinomycetemcomitans has been frequently isolated from actinomycotic lesions of bone where it is usually a component of a mixed infection with *Actinomyces israelii* (hence the name "actinomycetemcomitans" which means "with actinomyces"). H. actinomycetemcomitans is occasionally isolated from cases of endocarditis and brain abscess, where it is thought to spread from the oral cavity by hematogenous dissemination. Most cases of *H. actinomycetemcomitans* endocarditis occur in subjects with rheumatic heart disease or heart valve replacements.

H. actinomycetemcomitans is frequently isolated from human dental plaque, where it is readily distinguished from the closely related organism, *H. aphrophilus*, by its ability to decompose hydrogen peroxide (catalase-positive). *H. actinomycetemcomitans* has been found in larger numbers in subgingival plaque than in supragingival plaque and is not commonly isolated from saliva. The subgingival plaque from patients with juvenile periodontitis usually contains high numbers of this organism, and there is considerable evidence that *H. actinomycetemcomitans* may play an important role in this disease (see Chapter 28).

Table 9–4 ■ Haemophili in saliva and plaque

Species*	% Haemophili in Saliva†	% Haemophili in Mature Plaque‡
H. parainfluenzae	85	57
H. segnis	9	33
H. influenzae	2	0
H. aphrophilus	0	7
H. paraphrophilus	2	3

*Total haemophili did not include *H. actinomycetemcomitans* in this analysis.

†Haemophili comprised 10% of total salivary anaerobes.

‡Haemophili comprised 2% of total plaque anaerobes.

HAEMOPHILUS PARAINFLUENZAE

H. parainfluenzae is the most ubiquitous of the oral haemophili. It is the only species of haemophili routinely isolated from saliva, where it constitutes about 10 percent of the anaerobic flora. In one study, *H. parainfluenzae* accounted for 85 percent of the haemophili isolated from salivary samples, and for 57 percent of the haemophili found in mature dental plaque (Table 9–4). Haemophili, however, represent only 2 percent of the total anaerobic flora found in mature dental plaque. When smooth-surface plaque was allowed to accumulate for 18 hours, the proportion of haemophili in this early plaque was significantly higher than in mature dental plaque, but still represented only 10 percent of the cultivable anaerobic flora.

H. parainfluenzae is of medical importance in the etiology of bacterial endocarditis. It is not associated with any dental diseases. The widespread prevalence of *H. parainfluenzae* in the oral microflora may reflect its affinity for salivary glycoproteins, and indeed, the presence of neuraminidase may play a role in the adhesion of these organisms to the sialic acid residues found on salivary glycoproteins.

HAEMOPHILUS INFLUENZAE

Haemophilus influenzae is the most medically significant species of haemophili. In the United States, it is the most common cause of meningitis during the first 4 years of life and is frequently associated with epiglottitis in children between 2 and 7 years of age.

There are six antigenic types of *Haemophilus influenzae* capsular carbohydrates (a, b, c, d, e, f). Only the encapsulated form of the serotype b organism is commonly associated with meningitis and epiglottitis. The other five capsulated types are rarely pathogenic. Nonencapsulated forms of *H. influenzae* are common in the upper respiratory tract and should be regarded as part of the normal nasopharyngeal flora. They are, however, commonly associated with acute exacerbations of chronic bronchitis.

Haemophilus influenzae is occasionally isolated from the oral cavity, probably as a contaminant from the nasopharynx. The high degree of ecologic specificity exhibited by this organism may be related to its high affinity for glycoproteins of the respiratory mucosa.

HAEMOPHILUS AEGYPTIUS

Haemophilus aegyptius is the name traditionally given to all haemophili isolated from the conjunctiva. However, this species is difficult to distinguish from *H. influenzae,* and on the basis of genetic data should be placed within the same species. Many of the conjunctival isolates do possess hemagglutinating activity and are more fastidious and slower growing than *H. influenzae. H. aegyptius* is the causative agent for purulent conjunctivitis and is associated with epidemic conjunctivitis in warmer climates.

HAEMOPHILUS DUCREYI

H. ducreyi is the causative agent for the venereal disease soft chancre, which is endemic in parts of the world. However, the clinical and epidemiologic investigation of this disease has been hampered by the stringent growth requirements of this organism. *H. ducreyi* requires blood for growth, and recovery is improved by the addition of fetal calf serum.

The lesions of soft chancre (chancroid) consist of ulcerations on the genitalia accompanied by swelling and tenderness. A marked regional lymphadenopathy is apparent, with pain elicited upon palpation of the nodes.

The Genus Pasteurella

The genus *Pasteurella* has changed significantly in the recent past with the transfer of *Pasteurella pestis* and *Pasteurella pseudotuberculosis* from this genus to the genus *Yersinia,* and transfer of *Pasteurella tularensis* to the genus *Francisella.* These changes have substantially reduced the importance of the Pasteurella genus in the etiology of human dis-

ease. *Yersinia pestis* is responsible for bubonic plague and is of considerable medical and historic interest, as is *Francisella tularensis,* the causative agent of tularemia.

The *Pasteurella* species are gram-negative, nonmotile, coccobacillary organisms that frequently show bipolar staining. The organisms are oxidase positive and are best cultured on media containing blood. Of the species remaining in this genus, the two most important are *Pasteurella ureae* and *Pasteurella multocida.* Both are primarily associated with infections in medically compromised patients.

PASTEURELLA UREAE

Pasteurella ureae is the only species in this genus found solely in humans. Its frequency of occurrence as a member of the normal respiratory flora is unknown. *P. ureae* has been isolated from the respiratory tract of patients afflicted with respiratory diseases such as chronic bronchitis and chronic bronchiectasis. Since *P. ureae* is frequently isolated with *H. influenzae* or pneumococci as a mixed respiratory infection, its role in the pathogenesis of respiratory diseases is unclear. There have been very few instances of severe infections due to *P. ureae,* and these have primarily been cases of meningitis associated with predisposing conditions such as trauma to the skull.

PASTEURELLA MULTOCIDA

Pasteurella multocida is a member of the normal flora of many domestic and wild animals including cats, dogs, cattle, sheep, horses, rabbits, and birds. *P. multocida* is the causative agent of hemorrhagic septicemia in several different animal species. A polysaccharide capsule of variable chemical composition is associated with this organism. *P. multocida* has been isolated from the saliva of healthy domestic animals and birds and commonly infects humans as the result of dog and cat bites and cat scratches. Local abscess formation usually follows the animal bite, and in deep wounds, osteomyelitis in underlying bone may ensue.

P. multocida is occasionally isolated from human sputum samples, and the majority of isolations are from patients in contact with animals or animal products. Many times the organism is associated with chronic respiratory tract disease and can cause severe infections including meningitis and septicemia.

REFERENCES

Carter, G. R.: Genus I. Pasteurella. In Krieg, N. R. (ed.): Bergey's Manual of Systemic Bacteriology. Williams and Wilkins, Baltimore, 1984, p. 552.

Kilian, M.: A taxonomic study of the genus *Haemophilus*, with the proposal of a new species. J. Gen. Microbiol. 93:9, 1976.

Kilian, M., and Biberstein, E. L.: Genus II. Haemophilus. In Krieg, N. R. (ed.): Bergey's Manual of Systemic Bacteriology. Williams and Wilkins, Baltimore, 1984, p. 558.

Kilian, M.: Haemophilus. In Lennette, E. H., Belows, A., Hausler, W. J. Jr., and Shadomy, H. J. (eds.): Manual of Clinical Microbiology, ed. 4. American Society of Microbiologists, Washington, DC, 1985, p. 387.

Potts, T. V., Mitra, T. O., O'Keefe, T., Zambon, J. J., and Genco, R.: Relationships among isolates of oral haemophili as determined by DNA-DNA hybridization. Arch. Microbiol. 145:136, 1986.

Weaver, R. E., Hollis, D. G., and Bottone, E. J.: Gram-negative fermentative bacteria and *Francisella tularensis*. In Lennette, E. H., Belows, A., Hausler, W. J. Jr., Shadomy, H. J. (eds.): Manual of Clinical Microbiology, ed 4. American Society of Microbiologists, Washington, DC, 1985, p. 309.

chapter 10

Neisseria

Michael A. Apicella, M.D.

Our knowledge of the genus *Neisseria*—in particular, its two important members, the meningococcus and the gonococcus—has increased greatly over the past 20 years. The stimulus for the renewed interest in these microorganisms is related to two events that occurred in the early 1960s. In 1963, at the United States Army Recruit Training Base at Fort Ord, California, group B meningococci that were resistant to sulfonamides were isolated during an epidemic. The use of sulfa prophylaxis had failed to abort this epidemic, and the clinically significant emergence of sulfonamide-resistant meningococci heralded the end of a 20-year period when sulfa drugs could be used effectively to prevent meningococcal disease in susceptible populations. The subsequent failure to develop new and effective prophylactic measures and the increasing incidence of meningococcal disease in military recruit camps led to the study of the immunologic factors involved in human meningococcal defenses and to the development of an effective vaccine for the prevention of meningococcal serotype A and C disease.

At approximately the same time, a dramatic increase in the incidence of gonococcal infection occurred. Because of the epidemic nature of this increase and the failure of available methods to contain the spread of infection, renewed interest in understanding the basic immunobiology of the gonococcus was initiated.

Neisseria gonorrhoeae

MORPHOLOGIC, CULTURAL, AND BIOCHEMICAL CHARACTERISTICS

Neisseria gonorrhoeae is a gram-negative diplococcus measuring approximately 0.8 to 0.6 μm in size. The organism will not grow at 22°C and flourishes optimally at 35°C in a humid atmosphere containing from 2.5 to 5 percent carbon dioxide. The organism grows on chocolate media that has been supplemented with co-carboxylase, cysteine, and glutamine, Columbia media, and supplemented Mueller-Hinton media.

The use of Thayer-Martin media has dramatically improved the ability to isolate the gonococcus and the meningococcus from areas where it competes with other faster-growing microbes and subsequently becomes overgrown on culture. This medium contains standard chocolate agar and the antibiotics vancomycin (3 μg/ml), colistin (7.5 μg/ml), and nystatin (12.5 units/ml). All other competing organisms are suppressed and this selective medium for the growth of the gonococcus has greatly enhanced the isolation of the organism from the cervix, pharynx, and rectum.

The gonococcus produces acid in the presence of glucose without gas formation, and will not ferment maltose or sucrose (Table 10–1). These fermentation characteristics are used for its differentiation from the meningococcus. Like all species of *Neisseria*, the gonococcus oxidizes dimethylparaphenylene diamine. This so-called oxidase test causes a conversion of a colorless dye to pink and then dark-purple. It is useful in the early identification of *Neisseria*.

ANTIGENIC AND CELL SURFACE STRUCTURES

Intense interest has been generated in the last decade over the antigenic structure of the outer membrane of the gonococcus. The gonococcus contains a gross outer membrane structure that is identical to that found in the *Enterobacteriaceae*. The outer membrane contains lipopolysaccharide and a series of proteins, including the principal outer membrane protein. This structure rests on an inner membrane composed of peptidoglycan. Principal outer membrane proteins are a series of hydrophobic proteins present in the outer membrane which have been shown to be antigenically distinct and of differing molecular couplets. Gonococci can be segregated into different antigenic types based upon the outer membrane proteins that the individual strain contains.

The lipopolysaccharide (LPS) of the gonococcus is very similar to that isolated from other gram-negative organisms. The polysaccharide portion contains a series of antigens that can be utilized to serotype the gonococcus. It appears that the gonococcus contains common, as well as serotypically distinct, LPS polysaccharide antigens. The lipid A of the gonococcal LPS has been studied and shown to contain the 14-carbon major fatty acid, myristic acid, as its major component. It is the principal toxin of the organism.

The pilus is the membrane structure that has gained the most recent attention. It is believed that the structure gives the organism an environmental advantage because it allows more ready adherence to the mucosal surface of the cervix and urethra. This structure may also have some effect on preventing phagocytosis of the organism by neutrophils. The pilus is composed of proteins designated pilin, which are approximately 19,000 molecular weight (MW) in size. The pilus antigens are extraordinarily heterogeneous, and large numbers of pilus serotypes exist. There appears to be a common pilus antigen, and it has been estimated that approximately 10 percent of the pilus is composed of an antigen structure common to most gonococci. This latter factor may be important in the future development of a pilus vaccine, since, if a common antigen could be identified and an antibody to it developed, this antibody could be potentially protective.

Gonococcal Infection

While a number of animal models have recently been developed, naturally occurring gonococcal infection is found only in the human host. Studies performed by epidemiologists in the United States Navy indicate that the risk of infection following a single exposure is approximately 20 to 30 percent. The incubation period is usually between 3 and 10 days, but occasionally intervals of up to 30 days can occur between the time of infection and the onset of symptoms.

In many women (up to 75 percent) and some men (1 to 2 percent of all infected), the disease can be asymptomatic for long periods of time. The asymptomatic woman has been

Table 10–1 ■ Characteristics of *Neisseria* species

Species	Oxidase	Growth at 22° C	Produce IgA Protease	Fermentations Glucose	Maltose	Sucrose
N. meningitidis	+	−	+	+	+	−
N. gonorrhoeae	+	−	+	+	−	−
N. sicca	+	+	−	+	+	+
N. flavescens	+	+	−	−	−	−
N. subflava	+	+	−	+	+	V*

*V = variable.

long recognized as a serious problem in achieving eradication of this disease. The presence of the asymptomatic man has also been shown.

In men, the characteristic symptomatology of acute infection is dysuria, urethritis, and a purulent discharge. In women, changes in color and odor of vaginal discharge and abdominal pain are the primary symptoms of cervical infection. Using punch biopsies in patients with acute gonococcal infection, the electron microscopic picture of cervical gonococcal infection has been studied. Gonococci were ingested by the stratified squamous epithelial cells on the cervical surface, present in cells shed from the surface, and appeared to be repeatedly rephagocytosed by leukocytes in the cervical secretions. This ability of squamous cells to ingest gonococci may be important in the asymptomatic state, since the organism would be relatively protected from the effects of antibiotics and ingestion by macrophages.

Pelvic inflammatory disease (PID) in the woman is a serious consequence of gonococcal infection. Approximately half the cases of PID are caused by *Neisseria gonorrhoeae*. The mechanisms of this infection are not known, but it appears that the gonococcal LPS alters the mucosal surface of the fallopian tubes, permitting the invasion by aerobic gram-negative and anaerobic organisms. Studies have demonstrated that early after the onset of symptoms, the gonococcus is isolatable from the cul de sac. As the period of time increases between the onset of symptoms and the attempted culture, the ability to isolate the gonococcus decreases remarkably. In all of these patients, the cervical culture was positive for *Neisseria gonorrhoeae*.

Disseminated gonococcal infection is characterized by fever, arthralgias, arthritis, tenosynovitis, and a skin eruption. This disease occurs in approximately 1 in 300 to 1 in 600 cases of genital gonorrhea. Recent studies have indicated an association between disseminated gonococcal infection and a specific biotype. Organisms that cause this form of gonorrhea usually are exquisitely penicillin sensitive, are resistant to killing by normal human serum, are of the AHU auxotype, and may be one specific POMP serotype. This form of gonococcal disease occurs six times more frequently in women than in men. In over half the cases, it occurs within 1 week of menses, and there appears to be a relationship between this disease and the third trimester of pregnancy, since there is a higher disease frequency than in the general population. There also appears to be an association between disseminated gonococcal disease in men and homosexual preference.

Pharyngeal infection by the gonococcus can occur. It is associated with fellatio and tends to be self-limiting. Symptomatic infection can occur and should be treated with appropriate antibiotics.

TREATMENT OF GONOCOCCAL INFECTION

Penicillin G is still the principal antibiotic agent used in the treatment of gonococcal infection. As the increasing resistance of the gonococcus to penicillin became apparent, increasingly larger doses of drug have been employed to achieve success in single-dose regimens. In addition, it has become important that therapeutic levels of drug be maintained for periods up to 8 hours after administration to optimize the cure rates. For this reason, Benemid (probenecid) is administered with the penicillin in the single-dose schedule. Using 4.8 million units of aqueous procaine penicillin intramuscularly and 1 g of Benemid orally, cure rates in the range of 95 percent can be expected with patients with uncomplicated genital gonorrhea. Similar outcomes can be anticipated when penicillin-allergic patients with the same type of disease process are treated with 2 g of spectinomycin intramuscularly. The treatment of extragenital and fallopian tube gonorrhea may require longer courses of therapy and may sometimes necessitate hospitalization of the patient.

Therapy of gonococcal infection has been recently complicated by the emergence of penicillinase-producing gonococcal strains. These first appeared in 1974, in California and Liverpool, England, and appear to have arisen independently. Both contain a plasmid that codes for the production of penicillinase. This plasmid is similar, if not identical, to the TNA plasmid found in enteric species and in *Haemophilus influenzae*. These strains have had limited frequency among the general population, but therapeutic failures to penicillin should always be examined for the possibility of penicillinase-producing strains as the etiologic agent. Treatment of these strains with spectinomycin is recommended.

Drugs to prevent gonococcal infection have been universally unsuccessful, with one exception. During passage down the birth canal, newborns can develop gonococcal conjunctivitis if the mothers' genital secretions are infected. Prophylactic treatment by the installation of 1 percent silver nitrate into the conjunctival space immediately after birth has markedly reduced this complication of gonococcal infection.

Neisseria Meningitidis

MORPHOLOGIC, CULTURAL, AND BIOCHEMICAL CHARACTERISTICS

Neisseria meningitidis is a gram-negative diplococcus ($0.6 \times 0.8\mu$). The adjacent sides are flattened to produce the typical "biscuit" shape. Because the organism tends to readily undergo autolysis, considerable size and shape variation can be seen in older cultures. The organism is considered fastidious in its growth conditions, necessitating the use of appropriate media and growth conditions. These problems in reliable growth may relate as much to nutritional factors as to the presence of substances toxic to the meningococcus in the medium. On solid media, the meningococcus grows as a transparent, nonpigmented, nonhemolytic colony, approximately 1 to 5 mm in diameter. Colonies are convex and, if large amounts of polysaccharide are present, will appear mucoid rather than smooth. Optimal growth conditions are achieved in a moist environment at 35 to 37°C under an atmosphere of 5 to 10 percent carbon dioxide. The organism will grow well on a number of medium bases, including blood agar base, trypticase soy agar, supplemented chocolate agar, and Mueller-Hinton agar. Confirmation of the presence of this organism in clinical specimens is dependent on a series of carbohydrate fermentations (Table 10–1). The meningococcus will ferment glucose and maltose to acid without gas formation and fails to ferment sucrose or lactose. Indole and hydrogen sulfide are not formed. In addition, the organism contains the enzyme cytochrome oxidase in its cell wall which will oxidize the dye tetramethyl-phenylene-diamine (TMPD) from colorless to deep pink. This latter test was initially considered specific for gonococci, but subsequent studies have shown that other genera, as well as *Neisseria*, exhibit TMPD-oxidase activities, including *Pseudomonas, Aeromonas,* and *Moraxella*.

Meningococci can be segregated by seroagglutination into nine serogroups, A, B, C, D,

Table 10–2 ■ Chemical composition of meningococcal capsular polysaccharides

Capsular Serogroup Antigen	Chemical Composition of Capsular Polymer
A	N-acetyl mannosamine phosphate
B	N-acetyl neuraminic acid
C_{+1}	O,N-acetyl neuraminic acid
C_{1-}	N-acetyl neuraminic acid
X	2-acetamido-2 deoxy-D-glucose 4-phosphate
Y	D-glucose N-acetylneuraminic acid, 1:1

X, Z, (Z'), W-135, and 29E. Capsular polysaccharides responsible for the serogrouping specificity of the groups A, B, C, X, and Y have been purified. Chemical analysis of these five polysaccharides has been completed (Table 10–2). Group C polysaccharides can be biochemically divided into neuraminidase-sensitive and neuraminidase-resistant polysaccharides. The C strains producing the neuraminidase-sensitive polysaccharide have been designated C variant strains and have been given the designation C_{1-}.

Noncapsular cell wall antigens appear to be important in understanding the immunobiology of the meningococcus. The antigen responsible for the noncapsular meningococcal serotyping system is protein in nature and resides in the outer membrane as part of a lipoprotein-lipopolysaccharide complex.

THE HUMAN IMMUNOBIOLOGY OF NEISSERIA MENINGITIDIS

At birth, due to maternal transfer of antibodies, approximately 50 percent of the infants have bactericidal antibody titers. The prevalence of bactericidal antibody decreases after birth and reaches its nadir between 6 and 24 months of age. Thereafter, a linear incidence increase in antibody occurs until age 12. In early adulthood, the prevalence of bactericidal antibody varies with the serogroup but ranges from 67 percent for group A to 86 percent for group B. The protective nature of bactericidal antibody against homologous serogroups has been demonstrated during epidemics. In a group that became infected, only 3 of 54 previously had bactericidal antibody, while 444 of 550 uninfected controls had homologous bactericidal antibody. Based on their observations, 38.5 percent of the persons who lacked bactericidal antibody and who acquired the epidemic strain in their nasopharynx in the military recruit environment developed systemic meningococcal disease. The conclusion was that deficiency of circulating antimeningococcal antibodies is firmly associated with the establishment of meningococcemia. It appears that bactericidal antibodies are directed against both the capsular polysaccharide and other cell wall antigens that may cross-react within the family *Neisseria* and with other bacterial genera. The meningococcal carrier state is an immunizing process and that within 2 weeks of colonization production of antibodies to meningococci can be identified. Nontypable meningococcal strains, which are seen in carrier studies in children, contain cross-reacting antigens with the encapsulated strains, and bactericidal antibody to these strains develops after nasopharyngeal colonization.

Studies indicate that serologic cross reactions between the meningococcal group A polysaccharide occur with *B. pumilis* and that the *E. coli* K1 antigen is immunologically and chemically identical to the group B capsular polysaccharide. These unrelated yet immunologically similar antigens may play a very important role in the development of natural immunity to the meningococcus and ultimately in protection against virulent meningococci.

Antibodies to the meningococcus may also enhance susceptibility to infection. Using immunoabsorbent columns to remove serum IgA demonstrated that bactericidal activity was deficient in the acute sera of 24 of 28 patients with meningitis or meningococcemia before absorption, but that it was uniformly present after removal of IgA. These investigators speculate that susceptibility of meningococcal disease may be affected by blocking of bactericidal IgM by circulating IgA.

Meningococcal Infection

EPIDEMIOLOGY

Meningococcal disease is a major worldwide health problem. Feldman estimates that during the period 1939 to 1962 there were almost 600,000 cases in the world, and more than 100,000 of them were fatal. The greatest percentage of cases was and still is in children. In 1975, there were 1478 cases reported to the Centers for Disease Control; 333 (22.5 percent) were in infants and 358 (24.2 percent) were in children between 1 and 4 years of age. The case rate in the United States has been decreasing since 1969, and, based on 1970 census estimates, there is approximately 0.68 reported case per 100,000 population. The case fatality rate during a surveillance of 512 endemic cases in 1973 and 1974 was 19 percent. This is higher than the 8 percent case fatality rate that has been reported previously from major medical centers in the United States in endemic areas.

In epidemics, the case rate rises dramatically. During an epidemic in Chile from 1940 to 1943, the case rate in the province of Valparaiso during 1942 was 188.1 per 100,000 population. In 1966, an epidemic was reported in Holland that was caused primarily by group B meningococci. There were 516 cases, with a case fatality rate of 8.5 percent. From 1974 to 1975, an epidemic in Brazil due to group A and C strains had a case fatality rate of less than 10 percent.

THE CARRIER STATE

The carriage of *Neisseria meningitidis* in the nasopharynx of otherwise healthy humans has been recognized since 1896. In 1908, Bruns and Hohn noted a close relationship between the carrier rate in a population and the onset, rise, and decline of an epidemic. Glover noted the same association in the British Army military camps of the First World War and felt that when the carrier rate exceeded 20 percent the community was in danger of an epidemic, usually caused by the predominant carrier serotype. Many of Glover's concepts have prevailed until today, despite considerable data that fail to support them.

The transmission of the meningococci from carrier to carrier is probably via the respiratory route, but precise data supporting this thesis or the mechanisms involved are not available. The rate of spread of the carrier state through a population has been the subject of a number of studies. During epidemics in military camps, the rate of new carrier acquisition can be very rapid, while in nonepidemic situations, both military and civilian, the rate of new carrier acquisition can be considerably slower and the state of carriage can exist for prolonged periods of time. The carrier rates in families not exposed to clinically important meningococcal infection during a nonepidemic period have been studied. The rate of transmission in these circumstances was considered low in comparison to most communicable pathogens, and it was estimated that at this level a susceptible person would have more than a 50 percent chance of escaping carriage, even if exposed continually to household carriers for a 5-year period.

The carrier state is an immunizing process. Indirect evidence for this phenomenon is the fact that while military recruits have a high frequency of meningococcal carriage disease, seasoned veterans have a much lower carriage rate and a disease incidence no different than the civilian population. In military recruits, antimeningococci antibodies have been shown to persist for a minimum of 4 to 6 months after exposure. These antibodies are of the three major immunoglobulin classes and react with group-specific and cross-reactive antigens.

MENINGOCOCCAL DISEASE

The clinical manifestations of meningococcal disease can be quite varied. This can range from transient fever and bacteremia to fulminant disease with death ensuing within hours of the onset of clinical symptoms. Four clinical situations have been described:

1. *Bacteremia without sepsis.* Admission is for an upper respiratory illness or viral exanthem. After recovery and frequently after discharge without specific antimicrobial therapy, the results of blood cultures are reported as positive for *Neisseria meningitidis.*

2. *Meningococcemia without meningitis.* In these cases, the patient is septic, and the signs of leukocytosis, skin rashes, generalized malaise, weakness, headache, and hypotension develop on admission or shortly thereafter.

3. *Meningitis with or without meningococcemia.* In these patients, headache, fever, and meningeal signs, as well as a cloudy spinal fluid, are present. The state of the sensorium may vary widely from fully alert to completely depressed. The deep tendon and superficial reflexes are present. There are no pathologic findings.

4. *The meningoencephalitic presentation.* These patients are profoundly obtunded with meningeal signs and septic spinal fluid. The deep tendon reflexes and superficial reflexes are altered (either are absent or, rarely, are hyperactive). Pathologic reflexes are frequently present.

Variations of these manifestations can oc-

cur, and the patient can progress from one to the other during the course of disease.

Persistent meningococcal bacteremia associated with low-grade fever, rash, and arthritis has been reported. The distribution and appearance of the cutaneous lesions are identical to those seen in chronic gonococcemia, for which it is mistaken. Feldman has commented on a patient with chronic meningococcemia who appeared normal in every respect, including the ability to produce antibodies against the capsular polysaccharide of the infecting organism. The syndrome of chronic meningococcemia must be distinguished from the problem of recurrent episodes of meningococcal meningitis. Studies have recently demonstrated the absence of the sixth complement component in such a patient. In addition, at least one of the patients with recurrent meningococcal disease lacked C3. Studies by Petersen and associates indicated that human deficiency of C8 has been found in some persons with disseminated gonococcal infections and that this complement component is required for serum bactericidal activity against the gonococcus. These studies would stress the previously unrecognized importance of the complement system in protection against neisserial infections, particularly of the chronic or recurrent variety.

Meningococcal pneumonia has been a recognized clinical syndrome for over 60 years. Because of the nasopharyngeal carriage of the meningococcus, the ability to establish the diagnosis based on the sputum culture alone is hazardous. The incidence of sepsis associated with this type of meningococcal infection appears to be quite low. Therefore, blood cultures may not be of value. Transtracheal cultures have been used to establish the diagnosis in 68 Air Force recruits with group Y meningococcal pneumonia; the prognosis was good with no deaths occurring in these patients. The association of meningococcal infection with preceding viral respiratory infections has been reported.

Meningococcal upper respiratory tract infections (pharyngitis) associated with contacts of cases and as a prior symptom and sign in cases of serious meningococcal disease has been described by several authors. Suggestions that pharyngeal inflammation is the predecessor to bacteremic dissemination have been made but are unsubstantiated.

The definite diagnosis of serious meningococcal infection has as a prerequisite the bacteriologic isolation of *Neisseria meningitidis* from a usually sterile body fluid such as blood, cerebrospinal fluid, synovial, pleural, or pericardial fluids. In 727 cases of meningococcal disease, Hoyne and Brown described the results of 400 blood cultures in which 51.4 percent were positive for meningococci. Spinal fluid examination of 423 patients from the same series indicated that 94 percent were positive for gram-negative diplococci by either smear or culture for the meningococci.

Recent studies using counterimmunoelectrophoresis have demonstrated the capability of detecting 0.02 to 0.5 μg of meningococcal antigens per milliliter of spinal fluid of infected patients. The technique offers rapidity in diagnosis and specificity providing organisms containing cross-reacting antigens are not involved (e.g., *E. coli* K1 and group B meningococcus). False-negative results occur commonly.

TREATMENT OF MENINGOCOCCAL INFECTIONS

Penicillin therapy for the treatment of meningococcal infections is safe and effective. The drug can be administered intravenously or intramuscularly. The intrathecal route is contraindicated because of the severe neurotoxicity of penicillin in high concentrations in the central nervous system. A dose of 200,000 units per kg per day is recommended with an upper limit of 20 million units per day total dose. Chloramphenicol is an effective substitute for use in the penicillin-allergic patient and should be administered intravenously in a dose of 100 mg per kg per day up to a maximum of 4 g per dose. Duration of antibiotic therapy will vary somewhat with the presentation and manifestation of the disease with the response of the patient. At present, the meningococcus is quite sensitive to the agents just mentioned, and 10 to 14 days of therapy is usually sufficient.

CHEMOPROPHYLAXIS

Treatment of patients carrying meningococcal infection with sulfonamides eradicated carriage quickly for prolonged periods. The length of time was a function of the initial dose of sulfonamides and with doses as high as 8 g the carrier rate was reduced from approximately 45 percent to less than 10 percent at 16 weeks. On military bases and in closed environments such as boarding schools, institutions, and family units, where cases arose, this form of chemoprophylaxis was effective in disrupting the spread of meningococcal infections.

With the recognition of widespread sulfonamide-resistant meningococci and the failure of sulfadiazine to affect the epidemic at Fort Ord, these agents have been abandoned for meningococcal chemoprophylaxis except in instances when the meningococcal case strains are known to be sulfa-sensitive.

The search for new agents for chemoprophylaxis has been extensive. Penicillin has proven ineffective for several reasons. Long-acting mixtures do not eradicate the nasopharyngeal carriage, and whereas massive doses cause persons to become noncarriers, the carrier state recurs promptly after discontinuation of the drug. At the present time, the recommended therapy for meningococcal prophylaxis is rifampin, 600 mg every 12 hours for 2 days for adults, and 10 mg per kg every 12 hours for 2 days for children.

The question as to who should receive prophylaxis has plagued public health officials since the advent of effective chemoprophylaxis. With sulfonamides, initially little discrimination between high-risk and low-risk populations was attempted, and the drug was administered very widely to persons without the remotest increased risk of disease. Since the clinical emergence of sulfa resistance and the problem in finding agents that are safe and effective, more attention has been paid to the populations at greatest risk who need chemoprophylaxis. During epidemics and in the endemic situations in civilian populations, household contacts have been shown to be at increased risk to infection. Analysis by the Centers for Disease Control Meningococcal Surveillance Group showed that the attack rate in this group was 500 to 800 times greater than for the general population. Similar high-risk situations exist in closed populations such as college dormitories, chronic care hospitals, nursery schools, and military barracks. Secondary cases usually occur within 10 days of exposure to the primary case, but longer intervals have occurred. Close surveillance of this group for at least 10 days would ensure prompt treatment of secondary cases in the absence of effective chemoprophylaxis. Hospital personnel are not at increased risk and, in general, should not receive chemoprophylaxis. Medical staff who have intimate exposure such as mouth-to-mouth resuscitation should receive treatment, not prophylaxis.

IMMUNOPROPHYLAXIS

After the emergence of sulfa-resistant meningococci, intense effort was directed at developing a vaccine to prevent meningococcal infections in high-risk populations. The result was two vaccine preparations derived from the capsular polysaccharide of the group A and C meningococci. The effectiveness of the group C vaccine has been demonstrated in studies of American Army recruits. Only one case of meningococcal disease occurred among 13,763 vaccinees, while 38 bacteriologically proven cases occurred in a control group of 68,072. This was an 87 percent reduction in disease and was statistically significant. Group A polysaccharide administered to Finnish military recruits also significantly lowered the incidence of disease due to this serogroup when compared with an unvaccinated control population. Studies from Finland during a group A epidemic demonstrated the effectiveness of this vaccine in children 3 months to 5 years of age. The immunologic response of the group C vaccine is not protective under the age of 24 months. Studies of the immune response to the A and C vaccine in infants have demonstrated that detectable levels of antibody are generated but that these levels are significantly lower than in older children. In adults, the group C antibody titer persisted for 2 to 4 years after vaccination, and in children vaccinated with group A polysaccharide protection has lasted at least 2 years.

There is no vaccine presently available for prevention of group B disease. The group B capsular polysaccharide is not sufficiently immunogenic to produce an effective antibody response in humans. Several solutions to this problem are being studied, including the chemical alteration of the capsular B antigen to make it more immunogenic and the search for other cell wall antigens capable of eliciting bactericidal antibodies against B meningococci with a minimum of side effects.

REFERENCES

Advisory Committee on Immunization Practices: Meningococcal polysaccharide vaccines. Ann. Int. Med. 84:179, 1976.

Artenstein, M. S., and Ellis, R. E.: The risk of exposure to a patient with meningococcal meningitis. Milit. Med. 133:474, 1968.

Eisenstein, B. I., and Masi, A. T.: Disseminated gonococcal infection (DGI) and gonococcal arthritis (GCA). I. Bacteriology, epidemiology, host factors, pathogen factors and pathology. Semin. Arthritis Rheum. 10:155, 1981.

Eschenbach, D. A.: Acute pelvic inflammatory disease: Etiology, risk factors, and pathogenesis. Clin. Obstet. Gynecol. 19:147, 1976.

Feldman, H. A.: Meningococcal infections. Adv. Int. Med. 18:177, 1972.

Griffiss, J. M.: Epidemic meningococcal disease: Synthesis of a hypothetical immunoepidemiological model. Rev. Infect. Dis. 4:159, 1982.

Hook, E. W., and Holmes, K. K.: Gonococcal infections. Ann. Int. Med. 102:229, 1985.

Hutt, D. M., and Judson, F. N.: Epidemiology and treatment of oropharyngeal gonorrhea. Ann. Int. Med. 104:655, 1986.

Peltola, H.: Meningococcal disease: Still with us. Rev. Infect. Dis. 5:71, 1983.

Peterson, B. H., Lee, T. J., Synderman, R., et al.: Neisseria meningitidis and Neisseria gonorrhoeae bacteremia associated with C6, C7, or C8 deficiency. Ann. Int. Med. 90:917, 1986.

Wiesner, P. J., Tronca, E., Bonin, P., et al.: Clinical spectrum of pharyngeal gonorrhoeae. N. Engl. J. Med. 288:181, 1973.

chapter 11

Corynebacterium and Mycobacterium

Joseph J. Zambon, D.D.S., Ph.D.

Corynebacterium

The Corynebacteria include a group of facultatively anaerobic pathogenic and saprophytic gram-positive, nonmotile, non–spore-forming rods (Table 11–1). The name "Corynebacteria" derives from the Greek "koryne," meaning club, and "bakterion," meaning small rod. Hence, these bacteria are small straight or slightly curved rods, some having club-shaped ends, that stain irregularly. Cell division results in right angle or palisade cell groupings. The Corynebacteria are related to the genera Mycobacterium, Nocardia, and Rhodococcus in that they possess a cell wall peptidoglycan containing mesodiaminopimelic acid; however, the latter three genera have n-glycolyl residues in their cell wall glycans, which are not found in Corynebacteria. Corynebacteria also possess arabinose and galactose as major cell wall sugars and have short-chain (22 to 36 carbon atoms) mycolic acids in the cell wall.

CORYNEBACTERIUM DIPHTHERIAE

The most important microorganism in this genus is *Corynebacterium diphtheriae*, which causes diphtheria (croup). This disease is named after the gray pseudomembrane composed of fibrin, bacteria, and trapped leukocytes (from the Greek "diphthera," meaning skin or membrane) that forms in the patient's throat during the course of the disease.

Characteristics of the Microorganism

These organisms are gram-positive, non–spore-forming, straight or slightly curved rods, with tapered ends but without flagella or capsule. The cells may have swollen or club-shaped ends and often have accumulations of polyphosphate in metachromatic granules (Babès-Ernst bodies), which stain bluish-purple with methylene or toluidine blue. The organism measures 0.3 to 0.8 μm wide by 1 to 8 μm long. *C. diphtheriae* multiplies by "snapping," resulting in accumulations of cells that are at right angles to one another and appear as Chinese or cuneiform characters. The term "diphtheroid" is used in medical microbiology to designate gram-positive rods resembling *C. diphtheriae*.

C. diphtheriae grows as an obligate aerobe at 30 to 37°C. Complex media such as Loeffler's coagulated serum medium are required for primary isolation. Colonies appear cream-

197

Table 11–1 ■ *Corynebacterium*

Characteristics	Facultative anaerobes
	Gram-positive, nonmotile, non–spore-forming, club-shaped rods with *metachromatic granules*
	Pathogens and saprophytes
	Cell wall with meso-diaminopimelic acid
Major species	*C. diphtheriae*
Growth	Loeffler's medium, medium containing 0.045% tellurite
	Colony morphologies include "gravis," "mitis," and "intermedius"
Disease	Diphtheria
Pathogenesis	Exotoxin
	β-prophage carries the structural gene for the toxin
	Clinically characterized by grayish pseudomembrane
	Schick test for circulating antibody to the toxin
Prevention	Vaccination with toxoid
Treatment	Penicillin, erythromycin, tetracycline

colored or grayish-white on Loeffler's medium but are characteristically dark gray or black on medium containing 0.045 percent tellurite, as a result of the organism's reduction of tellurite to tellurium. Three morphologically distinct types of colonies have been described. Each colony morphology was originally thought to relate to the patient's clinical condition, but today there is thought to be little such correlation. These morphologies include (1) "gravis" strains, which have short, irregular, rod-shaped bacterial cells and form, on tellurite medium, large, radially striated, flat gray to black colonies; (2) "mitis" strains, which have long, curved, rod-shaped cells and form colonies that are small, black, and convex with a glossy surface; and (3) "intermedius" strains, which have long, rod-shaped cells and form flat, creamy, transparent colonies.

Pathogenesis

Diphtheria is caused by an exotoxin produced by strains of *C. diphtheriae* that have been infected with a beta-prophage. This bacteriophage carries the structural gene (tox) for the toxin molecule. Toxigenic *C. diphtheriae* strains that are cured of the bacteriophage lose the ability to produce toxin and are avirulent. Furthermore, toxin production in toxigenic, lysogenic strains of *C. diphtheriae* is dependent upon environmental factors including iron. Toxin is produced at high levels when iron levels are low. The toxin is a heat-labile protein of 60,000 daltons molecular weight. It originates as a larger latent precursor molecule. Cleavage of a peptide linkage 194 residues from the N-terminus transforms the latent form to the active toxin. The active toxin itself is composed of two fragments—an N-terminal fragment A of 21,150 daltons, which carries the enzyme activity, and a larger fragment B of 39,000 daltons, which is responsible for binding to specific surface receptors on sensitive cells. Following this binding, fragment A is transported across the cell membrane, where it catalyzes the transfer of an ADP-ribosyl group from nicotinamide adenine dinucleotide (NAD) to elongation factor, EF2. This effectively blocks EF2 from carrying out its crucial role in cellular protein synthesis and the cell dies within a few hours.

C. diphtheriae is transmitted by droplet infection from asymptomatic carriers or active cases and by contact with cutaneous lesions. Human disease begins as an upper respiratory tract infection in which virulent *C. diphtheriae* multiply and secrete a toxin that causes cellular necrosis in the mucosa of the oropharynx—especially of the tonsils. The microorganism rarely invades the deeper tissues; however, the toxin can be carried via the blood to other parts of the body, causing a toxemia. At the site of infection, accumulations of necrotic epithelial cells, *C. diphtheriae*, fibrin, erythrocytes, and leukocytes form the characteristic grayish pseudomembrane. Patients usually have a moderate fever, chill, malaise, sore throat, and cervical lymphadenopathy, which may become so pronounced as to give the appearance of a "bull neck." Extension of the disease to adjacent areas of the larynx and trachea is known as laryngeal diphtheria, while extension into the nasal passages is known as nasopharyngeal diphtheria. Laryngeal diphtheria is associated with respiratory tract obstructions, which may necessitate tracheotomy. Nasopharyngeal diphtheria is associated with neurologic and cardiac complications due to circulating toxin. Cardiac complications of nasopharyngeal diphtheria appear within 2 weeks and involve myocardial degeneration. Neurologic complications appear within 3 to 5 weeks and produce paralysis of cranial nerves, which can lead to both paralysis of the soft palate and polyneuritis of peripheral nerves. In tropical areas, cutaneous diphtheria may occur as a secondary infection of pre-existing skin lesions. These appear as chronic, sometimes spreading, ulcers, which do not heal and which are covered by a grayish pseudo-membrane.

Immunity

As a result of transplacental transfer of maternal antibody to the C. diphtheriae toxin, newborn infants may have passive immunity for up to 2 years. However, after the first few months of life, maternal antibody levels are generally insufficient to prevent C. diphtheriae infection and the development of diphtheria. Children born to mothers who do not have antibody to C. diphtheriae likewise do not have this passive immunity. For these reasons, diphtheria toxoid is used to immunize infants as part of the DPT (diphtheria, pertussis, and tetanus) conbined vaccine. The toxoid is derived from formaldehyde treatment of the C. diphtheriae toxin, which results in the loss of toxicity but retention of antigenicity. Active immunization with DPT vaccine produces adequate antibody levels to the C. diphtheriae toxin for several years. Booster immunizations, however, are necessary to maintain antibody levels during childhood.

The Schick test identifies persons with circulating antibody to the C. diphtheriae toxin. A small amount of C. diphtheriae toxin is injected intradermally. Persons without antibody develop red to brown pigmented areas of swelling, redness, and necrosis at the site of injection within 4 to 5 days. Persons with enough circulating antibody to neutralize the injected toxin will not develop this "positive" Schick test result. Thus, a positive Schick test result identifies susceptible individuals, and a negative result identifies those with protective immunity. Often, intradermal injection with a C. diphtheriae toxoid preparation is used as a control to distinguish a true-positive reaction from delayed hypersensitivity reactions (allergy) to the toxin or to non-toxin antigens present in the same preparation.

Diagnosis and Treatment

The diagnosis of diphtheria is made by the identification of toxigenic C. diphtheriae. Swabs of throat lesions are cultured onto a Loeffler's slant, a blood agar plate, and a tellurite agar plate. Smears are made from colonies appearing 24 hours after incubation on any of the media. The smears are stained with methylene blue and microscopically examined for coryneform cell morphology. If colonies appear on the blood agar plate but not on the tellurite medium, the latter is reincubated for an additional 24 hours. Negative growth after the second incubation is used to rule out Corynebacterium infection.

After culture, C. diphtheriae isolates should be tested for toxin production by an in vivo assay in guinea pigs or rabbits or by in vitro gel diffusion assay. The in vivo test involves subcutaneous injections of the experimental animal with 0.2 ml of a 48-hour broth culture or 0.1 ml of a heavy bacterial suspension from the Loeffler's slant. After 4 hours, the animal is intraperitoneally injected with 500 units of diphtheria antitoxin, and after an additional 30 minutes the animal is reinjected with an additional sample of the bacterial suspension into a new site. If the C. diphtheriae strain is toxigenic, the site injected prior to administration of the antitoxin will have become necrotic within 48 to 72 hours, while the site injected after administration of the antitoxin will reveal only nonspecific inflammation.

The in vitro gel diffusion test involves pouring calf serum–peptone maltose agar into a Petri plate containing a filter paper strip impregnated with diphtheria antitoxin. The C. diphtheriae strain to be tested is streaked across the surface of the solidified agar at right angles to the paper strip and the plate is incubated for 24 hours. The appearance of an antigen-antibody precipitin line indicates that the C. diphtheriae strain produces toxin.

Since the diphtheria toxin can enter sensitive cells within a short period of time, suspected cases of diphtheria should be immediately treated with antitoxin—even before microbiologic assays are completed. Once the toxin has entered the target cells, the antitoxin is no longer effective in neutralizing it. A large single bolus of antitoxin is administered intramuscularly, 100 to 500 units per pound, in order to neutralize both circulating toxin and toxin that has bound to cell membranes but that has not yet entered the cell.

C. diphtheriae is susceptible to a number of antibiotics, including penicillin, erythromycin, and tetracycline. Therapy, however, should be first directed toward neutralization of the diphtheria toxin. Antibiotic therapy can then be useful in eliminating the primary C. diphtheriae infection.

Mycobacterium

This genus contains saprophytic and parasitic microorganisms including two major

Table 11–2 ■ *Mycobacterium*

Characteristics	Acid- and alcohol-fast bacilli Ziehl-Neelsen or fluorochrome stains
Major species	*Mycobacterium tuberculosis* 　　Obligate aerobe 　　Grows as serpentine cords *Mycobacterium leprae*— 　　noncultivable
Growth	Slow growth on egg yolk or oleic 　　acid agar
Disease	Tuberculosis and leprosy
Pathogenesis	Destructive granulomas with central 　　areas of necrosis
Prevention	Skin testing with a purified protein 　　derivative (PPD) or lepromin
Treatment	Streptomycin, isoniazid, para- 　　aminosalicylic acid for 　　tuberculosis Dapsone (diaminodiphenylsulfone) 　　for leprosy

human pathogens, *Mycobacterium tuberculosis* and *Mycobacterium leprae*, which cause tuberculosis and leprosy, respectively (Table 11–2). Diseases caused by mycobacteria are characterized by the development of destructive granulomas with central areas of necrosis. These organisms are classified in the order *Actinomycetales* and are closely related to the genera *Corynebacterium* and *Nocardia*. The group as a whole is sometimes referred to as the "CNM" group. The bacterial cells are slow-growing, nonmotile, non–spore-forming, acid- and alcohol-fast bacilli. They are slightly curved or straight rods, and range in size from 0.2 to 0.6 μm wide and 1 to 10 μm long. Bacilli stained with dyes during the Ziehl-Neelsen procedure or the fluorochrome technique are resistant to decolorization with acid or alcohol, owing to the high lipid content in the cell walls. Bacterial cells grow as branches, filaments, or mycelia, which can be dispersed into cocci. Microscopy is therefore a key test for identification of Mycobacteria in clinical specimens. Mycobacteria are similar to Corynebacteria and Nocardia in that they have arabinose, galactose, and mycolic acid in the cell walls. They are serologically similar, in that they have a common antigen.

MYCOBACTERIUM TUBERCULOSIS

Mycobacterium tuberculosis causes tuberculosis (consumption), a disease affecting mankind since ancient times. Radiographic examination of Egyptian mummies, for example, reveals evidence of tuberculosis.

This disease is associated with unsanitary and crowded living conditions. Until fairly recently, treatment involved isolation of tubercular patients for extensive periods of time in sanitariums. The discovery by Dr. Robert Koch of *M. tuberculosis* as the cause of this pulmonary disease stands as a landmark in the history of microbiology and led to the development of Koch's postulates. These have been extremely valuable in pinpointing the microbial etiology of other infectious diseases.

Cellular and Colonial Characteristics

M. tuberculosis is a slow-growing obligate aerobe. The bacterial cells are slender, slightly curved rods measuring approximately 0.3 to 0.6 μm wide by 1 to 4 μm long. The cell morphology may vary from cocci to filaments, depending on the growth medium. Bacterial cells often have a beaded or banded appearance due to polymetaphosphate accumulations and glycogen granules, which stain metachromatically. The cells may grow parallel to one another in long aggregated strands known as "serpentine cords" and may form adherent mold-like clumps.

The factor responsible for serpentine growth, the "cord factor," may also play a role in virulence. Highly virulent strains contain large amounts of cord factor, whereas cord factor–free cells are viable but avirulent. Cord factor is toxic, and immunization against cord factor can prevent the development of tuberculosis in experimental animals.

Dispersed growth of the bacterial cells will occur with the addition of a non-ionic detergent (such as Tween) to broth cultures. Cell walls contain a peptidoglycan and large amounts of glycolipid, including mycolic acids, which are unique to the CNM *(Corynebacterium-Nocardia-Mycobacterium)* group of organisms.

Bacterial colonies are slow to appear: generally 3 to 6 weeks may be required. The colonies are buff-colored, rough, and raised, with a wrinkled surface, and they produce niacin. Serpentine cord formation is seen in smears made from cultures.

Antigenicity

M. tuberculosis contains species-specific and strain-specific antigens as well as common antigens shared with Corynebacteria and Nocardia. Patients with tuberculosis due to *M. tuberculosis* or *M. bovis*, as well as nondiseased subjects who have been exposed to either of these microorganisms, can develop delayed hypersensitivity reactions to the organism. This can be detected by intradermal testing with a purified protein derivative (PPD) from *M. tuberculosis*. Patients with tuberculosis due to *M. bovis* also exhibit a positive reaction to this preparation.

Immunity

In addition to identifying the etiologic agent in tuberculosis, Koch also demonstrated the development of partial immunity to *M. tuberculosis* in an animal model. This is known as the "Koch phenomena." The first injection of *M. tuberculosis* into an experimental animal such as a guinea pig results in a large persistent ulceration at the site of injection, which appears after approximately 2 weeks. Subsequent challenge with another dose of *M. tuberculosis* in another site results in the rapid development of an ulceration at the site of injection, but this second lesion soon heals as a result of the partial immunity developed in response to the first injection.

Pathogenesis

The pathogenesis of *M. tuberculosis* in tuberculosis is a classic example of the relationship between microbial virulence on the one hand and host resistance on the other. Accordingly, there is a range of host responses to infection with *M. tuberculosis*. The microorganism is generally transmitted by droplet (as from coughing) from a person with an active case of tuberculosis. The microorganism is very stable in such sputum droplets and can remain viable in even dry sputum for as long as 6 weeks. *M. tuberculosis* in the droplets is then inhaled into the previously uninfected host and lodges in the highly aerobic environment of the lung, where it produces a nonspecific pneumonitis. Histologically, the initial response is exudative, followed by a granulomatous response, during which the patient develops the delayed hypersensitivity characteristic of tuberculosis. In pulmonary sites of infection, macrophages in contact with *M. tuberculosis* form complexes known as tubercles and may fuse to form giant cells. This initial infection of the lung and regional extension to the hilar lymph nodes is known as the primary complex. As the tubercular lesion progresses, there is often cheese-like necrosis in the center of the lesion, known as caseation necrosis.

If host resistance is adequate at this point, these caseous lesions heal by calcification to form Ghon's complexes, which are visible on chest radiographs as radiodensities. If host resistance cannot overcome this pathogenic process, then the caseation necrosis proceeds to frank liquefaction, that is, there is a liquid produced in the necrotic center. This liquefaction serves as the basis for cavity formation and rapid proliferation of *M. tuberculosis*. It is at this point that *M. tuberculosis* can again be spread by droplet infection. Coughing caused by the bronchial irritation of the infection brings up *M. tuberculosis*–infected sputum, which can then be transmitted to other persons. If the tubercular cavity in the lung becomes large enough, it may gain access to the vasculature and become disseminated (or miliary) tuberculosis. Within the same patient, there may, in fact, be both healing and active tubercular lesions.

There are several factors related to the pathogenesis of tuberculosis. The disease is associated with unsanitary and crowded living conditions and, accordingly, with low socioeconomic status, stress, and malnutrition. Genetics also appear to be important, as evidenced by the high prevalence of tuberculosis in American Indians and Eskimos. Age and hormonal status also appear to be important. Prior to the first half of this century, most children were exposed to *M. tuberculosis* and became skin test–positive. The high prevalence of this infection led many investigators to the conclusion that *M. tuberculosis* represented an "endogenous" infection. However, with improvements in living conditions and sanitation, children today are very rarely exposed to *M. tuberculosis*. At present, the typical tuberculosis patient in the United States is an elderly man who is malnourished and possibly alcoholic. These cases of tuberculosis may, in fact, represent recurrence of previously quiescent tuberculosis.

Diagnosis

Tuberculosis can be diagnosed in several ways. First, demonstration of acid-fast bacilli in smears made from sputum samples is indicative of tuberculosis. Second, *M. tuberculosis* can be cultured from sputum or other contaminated fluids onto egg yolk containing agar or onto oleic acid–albumin agar following 2 to 4 weeks of incubation. Finally, a positive skin test is indicative of tuberculosis. Previously, an old tuberculin (OT) preparation was used in skin testing. This consisted of autoclaved or boiled tubercle bacilli in which the bacterial cells were filtered away. Currently, as mentioned earlier, purified protein derivative (PPD) is used in skin testing. This is an ammonium sulfate precipitate from tubercle bacilli cultures. In what is known as the Mantoux test, 0.1 ml of appropriately diluted PPD is injected into the skin of the forearm. If a patient has been sensitized and has developed delayed hypersensitivity to *M. tuberculosis,* then a large area of induration and erythema will appear after 48 hours at the site of injection. These areas are measured with a ruler. A positive reaction, therefore, indicates sensitivity to *M. tuberculosis.* It does not distinguish between patients who currently have tuberculosis and those who have previously had tuberculosis. Delayed hypersensitivity becomes apparent 4 to 6 weeks following exposure to the organism and may remain apparent for months or years.

Treatment

Before the development of appropriate antibiotics in the 1940s, treatment for tuberculosis involved rest, proper nutrition, and sometimes artificial collapse of one lung. When tuberculosis was epidemic, large numbers of tuberculosis sanitariums were operated for this type of treatment and to sequester these patients from the general population. Streptomycin, developed in 1945, was the first useful antibiotic for treatment of tuberculosis. This antibiotic, however, is toxic and can cause eighth nerve deafness. Also, although bactericidal, streptomycin is not capable of killing *M. tuberculosis* located intracellularly. A much better drug for the treatment of tuberculosis is isoniazid (INH). This drug can kill *M. tuberculosis* in extracellular and intracellular sites. Its low toxicity, cost, and oral route of administration have revolutionized the treatment of tuberculosis. Tuberculosis is no longer treated by long periods of confinement in sanitaria. Isoniazid and other drugs have made it possible to treat tuberculosis on an out-patient basis. In fact, current drug therapy for tuberculosis involves a combination of antibiotics such as rifampin, para-aminosalicylic acid (PAS), ethambutol (EMB), kanamycin, capreomycin, cycloserine, ethionamide, and pyrazinamide. Even so, treatment for tuberculosis requires long periods of antibiotic therapy—as long as 18 to 24 months.

When tuberculosis was prevalent in the United States, mass screening by chest radiography and skin testing was commonplace for epidemiologic prevention. Since this disease is now relatively infrequent, these approaches have been abandoned. In their place have come prophylactic approaches targeted to household and familial contacts of tuberculosis patients. These subjects are placed on chemotherapeutic regimens similar to those of patients with tuberculosis.

MYCOBACTERIUM LEPRAE

Another important human pathogen in the genus *Mycobacterium* is *Mycobacterium leprae.* This microorganism, also known as Hansen's bacillus, causes leprosy, a grossly disfiguring and degenerative disease that was prevalent in Biblical times and that even today affects millions of subjects worldwide.

M. leprae is morphologically indistinguishable from *M. tuberculosis;* however, this microorganism has never been cultured. It can be found in high numbers of lepromatous lesions and propagated in mice foot pads and in the nine-banded armadillo. Even though *M. leprae* has not been cultured, an extract known as lepromin can be obtained by boiling *M. leprae*–rich human tissue, and this is used in skin testing.

Pathogenesis

M. leprae is apparently transmitted from infected cutaneous lesions through skin abrasions where it may lie dormant for months to decades. It then forms chronic granulomatous lesions similar to those of tuberculosis, with epithelioid and giant cells but without caseation necrosis. *M. leprae* affects mainly skin and nerve tissue. The cutaneous form of leprosy results in the production of numerous firm nodules. The neural form results in peripheral nerve paresthesia and anesthesia. Subjects with this form of leprosy are liable to injure their extremities, with the development of secondary infection and severe cosmetic defects.

Lepromin is useful in determining the prognosis and progression of the disease, similar to tuberculin skin testing. The development of a hypersensitive granuloma following injection of lepromin into a sensitized patient is known as a Mitsuda reaction.

There are three phases of leprosy. During the progressive phase, lesions exhibit macrophages with foamy cytoplasm, known as leprae cells, as well as acid-fast bacilli. There is a negative Mitsuda reaction during the progressive phase. During the intermediate phase, acid-fast bacilli are found in necrotic tissues, and there is a positive Mitsuda reaction. During the healing phase, fibrotic resolution of the lesions is evident and few leprae cells are evident. Patients do not die of leprosy per se but rather of secondary infections by other microorganisms and of a systemic disease known as amyloidosis, which results in the deposition of waxy substances in internal organs.

Diagnosis and Treatment

Leprosy can be diagnosed by the demonstration of acid-fast bacilli in skin lesions. Often there is a false-positive reaction to the serologic test for syphylis. Leprosy is treated with the drug dapsone (diaminodiphenylsulfone).

REFERENCES

Bailey, W. C., Albert, R. K., Davidson, P. T., Farer, L. S., Glassroth, J., Kendig, E., Loridan, R. G., and Inselman, L. S.: Treatment of tuberculosis and other mycobacterial diseases. Am. Rev. Respir. Dis. 127:790, 1983.

Dutt, A. K., and Snead, W. W.: Present chemotherapy for tuberculosis. J. Infect. Dis. 146:698, 1982.

Kim, T. C., Blackman, R. S., Heatwole, K. M., Kim, T., and Rochester, D. F.: Acid-fast bacilli in sputum smears of patients with pulmonary tuberculosis. Am. Rev. Respir. Dis. 129:264, 1984.

chapter 12

Enterobacteriaceae and Vibrionaceae

Eugene A. Gorzynski, Ph.D.

Enterobacteriaceae

During the past 30 years, there has been a decline in the frequency of infectious diseases caused by certain pathogenic bacteria—e.g., staphylococci, streptococci, and pneumococci. However, this decline has been offset by microorganisms previously judged to be less, if at all, pathogenic. Many of these microorganisms are present in the normal flora of the human host and always have the capacity to invade an individual sufficiently compromised to accept and succumb to an infectious agent. Today, however, in contradistinction to a generation ago, the average individual at risk is not only older, but inordinately compromised by an underlying disease or condition. Many invasive devices and heroic measures, both surgical and prosthetic, prolong life and, frequently, reduce competency to resist infection.

Normal Flora, Large Intestine

Microorganisms encountered in the colon (Table 12–1) of the healthy human being are responsible for many infections that ensue in the compromised individual. Significantly, by the second to third year of life, an individual has more bacteria per gram of feces (about 10^{11}) than found in any other site; 95 to 98 percent of these are anaerobes and outnumber by 1000:1 to 10,000:1 the facultative anaerobes (e.g., *Escherichia coli*) present. Of the microorganisms listed in Table 12–1, only members of the family *Enterobacteriaceae* will be considered in this chapter.

Taxonomy

Fifteen years ago, there were only 11 genera and 26 species in the family *Enterobacteriaceae*; at present, there are 22 genera and 69 species. The genera and clinically significant species are shown in Table 12–2. It is of interest that more than 99 percent of all clinical isolates belong to only 23 species; moreover, *Escherichia coli*, *Klebsiella pneumoniae*, and *Proteus mirabilis* are responsible for most infections caused by *Enterobacteriaceae*.

General Characteristics

The family *Enterobacteriaceae* is composed of gram-negative, aerobic and facultatively

Table 12–1 ■ Normal flora: large intestine

Staphylococcus epidermidis	Pseudomonas aeruginosa
Staphylococcus aureus	Alcaligenes faecalis
Viridans streptococci	Bacteroides spp.
Enterococci	Fusobacterium spp.
Streptococcus pyogenes*	Actinomycetes
Peptostreptococci	Candida spp.
Lactobacilli†	Protozoans
Corynebacteria	Viruses
Enterobacteriaceae	Bacteriophages
Mycobacteria	Mycoplasma spp.

*Occasionally.
†Especially in infants.

anaerobic, rod-shaped bacteria that do not produce spores. Many species have flagella; nonmotile variants of motile species may be encountered. Nitrates are reduced to nitrites and glucose is used fermentatively. The percentages of positive reactions to identifying or differentiating biochemical substrates are shown in Table 12–3.

REQUIREMENTS FOR PATHOGENICITY

Bacteria vary significantly in their capacity to cause disease (i.e., in their pathogenicity). The degree of pathogenicity or virulence reflects not only the microbial species or strain per se but also the number of these required to produce infection. To avoid confusion, the adjectives "pathogenic" and "virulent" may be used as synonyms. That is, one may characterize a microorganism as being either more or less pathogenic or more or less virulent under certain conditions. The major requirements for pathogenicity (virulence) can be addressed according to the microorganism's ability to (1) colonize the host, (2) penetrate mucous surfaces, (3) invade and multiply in tissue, (4) circumvent or inhibit local or systemic defense mechanisms, and (5) directly or indirectly cause damage. The requirements are summarized in Table 12–4.

DETERMINANTS OF PATHOGENICITY

Adhesins

These macromolecules are on the surface or appendages of many bacteria and promote attachment to specific receptors on some eukaryotic cells. Adhesins may reside on fimbriae (non-flagellar, proteinaceous, filamentous appendages), pili (filamentous appendages involved in the conjugative trans-

fer of DNA), or glycocalyx (a loose network of fibrils extending outward from the cell). The microbial flora identified as normal in certain body sites (skin, oral cavity, intestinal tract) reflects selective colonization by microorganisms bearing adhesins; a portion of the bacterium is adsorbed to the animal-cell surface while the remaining portion divides and releases its progeny. Studies in oral microbiology have contributed significantly to our knowledge of colonization and the persistence of microorganisms despite the flushing action of oral (saliva) and lumen (e.g., intestinal) contents. Desquamation of surface epithelial cells, releasing both cells and adherent bacteria, contributes to host defense against pathogens. Also, intercepting bacterial adsorption by blocking or neutralizing specific-receptor loci with antibodies, mannose-binding plant protein (concanavalin A), secreted glycoproteins, or antimicrobial agents has clinical applicability.

Endotoxins

The cell walls of gram-negative bacteria contain three components outside of the pep-

Table 12–2 ■ Family: Enterobacteriaceae

Genera	Most Significant Species in Human Infection*
Buttiauxella	
Cedecea	(5)*
Citrobacter	freundii and diversus (2)
Edwardsiella	(2)
Enterobacter	aerogenes and cloacae (5)
Escherichia	coli (4)
Ewingella	(1)
Hafnia	alvei
Klebsiella	pneumoniae and oxytoca (4)
Kluyvera	(2)
Moellerella	
Morganella	morganii (1)
Obesumbacterium	
Proteus	mirabilis and vulgaris (1)
Providencia	rettgeri, stuartii, and alcalifaciens (1)
Rahnella	(1)
Salmonella	typhi, paratyphi A, and most serotypes (8)
Serratia	marcescens (8)
Shigella	sonnei and serogroups A, B, and C
Tatumella	(1)
Yersinia	enterocolitica, pestis, and pseudotuberculosis (4)
Xenorhabdus	

*Number in parenthesis indicates additional strains, species, biogroups, or biotypes less frequently causing human infection.

Extracted from Farmer et al., J Clin Microbiol 21:46, 1985, with permission.

Table 12–3 ■ Percentages positive biochemical reactions of *Enterobacteriaceae* causing human infections most frequently

Enterobacteriaceae	Indole Production	Methyl Red	Voges Proskauer	Citrate (Simmons)	H$_2$S Production	Urea Hydrolysis	Lysine Decarboxylase	Arginine Dihydrolase	Ornithine Decarboxylase	Motility at 36°C	D-Glucose, Gas	Lactose Fermentation	Sucrose Fermentation	D-Mannitol Fermentation
Citrobacter freundii	5	100	0	95	80	70	0	65	20	95	95	50	30	99
Citrobacter diversus	99	100	0	99	0	75	0	65	99	95	98	35	45	100
Enterobacter aerogenes	0	5	98	95	0	2	98	0	98	97	100	95	100	100
Enterobacter cloacae	0	5	100	100	0	65	0	97	96	95	100	93	97	100
Escherichia coli	98	99	0	1	1	1	90	17	65	95	95	95	50	98
Hafnia alvei	0	40	85	10	0	4	100	6	98	85	98	5	10	99
Klebsiella pneumonia	0	10	98	98	0	95	98	0	0	0	97	98	99	99
Klebsiella oxytoca	99	20	95	95	0	90	99	0	0	0	97	100	100	99
Morganella morganii	98	97	0	0	5	98	0	0	98	95	90	1	0	0
Proteus mirabilis	2	97	50	65	98	98	0	0	99	95	96	2	15	0
Proteus vulgaris	98	95	0	15	95	95	0	0	0	95	85	2	97	0
Providencia rettgeri	99	93	0	95	0	98	0	0	0	94	10	5	15	100
Providencia stuartii	98	100	0	93	0	30	0	0	0	85	0	2	30	0
Providencia alcalifaciens	99	99	0	98	0	0	0	0	1	96	85	0	15	2
Salmonella typhi	0	100	0	0	97	0	98	3	0	97	0	1	0	100
Salmonella paratyphi A	0	100	0	0	10	0	0	15	95	95	99	0	0	100
Salmonella, most serotypes	1	100	0	95	95	1	98	70	97	95	96	1	1	100
Shigella sonnei	0	100	0	0	0	0	0	2	98	0	0	2	1	99
Shigella serogroups A, B, C	50	100	0	0	0	0	0	5	1	0	2	0	0	93
Yersinia enterocolitica	50	97	2	0	0	75	0	0	95	2	5	5	95	98
Yersinia pestis	0	80	0	0	0	5	0	0	0	0	0	0	0	97
Yersinia pseudotuberculosis	0	100	0	0	0	95	0	0	0	0	0	0	0	100

Extracted from Farmer et al., J Clin Microbiol 21:46, 1985, with permission.

Table 12–4 ■ Requirements for pathogenicity

Progression	Comments
Colonization	The establishment and growth of an exogenous microbial strain on or in a host; clinical manifestations or immune responses may or may not ensue.
Penetration	Whereas any microorganism can invade tissue damaged by burn or trauma, most gain access after initial colonization of mucosal surfaces of the respiratory, alimentary, and urogenital tract. Normally, mucosal surfaces are protected from invasion by the (1) normal microbial flora, (2) bactericidal or bacteriostatic influences present in mucous secretions, (3) mechanical flushing of lumen contents, including mucus. However, some bacteria produce substances that enhance adsorption to mucosal surfaces or promote phagocytosis by surface cells, which protects against the flushing action of lumen contents.
Multiplication in vivo	To produce infection, bacteria must multiply on mucosal surfaces or within the host's tissue. However, multiplication is initiated and continues only when the nutritional conditions are favorable and the microorganism either circumvents or fails to stimulate host defense mechanisms.
Inhibition of host defenses	Aggressins are products of bacterial growth that inhibit host defense mechanisms, e.g., bactericidal factors present in body fluids, action of phagocytes (mobilization, contact, ingestion, intracellular killing). In addition, cytoplasmic factors or endotoxins of gram-negative bacteria may interfere with humoral or cell-mediated immunity. The clinical outcome depends on the results of interplay between the microorganism and its host's or tissue environment.
Damage to the host	Species of *Enterobacteriaceae* can harm the host by one or several of the following: (1) production of exotoxin, (2) liberation of endotoxin, (3) elicitation of hypersensitivity responses to continued or subsequent infection by the identical pathogen.

tidoglycan layer: lipoprotein, outer membrane, and lipopolysaccharide. The lipoprotein stabilizes the outer membrane by anchoring it to the peptidoglycan layer; the outer membrane protects enteric bacteria from bile salts and hydrolytic enzymes of the host environment; the lipopolysaccharide (LPS) is composed of a polysaccharide attached to a potent nonprotein toxin, a complex lipid called lipid A. The polysaccharide of LPS represents the major surface (O) antigen of the bacterial cell; specificity of antigen is conferred by terminal repeat units (linear trisaccharides or branched tetra- or pentasaccharides) that branch from a core polysaccharide constant in all species of *Enterobacteriaceae*. The endotoxin moiety is stable at 100°C; it can be extracted with phenol water from intact cells and further separated into lipid A and polysaccharide components by mild acid hydrolysis. Significantly, both in vitro and in situ, LPS is liberated when bacteria lyse. The pathophysiologic effects are similar, independent of enterobacterial origin, and range from self-limited fever, at one extreme, to refractory endotoxic shock. Major biologic effects are presented in Table 12–5.

Enterotoxins

These are extracellular toxins (exotoxins), protein in character, and intrinsically different from cell-wall endotoxins. In contradistinction to the latter, enterotoxins

1. do not cause fever in the host
2. are unstable at temperatures above 60°C
3. stimulate the formation of enterotoxin-neutralizing antibodies (antitoxins)
4. are excreted by living cells
5. are toxic to laboratory animals in nanogram amounts
6. activate adenyl cyclase present in the intestinal epithelial membrane causing a rise in intracellular cyclic adenosine monophosphate (cAMP) levels and, accordingly, affect electrolyte transport

Exotoxin production has been demonstrated by many strains of enteric bacteria (*Vibrio cholerae*, *V. parahaemolyticus*, *Yersinia enterocolitica*, *Escherichia coli*, *Shigella dysenteriae*, *Klebsiella pneumoniae*, species of *Citrobacter* and *Enterobacter*) and even *Pseudomonas aeruginosa*. The exotoxins of *E. coli* and *V. cholerae* have characteristics in common and will be addressed later.

Capsular Polysaccharides

Certain species of *Enterobacteriaceae* have capsules composed of polysaccharide antigens that are external to the O antigens of LPS. The extracellular layer of capsule provides a good means of circumventing host defense and, as a result, contributes to the pathogenic asset of the microorganism per se

Table 12–5 ■ Biologic effects of enterobacterial lipopolysaccharide

Effect	Comment
Fever	Caused by release of endogenous pyrogen from polymorphonuclear leukocytes
Leukopenia	Within minutes after the administration of LPS, the number of leukocytes per mm³ may be reduced more than 70%, leukopenia is transient
Leukocytosis	Occurs after initial (transient) leukopenia
Phagocytosis	Enhanced by small doses; depressed by large doses
Complement activation	In vitro, via the alternative pathway; however, lysis of endotoxin coated erythrocytes likely does require the classical pathway
Macrophage activation	Results in markedly augmented, nonspecific microbicidal activity
Elicitation of Shwartzman phenomenon	Subcutaneous injection into a rabbit of a few micrograms of LPS causes slight inflammation at the site of administration. If, 24 hours later, the same amount of any LPS is injected intravenously, a hemorrhagic or necrotic lesion appears within a few hours at the skin site injected initially.
Activation of intravascular coagulation	A very serious consequence of endotoxin intoxication. Fibrin deposition in the microcirculation of vital organs contributes significantly to ensuing death. Heparin, administered prophylactically during sepsis, may ameliorate an untoward intravascular reaction.
Adjuvant activity	Similar to other adjuvants (Freund's, alum, aluminum hydroxide, dextran sulfate), LPS enhances the immunogenicity of adsorbed soluble proteins. Macrophage and T (helper) cell activities are increased by most adjuvants. LPS is a polyclonal B cell activator and, likely, promotes proliferation of B cells.
Altered resistance to infection	Endotoxin affects resistance to bacterial infection nonspecifically. Whereas large doses depress phagocytosis and resistance, small doses enhance both phagocytosis and synthesis of antibody. To an appropriate dose, the response is biphasic; i.e., depression followed by enhancement as the concentration in situ decreases.
Endotoxemia	Toxemia that follows the administration or acquisition of a large amount of LPS presents hypoglycemia, high blood lactate/pyruvate ratios, and decreased tissue oxygen utilization. As noted previously, other events occur simultaneously or progressively. Irreversible shock and death are predictable sequelae.

by shielding against the bactericidal action of complement and phagocytes. In *E. coli*, the capsular antigen is called K. Specific K determinants are numbered; K-12 antigen is often encountered in *E. coli* causing urinary tract infection; *E. coli* containing K-1 is a significant cause of neonatal meningitis. Certain K antigens of *E. coli* cross-react; e.g., K-12 with K-14. Also, other K antigens of *E. coli* bear strong similarities to polysaccharide antigens present in species of other genera; e.g., *E. coli* K-27 with *Klebsiella* K antigen; *E. coli* K-14 with the capsular polysaccharide of *Neisseria meningitidis* group 29-E. It is of interest to note that the capsular polysaccharide of *N. meningitidis* Group B and K-1 of *E. coli* have the identical structure and are inherent as etiologic agents of the same disease, neonatal meningitis. The latter is an excellent example of intergeneric identity (or structural relatedness) and pathogenicity.

Plasmids

Extrachromosomal genetic elements composed of circular, double-stranded DNA molecules, distinct from the chromosomes of the bacterial host, are called plasmids. The following are characters or markers attributable to plasmids:

1. production of enterotoxin
2. production of beta hemolysin
3. production of bacteriocins
4. resistance to antimicrobial agents
5. unique or altered metabolic activity
6. physiologic mechanisms that mediate bacterial mating (conjugation)

A plasmid may replicate autonomously, in synchrony with its bacterial-host chromosome, or integrate with the latter chromosome and replicate as a single unit (replicon) and, by conjugation, transfer donor characters or markers to recipients of the same or heterogeneric species.

Bacteriocins

These are proteins produced by many gram-negative microorganisms that have antimicrobial properties active against other strains of the same bacterial species. Bacteriocins are named according to respective bacterial hosts; for example, marcescins (*Serratia marcescens*), colicins (*Escherichia coli*), and pyocins (*Pseudomonas aeruginosa,* formerly *P. pyocyaneus*). Bacteriocins are encoded by plasmid genes and are nonconjugative. After release from host cells, bacteriocins attach to specific receptors on susceptible cells and induce a specific metabolic block, that is, cessation of nucleic acid or protein synthesis, or of oxidative phosphorylation; the recipient cell dies. Bacteria can be identified or "typed" according to their susceptibility to a specific bacteriocin.

Summary

Enterobacteriaceae vary in their capacity to cause infection; this variation occurs not only among species of the same genus but also among strains of the same species. Pathogenicity is highly polygenic. That is, it requires the action of several different genes and can be affected by mutation or changes in a microorganism's nutrition, growth rate, or environment. The degree of pathogenicity is determined by virulence factors, that is, by inheritable and/or transmissible toxins and by surface molecules that are antiphagocytic or promote adsorption to susceptible eukaryotic cells. Virulence can be quantitated under appropriately controlled laboratory conditions. As a result, by manipulating the physiologic requirements or determinants of a microbial strain and by addressing routes of administration to a suitable animal host, specific factors can be characterized, modes of action can be predicted, and modulation by chemotherapeutic intervention can be studied.

ANTIGENIC STRUCTURE

The etiologic agent of an enterobacterial disease can be identified with a measurable degree of certainty by biochemical tests (see Table 12–3). Usually, appropriate therapy and management of an infected patient will ensure identification made by biochemical profile. To confirm the identification of an isolate for therapeutic, epidemiologic, or academic reasons, an analysis of the bacterium's antigenic structure or composition may be required. This is accomplished by serologic typing; that is, by employing antisera containing antibodies directed against antigenic determinants on a microorganism, its fraction, or substrate. The antigens of *Enterobacteriaceae* are classified under three main groups: somatic (O antigens), flagellar (H antigens), capsular (K antigens).

Somatic (O) Antigens

These are complexes located on the most external part of the cell wall lipopolysaccharide. Specificity is determined by the nature of the terminal groups and the order in which these groups occur in the repeating units of the polysaccharide chain. Eighteen different monosaccharides have been identified in certain genera; some species have as many as nine.

Somatic antigens of *Enterobacteriaciae* are stable at 100°C and are resistant to ethanol and dilute acid. Whereas each genus of the family *Enterobacteriaceae* is characterized by the presence of certain O antigens, species may carry one or several additional O antigens. Moreover, species of different genera may share O (heterogeneric) antigens. For example, most *Enterobacteriaceae* share the O14 antigen with *E. coli*. Therefore, on the basis of determining the presence of both generic and species antigens, a miroorganism can be identified serologically to species level if one uses care to preclude or account for cross-reactions.

Flagellar (H) Antigens

These proteins, called flagellins, are found in flagella. Specificity is determined by amino acid content and by the order in which these acids occur in the flagellins. Flagellins are heat-labile, inactivated by ethanol, and form loosely knit floccular aggregates in the presence of anti-H antibodies. Unless removed chemically or destroyed by heat, H antigens may interfere with the serologic detection of the microorganism's O antigen. Uniquely, in the genus *Salmonella,* a reversible variation (phase variation) of H antigen(s) may occur. In phase variation, the antigenic identity of flagellin may shift during culture of a flagellated species, from a specific (homologous) to a nonspecific (heterologous) serotype. The shift designations are called phase 1 (specific) and phase 2 (nonspecific). On further subculturing the phases may shift back and forth. Not all salmonellae are diphasic; some are irreversibly monophasic, others are multiphasic.

Capsular (K) Antigens

Capsules, if present, are topographically external to the somatic antigens of *Enterobacteriaceae*. Most capsules are composed of polysaccharide that protect the bacterial cell against the bactericidal action of phagocytes and complement. Like flagellin, capsular antigen is heat-labile and may interfere with O agglutination by anti-O antibodies. Many antigenically different K antigens have been identified; they are labeled numerically. As noted earlier, certain K antigens are associated with virulence (e.g., *E. coli* with K1 antigen is a frequent cause of neonatal meningitis). Also, some species of *Salmonella* possess a capsular antigen, called Vi, that may be associated with invasiveness. Of note, a Vi-related antigen has been reported for certain serotypes of *Citrobacter*, a genus with species less frequently associated with invasive disease.

Enterobacterial Common Antigen (ECA)

This heat-stable, ethanol-soluble antigen exists in one or both of two forms in species of *Enterobacteriaceae*; one form is immunogenic in laboratory animals and the other is "nonimmunogenic," although both forms contain the identical antigenic determinant. The immunogenic form is present in only few bacterial species, probably covalently linked to LPS; *E. coli* O14 is the prototype. The "nonimmunogenic" form is present in most other species of *Enterobacteriaceae*. Significantly, after separation from LPS by ethanol extraction, the "nonimmunogenic" form elicits anti-ECA antibodies that may protect against infection induced against heterologous enteric species containing ECA. Taxonomically, a determination that a microorganism produces ECA may be a significant aid to assigning a new species to the family *Enterobacteriaceae*.

CLINICAL INFECTIONS

Whereas a few enterobacterial species have always been characterized as causes of overt intestinal infection, it is likely that all species of *Enterobacteriaceae* have the capability of causing infection outside of the intestinal tract. It is important to emphasize, however, that the mere presence of enteric microorganisms in urine, sputum, wounds, burns, or specimens obtained from normally sterile body fluid (e.g., blood, peritoneal, cerebrospinal) does not indicate the unequivocal cause of disease. These microorganisms may be contaminants or may represent a transient population of innocuous microbial strains. Definition of the (potential) role these microorganisms play requires clinical judgment supported by the careful and timely acquisition of appropriate specimens, and laboratory data obtained from tests that are sensitive and provide specific and quality-controlled information. In the subsequent sections, the *Enterobacteriaceae* most frequently encountered in human disease (see Table 12–2) will be addressed. General morphologic and physiologic attributes were presented in the previous section on General Characteristics in Table 12–3.

Escherichia coli

This is the most prominent aerobic species in the large bowel. Whereas more than 150 serotypes have been identified, only a few serotypes or strains have been shown to cause intestinal disease or to produce enterotoxin. The presence of *E. coli*, regardless of serotype, outside its host (e.g., food, water, soil, solutions, instruments, and devices) always indicates fecal contamination. The presence in clinical specimens may indicate contamination, colonization, or infection.

Intestinal disease

Infantile diarrhea ■ At least 12 antigenic types (e.g., O111, O55, O26, and O127) have been identified as causes of severe, life-threatening diarrhea in infants. Responsible strains are designated by the acronym EPEC (enteropathogenic *E. coli*). EPEC strains do not cause intestinal disease in older children or adults; therefore, except in outbreaks of infantile diarrhea, serotyping is not indicated.

Traveler's diarrhea ■ Enterotoxin-producing strains of *E. coli*, designated ETEC, are responsible for a diarrhea, milder than infantile diarrhea and usually self-limited, that may affect people traveling abroad or relocating to a different geographic area. ETEC strains produce one or each of two kinds of enterotoxins; a heat-labile toxin (LT), which resembles the toxin of *Vibrio cholerae*, and a heat-stable toxin (ST). LT activates adenyl cyclase; ST activates guanyl cyclase. The toxins are active in the small bowel and, likely, in the colon. Enterotoxin production is mediated by plasmids.

Extraintestinal infection ■ Of the more than 150 serotypes, about 10 percent are encountered most frequently in urinary tract, meningeal, wound, postsurgical, and peritoneal infections caused by *E. coli*. The presence of a particular capsular polysaccharide antigen (K-1) is associated with pyelonephritis and neonatal meningitis. Of interest are reports of immunochemical similarity between certain *E. coli* K antigens and capsular antigens of other invasive microorganisms, e.g., *Haemophilus influenzae* (serotype b), *Neisseria meningitidis* (serogroups B and C), and several serotypes of *Streptococcus pneumoniae*.

Shigella

This genus comprises four species. Significant characteristics are presented in Table 12–6. It is noteworthy that, in contradistinction to most other enterobacterial causes of intestinal infections, shigellae are not motile. All species are pathogens and cause bacillary dysentery (shigellosis) in humans. The infective dose is low, less than 10^3 microorganisms. Shigellosis is transmitted by the fecal-oral route, primarily by hand to mouth contact. Outdoor latrines and the density of flies can be related to the incidence of bacillary dysentery. Usually, infections are limited to the terminal ileum and the colon, where mucosal ulcerations, covered by a pseudomembrane, evolve after initial invasion of intestinal epithelial cells. Endotoxic lipopolysaccharide, released upon autolysis of shigellae, likely contributes to the death of epithelial cells. Rarely do *Shigella* species invade the blood stream or cause infection at sites other than the intestinal tract. *S. dysenteriae* produces a heat-labile exotoxin that is both neurotoxic and enterotoxic.

Bacillary dysentery has a brief incubation period (1 to 4 days) and is characterized by a sudden onset of abdominal pain, diarrhea, and fever. The loss of water and salts may cause dehydration and electrolyte imbalance. Mucus and blood in feces are common findings.

During convalescence, most persons develop fecal (copro) and humoral antibodies; these do not protect against reinfection.

Enterobacter

Species of this genus are found normally in 40 to 80 percent of fecal specimens obtained from human subjects. In examining food and water supplies for evidence of fecal contamination, it is important to distinguish *E. coli*, the index microorganism, from species of *Enterobacter*. The latter are found commonly on plants and can be differentiated from *E. coli* by biochemical tests (Table 12–7).

Enterobacter species may cause extraintestinal infections. Often they are isolated as secondary invaders or as opportunists from patients compromised by malignancy, instrumentation, or therapy. They have characteristics in common with species of *Klebsiella* (see next section), causes of respiratory and urinary tract infections, with major differences in susceptibility to antimicrobial agents.

Klebsiella

The most virulent species of this genus, *pneumoniae*, is encapsulated; variants (rough strains) are avirulent. Whereas *K. pneumoniae* may be found in the respiratory tract and feces of healthy individuals, it is a significant cause of acute bacterial pneumonias and, next to *E. coli*, the most common cause of urinary tract infections. Because of its capsule (K antigen), *K. pneumoniae* produces large, moist, mucoid colonies on nutrient media. In situ, these capsules preclude phagocytosis and interfere with antimicrobial therapy.

Unlike *K. pneumoniae*, *K. oxytoca* produces indole in media containing tryptophan. Although not a frequent pathogen, *K. oxytoca* has been recovered from blood, urine, wounds, and sputum; it may be found in feces of healthy hosts. Administration of an aminoglycoside or a cephalosporin or, in se-

Table 12–6 ■ Species and characteristics of Shigellae

Species	Motility	Groups	Types	Mannitol*	Ornithine Decarboxylase*
S. dysenteriae	−	A	1 to 10	−	−
S. flexneri	−	B	1 to 6	+	−
S. boydii	−	C	1 to 15	+	−
S. sonnei	−	D	1	+	+

*− = 95% or more negative in 24 to 48 hours; + = 95% or more positive in 24 to 48 hours.

Table 12-7 ■ Percentages positive metabolic reactions of *Escherichia coli* and species of *Enterobacter*

	Reactions			
	I	*MR*	*VP*	*C*
Escherichia coli	96.3	99.1	0	0.2
Enterobacter				
aerogenes	0.8	1.6	100	92.6
cloacae	0	3.3	100	98.9

I = Indole formation in media containing tryptophan

MR = Methyl red as indicator of mixed acid fermentation

VP = Voges-Proskauer reaction, a color test for acetoin, a product of butylene glycol fermentation

C = Citrate as the only source of carbon

Reprinted by permission of the publisher from Chapters 6, 9, and 14 by W.H. Ewing, Edwards and Ewing's Identification of Enterobacteriaceae, 4th edition. Copyright 1986 by Elsevier Science Publishing Company, Inc.

vere cases, a combination of both antimicrobic agents, remains the most effective therapy of klebsiellae infections. As a rule, antimicrobials should be used only after susceptibility tests have been performed and only when indicated.

Salmonella

This genus comprises three species: *typhi* (one serotype), *choleraesuis* (one serotype), and *enteritidis* (more than 1800 serotypes). Serotypes reflect the presence of from one to several major and from none to several minor O antigens. Serotypes with the same major O antigens are placed in the same lettered O serogroup. Representative antigenic formulas of salmonellae are shown in Table 12–8. Whereas *Salmonella* serotypes are not species, reporting these microorganisms as species is a convenient way to avoid long names; for example, *S. enteritidis* serotype Typhimurium may be reported simply as *S. typhimurium*.

Approximately 95 percent of the *Salmonella* species causing human infection belong to the five serogroups shown in Table 12–8; these serogroups are composed of fewer than 40 species. The 10 species isolated most frequently in 1981 are presented in Table 12–9 according to median age of persons from whom isolates were recovered. For diagnostic, management, and epidemiologic reasons, identifying *Salmonella* species by serotyping is important. The application of molecular and biologic methodologies to epidemiologic studies assists in tagging outbreaks caused by salmonellae of defined antigenic serotype.

In humans, species of *Salmonella* cause the clinical diseases summarized in Table 12–10. Independent of source or mode of transmission, the mean infecting dose usually is high, 10^6 to 10^8 microorganisms. As expected in individuals compromised by age, diet, underlying disease, or environment, the infectious dose may be low—for example, 10^3 or less. Additional salient features of salmonellosis are as follows.

Enterocolitis ■ This is the most common manifestation of infection by salmonellae (see Table 12–9). Although any serotype of *S. enteritidis* may cause this condition, *S. typhimurium* is responsible most frequently (about 34 percent).

Nausea, vomiting, profuse diarrhea, and low-grade fever are the most common symptoms. Most infections are self-limited; moreover, antimicrobial treatment may prolong excretion of the etiologic agent.

Enteric fever (typhoid) ■ After ingestion, etiologic microorganisms infect the small intestine and, through lymphatics, invade the blood stream. After infecting many organs and multiplying in lymphatic tissue, these microorganisms reach the intestine in large numbers and are expelled in the feces.

Usual symptoms include fever, constipation, prostration, abdominal tenderness, and frequently, distention; an enlarged spleen

Table 12-8 ■ Representative antigenic formulae of Salmonellae

Serogroup	Serotype ("species")	O	H1	H2
A	*S. paratyphi* A	1,2,12	a	—
B	*S. typhimurium*	1,4,5,12	i	1,2
C	*S. choleraesuis*	6,7	c	1,5
D	*S. typhi*	9,12,Vi*	d	—
E	*S. anatum*	3,10	e,h	1,6

H1: Phase 1 flagellar antigen(s).

H2: Phase 2 flagellar antigen(s).

*Vi may not be present.

Reprinted by permission of the publisher from Chapters 6, 9, and 14 by W.H. Ewing, Edwards and Ewing's Identification of Enterobacteriaceae, 4th edition. Copyright 1986 by Elsevier Science Publishing Company, Inc.

Table 12–9 ■ Serotypes of *Salmonella* isolated most frequently from humans (1981)

Serotype	No. of Isolates	Percentage of Total	Median Age of Persons From Whom Isolates Were Obtained
S. typhimurium	12, 176	34.2	8.0
S. enteritidis	2,554	7.2	19.0
S. newport	2,134	6.0	15.0
S. heidelberg	2,049	5.8	4.0
S. infantis	1,497	4.2	5.0
S. agona	1,205	3.4	2.0
S. saint-paul	861	2.4	17.5
S. montevideo	739	2.1	18.5
S. muenchen	644	1.8	15.5
S. typhi	604*	1.7	26.0
Subtotal†	24,463	68.8	
Total Salmonellae	35,625		12.0

*38 (6.3%) of the 604 isolates of *S. typhi* were from carriers, 195 (32.3%) from overt infections, and the remaining 371 (61.4%) undesignated.

†Most frequent isolates.

Reprinted by permission of the New England Journal of Medicine, from Morbidity and Mortality Weekly Report *31*/No. 45; November 1982.

and leukopenia are also common. Rarely, intestinal hemorrhage and perforation of the bowel with subsequent peritonitis may occur, with fatal sequelae.

Septicemia ■ This feature is characterized by an abrupt onset with high, remittent fever and bacteremia. Gastrointestinal involvement is not apparent. Focal suppurative lesions may develop in kidneys, heart, meninges, spleen, lungs and joints. The septicemia may be prolonged and is difficult to control by treating with antimicrobial agents effective in vitro.

Proteus

Species of this genus are found commonly in sewage, manure, soil, and normal human feces. Owing to peritrichous flagella, *Proteus* species are actively motile; unless inhibited by chemicals (such as phenylethyl alcohol)

incorporated in a medium, "swarming" on the medium's surface will occur, masking or covering colonies of other bacterial species that may be present.

Proteus species are frequent causes of urinary tract infection; the urine becomes alkaline, promoting stone formation and making acidification very difficult. The high pH results from the liberation of ammonia that occurs after the hydrolysis of urea by urease-producing species. Outside of the intestinal tract, species of *Proteus* may cause wound infections, pneumonia, and focal infections in debilitated patients. Although not an established cause of diarrhea, *Proteus* species are often found in increased numbers in patients receiving antimicrobial therapy or during diarrheal diseases caused by other microorganisms. *P. vulgaris*, which usually produces indole, is more resistant to antimicrobial agents than is *P. mirabilis*. The latter

Table 12–10 ■ Clinical diseases caused by Salmonellae

Observation	Enterocolitis	Enteric Fever	Septicemia
Etiology	S. typhimurium	S. typhi†	S. choleraesuis
Source	Animals*	Humans‡	Animals (swine)
Modes of transmission	Contaminated food, drink, direct contact, and insects (flies) as couriers		
Incubation period	1–2 days	7–14 days	Variable
Duration	2–5 days	18–32 days	Variable
Blood cultures	Negative	Positive during the initial 12–14 days	Positive
Stool cultures	Usually positive	Negative early in disease; positive after blood cultures become negative	Usually negative

*Turtles, poultry, pigs, rodents, and so on.

†*S. paratyphi* A causes less grave enteric fever with a briefer incubation period.

‡Most laboratory animals are resistant, unless the infectious dose is suspended in mucin.

may be inhibited readily by a cephalosporin or an aminoglycoside; even a penicillin-like agent may be effective.

Morganella

The single species of this genus, *morganii*, has been implicated as a cause of diarrhea. More significantly, it causes urinary tract infections and is recovered as a potential pathogen from many other body sites. Tests for indole, H_2S production, and ornithine decarboxylase activity are useful for separating *M. morganii* from species of *Proteus*.

Providencia

Hospital-borne infections of the urinary tract occasionally are caused by a species of *Providencia,* either *stuartii* or *alcalifaciens.* The latter is present in the feces of healthy individuals. Whereas *P. alcalifaciens* is frequently isolated from feces of children with diarrheal gastroenteritis, its etiologic role has not been established. In contrast, *P. stuartii,* rarely found in feces, is a cause of infection in patients compromised by instrumentation, intensive antimicrobial treatment, or burns. In burn patients, septicemia and pneumonia are frequent complications.

Yersinia

This genus, comprising three clinically significant species (*pestis, enterocolitica,* and *pseudotuberculosis*), is a recent addition to the family *Enterobacteriaceae*. Animals are the natural hosts of yersiniae.

Y. pestis ■ This is the etiologic agent of plague (black death), a disease that killed millions of people during pandemics of the 6th century A.D., of the 14th century, and at the close of the 19th century. Although plague declined worldwide during the first half of the 20th century, there has been a gradual increase recently on various continents. In the United States, sylvatic (wild) plague is epizootic among pack rats, prairie dogs, squirrels, and rabbits. As a result, sporadic cases in humans do occur, especially in many western states where sylvatic plague is epizootic.

Plague is transmitted among rodents and from rodents to humans through the bite of fleas infected by blood sucked from their infected hosts. From the bite, *Y. pestis* extends to regional lymph nodes via lymphatic channels. There is rapid and progressive hemorrhagic inflammation at the bite site, along the lymphatic channels, and in the infected lymph nodes. The nodes, most frequently located in the axilla or groin, become very large "bubos." This phase of infection is called bubonic plague. Often, infection progresses via efferent lymphatics and the thoracic duct to the blood and, as a consequence, to all organs of the host. Rapid proliferation in the blood is the septicemic form of plague. The parenchymatous lesions produced in infected organs are hemorrhagic; disseminated intravascular coagulation may ensue. If metastatic pneumonia (pneumonic plague) develops, the infection may be transmitted readily by droplets from the respiratory tract. Pneumonic plague is extraordinarily malignant and resistant to therapy, and prognosis is poor.

Strains of *Y. pestis* produce the following factors which significantly influence virulence:

1. fraction 1 (F1), an envelope (heat-labile protein) antigen
2. VW antigen, comprising a protein (V) and a lipoprotein (W)
3. lipopolysaccharide (endotoxin)
4. murine toxin, lethal to mice and rats but not to rabbits or monkeys
5. enterobacterial common antigen (ECA)

It is important to note that both F1 and VW are antiphagocytic antigens; effective vaccines must contain both complexes.

Y. enterocolitica ■ This enterotoxigenic microorganism causes in humans a diffuse and severe enterocolitis with mucosal ulcers and mesenteric lymphadenitis. Symptoms simulate appendicitis and include fever, severe abdominal pain, and diarrhea. An outbreak affecting 218 children in Oneida County, New York, was traced to the consumption of contaminated chocolate milk (*Morbidity and Mortality Weekly Report,* a publication of United States Public Health Service, 18 February 1977).

Y. pseudotuberculosis ■ This microorganism, which has an extensive animal reservoir, may cause mesenteric lymphadenitis in children and young adults. Food and water contaminated by animal excreta appear to be the main modes of transmission. However, institutional outbreaks suggest transmission also through direct contact with infected patients.

Hafnia alvei

Compared with other *Enterobacteriaceae,* this microorganism is less frequently encountered as a cause of extraintestinal infection. Until recently, the species *alvei* was classified under the genus *Enterobacter*.

Citrobacter

The two species, *freundii* and *diversus*, are well-recognized human pathogens found to be primary or secondary causes of a variety of diseases in humans compromised by age or invasive procedures. Certain strains of *C. freundii* produce H_2S and therefore may be confused with species of *Salmonella*. Differentiation is made by biochemical tests.

Serratia marcescens

This microorganism, long considered a harmless saprophyte, has emerged as a significant cause of opportunistic, nosocomial, and iatrogenic infections, with bacteriuria, wound infections, pneumonia, and septicemia as serious sequelae, especially in patients compromised by age, malignancy, or therapy. Its relative frequency as a cause of sepsis is 5 to 7 percent. *S. marcescens* may produce an intense red pigment in culture; more frequently, nonpigmented variants are isolated as etiologic agents.

Highlights of the *Enterobacteriaceae* associated with diarrhea are presented in Table 12–11.

Vibrionaceae

This family is composed of gram-negative, facultative, oxidase-positive, motile bacilli with predominantly polar flagellation when grown in a liquid medium and, frequently, peritrichous flagella when grown on a solid medium. Water sources are the normal habitats of representatives of this family. Several species of *Vibrio* and *Aeromonas* have clinical significance.

Vibrio

Species are curved rods on initial culture and become straight, resembling *Enterobacteriaceae*, after prolonged or repeated cultivation. The microscopic recognition of curved gram-negative bacilli in a fresh, appropriately collected diarrheal sample may guide a preliminary report and subsequent speciation. *Vibrio* species are uncommon isolates in most inland laboratories in the United States; strains are encountered more frequently in laboratories serving coastal areas. Whereas 28 species of *Vibrio* have been characterized, 10 are considered human pathogens. Two, *V. cholerae* and *V. parahaemolyticus*, are encountered most frequently.

V. cholerae ■ This is the etiologic agent of cholera, endemic in India for centuries with periodic epidemics in Southeast Asia and China. Seven pandemics have been recorded

Table 12–11 ■ Bacterial causes of diarrhea: highlights

Etiologic Agent	Site	Salient Characteristics
Invasive		
Escherichia coli	Small bowel? colon?	EPEC; >12 antigenic types
Salmonella spp	Small bowel, colon	*S. typhimurium* causes self-limiting gastroenteritis
Proteus spp	?	May be responsible for diarrhea in patients receiving antibiotics
Noninvasive		
Shigella spp	Ileum, colon	Infecting dose, <10^3; ulcers covered by pseudomembrane
Vibrio cholerae	Large bowel	Massive loss of fluid and electrolytes
Vibro parahaemolyticus	Large bowel	Self-limiting enteritis requiring restoration of fluid and electrolytes
Enterotoxin Producers		
Escherichia coli	Small bowel, colon?	ETEC strains producing LT and/or ST; cause of traveler's diarrhea
Shigella dysenteriae	Small bowel, colon	Infecting dose, <10^3; neurotoxic
Yersinia enterocolitica	Intestinal lymph nodes	Cause mucosal ulcers and mesenteric lymphadenitis; symptoms simulate appendicitis
Campylobacter jejuni	Proximal small intestine	Causes acute diarrhea; stools may contain blood and inflammatory cells

since 1817; the most recent, in the 1960s, spread from Indonesia to the Fast East, India, the Middle East, and Africa. Later, sporadic outbreaks were reported in several European nations bordering the Mediterranean Sea. In the United States, during recent years, sporadic cases and minor outbreaks have been reported from Louisiana, Florida, and Texas. Likely, *V. cholerae* now is endemic in the coastal waters of the Gulf of Mexico. Whereas the diagnosis of cholera during an epidemic presents no problem on the basis of clinical findings alone, sporadic or mild cases are not readily differentiated from other diarrheal infections. The high infecting dose (more than 10^8) required for infection likely contributes to its low prevalence in industrialized areas where water contaminated with feces, the primary mode of transmission, is monitored and controlled.

Cholera is not an invasive infection. Enterotoxigenic strains of *V. cholerae*, present in contaminated water supplies and marine food, multiply and remain localized in the intestinal tract; they do not invade the bloodstream. In the intestines, enterotoxin, endotoxin, and, likely, mucinases are released by the rapidly multiplying *V. cholerae*. The enterotoxin is adsorbed by epithelial cell gangliosides; absorption of sodium is inhibited. Owing to a hypersecretion of water and chloride, and the elution of fluid and electrolytes into the small intestine, massive diarrhea results 2 to 5 days after consuming a toxigenic dose of *V. cholerae*. The loss of luminal fluid, rice water–like in appearance, may reach 10 to 15 liters per day; without intervention, dehydration, acidosis, shock, and death ensue. The prompt and adequate replacement of fluid and electrolytes is life-saving. Whereas the administration of antimicrobial agents may eliminate intestinal *V. cholerae*, only heroic rehydration and infusion of electrolytes will preclude shock and death.

V. parahaemolyticus ■ This is a halophilic microorganism (requiring 3 to 7 percent sodium chloride for growth) found in marine water and fauna throughout the world. It has been recovered from seafood (e.g., plankton, shellfish, and crustaceans) and in Japan accounts for at least 70 percent of all cases of bacterial food poisoning. In the United States, *V. parahaemolyticus* is isolated from feces with increasing frequency as a cause of vomiting and diarrhea. The incubation period is brief: 12 to 24 hours after ingestion of contaminated seafood. The en-

teritis is self-limiting, usually requiring only the restoration of fluids and electrolytes.

Aeromonas hydrophilia

This microorganism, classified in the family *Vibrionaceae* because of its characteristic morphology, biochemical reactions, and ecology, may cause serious human infection. Although *A. hydrophilia* has been isolated from many body fluids without evidence of pathogenicity, it has been reported as a cause of septicemia, pneumonia, and gastroenteritis. Patients with severely impaired host defenses are most vulnerable.

CAMPYLOBACTER

Formerly, on the basis of gram-negative, slightly curved, monotrichous morphology, species of this genus were considered vibrios that infected various animals, including sheep, cattle, poultry, and wild birds. During the past decade, classification at the species level has been undergoing changes. These changes reflect, in part, the fact that certain *Vibrio* species have different nucleotide-based compositions and are not able to use sugars either oxidatively or fermentatively. Accordingly, these species were placed in a new genus, *Campylobacter*, and divorced from the family *Vibrionaceae*. At present, at least seven species of *Campylobacter* have been identified on the basis of DNA hybridization studies. At least two, *C. jejuni* and *C. fetus* subspecies *fetus* (formerly called subspecies *intestinalis*), are unequivocal human pathogens acquired by direct contact with infected animals or by consuming contaminated water or food. Human campylobacteriosis is manifested most frequently as a self-limiting gastroenteritis, usually due to *C. jejuni*, and infrequently as a systemic disease (bacteremia, endocarditis, pericarditis, arthritis), usually caused by *C. fetus* subspecies *fetus*. Recent reports implicate additional species of *Campylobacter* as causes of disease in humans.

Campylobacteria will not grow on simple nutrient media; they are fastidious and require enriched media supplemented with hemin, vitamin K, and 5 percent defibrinated sheep blood. A microaerophilic atmosphere (5 percent O_2, 5 percent CO_2, and 90 percent N_2) is required for growth. Duplicate sets of media should be inoculated for incubation in parallel at 35°C and 42°C; *C. fetus* subspecies *fetus* grows at 35°C and not 42°C, *C. jejuni* thrives better at 42°C than at 35°C.

The highlights of the bacterial causes of diarrhea addressed in this chapter are presented in Table 12–11.

Laboratory Diagnosis of Gram-Negative Infections

Diagnosis of an infectious disease starts in the clinic or at the patient's bedside where a history is recorded, physical examination is undertaken, (tentative) diagnosis is made, and orders for specimen acquisition are written. Laboratory diagnosis ends when the primary care physician or dentist receives and assesses data or results from specimen analysis. It is obvious that the length of time between history-taking and the receipt of laboratory results depends on factors directly controlled by the clinician, health-care personnel (including couriers of specimens), laboratorians, and communication system. With certain exceptions, the laboratorian is unable to measure the integrity of a specimen; that is, whether or not the specimen was obtained from the proper site and under conditions that exclude or minimize contamination. The specimen will be examined and results reported according to routine protocol of the testing laboratory.

The most convincing way of identifying the etiologic agent of an infection is initiated by separating the (potential) pathogen from other microorganisms that may be present as contaminants or representatives of a normal flora. Usually, this is accomplished by spreading a minute sample of specimen over the surface of a nutrient agar medium. Frequently, on the basis of the morphology, color, and texture of bacterial colonies that form after the required period of incubation, and stained, microscopic characteristics of the microbial population, an experienced technologist can provide a presumptive identification to genus level. In many cases, knowledge of genus alone is sufficient for clinical decision making. Speciation, if required, is accomplished by interpreting the isolated microorganism's phenotypic characteristics, including biochemical and antigenic profiles.

The *Enterobacteriaceae* grow readily on simple nutrient media; isolation of species from normally sterile body sites presents no problem. However, media for specimens likely to contain mixtures of microorganisms (feces, sputum, urine, wound) should be selected on the basis of their ability to enhance growth when small numbers of *Enterobacteriaceae* are present, eliminate or reduce growth of normal flora or saprophytes, or provide distinguishing characteristics to bacterial colonies that form during incubation at an appropriate

Table 12–12 ■ Media for primary isolation of gram-negative enteric bacilli

Micoorganism	Media*	Incubation T° (C)	Days	Remarks
Escherichia, Enterobacter,	BA	35	1	
Klebsiella, Serratia	MC	35		On MC, colonies, of lactose fermenting bacteria are pink to red.
Proteus	PEA	35	1	Gram-negative microorganisms other than *Proteus* are markedly or completely inhibited.
Salmonella, Shigella	BA	35	2	
	MC	35	2	Colorless colonies on MC.
	XLD	35	2	Red colonies on XLD; may have black center.
	HEK	35	2	Blue or blue-green colonies on HEK; may have black center.
Vibrio	TCBS	35	2	Yellow or blue colonies.
Yersinia enterocolitica	YSAB†	25	2	Red colonies.
	S	4	21	Transfer from S to YSAB once each week.
Campylobacter				
jejuni	CBA(B)	42	2	Requires atmosphere of 5% O_2, 5% CO_2,
fetus subsp. *fetus*	CBA(B)	35	2	and 90% N_2; only *C. jejuni* will grow at both 25° C and 42° C

*BA, blood agar; MC, MacConkey; PEA, phenylethyl alcohol agar; XLD, xylose-lysine-deoxycholate agar; HEK, hektoenteric agar; TCBS, thiosulfate-citrate-bile-sucrose agar; YSAB, yersinia selective agar base; S, saline; CBA(B), campy blood agar (Blaser)

†Preferably supplemented with cefsulodin and novobiocin to improve inhibition of normal enteric bacteria

temperature. Media that may be employed to grow microorganisms addressed in this chapter are presented in Table 12–12.

Less sensitive and more costly, albeit more rapid, methods are available for detecting the presence of certain bacteria in selected specimens. Dedicated antisera or monospecific antibodies are used; detection is on the basis of recognizable antigen-antibody reactions. Whereas positive data may have clinical significance, if quality controlled reagents and protocols are employed, negative data do not rule out the presence, in small numbers, of a specified microorganism.

A retrospective diagnosis of a specific cause of infection, in the absence of successful culture, may be feasible by using serologic techniques; i.e., testing serum samples for the presence and concentration (titer) of antibodies against known antigens. However, resulting data may be difficult to interpret because of unaccountable or uncontrollable variables. For example, in the serodiagnosis of typhoid fever (Widal test) the following must be considered: (1) *Salmonella typhi* shares antigens with other *Enterobacteriaceae*; (2) anti-O and anti-H antibody titers to typhoid and other antigens may rise during unrelated febrile illness or in recently immunized individuals; (3) the predictive values of both elevated and low or unchanged titers depend upon the prevalence of similar titers in a given population or geographic area; (4) *S. typhi* antibodies may be absent or in low titer owing to the stage of infection, poor antigenic stimulus, immunoincompetence of the host, or nutritional hypoprotei-nemia; (5) the patient may have a history of typhoid infection or may have been specifically immunized; and (6) in endemic areas, significantly elevated titers are encountered during early stages of typhoid.

After the microbiologic cause of an infection is established by employing parameters addressed, multiple antibiotics with specific or broad-spectrum designations are available for judicious use. However, the empirical or arbitrary use of a chemotherapeutic agent is never justified without knowledge of its potential efficacy and without considering its pharmacokinetics, effect on normal microbial flora, and cost.

REFERENCES

Brenner, D. J., Farmer, J. J. III, Hickman, F. W., Asbury, M. A., and Steigewalt, A. G.: Taxonomic and Nomenclature Changes in Enterobacteriaceae. Centers for Disease Control, Atlanta, 1977, pp. 1–15.

Edwards, P. R., and Ewing, W. H.: Identification of Enterobacteriaceae. 4th ed. Elsevier Science Publishing Co., New York, 1986.

Farmer, J. J. III, Davis, B. R., Hickman-Brenner, F. W., McWhorter, A., Huntley-Carter, G. P., Asbury, M. W., Riddle, C., Wathen-Grady, H. G., Ellis, C., Fanning, G. R., Steigerwalt, A. G., O'Hara, C. M., Morris, G. K., Smith, P. B., and Brenner, D. J.: Biochemical identification of new species and biotypes of *Enterobacteriaceae* isolated from clinical specimens. J Clin Microbiol 21:46, 1985.

Lennette, E. H., Balows, A., Hausler, W. J. Jr., and Shadomy, H. J.: Manual of Clinical Microbiology. American Society for Microbiology, Washington, DC, 1985, pp 263–308.

Urbaschek, B., Urbaschek, R., and Neter, E.: Gram-Negative Bacterial Infections. Springer-Verlag, New York, 1975, pp 8–15.

chapter 13

Pseudomonadaceae

Bernard J. Moncia, B.S., M.S., Ph.D.

The family of the *Pseudomonadaceae* is one of the most diverse in the microbial world. Phenotypically, the members resemble many other groups of bacteria. Overall, they have very simple growth requirements and can be isolated from a multitude of sources.

The family consists of four genera of bacteria: *Pseudomonas, Xanthomonas, Frateuria,* and *Zoogloea* (Table 13–1). *Pseudomonas* species are the most important members of this family because they are pathogenic to humans, animals, and plants. *Xanthomonas,* while not pathogenic to humans, is an important plant pathogen. *Zoogloea* is found in water heavily polluted with organic material. The correct placement of this genus is debatable and the reader is referred to *Bergey's Manual of Systematic Bacteriology* for further discussion. *Frateuria* species are associated with plants.

The organisms of the Pseudomonadaceae family are straight or curved gram-negative rods, motile via polar flagella, strictly aerobic chemo-organotrophs with a respiratory metabolism. They grow at temperatures ranging from 2 to 45°C and are capable of utilizing an amazing diversity of organic compounds as carbon and energy sources. They are cat-alase-positive and usually oxidase-positive. As already mentioned, the most important genus is *Pseudomonas,* and the discussion here will concentrate on these organisms, with special emphasis on *P. aeruginosa.*

Characteristics

Pseudomonas aeruginosa is a gram-negative rod, 0.5 to 1.0 µm wide by 3 to 4 µm long, motile by means of one to three polar flagella. The cell wall structure is similar to *Escherichia coli* except the lipid A moiety lacks β-hydroxymyristic acid and the carbohydrate side chain consists of amino rather than neutral sugars. The organism is a strict aerobe but can grow anaerobically if provided with an alternate electron acceptor (such as nitrate or arginine). Like other members of the family, it is catalase-positive and usually oxidase-positive and produces a variety of water-soluble pigments. It is, however, the only pseudomonad that produces a chloroform-soluble pigment (pyocyanin).

Clinical identification is based on cell and colony morphology, Gram-stain reaction, odor (often described as a sweet, fruity odor),

Table 13–1 ■ Family Pseudomonadaceae

Genus	Importance
Pseudomonas	Human pathogens,
Xanthomonas	plant pathogens
Frateuria	Plant organisms
Zoogloea	Polluted water

pigmentation, absence of spores, motility, mode of glucose utilization, production of certain enzymes, hydrogen sulfide production, carbohydrate utilization patterns, and growth temperature.

Habitat

The "natural habitat" of *P. aeruginosa* is not clear. For years it has been debated whether it is a "soil organism" or an "aquatic organism." *Pseudomonas* can easily and routinely be isolated from a wide range of sources: soil, ground water, many fruits and vegetables, a variety of foods, house plants, animals, humans, jet fuel, and various medical instruments (Table 13–2). It is safe to assume that any moist environment can harbor *P. aeruginosa*. The ubiquitous nature of this organism is the result of many features that are essential for survival in diverse environments. The organism's simple metabolic requirements enable it to grow in aquatic environments where substrates are often very dilute and of limited assortment. In fact, the organism can grow to substantial numbers in distilled water in a very short time. The organism produces many extracellular enzymes, a characteristic of successful soil microorganisms, which would enable it to

Table 13–2 ■ Sources from which *Pseudomonas aeruginosa* has been isolated

Hospitals	Other
Sink traps and drains	Faucet aerators
Ice machines	Water filters
Water pitchers	Soap dishes
Mops	Hand creams
Soiled linen	Medications
Respiratory equipment	Heated whirlpools
Turbo jets	Swimming pools
Nebulizers	Water filters
Medications	Water deionizers
	Disinfectants
	Hexachlorophene soaps
	Milk

take advantage of the great diversity of components in soil. The pigments of *P. aeruginosa* are potent antimicrobials. One pigment, pyocyanin, also decreases oxygen consumption by several tissues and leukocytes. This organism is notorious for its antibiotic resistance, not surprising in view of the fact that the vast majority of the known antibiotics have been isolated from soil organisms. The organism has had a very long time to evolve survival mechanisms for dealing with such compounds. The slime layer of *P. aeruginosa* is protective against amebic predators and hydraulic forces and is antiphagocytic.

P. aeruginosa is genetically very promiscuous; that is, it may act as either a donor or a recipient for a large number of bacteriophages and plasmids. These plasmids contribute significantly to the wide range of habitats of this organism. The plasmid can confer new characteristics offering survival benefits. Plasmids have been identified that transfer biochemical abilities such as the ability to grow on unusual energy/carbon sources (toluene, naphthalene octane, and xylene) as well as their resistance to antibiotics and disinfectants. The genetics of this organism have been extensively studied. For a deeper understanding of the role of various pathogenic factors and the use of genetics to study this organism, see the Lory and Tai chapter in Goebel's *Current Topics in Microbiology and Immunology*. Many of these properties that make this organism so adaptable in nature also contribute to this opportunistic pathogen's ability to cause disease in humans.

Clinical Significance

Traditionally, *P. aeruginosa* has not been considered a significant pathogen; however, recently there has been a significant increase in the number of infections involving this organism, especially nosocomial infections. In fact, *P. aeruginosa* has now replaced *Staphylococcus aureus* as the primary cause of nosocomial infection. This rise in importance is due to several factors, one of the most important being the inappropriate use of antibiotics over the past 30 years. During antibiotic therapy a pressure is created for the selection of resistant organisms. *P. aeruginosa* is notorious for its resistance to many antibiotics, which could contribute to its increased colonization. This organism also acquires antibiotic resistance genes easily, a contributing factor in the difficulty in treating such patients.

Another factor relative to nosocomial infection is the fact that *P. aeruginosa* is very resistant to many disinfectants, particularly the phenolic-based disinfectants. The extensive use of disinfectants in the hospital setting, where antibiotic use is also high, favors colonization by resistant organisms. Changing hospital populations also contribute to the rise of infection. Because better treatments enable compromised patients to live longer, there is now a larger number of patients susceptible to *Pseudomonas* infection. The changing American lifestyle also contributes to increased rates of infection. The increased use of "hot tubs" has given rise to a much greater number of cases of *Pseudomonas* folliculitis. The use of extended-wear contact lenses also has given rise to increased frequency of ocular infection.

Management of *Pseudomonas* infection is a major problem in dealing with immunocompromised patients. High-risk patients include those who are immunosuppressed (either acquired or natural) or neutropenic; who have suffered thermal injury, severe trauma, or postoperative complication; or who have cystic fibrosis. *P. aeruginosa* bacteremias have the highest mortality rate, and bacteremias associated with *P. aeruginosa* pneumonia are fatal in 95 percent of the cases. *Pseudomonas* infections have been associated with some oral surgical and endodontic procedures. About 1 percent of all oral infections involve *Pseudomonas* species, and such infections are usually mixed. *Pseudomonas* infections have been reported in open root canals, after removal of impacted molars, and after oral surgery in the soft tissue and bones. They have also been associated with osteomyelitis of the mandible and maxilla. Virtually every tissue of the body is susceptible to infection by this organism. If the practicing dentist suspects a *Pseudomonas* infection, cultures should be taken and an infectious disease specialist or clinical microbiologist consulted for the most appropriate therapy.

Other species of *Pseudomonas* are known pathogens, including *P. cepacia, P. maltophilia, P. mallei, P. pseudomallei,* and *P. fluorescens. P. mallei* causes glanders in horses and donkeys and can be transmitted to humans through abrasions or cuts. *P. pseudomallei* causes a glanders-like disease in humans; however, it has rarely been observed in the western hemisphere.

Transmission

Epidemics involving *Pseudomonas aeruginosa* are extremely rare since this organism is an opportunistic pathogen. As with many organisms, colonization is a prerequisite to subsequent infection. Once established, the organism may persist indefinitely without causing ill effects until an opportunity arises for extensive proliferation and invasion. Many properties that enable the organism to survive in nature also become important virulence factors in the susceptible host.

The prevalence in normal human adults varies and has been reported to range from 3 to 19 percent. It can be isolated from skin, throat and nasal mucosa, and stools, and colonizes the gingival sulcus of a small percentage of the normal adult population. After admission to the hospital, certain groups show a marked increase in the prevalence rate. The source of exposure is uncertain. Transmission among patients is extremely rare, with the exception of cystic fibrosis patients, in whom long-term exposure or contact can result in colonization. By the time cystic fibrosis patients reach adulthood, greater than 90 percent are colonized. Reservoir-to-patient transmission has been reported—for example, from respiratory equipment. Personnel-to-patient transmission has not been fully documented. The best mode of transmission appears to be food-borne, and *Pseudomonas* can be found in many fresh fruits and vegetables. Some studies suggest that patients become colonized after eating hospital food. It has been shown that colonization is an extremely important factor in subsequent infection with this organism.

Colonization of most human tissue is poorly understood; however, some mechanisms are known. Colonization of the upper and lower respiratory tract has been studied extensively because of its importance in cystic fibrosis treatment. The first step in colonization is attachment to tissues. Fibronectin usually coats the epithelial cells in the respiratory tract. Attachment of *P. aeruginosa* is prevented by the fibronectin. If the fibronectin is damaged, the pili of *P. aeruginosa* can mediate attachment. The damage can result from illness (such as influenza), mechanical insult (endotracheal intubation), or other factors in hospitalization. Host factors may also be important. For example, increased colonization has been associated with increased loss of fibronectin owing to increased salivary protease activity. Other factors may also be important in the initial adherence of this organism to tissue. *P. aeruginosa* is known to have specific lectin-like molecules on its surface that can specifically bind galactose, mannose, and sialic acid residues. These sugars are important moieties of many glycoproteins on the surfaces of most human or animal cells and are found in very high concentration in mucins. It is believed that mucins may function as receptors for this organism. Recent work has demonstrated that sialic acid moieties are required for colonization of corneal epithelial cells.

After colonization the organism persists until the opportunity arises for infection. This process is not well understood in *Pseudomonas*, but several factors are known that have been suggested to play a role in pathogenesis.

One of the most extensively studied factors is the proteases of *P. aeruginosa*. Three distinct proteases have been characterized; the two most studied are elastinase (neutral protease) and alkaline protease. None is lethal upon injection but both may contribute to invasion by causing generalized tissue damage, inhibiting host immune function, contributing to breakdown of physical barriers, and providing bacterial nutrients. Loss or reduction of protease activity has been correlated with decreased virulence. The elastinase is a heat-stable zinc containing metaloprotease, which preferentially cleaves phenylalanine and leucine adjacent residues. It is inhibited by α_2-macroglobulin. The elastinase causes the hemorrhagic lesions observed in *Pseudomonas* infection by attacking the elastic lamina of the blood vessels. The enzyme appears to cleave and inactivate IgG antibodies and certain complement components as well as causing disruption of the connective tissue components fibrin and elastin. The alkaline protease is believed responsible for the necrosis of various other tissues. *Pseudomonas* proteases can be extremely potent and are responsible for the corneal damage during eye infections.

Pseudomonas aeruginosa (also *P. fluorescens* and *P. aureofaciens*) produces an extracellular phospholipase C (PLC). This enzyme hydrolyzes phospholipids to yield an α,β-diglyceride and a phosphoryl-nitrogenous alcohol (e.g., phosphoryl choline). Similar enzymes have been demonstrated as important virulence factors in other organisms such as *Clostridium perfringens* and *Staphylococcus aureus*. Their role in pathogenesis is best understood by a consideration of basic cellular structure. Virtually every cell membrane comprises a lipid bilayer composed of various lipids (phospholipids) and proteins. The composition of the lipids is species- and tissue-specific. Furthermore, each half of the lipid bilayer is made up of a unique mixture of phospholipids. For example, a cell may be composed primarily of four or five phospholipids with specific types concentrated on the outer cell surface, while others are located on the inner surface. Specific PLCs have different substrate specificities. For example, *S. aureus* PLC will hydrolyze sphingomyelin but not phosphatidyl choline, whereas *C. perfringens* will attack both. Tissue destruction by this enzyme is therefore a function of cellular or tissue lipid composition and enzyme specificity. The PLC of *P. aeruginosa* has a rather large range of lipid species that can act as substrate, allowing it to play a role in the damage of many different tissues. The enzyme is coregulated with the enzyme phosphatase, suggesting these two provide the organism with phosphate, which is limiting both in the body and in nature. In vivo it probably functions in a similar fashion, and combined with the proteases would cause considerable necrosis. Interestingly, the PLC is believed to contribute to pneumonia by attacking the pulmonary surfactant and tissues leading to atelectasis (incomplete expansion of the lungs) and necrosis.

Pseudomonas aeruginosa also produces two glycolipids called hemolysins that can cause tissue damage via action against membrane lipid. About 80 percent of clinical isolates produce one or both of these hemolysins, which appear to act in a detergent-like manner. This perturbation of the membranes can (1) directly cause lysis or death of cells such as red blood cells, and (2) indirectly make membrane lipids accessible to the action of phospholipase C.

Pseudomonas aeruginosa produces three potent exotoxins (A, B, and C) that are lethal when injected into mice and dogs and cause hypotensive shock in monkeys. Exotoxin A is the best understood. It is the most potent toxin produced by *P. aeruginosa* and is found in 90 percent of the clinical isolates. This toxin is produced in vivo under conditions of little or no available iron. This is consistent with the in vivo observation, as iron is a limiting nutrient for bacterial growth in vivo. The toxic activity appears to be identical to that of the diphtheria toxin—that is, it causes ADP-ribosylation of elongation factor 2 and therefore inhibits protein synthesis. The protein toxin is produced as a protoxin that is activated by proteases, has a molecular weight of about 70,000 daltons, and is antigenically distinct from the diphtheria toxin. It causes necrosis locally in tissues and inhibits granulocytic and macrophage progenitor cells in the bone marrow. Its primary target appears to be the liver. *P. aeruginosa* produces another ADP-ribosylating enzyme exoenzyme S, which does not ribosylate EF-2 or EF-1. It is observed in about 40 percent of clinical isolates. Loss of this characteristic results in decreased virulence. Its role in pathogenesis is unknown.

Lipopolysaccharides (LPS), or endotoxins, in *P. aeruginosa,* as in all gram-negative organisms, are very potent toxins that become important when significant numbers of organisms are present. Circulating endotoxins are responsible for many of the toxic effects observed in gram-negative sepsis: adult respiratory distress syndrome, fever, oliguria, hypotension leukopenia/leukocytosis, and disseminated intravascular coagulation. The LPS activates the complement, fibrinolytic and clotting systems, as well as stimulating release of vasoactive peptides.

The Slime Layer

Many clinical isolates of *P. aeruginosa* possess an external polysaccharide layer referred to as "the slime layer," "mucoid substance," or "glycocalyx."

The slime appears to be composed of repeating sugar chains in the outermost layer of the bacteria. This layer is not considered a capsule because it is amorphous and is easily dispersed or removed from cells. In contrast, capsules are very distinct layers that are not easily removed. As with many so-called virulence factors, the function of this entity is unknown. Because this structure is at the outermost portion of the bacterium, it may affect the interaction of the bacterium with its immediate environment, for example, in attachment or protection from deleterious agents. The slime layer is antiphagocytic, is a permeability barrier to certain antibiotics, and reduces susceptibility to opsonizing antibody.

It is important to note that isolates from cystic fibrosis patients are characterized by an overproduction of the slime layer, which is easily recognized by the mucoid appearance on culture.

Leukocidin

Pseudomonas aeruginosa produces a leukocidin. This toxin destroys PMNs without lysis. Since PMNs are the body's main defense against *Pseudomonas*, the importance of this toxin is obvious. Unfortunately, little is known about this substance. It is cell-associated and is activated and released via the action of proteases (elastinase).

Control

The ubiquitous nature of *Pseudomonas* species makes eradication of these organisms from the clinical setting an impossibility. Control of *Pseudomonas* in the environment is therefore a more realistic goal for the practicing dentist. Dilute acids have been recommended, even though these agents are not bacteriocidal for *P. aeruginosa,* but only bacteriostatic. The organism is capable of a wide array of resistances to deleterious agents. Free chlorine and hydrogen peroxide may be of some use in controlling the numbers of these bacteria. If the clinician suspects a problem with pseudomonads, a thorough treatise on disinfection must be consulted (see Block's *Disinfection, Sterilization, and Preservation,* 1977). The best advice is to keep your equipment and work area clean and dry. Complete desiccation may well be the best means of controlling this organism.

SUGGESTED READING

Block, S. S.: Disinfection, sterilization, and preservation. Lea and Febiger, Philadelphia, 1977.

Doggert, R. G.: *Pseudomonas aeruginosa* clinical manifestations of infection and current therapy. Academic Press, San Francisco, 1979.

Lory, S., Tai, P. C.: Biochemical and genetic aspects of *Pseudomonas aeruginosa* virulence. In Goebel, W. (ed.): *Current Topics in Microbiology and Immunology.*

Palleroni, N. J., Family 1. *Pseudomonadaceae.* Winslow, Broadhurst, Buchanan, Krumwiede, Rogers and Smith, 1917. In Krieg, N. R., and Holt, J. G. (eds.): *Bergey's Manual of Systematic Bacteriology.* Williams and Wilkins, Baltimore, 1984.

Reviews of Infectious Diseases 6 (Suppl. 3), 1984. (Special issue on *Pseudomonas* infection.)

Young, V. M.: *Pseudomonas aeruginosa*: Ecological aspects and patient colonization. Raven Press, New York, 1977.

chapter 14

Brucella, Yersinia, and Francisella

Joseph J. Zambon, D.D.S., Ph.D.

CHAPTER OUTLINE

Brucella

The bacterial genus *Brucella* is composed of a group of gram-negative bacterial species that exist as obligate parasites in a variety of animal hosts (Table 14–1). The genus is named after Sir David Bruce, who isolated *Brucella* from the spleens of British soldiers who had died of *undulant fever* on the island of Malta *(Malta fever)* after drinking contaminated goat's milk. Three species of *Brucella* have special importance as human pathogens in causing acute or chronic brucellosis characterized by an acute or relapsing (undulant) fever. These bacterial species are classified on the basis of their animal reservoirs: *B. melitensis,* derived from goats and sheep; *B. abortus,* derived from cattle; and *B. suis,* derived from swine (also hares and reindeer). Three other species—*B. ovis,* found in sheep; *B. neotomae,* found in desert wood rats; and *B. canis,* found in dogs—are not usually associated with disease in humans.

CHARACTERISTICS OF BACTERIAL CELLS AND COLONIES

Microorganisms in the genus *Brucella* are nonmotile, short, slender bacilli, sometimes appearing as cocci, coccobacilli, or short rods, and are 0.5 to 0.7 μm in diameter. The cells generally have slightly convex sides and rounded ends, and usually are found singly but sometimes may occur in pairs, short chains, or small clusters. The bacterial cells sometimes exhibit *bipolar staining.* Bacterial colonies are small, moist-appearing, translucent, convex, and raised, with an entire edge and a smooth, shiny surface. The *Brucella* are generally *aerobic* but can utilize nitrate anaerobically. Optimum growth is at 36 to 38°C but can occur over the range of 20 to 40°C. Primary cultures are slow growing and fastidious, with colonies rarely visible before 48 hours, at which time they are 0.5 to 1.0 mm in diameter. Of all the *Brucella* species, only *B. abortus* requires 5 to 10 percent CO_2 for primary isolation. These microorganisms grow on media containing special dyes, thionine, and basic fuchsin. They produce catalase and decompose urea but, with the exception of *B. neotomae,* do not ferment sugars. Initial isolates of *Brucella* exhibit a smooth colony morphology, which is indicative of a highly virulent form. The organism undergoes change in colony morphology from the original smooth (S) form through an intermediate (I) form to a mucoid (M) or a rough (R) colony that is less virulent than

Table 14–1 ■ Brucella

Characteristics	Nonmotile, short, slender bacilli, cocci, or coccobacilli; or short rods
	Bipolar staining
	Aerobic but *B. abortus* requires 5 to 10 percent CO_2 for primary isolation
Major species	*B. melitensis* from goats and sheep—relapsing fever
	B. abortus—abortions in cattle
	B. suis from swine
	B. ovis in sheep
	B. neotomae in rats
	B. canis in dogs
Growth	Media containing special dyes, thionine, and basic fuchsin
Disease	Brucellosis
Pathogenesis	Contaminated milk, cheese, or animal tissues
	Viscerotropism based on erythritol
	Intracellular parasites
	Granuloma formation
Prevention	Vaccination of cattle
Treatment	Ampicillin, chloramphenicol, erythromycin, kanamycin, novobiocin, tetracycline, and streptomycin

the original and that also exhibits less agglutination. For example, the smooth form, unlike the rough form, is able to multiply in nonimmune monocytes. Transformations in colony morphology are thought to occur as a result of production and accumulation of D-alanine, as well as reduction in the pO_2 by the smooth form. Both factors produce a selective pressure on the microorganism favoring the emergence of the rough form.

There are two major antigens shared among the *Brucella* species, A and M, which are part of the protein-lipopolysaccharide complex. The A antigen is a major antigen in *B. abortus* and *B. suis* but only a minor antigen in *B. militensis*. The M antigen is a major antigen in *B. militensis* but is minor in the other two species. Brucella species also have antigens that cross-react with *Escherichia coli, Francisella tularensis, Vibrio cholerae,* and *Yersinia enterocolitica*. Brucella species do not exhibit antiphagocytic factors or exotoxins. In fact, the pathogenesis of the organism is partly dependent on its ability to undergo phagocytosis as a means of gaining access to the host lymphatic tissues.

THE PATHOGENESIS OF BRUCELLA INFECTIONS

Brucella often produces a generalized infection and bacteremia in animal hosts and then localizes in the reproductive and reticuloendothelial systems. This is an example of *viscerotropism*—a specific infection of certain tissues by a bacterial pathogen. *Brucella* viscerotropism is dependent on the presence of *erythritol*, a four-carbon polyhydric alcohol, found in high concentrations in bovine allantoic and amniotic fluids as well as in the chorion, cotyledons, and fetal fluids of other animals. *Brucella* infection in pregnant animals often results in abortion; hence, the name *B. abortus* for the organism responsible for abortions in cattle. Animal infection can also localize in the mammary glands, resulting in contaminated milk. Humans become infected by ingesting contaminated milk and animal tissues or by handling contaminated animal tissue. The organism enters the host through breaks in the skin or mucosa of the gastrointestinal tract, through the conjunctiva, and possibly by inhalation of contaminated aerosol sprays. Once the organism gains entrance, the bacterial cells are phagocytosed by polymorphonuclear leukocytes and monocytes, which provide the setting for intracellular growth by the organism. As *intracellular parasites*, they can be transported to regional lymph nodes, liver, spleen, bone marrow, and kidneys, where they form granulomas.

Following infection, clinical symptoms of human brucellosis appear only after a long incubation period of weeks or months. This is followed by an insidious onset. Symptoms include malaise, chills, fever, sweats, weakness, myalgia, and headache, as well as vague gastrointestinal and nervous complaints. Clinical examination of these patients reveals enlarged lymph nodes, spleen, and liver, with approximately 20 percent of the subjects demonstrating bacteremia. Liver involvement is common and characterized by small noncaseating granulomas, which become larger, sometimes calcify, and develop suppurative abscesses. This is especially true in chronic brucellosis due to *B. suis*. *B. melitensis* causes a form of brucellosis characterized by relapsing fever, diffuse hepatitis with focal areas of necrosis in the liver, and occasionally epididyorchitis. Brucellosis can also result in acute meningoencephalitis, osteomyelitis, endocarditis, and interstitial nephritis with focal glomerular lesions.

Humoral immunity in patients with brucellosis is detected by agglutination, precipitin, opsonization, and bactericidal tests. However, these antibodies do not appear to confer protection against infection by the organism. On the other hand, exposure to contaminated animal tissues appears to produce relative immunity in slaughterhouse workers. Cellular immunity appears to be important in resistance to *Brucella* infection as demonstrated by the fact that brucellae in macrophages taken from actively immunized animals appear to survive for shorter periods of time in culture than in macrophages taken from nonimmunized animals.

DIAGNOSIS AND TREATMENT

Diagnosis of brucellosis is based on history, clinical findings, and laboratory examinations. The patient typically has a history of unexplained fever. The organism can be identified from blood or biopsy specimens cultured on *Brucella* agar, on trypticase soy broth in 10 percent CO_2, or by serologic tests for antibodies to *Brucella*. Since there is a long incubation period before symptoms become apparent, serum antibodies to the organism are generally present at the time of initial examination. As with other humoral immune responses, there is an initial elevation in IgM antibody titers to *Brucella* followed by an elevation in IgG titers.

Agglutination assays for serum antibodies utilize phenol-killed suspensions of *B. abortus*. The presence of IgG titers between 1:640 and 1:2560, as well as the presence of IgG agglutinins resistant to degradation with 2-mercaptoethanol, suggests that the patient has an active *Brucella* infection. Chronic active brucellosis is similarly associated with elevated IgG titers. There can be cross-reaction between serum antibodies to *F. tularensis*, *V. cholerae*, *V. fetus*, or *Y. enterocolitica* and *Brucella* in serologic assays.

Most *Brucella* species are sensitive to ampicillin, chloramphenicol, erythromycin, kanamycin, novobiocin, tetracycline, and streptomycin. Combinations of these drugs are most effective. Streptomycin does not eliminate brucellae in monocytes. Most of these organisms are resistant to penicillin, cephalosporins, clindamycin, lincomycin, polymyxin, nalidixic acid, and nystatin. Since these microorganisms can exist intracellularly, it is important that antibiotic therapy be continued for 3 to 4 weeks, or relapse is likely to occur.

The incidence of brucellosis in cattle and subsequent transmission to humans can be reduced by vaccination with live attenuated *B. abortus* strain 19. Such vaccination produces partial immunity and limits *Brucella* infection.

Similar to diagnosis of brucellosis in humans, detection of infected cattle can be performed by agglutination assays on serum or milk. Alternatively, the organism can be directly detected in animal tissues such as abortion material by immunofluorescence. If detected, infected animals are destroyed. *Brucella* infection is also limited by vaccination of calves and pasteurization of milk. At present, human brucellosis is seen primarily in persons who work with animals or animal tissues, including veterinarians and workers in meat-packing plants, although 10 percent of cases are associated with ingestion of raw milk or imported cheese.

Yersinia

Yersinia species cause a group of infections in which the microorganism normally resides in a lower vertebrate host and is transmitted to humans (Table 14–2). These types of infections are known as *zoonoses*. Bubonic plaque is the best known of the *Yersinia* infections and is caused by *Y. pestis* (formerly classified as *Pasteurella pestis*). This disease is the "Black Death" of the Middle Ages, which was responsible for the death of approximately one quarter of the inhabitants of Europe. Even today, there are significant numbers of cases of bubonic plaque—881 cases in 1979.

Table 14–2 ■ Yersinia	
Characteristics	Gram-negative, nonmotile, short, ovoid bacillus
Major species	*Yersinia pestis*—bubonic and other forms of plague
	Yersinia pseudotuberculosis—acute mesenteric lymphadenitis
	Yersinia enterocolitica—enterocolitis
Pathogenesis	Plague—transmitted from rats and rat fleas, invades vasculature, proliferates in lymph nodes to form buboes
	Other yersinioses—ingestion of contaminated food or water, invasion of the gastrointestinal tract
Prevention	Plague—control of rat and invertebrate populations
	Other yersinioses—proper cooking of animal products and sanitation
Treatment	Streptomycin, tetracycline, chloramphenicol

YERSINIA PESTIS

Y. pestis is a gram-negative, nonmotile, short, ovoid bacillus named after Alexandre Yersin (1863–1943), who is credited with the discovery of this microorganism as the causative agent of plague during the 1884 epidemic in Hong Kong. Yersin describes bubonic plague in his book, *La peste bubonique à Hong Kong*:

The onset (of the disease) is rapid, with an incubation period of 4½ to 6 days. The patient is prostrated. Abruptly a high fever sets in, often accompanied by delirium. On the very first day a discrete bubo usually appears. In 75 percent of the cases it is located in the inguinal region, in 10% of the cases in the axillary region, and occasionally at the back of the neck or in other regions. The nodule rapidly reaches the size of an egg. Death occurs after 48 hours and often sooner. If the patient manages to survive 5 to 6 days, the prognosis is better, the bubo softens and one can operate to drain the pus. . .

He also described his isolation of *Y. pestis*;

It seemed logical to start first by looking for a microbe in the blood of patients and in the pulp of the buboes. The pulp of the buboes always contains masses of short, stubby bacilli which are rather easy to stain with aniline dyes and are not stained by the method of Gram. The ends of the bacilli are colored more strongly than the center. Sometimes the bacilli seem to be surrounded by a capsule. One can find them in large numbers in the buboes and the lymph nodes of the diseased persons. They are seen in the blood from time to time, but less abundantly than in the buboes and lymph nodes, and only in very serious and rapidly fatal cases.

Y. pestis infects the gastrointestinal tract of the fleas *Xenopsylla cheopis* and *Xenopsylla brasiliensis*, which reside on urban and domestic rats (*Rattus rattus* and *Rattus norwegicus*) and on sylvatic rodents such as squirrels and prairie dogs. The fleas are, in turn, transmitted to humans from the rodents.

Initially, the fleas become infected with *Y. pestis* by feasting on blood from infected rats. The microorganism multiplies and finally blocks a part of the insect's gastrointestinal tract, the proventriculus. When the infected flea next bites the rodent vector, it cannot eat because of the blockage. It does, however, regurgitate *Y. pestis* cells into the wound. The microorganism can also be transmitted through contamination of abraded skin with flea feces. Epidemics of plague are thus associated with increases in the rodent population and reflect the intimacy with which

people live with these infested animals. Even today, *Y. pestis* infection and plague are endemic in areas such as Vietnam.

Y. pestis exhibits a capsule on initial isolation. The microorganism also exhibits bipolar staining using Wayson's stain, which consists of methylene blue and carbol-fuchsin, as well as with Giemsa's stain. After 2 days' growth at 28°C on blood agar, the colonies appear brown and without hemolysis. The organism ferments glucose and mannitol with gas production but does not ferment lactose, sucrose, rhamnose, or adonitol.

Antigens

The *capsular* or envelope antigen (also known as fraction 1, or F1) is a glycoprotein that enables *Y. pestis* to resist complement-mediated phagocytosis. Even in the absence of a bacterial capsule, this microorganism can resist phagocytosis by means of the VW antigen system, which consists of a 90 kilodalton, cell-bound protein *V antigen* and a 90 kilodalton lipoprotein *W antigen*. These factors, which are produced at 37°C but not at 28°C, are not only responsible for resistance to phagocytosis but are also responsible for infectivity.

Another factor associated with *Y. pestis* infectivity and the microorganism's ability to invade the deep tissues is a monomeric 63 kilodalton protein known as *pesticin*. This factor is an N-acetylglucosaminidase, which hydrolyzes bacterial cell wall lipoproteins and acts as a bacteriocin against other species in this genus, including *Y. pseudotuberculosis* and *Y. enterocolitica*.

There are several other *Y. pestis* toxins that are involved in the pathogenesis of plague, including a *murine toxin* and a *lipopolysaccharide endotoxin*. The murine toxin is a protein composed of a 240 kilodalton toxin A and 120 kilodalton toxin B. As the name indicates, the murine toxin is highly lethal for mice and rats but less toxic for other species. Less than 1 μg can cause death in mice and rats. The murine toxin acts as an antagonist of adenosine 3':5'-cyclic monophosphate and causes beta-adrenergic blockade. The lipopolysaccharide endotoxin is similar to that produced by other enteric bacilli.

Pathogenesis

As previously described, the primary reservoir of *Y. pestis* is the gastrointestinal tract of wild and domestic rats. It can cause the death of these animals usually in the form of an acute bacteremia, or it can remain as a chronic infection. In the rat flea, *Y. pestis* is found in the gut and has neither a capsule nor the VW antigens. The microorganism is apparently nonvirulent in the flea, owing to its normally low body temperature (25°C), but the organisms can proliferate at this temperature and cause blockage of the proventriculus. *Y. pestis* multiplies in the flea, which then transmits the organism to other rats or to human beings through bites. *Y. pestis* can also be transmitted to humans through infected meat, through contact with other infected humans via droplet infection, or by means of a bite from the human flea, *Pulex irritans*.

Once transmitted to humans, the organism makes its way to the lymphatic system and to the regional lymph nodes, where it proliferates and after 2 to 8 days forms a large oval swelling known as a bubo—hence the name "bubonic plague." Although buboes may develop in the axilla or neck, they most frequently are found in the groin and are accompanied by intense pain. If the bacilli are not confined to the lymph nodes, they will extend through the efferent lymphatics to the vasculature, resulting in "septicemic plague," which may occur without formation of buboes. The microorganism can then seed to internal organs such as the lungs and spleen. Septicemia can develop into disseminated intravascular coagulation, which may be characterized by skin lesions (purpura), high fever, tachycardia, pain in the limbs and back, and gangrenous necrosis of distal extremities—the "black" in the "black death." Plague septicemia can also result in infection of the meninges *(meningeal plague)* and of the pharynx *(plague pharyngitis)*, the latter clinically resembling acute tonsillitis. After 3 to 5 days, the patient may die.

Secondary involvement of the lungs can result in *pneumonic plague*, which carries a very high mortality rate. This is the most fulminant form of the disease. Patients with pneumonic plague produce large amounts of bloody, frothy sputum. This form is so virulent that patients can die of pneumonic plague on the very same day that they develop symptoms. Pneumonic plague produces infected sputum and other bronchial secretions, which may be transmitted to uninfected persons by droplet infection.

Exposure to *Y. pestis* may produce immunity to the antiphagocytic F1 and VW antigens; however, antisera to the toxins is not protective.

Diagnosis

Bubonic plague can be diagnosed by culture of *Y. pestis* from aspirates taken of the buboes as well as from sputum, throat swabs, and autopsy material plated onto blood agar or into infusion broth. The resulting colonies can be identified by colony and biochemical characteristics. Inoculation of the suspected microorganism into animals such as mice or guinea pigs can also differentiate *Y. pestis* from other *Yersinia* species. Serologic tests including identification of the microorganism by means of fluorescent antibody staining, agglutination by specific antiserum, or lysis with a specific bacteriophage can also be useful.

Antibody assays of human or animal sera can be useful for retrospective diagnostic confirmation, seroepidemiology, and for monitoring *Y. pestis* in animals. Serum antibodies to the F1 antigen can, for example, be detected by passive hemagglutination.

Treatment

There is an extremely high mortality rate associated with plague. More than 50 percent of patients with untreated bubonic plague, and almost 100 percent of those with pneumonic plague, will die. With antibiotic treatment, however, the mortality rate can be brought down to 5 to 15 percent. Streptomycin is the drug of choice, and the dosage is 30 mg per kg of body weight administered intramuscularly for 10 days. Tetracycline is useful in patients who are allergic to streptomycin or when an orally administered drug must be used. Tetracycline is administered at a dosage of 2 to 4 gm per day for 10 days. Intravenous chloramphenicol is used in patients with meningeal plague.

Prevention

Bubonic plague will likely always be with us, as it is impossible to eliminate the animal reservoir or the vector. However, the prevalence of the disease can be kept in control, first by the use of insecticides to kill the rat flea and the human flea; second, by the isolation of patients with pneumonic plague; and third, by immunization with killed or attenuated microorganisms to provide short-term immunity.

OTHER *YERSINIA* SPECIES

There are two other *Yersinia* species—*Y. pseudotuberculosis* and *Y. enterocolitica*—that can cause disease in humans. These diseases are known as yersinioses. Both microorganisms are gram-negative coccobacilli that are found in domestic and wild mammal and bird reservoirs.

Y. pseudotuberculosis is found in rabbits, deer, racoons, turkeys, ducks, geese, pigeons, pheasants, and canaries and only rarely infects humans. The microorganism is transmitted by ingestion of improperly cooked and contaminated food or by direct contact with infected animals. This microorganism causes a yersiniosis characterized by acute mesenteric lymphadenitis. *Y. pseudotuberculosis* is highly invasive; it enters humans usually through the gastrointestinal tract and spreads to the mesenteric lymph nodes and bloodstream. It has a lipopolysaccharide endotoxin and VW antigens as does *Y. pestis* but, in contrast to *Y. pestis,* it lacks fibrinolysin and coagulase. There are six serotypes of *Y. pseudotuberculosis* (I through VI) and eight subtypes based on combination of 15 heat-stable somatic O antigens and heat-labile H antigens. Serotype I *Y. pseudotuberculosis* is the most prevalent serotype and is found in about 90 percent of human yersiniosis due to *Y. pseudotuberculosis*. Several of these antigens cross-react with antigens present on salmonella. *Y. pseudotuberculosis* infection is effectively treated by several antibiotics including kanamycin, tetracycline, and chloramphenicol.

The other organism responsible for the nonplague yersinioses is *Y. enterocolitica*. Humans and pigs are the main reservoirs for this microorganism. The organism is transmitted mainly in rural areas through food, especially improperly cooked meat; through feces-contaminated water; and through person-to-person contact. There is no known invertebrate vector. Once the organism is ingested, it proliferates in the bowel lumen and in the associated lymphoid tissue. It is highly invasive and can invade cells in culture. The organism's pathogenicity is also temperature dependent. Strains of *Y. enterocolitica* grown at 37°C are much less pathogenic than strains cultured at 25°C. A key feature in this disease is the enterotoxin produced by *Y. enterocolitica*. This enterotoxin is a 9000 dalton, heat-stable protein consisting of two toxic components, ST-1 and ST-2.

An acute gastroenteritis or enterocolitis is produced. This occurs predominantly in young children and may be clinically indistinguishable from gastroenteritis due to salmonella, shigella, or toxigenic *E. coli*. The patients experience considerable pain, which resembles acute appendicitis, as well as acute nonsuppurative polyarthritis, erythema nodosum, and Reiter's syndrome (arthritis with urethritis and conjunctivitis) in adults.

There are 34 serotypes of *Y. enterocolitica* based on somatic O antigens. The predominant human isolate in the United States is serotype 8. Serotypes 3 and 9 are predominant in Europe, Africa, Japan, and Canada. Antibodies to these O antigens are usually absent at the onset of the disease but may be demonstrated by hemagglutination at the peak of the disease and during convalescence. There is cross-reaction between *Y. enterocolitica* serotype 9 and *Brucella abortus,* which can be shown in coagglutination assays. There are also a number of biotypes of *Y. enterocolitica* based on reactions with indole, xylose, and trehalose and on the presence of lipase and DNAse. The prevalent human biotype is biotype 4.

Yersinial enterocolitis due to *Y. enterocolitica* can be diagnosed by identification and culture of the organism. *Y. enterocolitica* is distinguished by biochemical tests and agglutination with specific antisera. The organism is also identified by susceptibility to specific bacteriophages. *Y. enterocolitica* can be distinguished from *Y. pestis* and other *Enterobacteriaceae* on the basis of cellular motility, which is apparent at from 22 to 28°C but not at 37°C.

Other *Yersinia* species include *Y. intermedia, Y. frederiksenii,* and *Y. kristensenii* (formerly *Y. ruckeri*), which is the cause of red mouth disease in salmon and trout.

Francisella

Francisella contains two species: *F. tularensis,* which is responsible for tularemia in humans and animals, and *F. novicida,* which causes experimental infections in laboratory animals (Table 14–3). The genus is named after the American microbiologist Edward Francis, who extensively studied tularemia.

CHARACTERISTICS OF BACTERIAL CELLS AND COLONIES

These microorganisms are gram-negative, short, nonmotile, non–spore-forming, obli-

Table 14–3 ■ Francisella

Characteristics	Gram-negative, short, nonmotile, non–spore-forming, obligately aerobic rods
Major species	*Francisella tularensis* *Francisella novicida*
Growth	Sulfhydryl compound–containing medium, such as glucose-blood agar, coagulated egg yolk medium, or thioglycolate broth

Disease	Tularemia in humans and animals
	 Experimental infections in laboratory animals
	 Forms
	   ulceroglandular
	   oculoglandular
	   pneumonic
	   typhoidal

Pathogenesis	Infected rabbits, deer flies, ticks, infected muskrats Headache, fever, and general malaise Intracellular parasite spread through lymphatics Transitory bacteremia, spread to lungs, liver, and spleen Abscesses, granulomatous, caseating nodules
Prevention	Attenuated live vaccine Mechanical barriers
Treatment	Streptomycin, tetracycline and chloramphenicol

gately aerobic rods that occur singly and stain poorly. *F. tularensis* measures 0.2 μm by 0.2 to 0.7 μm, while *F. novicida* measures 0.7 μm by 1.7 μm. Older cultures of either organism exhibit significant pleomorphism with coccoid, bacillary, and filamentous forms. Virulent *F. tularensis* possesses a thick capsule; loss of virulence is associated with loss of the capsule. Culture of *F. tularensis* requires special media such as cysteine-glucose-blood agar, coagulated egg yolk medium, or thioglycolate broth, all of which contain sulfhydryl compounds. *F. novicida* does not require these same compounds but growth is stimulated by their addition. Primary isolates are visible after 2 to 10 days of culture at 37°C as smooth (S), gray, minute (1 to 4 mm diameter for *F. tularensis* and 6 to 8 mm diameter for *F. novicida*), transparent, easily emulsified colonies. They are catalase-positive, oxidase-negative, and slowly ferment carbohydrates, producing acid but not gas. *Francisella* species can be distinguished on the basis of carbohydrate fermentations. *F. tularensis* ferments maltose, whereas *F. novicida* ferments sucrose. Hydrogen sulfide gas is produced. Smooth forms are transformed to rough (R) forms, which are less virulent. Highly virulent strains of *F. tularensis* ferment glycerol

and are generally isolated from tick-borne tularemia in rabbits, whereas less virulent strains do not ferment glycerol and are associated with water-borne disease of rodents.

PATHOGENESIS

F. tularensis was first isolated from squirrels in Tulare County, California, in 1912. Francis cultured this microorganism from jack rabbits and showed them to be an important source of human tularemia. The organism can be transmitted from deer flies, ticks, infected muskrats, and polluted water in North America, Europe, USSR, and Japan. While *F. tularensis* can be found everywhere except Antarctica and Australia, tularemia is generally considered a disease of the Northern hemisphere. There are several types of human tularemia, each of which is related to the primary route of infection:

1. An *ulceroglandular* form, in which an ulcerating papule develops at the site of the primary skin lesion. This form occurs by transmission through abraded skin or through bites from infected animals.

2. An *oculoglandular* form, in which the initial infection occurs through the conjunctivae.

3. A *pneumonic* form, resulting from inhalation of infected droplets during processing of animal products or by hematogenous dissemination from the site of local infection.

4. A *typhoidal* form, caused by ingestion of contaminated meat. Patients with the typhoidal form exhibit gastrointestinal symptoms, toxemia, and fever similar to typhoid fever.

Symptoms usually appear 3 to 4 days after infection, but the incubation period can range from 2 to 10 days. Tularemia is an acute disease with symptoms including headache, fever, and general malaise. As the disease progresses, the patient may experience delirium and coma, and may die. The mortality rate in untreated ulceroglandular tularemia is 5 percent, and in typhoidal and pneumonic tularemia 30 percent.

Once the organism infects the host, it is phagocytized by monocytes and remains alive as an *intracellular parasite* for extended periods of time, which explains why patients have occasional relapses and a persistent immune response. The organism is transported within monocytes throughout the lymphatics to regional lymph nodes. From there, the organism can cause transitory bacteremia and spread to the lungs, liver, and spleen, where it can form abscesses and granulomatous, caseating nodules.

DIAGNOSIS AND TREATMENT

F. tularensis has a single serologic type. The cell wall antigens include an endotoxin, a polysaccharide antigen, and a protein antigen that cross-reacts with *Brucella* species. Skin tests with the polysaccharide antigen in convalescent patients elicit characteristic delayed hypersensitivity reactions transferable with spleen cells. Agglutinating serum antibodies are also demonstrable in convalescent sera by the second week of the infection and may persist for years. Since *F. tularensis* is an intracellular parasite, however, exacerbations of the disease can occur even in the presence of high serum antibody titers.

Laboratory diagnosis of tularemia is based on the identification of *F. tularensis* either by culture of clinical specimens such as gastric washings, sputum, and tissue specimens or by fluorescent antibody tests on smears. The microorganisms cultured on special sulfhydryl-containing media are often confirmed by fluorescent antibody tests. The presence of serum antibodies to *F. tularensis* is also useful in the diagnosis and treatment of tularemia. A rise in antibody titer indicates a recent infection, while a positive skin test reaction to polysaccharide antigen suggests either a present or a past infection.

Streptomycin is the drug of choice for treatment of tularemia, but bacteriostatic drugs such as tetracycline and chloramphenicol are also effective. Antibiotic treatment reduces the mortality of tularemia to approximately 1 percent. Patients may relapse if antibiotic therapy is not continued for a sufficient period of time or if the antibiotic is not able to eliminate the intracellular infection.

An attenuated live vaccine is available for laboratory workers and other persons likely to come into contact with infected material. Mechanical barriers such as gloves and face masks are also recommended for persons who skin and dress rabbits.

REFERENCES

Brucella

McAllister, T. A.: Laboratory diagnosis of human brucellosis. Scot Med J 21:129, 1976.
Schirger, A., Nichols, D. R., Martin, W. J., Wellman, W. E., and Weed, L. A.: Brucellosis: experiences with 224 patients. Ann Intern Med 52:827, 1960.

Yersinia

Yersin, A.: Ann Pasteur Inst (Paris) 8:662, 1894.
Pollitzer, R.: Plague. W. H. O. Monograph Series No. 22, World Health Organization, Geneva, 1954.

Francisella

Owen, C. R.: Francisella infections. In Bodily, H. L., Updyke, E. L., and Mason, J. O. (eds.): Diagnostic Procedures for Bacterial, Mycotic and Parasitic Infection, ed 5. American Public Health Association, New York, 1970.

chapter *15*

Bacillus and Clostridium

Sydney M. Finegold, M.D.

CHAPTER OUTLINE

- BACILLUS
- CLOSTRIDIUM

Bacillus

The ninth edition of *Bergey's Manual of Systematic Bacteriology* lists 34 species of *Bacillus*; four of these are found in infectious processes in humans on occasion and a few other species are encountered in infection very rarely. *Bacillus* species are widely distributed in nature and are relatively common contaminants in laboratory cultures. Contamination of alcohol swabs and of radiometric blood culture apparatus has led to falsely positive blood cultures, sometimes in clusters. Many or most of the true infections involving this genus are in immunocompromised hosts, including patients with implanted devices of one type or another.

DESCRIPTION AND GENERAL CHARACTERISTICS

Most organisms in the genus *Bacillus* are gram-positive, rod-shaped, obligately aerobic bacilli that produce endospores. Occasionally, species or strains are gram-negative or facultatively anaerobic. They closely resemble *Clostridium,* but the latter is characteristically obligately anaerobic. *Bacillus* species may be differentiated from each other on the basis of morphologic and biochemical characteristics, but speciation is not important for routine clinical purposes except for *B. anthracis*, the causative agent of anthrax. Most strains of *Bacillus* produce characteristic large, flat colonies with beta hemolysis.

PATHOGENESIS OF BACILLUS INFECTIONS

Capsules and **exotoxins** are the primary features in *Bacillus* strains that account for pathogenicity. The capsule permits strains to resist phagocytosis and the exotoxins are responsible for the pathology produced. *B. anthracis,* the prime pathogen in the genus, produces both capsule and toxin, the latter perhaps mediated by a plasmid. Other species may also produce capsule or exotoxin or both. The exact mode of action of the toxins is not known, but adenylate cyclase appears to be involved in the case of some toxins, including the exotoxin (enterotoxin) produced by *B. cereus,* a cause of food poisoning (an intoxication rather than an infection). *B. cereus* is also involved in true infection.

HOST DEFENSE MECHANISMS

Certain species, such as rats, chickens, and dogs, are relatively resistant to anthrax, compared with many other warm-blooded animals; this is at least partly due to a high degree of phagocytic activity against *B. anthracis*. Development of antibodies to the exotoxin of this organism leads to specific immunity. Vaccines have been developed.

CLINICAL FEATURES

The most serious *Bacillus* infection is **anthrax.** This disease is seen in three forms in humans. **Cutaneous anthrax** (malignant pustule) is the most common type seen in the United States. The organisms gain entrance and set up infection via an abrasion of the skin, usually on the hands or forearms. There is a serosanguinous discharge in which the organisms may be readily recognized. A second form of the disease is **pulmonary anthrax** or **woolsorter's disease;** the infection is acquired by inhalation of spores during shearing or handling of animal hair. Bacilli are found in large numbers in the sputum. The most severe and rarest form of anthrax is gastrointestinal anthrax. Infection is initiated by swallowing of the organism or its spores.

B. cereus is the cause of a variety of infections, often serious, particularly in immunocompromised hosts. Other predisposing factors include surgery, trauma, burns, intravenous drug abuse, implanted prosthetic devices, indwelling catheters, and use of hemodialysis and peritoneal dialysis. Types of infections encountered include septicemia, endocarditis, necrotizing pneumonia, empyema, meningitis, destructive ophthalmitis, peritonitis, wound infection, myonecrosis (which may simulate gas gangrene but is usually less rapidly progressive), and osteomyelitis. This organism, as noted before, is an important cause of food poisoning. A short-incubation-period type of food poisoning is most often associated with fried rice that has been held warm for extended periods; this is due to preformed toxin and is characterized primarily by vomiting. The long-incubation variety of food poisoning due to this organism is often associated with meat or vegetable dishes; toxin is formed in vivo, and the disease is characterized chiefly by diarrhea.

IDENTIFICATION

The clinical picture of many cases of anthrax is distinctive enough to suggest the diagnosis. *B. anthracis* is a facultative, large, square-ended, gram-positive rod with a centrally located spore that is ellipsoidal to cylindrical and does not cause the cell to bulge. Frequently, the bacterial cells occur in long chains with a bamboo-like appearance. Capsules may be evident. Spores are noted only on culture. Colonies are 4 to 5 mm in diameter, opaque, raised, and irregular with a curled margin. The organism is nonhemolytic on sheep blood agar. In broth, growth occurs in the form of a heavy surface pellicle. The organism is dangerous to work with; all work should take place in a bacteriologic safety hood. All areas should be decontaminated with a sporicidal germicide. The "string of pearls" test is a simple presumptive identification test based on penicillin susceptibility. A single streak of the organism is made on Mueller-Hinton agar, a 10 unit penicillin disk is placed on the streak, and a coverslip is placed. After 3 to 6 hours' incubation at 37°C, growth from beneath the coverslip is examined microscopically for the presence of strings of spherical forms of the organism. Specific identification can be made by public health laboratories using a gamma bacteriophage.

The clinical picture of *B. cereus* infection is usually not distinctive. Colonies of this organism vary from small, shiny, and compact to large, spreading, and feathery; on sheep blood agar, one sees a lavender colony with beta hemolysis. In contrast to *B. anthracis*, *B. cereus* is resistant to gamma phage, is usually resistant to penicillin, does not form capsules on bicarbonate agar, does not exhibit fluorescence of both cell wall and capsule, and produces lecithinase and hemolysin.

THERAPY

Penicillin G is the drug of choice for the treatment of anthrax. In systemic forms of the disease, the mortality may be significant if treatment is delayed. Alternative drugs for the penicillin-allergic patient include tetracycline, erythromycin, and chloramphenicol.

B. cereus food poisoning is of short duration and requires no specific therapy. Infections involving this organism cannot reliably be treated with penicillin G or other beta lactam drugs. Clindamycin and vancomycin should generally be effective. In certain situations, surgical drainage or debridement may be important considerations. The type and location of infection will influence the choice of therapy.

Clostridium

There are 85 species of *Clostridium* recognized in the ninth edition of *Bergey's Manual of Systematic Bacteriology*. Of these, 20 species are important human pathogens involved in infections or intoxications. Clostridia are widely distributed in nature, but most disease due to them in humans is of endogenous origin; exceptions include intoxications such as *C. perfringens*–induced food poisoning, tetanus, and botulism, and a small percentage of cases of gas gangrene (clostridial myonecrosis). The endogenous infections derive primarily from the clostridia present as normal intestinal flora and, to a lesser extent, the indigenous flora of the female genital tract or other mucosal surfaces.

DESCRIPTION AND GENERAL CHARACTERISTICS

Clostridia are chiefly anaerobic, gram-positive rods that are spore-formers. However, some species become aerotolerant on subculture, and some species (*C. carnis*, *C. histolyticum*, and *C. tertium*) grow aerobically. Differentiation between aerotolerant clostridia and *Bacillus* species is based on the findings that *Clostridium* species sporulate anaerobically only, grow much better anaerobically, and are almost always catalase-negative, whereas *Bacillus* species sporulate aerobically only, usually grow better aerobically, and are usually catalase-positive. A few species of clostridia are gram-negative, and older cultures may appear gram-negative. Sporulation may be difficult to demonstrate in some species. Differentiation between species of clostridia is based on the shape and location of spores and a number of biochemical tests; Table 15–1 lists the characteristics of the clostridia most often encountered in the clinical setting.

PATHOGENESIS OF CLOSTRIDIAL INFECTIONS

Clostridial infection of wounds or soft tissue, like other anaerobic infections, occurs primarily in an anaerobic tissue environment due to impaired circulation (arterial or venous), trauma, surgery, and malignant or other disease. The various factors listed previously may also account for the breach in the mucosal surface of the intestinal or female genital tract that permits the endogenous clostridial flora to enter the tissues that ultimately become infected. The vast majority of clostridial infections, like anaerobic infections in general, are mixed infections involving other anaerobes as well as aerobic and/or facultative bacteria.

Capsules may be important in protecting clostridia from the body's host defenses, particularly with *C. perfringens*. The major virulence factors, however, are **exotoxins** produced by many clostridial species. The toxins produced by *C. tetani* and *C. botulinum* are among the most potent poisons known to mankind (one million times as potent as rattlesnake poison). **Tetanus toxin (tetanospasmin)** binds to gangliosides in the central nervous system and acts in the manner of strychnine to suppress the central inhibitory balancing influences on motor neuron activity; this leads to spasticity and convulsions and intensified reflex responses to various stimuli. This toxin also acts on the sympathetic nervous system and on the neurocirculatory and neuroendocrine systems. **Botulinal toxin** attaches to individual motor nerve terminals to prevent acetylcholine release at the nerve endings. Other species of clostridia produce numerous toxins. For example, *C. perfringens* produces an alpha toxin (a lecithinase, phospholipase C); this toxin is a hemolysin and is also active against white blood cells and platelets and has necrotizing activity. The lambda toxin of this organism is a weak proteolytic enzyme. The nu toxin is an RNAse. The theta toxin is a hemolysin. The kappa toxin is a collagenase that is also active in breakdown of gelatin. The mu toxin is a hyaluronidase. The epsilon and iota toxins lead to increased capillary permeability. This organism also produces a neuraminidase and an enterotoxin, the latter acting very much like the enterotoxin of the cholera vibrio. The beta toxin of type C *C. perfringens* is the key factor in necrotizing enterocolitis and can be protected against with antitoxin. *C. difficile* produces at least three toxins—a cytotoxin, an enterotoxin, and a motility-altering toxin. A number of other clostridia produce important toxins.

HOST DEFENSE MECHANISMS

The normal intestinal flora is clearly an important defense mechanism against infant (and perhaps some cases of adult) botulism and against pseudomembranous colitis due

Table 15–1 ■ Characteristics of clostridial species

Species	Gelatin hydrolysis	Glucose fermentation	Lecithinase	Lipase	Indole	Butyric acid produced in PYG	Isoacids produced in PYG	Aerobic growth	Urease	Milk Reaction	Lactose	Maltose	Fructose	Cellobiose	Arabinose	Mannose	Xylose	Nitrate reduction	Spore location	End products from PYG
Saccharolytic—proteolytic																				
C. bifermentans	+	+	+	–	+	(+)	(+)	–	–	d	–	W	>	–	–	–	–	–		A B L
C. sordellii	+	+	+	–	+	(+)	–	–	+	d	–	W	>	–	–	–	–	–		A (p ib b iv iC l)
C. perfringens	+	+	+	–	–	+	–	–	–	d	+	+	+	–	–	+	–	–		A B L (p s)
C. novyi type A	+	+	+	+	–	+	–	–	–	c	–	>	–	–	–	–	–	–	OS	A P B
C. sporogenes	+	+	–	+	–	+	(+)	–	–	cd	–	+	>	–	–	–	–	–	OS	A B ib iv (p v ic l s)
C. cadaveris	+	+	–	–	+	+	–	–	–	cd	–	–	+	–	–	–	–	–	OT	A b
C. septicum	+	+	–	–	–	+	–	–	–	–	+	+	+	–	–	+	–	>	OS	A B (p)
C. difficile	–	+	–	–	–	+	+	–	–	–	–	+	+	–	–	+	–	–	OS	A ib B iv ic (v)
C. putrificum	+	+	–	–	–	+	+	–	–	d	+	+	+	–	–	+	–	–		A ib B iv (p v ic l s)
Saccharolytic—nonproteolytic																				
C. baratii	–	+	+	–	–	+	–	–	–	c	+	+	+	+	–	+	+	>	OT	A B L (s)
C. tertium	–	+	–	–	–	+	–	+	–	c	+	+	+	+	–	+	+	+	OS	A B F (l s)
C. butyricum	–	+	–	–	–	+	–	–	–	c	+	+	+	+	+	+	+	+	OT	A B L (s)
C. innocuum	–	+	–	–	–	+	–	–	–	–	–	+	+	+	–	+	–	–	R/OT	a L (s)
C. ramosum	–	+	–	–	–	–	–	–	–	c	+	+	+	+	>	+	–	–	OS	A (l s)
C. clostridioforme	–	+	–	–	–	–	–	–	–	c	+	+	+	+	>	+	+	+		
Asaccharolytic—proteolytic																				
C. tetani	+	–	–	–	>	+	–	–	–	d	–	–	–	–	–	–	–	–	RT	A B (l s)
C. hastiforme	+	–	–	–	–	+	+	–	–	–	–	–	–	–	–	–	–	–	S	A B ib iv (p ic)
C. subterminale	+	–	–	–	–	+	+	–	–	d	–	–	–	–	–	–	–	–	OS	A B ib iv (p ic l s)
C. histolyticum	+	–	–	–	–	–	–	+	–	d	–	–	–	–	–	–	–	–	OS	A (l s)
C. limosum	+	–	+	–	–	–	–	–	–	d	–	–	–	–	–	–	–	+	S	A (l s)

Note: *C. botulinum* types vary in proteolytic, saccharolytic, and lipase reactions. Send suspected isolates or suspected *C. botulinum*–containing material to the appropriate local or state agency. (From Sutter et al., with permission.)

Reactions

- = Negative reaction
+ = Positive reaction for majority of strains; includes weak as well as strong acid production from carbohydrates in saccharolytic organisms
V = Variable reaction
(+) = Delayed reaction
c = Clot formed in milk
d = Milk digested

PRAS carbohydrate fermentation:

+ = pH <5.5
W = pH 5.5–5.7
- = pH >5.7
V = variable

Fatty acid end products from PYG

A = Acetic
P = Propionic
IB = Isobutyric
B = Butyric
IV = Isovaleric
V = Valeric
IC = Isocaproic
L = Lactic
S = Succinic

Note: (1) Capital letters indicate major metabolic products; (2) lower case letters indicate minor products; (3) Parentheses indicate a variable reaction; (4) Isoacids are primarily from carbohydrate-free media (such as PY) in the case of saccharolytic organisms.

239

to *C. difficile* and certain other enteric infections or intoxications involving clostridia. Infant botulism is not seen after the age of eight months, by which time the normal intestinal flora is well established. Antitoxic immunity is clearly important in preventing tetanus, botulism, and necrotizing enterocolitis due to type C *C. perfringens* and may operate in other situations as well. Active immunization is useful in these settings.

CLINICAL FEATURES

The classic infections involving *C. perfringens* are clostridial myonecrosis (gas gangrene), gangrenous cholecystitis (with or without visceral gas gangrene), and post-abortal sepsis with intravascular hemolysis. **Clostridial myonecrosis** is a rapidly advancing infection, which may prove rapidly fatal. Onset is characterized by sudden pain in the region of a wound. The pain steadily increases in severity and remains localized to the area of the spreading infection. Soon there is local swelling and edema, and a thin hemorrhagic exudate may be apparent. There is relatively little fever but a disproportionately rapid pulse rate. There is tenderness of the wound and the skin is tense, white (with areas of blue discoloration at times), and colder than normal. Bronzed discoloration appears and increases with time. Swelling, edema, and toxemia increase rapidly; the serous discharge becomes more profuse; the skin becomes dusky; and bullae filled with dark red or purplish fluid appear. Gas is usually present, but only in limited amounts in the early stages of the infection. Despite toxic delirium, there may be sufficient mental clarity to allow the patient to appreciate the gravity of the disease process. Although the changes apparent at the skin surface may be impressive, the involvement of the underlying muscle (which may be apparent only at the time of its exposure during surgery) is the major pathology and the hallmark of the disease. Early changes in the muscle include pallor and edema, but there is progression to marked change in color, loss of contractility and then frank gangrene to liquefaction. *C. perfringens* is involved in 80 to 95 percent of cases, with *C. novyi* and *C. septicum* other important causes in civilian cases of clostridial myonecrosis.

Clostridia account for only a small percentage of postabortal infections, but often produce the most dramatic and severe illnesses of this type. With severe clostridial sepsis due to *C. perfringens*, there is a very dramatic clinical picture consisting of hemolytic anemia, hemoglobinemia, hemoglobinuria, disseminated intravascular coagulation, hyperbilirubinemia, shock, and anuria.

The clinical pictures just described are very dramatic and the illnesses are life-threatening. However, *C. perfringens* and a number of other clostridia are more commonly involved in infections of diverse types throughout the body, of the type caused by non–spore-forming anaerobes and other bacteria. Included are such entities as brain abscess, subdural empyema, aspiration pneumonia, thoracic empyema, intra-abdominal infection, infection related to gynecologic disease or surgery, wound infection following other types of surgery, and soft tissue infection. Bacteremia may be seen as a complication of some of these types of infection. There is a distinct association between infection involving *C. septicum* and malignancy and other diseases of the cecum.

Clostridia are not often involved in dental or oral infections but may be on occasion. There are reports of involvement of *C. perfringens*, in mixed culture, in a case of pyogenic granuloma and two cases of periostitis with subperiosteal abscess, of clostridia in mixed culture in gingival abscess, and of *C. sporogenes* along with other organisms in a case of cervical actinomycosis of buccodental origin.

Tetanus and **botulism** are classic clostridial intoxications, although, as indicated earlier, colonization with *C. botulinum* and subsequent toxin production in vivo are responsible for infant botulism and probably for some cases of botulism in adults. Adult botulism may also be secondary to wound infection with *C. botulinum* and absorption of toxin from that site. It is important to note that tetanus may result from infected gingiva or teeth or from surgery for such problems. Dental sources accounted for 1.2 percent of cases of tetanus in the United States in 1970–1971. It is also important to note that trismus related to dental problems may be confused with tetanus, and vice versa.

Early findings in tetanus include tension or cramps and twitching in muscles about a wound and stiffness of the jaw muscles with mild pains in facial muscles. In full-blown tetanus, the most typical complaint is **lockjaw** or **trismus**—inability to open the mouth because of spasm of the masseter muscles. Spasm of facial muscles leads to risus sardonicus, the characteristic grotesque, grinning facial expression. Spasms or contractions of the muscles of the trunk and extremities may be widespread and result in board-like rigidity, in painful intermittent tonic convulsions and opisthotonos, a condition in which the back is bowed backward so that the back of the head and heels approach each other. This is a very painful condition. External stimuli of even minor degree may precipitate extended painful tonic convulsions. Spasm of pharyngeal and laryngeal muscles may lead to difficulty in swallowing, cyanosis, and even respiratory arrest and death.

Botulism also has a distinctive clinical picture. As with tetanus, fever is absent and the patient's mentation is clear. There is a descending symmetrical motor paralysis first affecting muscles supplied by the cranial nerves. Common symptoms include diplopia, dysarthria, and dysphagia. Pupils are often dilated and fixed. Mucous membranes of the mouth, tongue, and pharynx may be extremely dry and even painful. Gastrointestinal symptoms are variable and are seen in about one third of patients.

Food poisoning due to certain serotypes of type A *C. perfringens* is common. It is a benign, self-limited process typically lasting only 24 hours. Symptoms include abdominal pain, nausea, and acute watery diarrhea without fever. Outbreaks are common and follow ingestion of contaminated foods, notably meat, poultry, or gravy.

Enteritis necroticans, known as "pig-bel" in New Guinea, where the disease has occurred with relative frequency, is a severe enteric infection due to type C *C. perfringens.* The disease is often fulminant with abdominal pain, bloody diarrhea, vomiting, peritonitis, and shock. There may be gangrene of the bowel.

It is now known that *C. difficile* is the primary cause of **pseudomembranous colitis** related to antimicrobial therapy and certain antineoplastic agents. Rare cases of this problem are caused by type C *C. perfringens* and other clostridia as well as by *Staphylococcus aureus.* Nonspecific colitis also appears to be due to *C. difficile* not uncommonly. Diarrhea without colitis that follows antimicrobial therapy may also involve *C. difficile* on occasion, and there is evidence to implicate type A *C. perfringens* in some of these cases as well. The hallmark of pseudomembranous colitis is a characteristic yellowish elevated plaque that may be seen by endoscopic examination

of the colon. Nonspecific colitis may involve various nonspecific inflammatory changes.

On the basis of the disease syndromes they produce or are involved in, clostridia may be placed in five groups:

Group 1—the **gas gangrene group.** This includes type A *C. perfringens, C. novyi, C. septicum, C. bifermentans, C. histolyticum, C. sordellii, C. sporogenes,* and others.

Group 2—*C. tetani,* the etiologic agent of **tetanus.**

Group 3—the **botulism group.** This includes various types of *C. botulinum,* as well as strains of *C. barati* and *C. butyricum* that produce an identical toxin.

Group 4—the **enteric group.** This includes *C. difficile,* responsible for most cases of pseudomembranous colitis related to antimicrobial and antineoplastic therapy, as well as other clostridia that may be involved in this process, including type C *C. perfringens, C. sordellii,* and others. In addition, type A *C. perfringens* is included as a cause of antibiotic-associated diarrhea without colitis and as a cause of food poisoning. Type C *C. perfringens* is the cause of enteritis necroticans.

Group 5—the miscellaneous infection group (wound infection, abscesses, bacteremia, and so forth). This group includes *C. perfringens, C. ramosum, C. bifermentans, C. sphenoides, C. sporogenes,* and a number of others.

IDENTIFICATION

The clinical picture of certain entities such as gas gangrene, tetanus, botulism, and post-abortal *C. perfringens* sepsis is usually distinctive enough to permit definitive diagnosis. The diagnosis is made by nonbacteriologic means in other cases—for example, by detection of the pathognomonic plaques in the colon of patients having pseudomembranous colitis.

The colonial and microscopic morphology of clostridia vary widely. As noted earlier, it may be difficult to determine that they are anaerobes, that they are gram-positive, and that they are spore-formers. In some cases, however, the morphology is distinctive enough to suggest that a clostridium is involved and even to indicate a particular species. Examples of such unique morphology include medusa-head colonies, the double zone of hemolysis around colonies of *C. perfringens* on sheep blood agar, lipase- and lecithinase-positive colonies on egg yolk agar, the large colonies that fluoresce chartreuse on cycloserine cefoxitin fructose agar (a highly selective medium for *C. difficile*),

Table 15–2 ■ In vitro susceptibility of clostridia to antimicrobial agents

Bacteria	Chloram-phenicol	Clinda-mycin	Erythro-mycin‡	Metro-nidazole	Cefoxitin	Ureido- and carboxy-penicillins*	Peni-cillin G§	Tetra-cycline	Vanco-mycin‡
C. perfringens	+++	++++†	+++	+++	+++	+++	+++	++	+++
Other Clostridium spp.	+++	++	+++ to +++	+++	+ to ++	+++	+++	++	++ to +++

Key: + = Poor or inconsistent activity; ++ = moderate activity, +++ = good activity; ++++ = good activity, good pharmacologic characteristics, low toxicity, drug of choice.
*Piperacillin, mezlocillin, azlocillin, carbenicillin, ticarcillin.
†Rare strains are resistant.
‡Not approved by FDA for anaerobic infections.
§Other penicillins and cephalosporins are frequently less active. Ampicillin and amoxicillin are roughly comparable to penicillin G in activity. Addition of beta-lactamase inhibitors, such as clavulanic acid and sulbactam, remarkably increase the activity against beta-lactamase producers.

the box car–like shape of *C. perfringens* (particularly in a clinical Gram stain in which the white blood cells have been severely damaged or destroyed by the organism's toxin), and gram-positive rods whose cells clearly contain spores. There are tests available for detection of toxins or other products of *C. difficile*, such as the cytotoxicity test in tissue culture and a latex agglutination test. There is a mouse lethality test and also an ELISA procedure for detection and confirmation of botulinal toxin in gastrointestinal contents and in implicated food specimens. Culture and biochemical reactions, as indicated in Table 15–1, are useful for diagnosis and identification in the vast majority of commonly encountered clostridial infections. It should be noted that collection of specimens so as to avoid indigenous flora and transport of such specimens in a manner designed to avoid exposure to air are very important for success in recovery of clostridia, as with all anaerobes.

THERAPY

Antitoxin therapy is important in intoxications such as tetanus and botulism, and toxoids may be used to induce immunity prophylactically. Surgical debridement and drainage are of particular importance in the management of clostridial infections, especially the more serious ones such as clostridial myonecrosis.

Antimicrobial therapy is also important in the proper management of most clostridial infections. Penicillin G is an excellent drug against clostridia but some strains, including some of *C. perfringens*, are resistant and others, such as some strains of *C. ramosum*, are relatively resistant (minimal inhibitory con-

centrations as high as 8 units per ml). *Clostridium ramosum*, often overlooked or misidentified, is commonly encountered in infection and is relatively resistant to antimicrobial agents. About 15 percent of strains of this species are highly resistant to clindamycin, and many strains are resistant to tetracycline and erythromycin. About 20 to 30 percent of strains of a number of clostridial species other than *C. perfringens* are resistant to clindamycin. One third of clostridia other than *C. perfringens* are resistant to cefoxitin. Metronidazole and chloramphenicol are essentially always active against clostridia. Table 15–2 summarizes the in vitro susceptibility of clostridia to some of the agents commonly employed in anaerobic infections or in infections of uncertain cause. For pseudomembranous colitis due to *C. difficile*, oral metronidazole, vancomycin, or bacitracin is the preferred antimicrobial agent. Some workers feel that bile acid–binding resins such as cholestyramine may be useful in the management of this disease as well, but controlled studies have not been carried out.

BIBLIOGRAPHY

Finegold, S. M.: Anaerobic Bacteria in Human Disease. Academic Press, New York, 1977.
Finegold, S. M., and Baron, E. J.: Bailey and Scott's Diagnostic Microbiology, ed. 7. C. V. Mosby, St. Louis, 1986.
Finegold, S. M., George, W. L., and Mulligan, M. E.: Anaerobic Infections. Year Book Medical Publishers, Chicago, 1986.
Sneath, P. H. A., Mair, N. S., Sharpe, M. E., and Holt, J. G.: Bergey's Manual of Systematic Bacteriology, Vol. 2. ed. 9. Williams and Wilkins, Baltimore, 1986.
Sutter, V. L., Citron, D. M., Edelstein, M. A. C., and Finegold, S. M.: Wadsworth Anaerobic Bacteriology Manual, ed. 4. Star Publishing, Belmont, CA, 1985.
Willis, A. T.: Clostridia of Wound Infection. Butterworths, London, 1969.

chapter 16

Bacteroides

K. Kornman, D.D.S., Ph.D.

Bacteroides species are the most commonly isolated anaerobes in clinical infections. These microorganisms are gram-negative, obligately anaerobic, nonmotile, non–spore-forming rods. The natural habitat of most *Bacteroides* species appears to be the mucous membranes of humans and other animals. Some of these species have been associated with diseases of the colon, oral cavity, upper respiratory tract, and female genital tract.

Classification

Recent studies of 16S ribosomal RNA suggest that *Bacteroides* are phylogenetically quite distinct from most other gram-negative bacteria. Catalogues of ribosomal RNA place oral and colonic *Bacteroides* species in a phylogenetic group that also contains *Fusobacterium*, another genus of gram-negative anaerobes, cytophages, and flavobacteria. Some rumen *Bacteroides* species such as *B. succinogenes* are not included in this grouping. Unfortunately,

speciation of **Bacteroides** may be difficult and may easily result in a misidentification. Isolates of other genera that are misidentified as *Bacteroides* are usually a result of failure to confirm obligate anaerobiosis or failure to detect spore formation.

The *B. fragilis* group, which includes the former subspecies of *B. fragilis* and additional new species, are the most frequently recovered anaerobes from the colon, intra-abdominal infections, and many other infections throughout the body. They are of added importance because of resistance to a variety of antimicrobial agents.

The black-pigmented *Bacteroides* species, or *B. melaninogenicus* group, are important pathogens in oral and respiratory infections. Other bile-sensitive nonpigmented *Bacteroides* species are similar to *B. oralis* and are found in the same environments as the black-pigmented *Bacteroides*. Two species, *B. bivius* and *B. disiens*, are found primarily in the female genital tract.

Bacteroides species may be best divided initially by the presence or absence of pigmented colonies and by their fermentative ability (Table 16–1). Pigmentation by *Bacteroides* species may range from a light coffee color to a deep brick-red or black and depends to a great extent on the growth medium and incubation time. In general, pigmentation develops more predictably on media with rabbit blood than on media with sheep or horse blood, but strains may vary in this regard. Fermentative ability of a microorganism refers to the lowering of the pH of basal broth medium containing glucose of 0.5 to 1.0 pH unit. The measurement of pH changes following bacterial growth in broth may commonly lead to erroneous conclusions with some anaerobes. The measurement of pH should be performed only where there is bacterial growth and within 24 to 48 hours of inoculation. In addition, it is essential to make a Gram stain from the broth culture to confirm that the pH change is due to pure culture rather than to a mixed culture. Thus, fermentative strains may be misread as nonfermentative if there is insufficient

growth in the broth tube, and nonfermentative strains may be read as fermentative if the culture is mixed or if the pH is not read for several days. The latter is a result of some nonfermentative *Bacteroides* species, which upon cell lysis lower the pH of certain media, especially those with added fumarate.

Black-Pigmented Bacteroides Species

The pigmented *Bacteroides* species have recently been termed "black-pigmented bacteroides," or **BPBs**. While this terminology is not an approved designation, it has descriptive value in referring to all *Bacteroides* species which grow as brown- or black-pigmented colonies on blood-containing media. It must be noted that not all pigmented colonies are *Bacteroides* species. For example, *Actinomyces odontolyticus* may be easily confused with BPB on some media. Likewise, some BPB may appear nonpigmented on certain growth media.

BPBs were first described as *Bacterium melaninogenicum* in 1921 (Oliver and Wherry) but were poorly defined until 1939 when Roy and Kelly classified these microorganisms as *Bacteroides melaninogenicus*. This designation was the same as "BPB," in that it referred to any *Bacteroides* that formed pigmented colonies. Several investigators noted the diversity of this group of bacteria and originally divided it into nonfermentors, weak fermentors, and strong fermentors. These groups later (Holdeman and Moore, 1970) became three subspecies: *B. melaninogenicus* subsp. *asaccharolyticus* (nonfermentors), *B. melaninogenicus* subsp. *melaninogenicus* (strong fermentors), and *B. melaninogenicus* subsp. *intermedius* (weak or "intermediate" fermentors).

Since 1979, we have greatly extended our understanding of black-pigmented *Bacteroides* and have reclassified them as shown in Figure 16–1. Thus, there are currently 10 recognized species of BPB, and recent work suggests that *B. intermedius* is heterogeneous and will probably be divided into two to three groups. Figure 16–1 demonstrates that depending on when an article was published, the name of the microorganism may refer to several different species that are not included in that designation today.

The major characteristics for differentiating the black-pigmented *Bacteroides* species commonly encountered in humans are listed in

Table 16–1 ■ *Bacteroides* species from human sources

I. Black-pigmented
  A. Fermentative
    B. denticola
    B. intermedius
    B. melaninogenicus
    B. loescheii
  B. Nonfermentative
    B. asaccharolyticus
    B. endodontalis
    B. gingivalis
II. Nonpigmented
  A. Fermentative
    B. bivius
    B. buccae
    B. disiens
    B. capillus
    B. distasonis
    B. eggerthii
    B. fragilis
    B. multiacidus
    B. oralis
    B. oris
    B. ovatus
    B. splanchnicus
    B. thetaiotaomicron
    B. uniformis
    B. vulgatus
    B. zoogleoformans
  B. Nonfermentative
    B. coagulens
    B. forsythus
    B. gracilis
    B. pneumosintes
    B. praeacutus
    B. ureolyticus

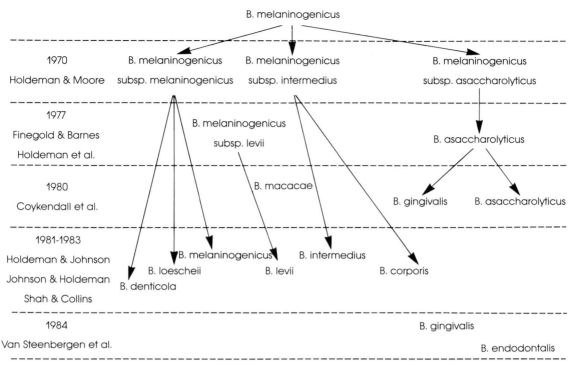

Figure 16-1 ■ Nomenclature of black-pigmented *Bacteroides* species.

Table 16-2 ■ Black-pigmented *Bacteroides* species: key identification characteristics of common human isolates

	B. mel.	B. loesch.	B. denticola	B. int.	B. corp.	B. g.	B. endo.	B. asacch.
Pigmented blood agar	+	+	+	+	+	+	+	+
End products* from PYG	SA	SA	SA	SA	SA	Biv apibs pa	A Biv absp	A Bivs pib
Esculin hydrolysis	−/+	+	+	−	−	−	−	−
Indole produced	−	−	−	+	−	+	+	+
Nitrate reduced	−	−	−	−	−	−	−	−
Acid from:								
Arabinose	−	−	−	−	−	−	−	−
Cellobiose	−	+	−	−	−	−	−	−
Glucose	+	+	+	+	+	−	−	−
Lactose	+	+	+	−	−	−	−	−
Ribose	−	−	−	−	−	−	−	−
Sucrose	+	+	+	+	−	−	−	−
Enzymes:								
Alkaline phosphatase	+	W	+	+	+	+	+	+
Trypsin	−	−	−	−	−	+	−	−
Acid phosphatase	+	+	W	+	+	+	+	+
A-galactosidase	W	−	W	−	−	−	−	−
B-galactosidase	+	W	+	−	−	−	−	−
B-glucuronidase	−	−	−	−	−	−	−	−
A-glucosidase	+	−	+	+	+	−	−	−
B-glucosidase	−	−	−	−	−	−	−	−
N-acetyl-B-glucosaminidase	+	+	+	−	−	+	−	−
A-fucosidase	+	−	W	W	−	−	−	W

*End products from PYG:
Capital letters indicate that the following are found as major components: A = acetic acid; B = butyric acid; Ib = isobutyric acid; Iv = isovaleric acid; Pa = phenylacetic acid; P = propionic acid; S = succinic acid.
Lower-case letters indicate that the same compounds are found as minor components in the end products.

Table 16–2. In general, once an organism has been identified as a BPB it may be classified as fermentative or nonfermentative. The fermentative BPBs all produce predominantly succinate and acetate from peptone yeast glucose broth (PYG) and are differentiated in the laboratory based on fermentation patterns; however, *B. melaninogenicus, B. denticola,* and *B. loescheii* are not reliably differentiated by phenotypic tests. The nonfermentative species are very important pathogens but also present identification difficulties. *B. gingivalis* may be distinguished from *B. endodontalis* and *B. asaccharolyticus* by means of trypsin-like enzyme activity and the presence of phenylacetic acid as an end product from glucose broth. *B. endodontalis* and *B. asaccharolyticus* are not readily differentiated by phenotypic tests but are distinct serologically and by electrophoretic patterns of cell wall proteins.

All BPB species require hemin and vitamin K_1 for growth. This requirement varies among species, as well as among strains of a single species, and the concentration range of these compounds for growth stimulation appears to be very narrow. Estradiol and progesterone have been shown to substitute for vitamin K in the growth of *B. intermedius* and some strains of *B. melaninogenicus* and *B. gingivalis*. Succinate appears to substitute for hemin in the growth of some BPB species.

Nonpigmented Bacteroides Species

There are currently over 30 species of nonpigmenting *Bacteroides*, which are differentiated primarily by means of indole production from tryptophan, acid production from various sugars, and growth in the presence of 20 percent bile. Many of the short identi-

fication schemes or commercially available test kits are designed to have high sensitivity in the identification of certain major medical pathogens. As such, these tests may have rather low specificity in differentiating less commonly encountered *Bacteroides* species. In the case of oral isolates, these schemes, often designed for intestinal anaerobes, may result in rather frequent misidentifications. In addition, since almost all of the fermentative *Bacteroides* species produce succinate and acetate as the primary end products from glucose, gas chromatography is of little value in the identification of the nonpigmented species. Some commercially available systems that use chromogenic substrates to assess a relatively large number of aminopeptidase or hydrolase enzymes have been shown to be reliable in differentiating many of the *Bacteroides* species.

For practical purposes, the nonpigmented fermentative *Bacteroides* species found in humans may be divided into species routinely isolated from the intestinal tract, species routinely isolated from the oral cavity, and urogenital species as shown in Table 16–3. Most of the human isolates of the intestinal fermentative nonpigmented *Bacteroides* species grow well in the presence of 20 percent bile and hydrolyze esculin. Most of the oral fermentative nonpigmented *Bacteroides* species are inhibited by bile, hydrolyze esculin, and do not produce indole from tryptophan. The fermentative nonpigmented *Bacteroides* species from the urogenital area are inhibited by bile and do not hydrolyze esculin or produce indole from tryptophan.

The nonfermentative, nonpigmented *Bacteroides* species routinely isolated from humans (Table 16–4) are often difficult to grow and to identify. Owing to the growth characteristics, end products from glucose broth may be minimal. Microorganisms such as *B. ureolyticus* and *B. gracilis* (which are nitrate

Table 16–3 ■ Nonpigmented fermentative *Bacteroides* species from humans			
	Intestinal	Oral	Urogenital
	B. fragilis	*B. oris*	*B. bivius*
	B. vulgatus	*B. buccae*	*B. disiens*
	B. distasonis	*B. oralis*	
	B. multiacidus	*B. zoogleoformans*	
	B. ovatus		
	B. thetaiotaomicron		
	B. uniformis		
	B. eggerthii		
	B. splanchnicus		
Growth in 20% bile	+	–	–

Table 16–4 ■ Differentiation of nonpigmented nonfermentative *Bacteroides* species

	B. coagulans	*B. forsythus*	*B. gracilis*	*B. pneumosintes*	*B. praeacutus*	*B. ureolyticus*
Indole produced	+	−	−	−	−	−
Nitrate reduced	−	*	+	−	+	+
Urease produced	−	−	−	−	−	+
Require hydrogen and fumarate			+			+

*Has not been reliably determined owing to poor growth in broth.

reductase–positive) are nonfermentative, require hydrogen and fumarate for growth, and are difficult to distinguish from *Campylobacter concisus* and *Wolinella recta*.

Bacteroides Species in the Oral Cavity

Although some *Bacteroides* species are indigenous members of the oral microbiota, the normal habitat of individual species and their association with oral diseases is not well defined. Most of the studies of the epidemiology of *Bacteroides* preceded current understanding of the speciation of these microorganisms. The fermentative pigmented *Bacteroides* species, *B. melaninogenicus*, *B. intermedius*, *B. loescheii*, and *B. denticola* may be routinely isolated from dental plaque and tonsils of individuals with periodontal health or with gingivitis. Although these species are present in most dentulous children, their rate of detection appears to increase around the time of puberty. *B. intermedius* is a predominant component of the subgingival microbiota in acute necrotizing ulcerative gingivitis and pregnancy gingivitis. This finding may relate to the effect of steroid hormones on stimulation of growth of *B. intermedius*. The microorganism has also been associated with progressing periodontitis in some cases.

The fermentative nonpigmented *Bacteroides* species *B. buccae*, *B. oris*, *B. oralis*, and *B. zoogleoformans* are also present in the oral cavity. *B. buccae* (*B. capillus*) has been associated with severe periodontitis, but little is known about its site or disease distribution.

The nonfermentative pigmented *Bacteroides* species *B. gingivalis* and *B. endodontalis* have not been reported in mouths without periodontal or endodontic diseases, but there are very few studies that used appropriate isolation techniques and identification procedures. Even in the presence of periodontitis, these two microorganisms are rarely isolated from oral mucosa or tonsils and appear to reside primarily in dental plaque.

B. gingivalis has been closely associated with periodontal pockets and progressing periodontitis. The prevalence of this microorganism in periodontal pockets has been reported to range from nondetectable to 81 percent, and approximately 50 to 60 percent of adults with periodontitis have elevated antibody levels to *B. gingivalis*. The great variability in its recovery rate is most likely due to variations in growth media, since relatively consistent recovery rates have been reported by groups that use similar growth media. Little is currently known about the origin, reservoirs, and transmission of *B. gingivalis*.

B. endodontalis has been strongly associated with symptomatic endodontic lesions. The distribution of this microorganism has not been well studied.

The nonfermentative nonpigmented *Bacteroides* species in the oral cavity, *B. forsythus* and *B. gracilis*, are found in subgingival plaque and have been associated with periodontitis. Although limited data are available, *B. forsythus* appears in cases of periodontitis that are progressing. In one recent report of 23 *B. gracilis* isolates submitted to a clinical microbiology laboratory, 83 percent were associated with serious visceral or head and neck infections. Since these microorganisms have only recently been described, their normal habitat and distribution are not known.

B. fragilis has been reported in some head and neck abscesses, especially those associated with bone fracture sites. This microorganism is not indigenous to the oral cavity. Other *Bacteroides* species may be isolated as transients in dental plaque but do not have a normal ecologic niche and are not routinely isolated from the mouth.

Bacteroides Species in the Intestinal Tract

The human colon is thought to contain more than 400 microbial species. *Bacteroides* is the most prevalent genus isolated from the colon and has been found in 100 percent of fecal samples from healthy individuals, with the exception of some Japanese. *Bacteroides* viable counts range from 10^9 to 10^{13} organisms per gram dry weight of feces and account for approximately 30 percent of all fecal isolates. The most numerous *Bacteroides* species isolated from the colon are *B. vulgatus, B. distasonis, B. thetaiotaomicron, B. fragilis, B. ovatus, B. eggerthii,* and *B. uniformis.* Although *Bacteroides* species clearly are important to the ecologic balance in the intestinal tract, little is known about the mechanisms that control the levels of these microorganisms in the climax ecosystem. Some of the intestinal *Bacteroides* species such as *B. fragilis, B. distasonis, B. thetaiotaomicron,* and *B. ovatus* have been associated with a variety of infections, such as abscesses of the brain, lung, or abdominal cavity. Infections caused by intestinal *Bacteroides* are often difficult to treat owing to their resistance to many antibiotics.

Bacteroides Species in the Urogenital Tract

Bacteroides species are indigenous and prominent isolates of the vaginal tract. Various studies of the cervical or vaginal microbiota have reported the isolation of *Bacteroides* species in up to 87 percent of the normal, healthy individuals. The relative levels of different species is not entirely clear since many studies of the urogenital microbiota have used media with vancomycin at a level (7.5 μg per ml) that is now known to inhibit some of the pigmented *Bacteroides* species. The largest single group of *Bacteroides* routinely isolated from the urogenital tract is the *B. bivius/disiens* group. These microorganisms may be found in approximately 40 percent of the samples from normal, healthy subjects.

Black-pigmented *Bacteroides*, including both saccharolytic and asaccharolytic species, have been observed in approximately 60 percent of normal samples, with *B. oralis*–like species present in 40 to 50 percent of these healthy individuals.

Quantitative increases in the proportional levels of *Bacteroides* species in the vaginal area have been reported during pregnancy, postpartum, and in symptomatic vaginal infections. *B. bivius* is now considered one of the primary causative agents of vaginosis, and treatment directed toward the anaerobic component of the microbiota is successful in resolving the symptoms of this disease.

Bacteroides Species in the Respiratory Tract

The total indigenous microbiota of the respiratory tract is not well defined, yet it is clear that the mucosa of certain respiratory passages is lined with anaerobes similar to those in the oral, intestinal, and urogenital tracts. For example, the microbiota of non-inflamed maxillary sinuses is dominated by anaerobic bacteria with *Bacteroides* species being the most prominent isolates. BPBs were the most common group reported with other *Bacteroides* representing the *B. oralis*–like microorganism. It is reasonable to expect that viral infections or allergic responses that produce a hyperemia and closing of the sinus would alter intrasinus conditions such that the emergence of anaerobes would occur. This is consistent with the observation that *Bacteroides* species are prominent isolates from chronic sinusitis. Much more study of the anaerobe populations in the respiratory tract is needed to determine the actual distribution of *Bacteroides* species and the similarities and differences to the microbiota of the oral cavity.

Surface Characteristics

As with all bacteria, surface structures of *Bacteroides* species may mediate attachment or may be involved in activating host mechanisms resulting in soft tissue damage. These structures include external appendages such as fimbria, capsular material, external surface layers (S layers), lipopolysaccharide, and outer membrane vessels (blebs). These have been discussed in detail in Chapter 3.

Fimbria are proteinaceous, filamentous, nonflagellar appendages that project from the surface and often are an important virulence factor in that they facilitate bacterial attachment to host cells. All *Bacteroides* species that have been evaluated possess fimbria, but great species differences have been reported with respect to morphology, function, chemistry, and immunology.

For example, *B. gingivalis* has been reported to have fimbria subunits of apparently large molecular weight (43,000 versus 15,000 to 28,000 as reported for other bacteria) and

B. gingivalis fimbria do not appear to have the capacity to hemagglutinate or block hemagglutination by whole cells of the microorganism. This suggests that *B. gingivalis* may have another fimbria of the lectin type, which mediates hemagglutination. Thus, *B. gingivalis* may have two distinctly different fimbria, one mediating attachment of the organism to other bacteria and the other to host cells.

Outer membranes of gram-negative microorganisms have been shown to act as antigens and mitogens, as well as activating various other host responses. These activities may allow the outer membrane to serve as a major virulence factor in many gram-negative species.

Studies of *Bacteroides* species have shown a pattern of outer membrane polypeptides which is substantially more complex than, for example, *Escherichia coli*. *B. intermedius*, both oral and nonoral strains, have a major outer membrane polypeptide of between 19 and 22 kD, and appears to also have a high molecular mass glycoprotein. *B. gingivalis* also had a distinctive, yet well conserved, polypeptide profile in the outer membrane. The profile of outer membrane polypeptides in *B. thetaiotaomicron* has also been found to be more complex than that usually seen in gram-negative bacteria.

Outer membrane fragments or "blebs" are commonly released from *Bacteroides* into the growth medium. Some species have been shown to release fragments that contain various enzymes. These fragments may be of importance to the virulence of these bacteria, since they may readily penetrate tissue and may also assist in evading certain host defense mechanisms.

Pathogenic Mechanisms of Oral Bacteroides

The association of certain *Bacteroides* species with abscesses, tissue destruction, and specifically periodontal diseases has led to extensive evaluations of pathogenic mechanisms in these microorganisms. The surface structures that are critical to attachment in *Bacteroides* have been discussed earlier. These structures may also interfere with host defense mechanisms.

Strict anaerobes cannot be routinely implanted in pure cultures into germ-free animals or sterile tissue spaces. For this reason, oral *Bacteroides* have been studied as mixed infections in animal models. Black-pigmented *Bacteroides*, when injected with certain other bacteria, produced severe subcutaneous abscesses that were transmissible. The BPBs were essential to the pathogenicity of the microbial mixture. The accompanying microbiota is essential to provide growth factors including vitamin K or succinate. In a mixed-infection abscess model, *B. gingivalis*, *B. intermedius*, and *B. endodontalis* exhibited substantial virulence. *B. melaninogenicus* and *B. loescheii* were the least virulent in the abscess model. Other oral *Bacteroides* species have not been well studied in a comparable manner.

Attempts to induce periodontitis in animal models with BPBs have been complicated by the difficulty of implanting the microorganisms and evaluating the role of a single species in a mixed infection. Recently, labeled pure cultures of *B. gingivalis* have been implanted into a stable subgingival microbiota in monkey, with resulting rapid loss of alveolar bone at the implanted sites.

B. gingivalis, therefore, and to some extent *B. intermedius* and *B. endodontalis* fulfill criteria for overt pathogens. These microorganisms have a variety of virulence factors that may contribute to pathogenicity. The surface structures, which are involved in the attachment of these bacteria to mucosa or other bacteria, have been described previously. In addition, these surface structures have the potential to alter the host response to either protect the microorganisms or to damage the tissue. For example, *Bacteroides* LPS activates the complement system and produces chemotactic factors for PMNs. However, capsular material and soluble extracellular products interfere with chemotaxis. In general, encapsulated strains of *B. gingivalis* and *B. endodontalis* appear to be more resistant to phagocytosis than less pathogenic strains.

A variety of soluble products may be produced by some of the oral *Bacteroides* species and damage the host directly or indirectly. Low molecular weight end products such as volatile sulfur compounds, ammonia, indole, and butyric and propionic acids are cytotoxic and may be specifically leukotoxic. The nonfermentative strains produce more of these substances than do fermentative species, but the in situ role of these compounds in periodontal disease has not been established.

Proteolytic enzymes are very characteristic of the *Bacteroides* species and these microorganisms are very active in degrading various peptides. Hyaluronidase, heparinase, nucleases, and fibrinolytic activities have been described for oral BPBs. Of particular interest is the presence of true collagenase and trypsin-like enzymes in *B. gingivalis*. In addition, *B. gingivalis* is capable of activating latent collagenase within the tissue. Recent interest has also focused on the ability of *B. gingivalis*, *B. intermedius*, and *B. endodontalis* to degrade IgA molecules. The presence of an IgA protease may be important in allowing the colonization and emergence of these microorganisms.

In general, the oral black-pigmented *Bacteroides* species—and *B. gingivalis*, *B. intermedius*, and *B. endodontalis* in particular—appear to have sufficient virulence factors to explain their observed pathogenicity.

References

Coykendall, A. L., Kaczmarek, F. S., and Slots, J.: Genetic heterogeneity in *Bacteroides asaccharolyticus* (Holdeman and Moore 1970) Finegold and Barnes 1977 (Approved Lists, 1980) and Proposal of *Bacteroides gingivalis* sp. nov. and *Bacteroides Macacae* (Slots and Genco) comb. nov. Int. J. Syst. Bacteriol. 30:559, 1980.

Finegold, S. M., and Barnes, E. M.: Report of the ICSB Taxonomic Subcommittee on Gram-Negative Anaerobic Rods. Proposal that the saccharolytic and asaccharolytic strains at present classified in the species *Bacteroides melaninogenicus* (Oliver and Wherry) be reclassified in two species as *Bacteroides melaninogenicus* and *Bacteroides asaccharolyticus*. Int. J. Syst. Bacteriol. 27:388, 1977.

Holdeman, L. V., and Moore, W. E. C.: *Bacteroides*, pp. 33–34. *In* Cato, E. B., Cummis, C. S., Holdeman, L. V., Johnson, J. L., Moore, W. E. C., Smibert, R. M., and Smith, L. D. (eds.): Outline of Clinical Methods in Anaerobic Bacteriology, 2nd rev. Virginia Polytechnic Institute and State University, Blacksburg, 1970.

Holdeman, L. V., Cato, E. P., and Moore, W. E. C. (eds.): Anaerobe Laboratory Manual, 4th ed. Anaerobe Laboratory, Virginia Polytechnic Institute and State University, Blacksburg, 1977.

Holdeman, L. V., and Johnson, J. L.: Description of *Bacteroides loescheii* sp. nov. and emendation of the descriptions of *Bacteroides melaninogenicus* (Oliver and Wherry) Ray and Kelly 1939 and *Bacteroides denticola* Shah and Collins 1981. Int. J. Syst. Bacteriol. 32:399, 1982.

Johnson, J. L., and Holdeman, L. V.: *Bacteroides intermedius* comb. nov. and descriptions of *Bacteroides carporis* sp. nov. and *Bacteroides levii* sp. nov. Int. J. Syst. Bacteriol. 33:15, 1983.

Shah, H. N., and Collins, M. D.: *Bacteroides buccalis*, sp. nov. *Bacteroides denticola*, sp. nov. new species of the genus *Bacteroides* from the oral cavity. Zentralbl. Bakteriol. Parasitenkd. Infektionskr. Hyg. Abt. 1 Orig. Reihe C 2:235, 1981.

Van Steenbergen, T. J. M., van Winkelhoff, A. J., Mayrand, D., Grenier, D., and de Graaff, J.: *Bacteroides endodontalis* sp. nov., an asaccharolytic black-pigmented *Bacteroides* species from infected dental root canals. Int. J. Syst. Bacteriol. 34:118, 1984.

chapter 17

Actinobacillus actinomycetemcomitans

Jørgen Slots, D.M.D., M.S., Ph.D. □ *Norton S. Taichman, D.D.S., Ph.D.*

CHAPTER OUTLINE

- MORPHOLOGY
- CULTIVATION AND METABOLISM
- ANTIGENIC COMPOSITION

- ORAL COLONIZATION
- POTENTIAL VIRULENCE MECHANISMS

Actinobacillus actinomycetemcomitans is a gram-negative, small, non–spore-forming, nonmotile, facultatively anaerobic rod. It represents the only *Actinobacillus* species that is regularly associated with human infections. Other *Actinobacillus* species are pathogenic in cattle, horses, and pigs. Coykendall and Potts and their colleagues established that *A. actinomycetemcomitans* is genetically more related to the *Haemophilus* genus than to *Actinobacillus lignieresii,* the type species of *Actinobacillus.*

Morphology

Fresh clinical isolates of *A. actinomycetemcomitans* appear as circular convex colonies, about 1.0 mm in diameter with slightly irregular edges (Fig. 17–1). Primary colonies are translucent and glistening, often exhibiting a star-like inner structure. They adhere to the agar surface and are difficult to break up. Growth in broth is granular with clumps of cell strongly adherent to the bottom of a test tube. The ability of the colonies to adhere to agar medium, the inner structure of the colonies, and the granular growth in broth disappear on repeated subculture.

A. actinomycetemcomitans cells are about 1.0 to 1.5 by 0.4 to 0.5 μm in size, and occur singly, in pairs, or in small clumps. In old cultures or after several transfers, some strains show longer cell forms.

Cultivation and Metabolism

A. actinomycetemcomitans grows best on serum or blood agar in an anaerobic atmosphere or in 10 percent CO_2. Cultures may be stimulated by 1 percent $NaHCO_3$. Growth is optimal at 37°C. Hemin (X-factor) and nicotinamide adenine dinucleotide (V-factor), which are important growth factors for the *Haemophilus* genus (*H. aphrophilus* exhibits no requirement for X and V factors), are not required by *A. actinomycetemcomitans.* Media for selective recovery of *A. actinomycetemcomitans* have been described.

251

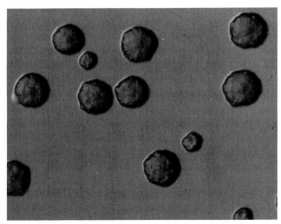

Figure 17–1 ■ Colonies of *Actinobacillus actinomyce-temcomitans* showing the characteristic star-shaped inner structure. (Courtesy of Dr. Joseph J. Zambon.)

Ten biotypes of *A. actinomycetemcomitans* have been identified on the basis of dextrin, maltose, mannitol, and xylose fermentation reaction patterns and three serotypes have been identified on the basis of heat-stable cell surface antigens. Determination of *A. actinomycetemcomitans* biotypes and serotypes (see further on) has helped delineate its mode of transmission among patients with localized juvenile periodontitis and infected family members.

Antigenic Composition

The three serotypes of *A. actinomycetemcomitans* defined by heat-stable surface polysaccharides are designated a, b, and c. These three serotype-determining antigens appear to be unique for the *A. actinomycetemcomitans* species. *A. actinomycetemcomitans* serotypes a and b occur with highest frequency in the human oral cavity. Serotype b is the most common serotype in localized juvenile periodontitis. The serotype c–determining antigen has been purified and is composed of 95 percent carbohydrate, mainly mannose, 2 percent protein, and 3 percent phosphate.

Common antigens also occur among the three *A. actinomycetemcomitans* serotypes and between *A. actinomycetemcomitans* and various *Actinobacillus* and *Haemophilus* species.

Oral Colonization

The establishment of *A. actinomycetemcomitans* in the human oral cavity can be assumed

to be dependent on appropriate attachment sites for initial colonization and to be influenced by factors pertaining to the interacting microflora and the host (Table 17–1).

A. actinomycetemcomitans is one of the few oral bacteria capable of colonizing buccal mucosa as well as dental plaque. It is of interest that freshly isolated *A. actinomycetemcomitans* strains are strongly adherent to agar, glass, and other surfaces, and that this adherent capability is lost on repeated subculture. It is not known if loss of attachment potential is caused by mutation or phenotypic regulation due to environmental changes.

Long thin surface appendages, termed fimbriae or pili, may mediate the initial attachment of *A. actinomycetemcomitans* to oral surfaces. Fresh isolates of *A. actinomycetemcomitans* produce an abundance of fimbriae, whereas established laboratory stains rarely do. *A. actinomycetemcomitans* also elaborate numerous vesicles, or "blebs," on the cell surfaces. Their role in initial colonization, if any, has not been determined.

Bacterial interactions also seem to be a determinant of oral colonization of *A. actinomycetemcomitans*. *Streptococcus sanguis*, *Actinomyces viscosus*, and *S. uberis* inhibit the in vitro growth of *A. actinomycetemcomitans*. That this antagonistic mechanism may operate in vivo is indicated from the finding that inhibitory organisms are frequently isolated from periodontal sites free of *A. actinomycetemcomitans* but are rarely recovered from localized juvenile periodontitis lesions infected with *A. actinomycetemcomitans*. On the other hand, *A. actinomycetemcomitans* also displays bacteriocin properties capable of inhibiting in vitro growth of *S. sanguis*, *A. viscosus*, and other common dental plaque microorganisms. This *A. actinomycetemcomitans*–mediated antagonism may explain, in part, why patients with localized juvenile periodontitis often exhibit relatively little supragingival plaque. In sum, mutual antagonism is possible between *A. actinomycetemcomitans* and various streptococcal and *Actinomyces* species, and both antagonistic mechanisms may occur in vivo. If the "protective" organisms are numerous, they may prevent *A. actino-*

Table 17–1 ■ *A. actinomycetemcomitans* colonization factors

Pili or fimbriae
Capsule
Interactions with other bacteria
Vesicles?

mycetemcomitans establishment and disease development. If *A. actinomycetemcomitans* happens to gain a foothold in the periodontal environment, it may suppress the "protective" organisms and disease may develop.

Potential Virulence Mechanisms

A. actinomycetemcomitans produces several biologically active substances that individually or collectively could be involved in the production of disease (Table 17–2). Of particular interest are those factors that seem to be unique to *A. actinomycetemcomitans* and are not shared by other putative periodontopathic bacteria. The *A. actinomycetemcomitans* leukotoxin and *A. actinomycetemcomitans* immunosuppressive factor have not, for example, been identified in other plaque organisms, whereas the capacity of *A. actinomycetemcomitans* to mediate bone resorption, depress fibroblast proliferation, or produce polyclonal B-cell activators is seen in many groups of bacteria. Differences in the biologic potentials of *A. actinomycetemcomitans* versus other bacteria may help to explain the peculiar features of periodontal lesions infected by *A. actinomycetemcomitans*.

A. ACTINOMYCETEMCOMITANS LEUKOTOXIN

A. actinomycetemcomitans kills human neutrophils and monocytes. The reaction is due to a proteinaceous, heat-labile leukotoxin. Although neutrophils and monocytes from several nonhuman primates are also destroyed by the leukotoxin, human leukocytes seem to be especially sensitive. Interestingly, other human cells (such as erythrocytes, fibroblasts, and endothelial and epithelial cells) as well as leukocytes from other species (such as dogs, rabbits, rats, and mice) are not affected by the leukotoxin. The mechanisms of leukotoxin-mediated killing of target

Table 17–2 ■ A. actinomycetemcomitans— host interactions

Leukotoxin
Inhibition of neutrophil functions
Immunosuppression via T-suppressor cell activation
Resistant to complement-mediated killing
Polyclonal cell activation
Endotoxin-mediated complement activation

cells are not completely understood, but the reaction is extremely rapid (a matter of minutes) and probably leads to pathologic changes in the cell membrane of the target cells. If the leukotoxin acts in vivo as it does in vitro, it could have profound effects on the course of *A. actinomycetemcomitans* infection by depleting neutrophils as they migrate into the area, thereby crippling innate resistance to bacterial attack. Furthermore, leukotoxin-damaged cells release lysosomal products into the extracellular milieu, and this may also contribute to tissue injury. Finally, killing of monocytes in the gingival tissues may perturb adaptive resistance (the immune response) and delay antibody synthesis against the leukotoxin or other bacterial antigens.

A. ACTINOMYCETEMCOMITANS IMMUNOSUPPRESSIVE FACTOR

Patients with localized juvenile periodontitis show a high incidence of infection by *A. actinomycetemcomitans,* and the vast majority also demonstrate antibodies to *A. actinomycetemcomitans*–derived antigens (including the leukotoxin) in serum and gingival exudates. Thus, there is a vigorous immune response to *A. actinomycetemcomitans* and this may be critical in limiting the extent of *A. actinomycetemcomitans* attack on the host. Very little is known, however, about the dynamics of the humoral immune response in *A. actinomycetemcomitans* infection, since the data currently available have been derived from patients with established (or advanced) disease. It is conceivable that *A. actinomycetemcomitans* may impede the local and/or systemic humoral immune response during early phases of infection and hence may provide *A. actinomycetemcomitans* with sufficient time to become "firmly" established in infected areas. As mentioned earlier, monocyte destruction by *A. actinomycetemcomitans* leukotoxin could contribute to this process. In addition, *A. actinomycetemcomitans* possesses a unique heat-labile immunosuppressive factor that inhibits various critical functions of lymphoid cells such as blastogenesis, antibody production, and lymphokine synthesis. The immunosuppressive factor does not kill cells but selectively activates T-suppressor cells. While several other plaque bacteria inhibit lymphoid responsiveness to antigens or mitogens, none appear to operate in this manner. The immunosuppressive factor, unlike the leukotoxin, can affect lymphoid cells from primates as well as other species and is also found in nonleukotoxic *A. actinomycetemcomitans* strains (see further on). Although its precise role in the development of *A. actinomycetemcomitans* infection is still to be elucidated, it is clear that this substance, together with the leukotoxin, may represent a potent mechanism for overwhelming local host defense systems.

A. ACTINOMYCETEMCOMITANS PERTURBATION OF NEUTROPHIL FUNCTIONS UNRELATED TO LEUKOTOXIN ACTIVITY

A. actinomycetemcomitans can affect neutrophil behavior without killing these cells. For example, strains of *A. actinomycetemcomitans* that lack the toxin (or have very low levels of leukotoxin) are not phagocytosed by neutrophils unless opsonized by antibodies or other serum components. Further, leukotoxic as well as nonleukotoxic strains contain unidentified substances that inhibit neutrophil chemotaxis. They also produce catalase and superoxide dismutase and seem to be relatively insensitive to hydrogen perioxide and superoxide anion. These data suggest that neutrophils may have difficulty dealing with *A. actinomycetemcomitans* even in the absence of leukotoxin. This might be relevant in situations when the host has formed neutralizing antibodies to the leukotoxin or in patients infected with nonleukotoxic *A. actinomycetemcomitans* strains. In this context, cross-sectional studies in patients with localized juvenile periodontitis suggest that there may be a shift from leukotoxic to nonleukotoxic *A. actinomycetemcomitans* during the course of infection. The basis for this change in biologic activity is not at present understood.

A. ACTINOMYCETEMCOMITANS INHIBITION OF FIBROBLASTS, ENDOTHELIAL CELLS, AND EPITHELIAL CELL ACTIVITIES

A. actinomycetemcomitans can modulate the behavior of fibroblasts, endothelial cells, and epithelial cells without actually killing these resident tissue cells (Table 17–3). The relevant factors have not been adequately defined but they are heat-sensitive and inactivated by proteolytic enzymes. For example,

Table 17–3 ■ *A. actinomycetemcomitans* effects on tissue

Inhibition of fibroblasts, endothelial cells, and
    epithelial cells
Endotoxin-mediated bone resorption
Endotoxin-mediated tissue toxicity
Collagenase
Invasion

extracts of either leukotoxic or nonleukotoxic *A. actinomycetemcomitans* can inhibit DNA, RNA, and protein synthesis in cultures of fibroblasts or endothelial cells. Likewise, epithelial cell proliferation and attachment to plastic tissue culture growth surfaces are depressed by *A. actinomycetemcomitans* extracts. Obviously, if the functions of resident tissue cells are compromised in vivo there are likely to be profound changes in the ability of infected tissues to resist or respond to injury.

A. ACTINOMYCETEMCOMITANS LIPOPOLYSACCHARIDE ACTIVITY

Bacterial endotoxic lipopolysaccharides have been advocated as important virulence factors in the pathogenesis of many forms of periodontal disease, and *A. actinomycetemcomitans* contains very potent lipopolysaccharides. These substances, for example, act as B-cell mitogens (see further on), produce hemorrhagic necrosis in the skin (local Shwartzman reaction), and activate the alternative complement pathway. In addition, endotoxin can stimulate bone resorption in vitro. In this context, *A. actinomycetemcomitans* also contains nonendotoxic factors that cause bone destruction in tissue cultures.

A. ACTINOMYCETEMCOMITANS POLYCLONAL CELL ACTIVATION

A. actinomycetemcomitans stimulates polyclonal antibody production as well as mitogenic responses in human blood lymphocytes. While not completely settled, stimulatory effects of *A. actinomycetemcomitans* on B cells seem to be mediated by both endotoxic as well as nonendotoxic components. Polyclonal cell activation could result in overproduction in immunologic effector molecules (e.g., antibodies, lymphokines) which may have potential beneficial and/or harmful effects on the host (e.g., hypersecretion of "osteoclast-activating factor" might lead to bone resorption; formation of "inappropriate" immune complexes could nonspecifically activate the complement system, stimulate neutrophil degranulation, and so forth).

A. ACTINOMYCETEMCOMITANS INVASION OF HOST TISSUES

A. actinomycetemcomitans appears to be localized at the "apical front" of subgingival deposits and is thus in a very strategic position to penetrate underlying soft tissues. Indeed, gram-negative organisms, including those resembling *A. actinomycetemcomitans*, have been identified in gingival specimens from patients with very severe localized juvenile periodontitis. Observation on whether *A. actinomycetemcomitans* also colonize soft tissues during initial or early phases of disease may help to settle whether *A. actinomycetemcomitans* invasiveness is a factor in the etiology of juvenile periodontitis.

From the foregoing it is apparent that *A. actinomycetemcomitans* possesses biologic properties that could allow it to attack the host. The capacity of *A. actinomycetemcomitans* to overwhelm or evade antibacterial defense systems in the gingival region may be particularly relevant in explaining how this organism causes disease.

REFERENCES

Berthold, P., and Listgarten, M.: Distribution of *Actinobacillus actinomycetemcomitans* in localized juvenile periodontitis plaque: An electron immunocytochemical study. J Periodont Res 21:473, 1986.

Coykendall, A. L., Setterfield, J., and Slots, J.: Deoxyribonucleic acid relatedness among *Actinobacillus actinomycetemcomitans*, *Haemophilus aphrophilus*, and other *Actinobacillus* species. Int J Syst Bacteriol 33:422, 1983.

Donaldson, S. L., Ranney, R. R., and Tew, J. G.: Evidence of mitogenic activity in periodontitis-associated bacteria. Infect Immun 42:487, 1983.

Hammond, B. F., Stevens, R. H., Bonner, P., and Lillard, S. E.: Toxicity of *Actinobacillus actinomycetemcomitans* (Aa) extracts for crevicular bacteria. J Dent Res 63:263, 1984.

Hillman, J. D., and Socransky, S. S.: Bacterial interference in the oral ecology of *Actinobacillus actinomycetemcomitans* and its relationship to human periodontitis. Arch Oral Biol 27:75, 1982.

Kamen, P. R.: Inhibition of keratinocyte proliferation by extracts of *Actinobacillus actinomycetemcomitans*. Infect Immun 42:1191, 1983.

Kiley, P., and Holt, S. C.: Characterization of the lipopolysaccharide from *Actinobacillus actinomycetemcomitans* Y4 & N27. Infect Immun 30:862, 1980.

Mandell, R. L., Tripodi, L. S., Savitt, E., Goodson, J. M., and Socransky, S. S.: The effect of treatment on *Actinobacillus actinomycetemcomitans* in localized juvenile periodontitis. J Periodontol 57:94, 1986.

McArthur, W. P., Tsai, C. C., and Taichman, N. S.: Non-cytolytic effects of *Actinobacillus actinomycetemcomitans* on leukocyte functions. In Genco, R. J., and Mergenhagen, S. E. (eds.): Host-Parasite Interactions in Periodontal Diseases. American Society for Microbiology, Washington, DC, 1982, p. 179.

Miyasaki, K. T., Wilson, M. E., Reynolds, H. S., and Genco, R. J.: Resistance of *Actinobacillus actinomycetemcomitans* and differential susceptibility of oral *Haemophilus* species to the bactericidal effects of hydrogen peroxide. Infect Immun 46:644, 1984.

Nowotny, A., Behling, U. H., Hammond, B., Lai, C. H., Listgarten, M. A., Pham, P. H., and Sanavi, F.: Release of toxic microvesicles by *Actinobacillus actinomycetemcomitans*. Infect Immun 37:151, 1982.

Potts, T. V., Zambon, J. J., and Genco, R. J.: Reassignment of *Actinobacillus actinomycetemcomitans* to the genus *Haemophilus* as *Haemophilus actinomycetemcomitans* comb. nov. Int J Syst Bacteriol 35:337, 1985.

Saglie, F. R., Carranza, F. A., and Newman, M. G.: The presence of bacteria within the oral epithelium in periodontal disease. J Periodontol 56:618, 1985.

Scannapieco, F. A., Kornman, K. S., and Coykendall, A. L.: Observation of fimbriae and flagella in dispersed subgingival dental plaque and fresh bacterial isolates from periodontal disease. J Periodont Res 18:620, 1983.

Shenker, B. J., Kushner, M. E., and Tsai, C. C.: Suppression of fibroblast proliferation and function by *Actinobacillus actinomycetemcomitans*. Infect Immun 38:986, 1982.

Shenker, B. J., Tsai, C. C., and Taichman, N. S.: Suppression of lymphocyte responses by *Actinobacillus actinomycetemcomitans*. J Periodont Res 17:462, 1982.

Slots, J.: Selective medium for isolation of *Actinobacillus actinomycetemcomitans*. J Clin Microbiol 15:606, 1982.

Slots, J., Reynolds, H. S., and Genco, R. J.: *Actinobacillus actinomycetemcomitans* in human periodontal disease: a cross-sectional microbiological investigation. Infect Immun 29:1013, 1980.

Taichman, N. S., Klass, J. E., Shenker, B. J., Macarak, E. J., Boehringer, H., and Tsai, C. C.: Suspected periodontopathic organisms alter in vitro proliferation of endothelial cells. J Periodont Res 19:583, 1984.

Taichman, N. S., Tsai, C. C., Shenker, B. J., and Boehringer, H. R.: Neutrophil interactions with oral bacteria as a pathogenic mechanism in periodontal diseases. In Weissman, G. (ed.): Advances in Inflammation Research. Raven Press, New York, 1984, p. 113.

Tsai, C. C., and Taichman, N. S.: Dynamics of infection by leukotoxic strains of *Actinobacillus actinomycetemcomitans* in juvenile periodontitis. J Clin Periodontol 13:330,, 1986.

Van Dyke, T. E., Bartholome, E., Genco, R., Slots, R. J., and Levine, M. J.: Inhibition of neutrophil chemotaxis by soluble bacterial products. J Periodontol 53:502, 1982.

Zambon, J. J., Christersson, L. A., and Slots, J.: *Actinobacillus actinomycetemcomitans* in human periodontal disease: prevalence in patient groups and distribution of biotypes and serotypes within families. J Periodontol 54:707, 1983.

Zambon, J. J., Slots, J., and Genco, R. J.: Serology of oral *Actinobacillus actinomycetemcomitans* and serotype distribution in human periodontal disease. Infect Immun 41:19, 1983.

Zambon, J. J., Slots, J., Miyasaki, K., Linzer, R., Cohen, R., Levine, M., and Genco, R. J.: Purification and characterization of the serotype *c* antigen from *Actinobacillus actinomycetemcomitans*. Infect Immun 44:22, 1984.

chapter 18

Veillonella, Wolinella, and Campylobacter

Joseph J. Zambon, D.D.S., Ph.D.

Veillonella Species

The *Veillonella* are gram-negative, anaerobic cocci found in the human intestinal and respiratory tracts as well as in some animals (Table 18–1). This genus is classified together with the genera *Acidaminococcus* and *Megasphaera* in the family *Veillonellaceae*. The genus name is derived from the name of the French bacteriologist A. Veillon, who first isolated the microorganism. The bacterial cells are cocci, 0.3 to 0.5 μm in diameter, which can be found as diplococci and in short chains. The organisms are nonmotile and grow best at 30 to 37°C. They are oxidase- and catalase-negative. The bacteria on agar may form lens-, diamond-, or heart-shaped colonies that are opaque, grayish white. One distinguishing feature is the ability of the bacterial colonies to exhibit a pink to red fluorescence when illuminated with a long-wave ultraviolet light. This fluorescence characteristic is shared with black-pigmented *Bacteroides* such as *B. intermedius*. The *Veillonella* can ferment pyruvate, lactate, malate, fumarate, and oxaloacetate but do not ferment carbohydrates. They exhibit between 36 and 43 mol% G + C.

Seven species of *Veillonella* have been identified—*V. parvula*, *V. rodentium*, *V. atypica*, *V. ratti*, *V. criceti*, *V. dispar*, and *V. caviae*—of which three species, *parvula*, *atypica*, and *dispar*, have been isolated from humans, especially from the human oral cavity. These species can be distinguished from one another only by DNA/DNA hybridization. There is at present no phenotypic scheme that can differentiate these species with a high degree of reliability. *V. parvula* and *V. dispar* have been isolated from human dental plaque in patients with periodontal disease. There is, however, no evidence to indicate

Table 18–1 ■ *Veillonella*

Characteristics	Gram-negative, anaerobic cocci Found in the human GI and respiratory tract Found in alimentary canal of animals
Major species	*V. parvula* *V. atypica* *V. dispar* } species found in humans
Growth	Anaerobic at 30–37° C
Disease	Possible association with human periodontal disease
Pathogenesis	Unknown

that these species are important in the etiology of human periodontal disease.

Wolinella Species

The *Wolinella* are gram-negative, motile anaerobes that can be found as helical, curved, or straight bacterial cells 0.5 to 1.0 μm by 2 to 6 μm with tapered or round ends (Table 18–2). These microorganisms can be found in large numbers in the subgingival dental plaque of adult periodontitis patients and may be involved in the pathogenesis of this form of periodontal disease. They are also found in infected root canals and in the gastrointestinal tract of cows. The genus is part of the family *Bacteroidaceae*, which includes other gram-negative microorganisms that can be found in subgingival dental plaque, such as the back-pigmented Bacteroides. *Wolinella* was named after the American microbiologist M. J. Wolin, who was the first to isolate it.

The *Wolinella* exhibit a rapid, darting type of bacterial motility by means of flagella located at one pole of the bacterial cell. This motility can be observed by phase contrast microscopy. The bacteria form three types of colonies on agar. One type is a pale, translucent, nonspreading yellow colony. Another type is a gray translucent colony, which may be mistaken for a water droplet on the agar. Another colony variant can, depending on the growth medium, pit the agar surface. The microorganism grows best at 37°C in an anaerobic environment of 85 percent N_2, 10 percent H_2, and 5 percent CO_2.

Many of the bacteria previously referred to as *Vibrio succinogenes* are now categorized in the genus *Wolinella*. The genus exhibits 42 to 48 mol% G + C. There are currently three species of *Wolinella*—*W. recta*, *W. succinogenes*, and *W. curva*—of which the former two have been best described. *W. succinogenes* appears as spiral or curved cells and thus can be distinguished from *W. recta*, which appears mainly as straight cells. *W. succinogenes*, as the name implies, also has a growth requirement for succinate or for compounds such as pyruvate and bicarbonate, which can be converted to succinate during bacterial metabolism. Electron microscopy demonstrates an unusual feature of *W. recta*. The outer cell membrane is covered by hexagonal subunits. The species can also be differentiated from the other *Wolinella* species on the basis of sensitivity to various dyes and antibiotics.

As previously mentioned, *W. recta* can be found in high numbers in subgingival dental plaque in adult periodontitis patients. In fact, this microorganism is, along with *Bacteroides* species, one of the predominant bacterial isolates from certain of these patients. For example, this is a predominant bacterial species in subgingival plaque from periodontitis patients with non–insulin dependent diabetes mellitus (Table 18–3). Of 392 bacterial isolates recovered from 8 patients, *Bacteroides intermedius* was the most frequently isolated microorganism, constituting 16 percent of the total isolates, while *W. recta* and *B. gingivalis* each accounted for 13 percent of the total. Data such as these point to the importance of *W. recta* in the etiology of adult periodontitis.

Campylobacter Species

The *Campylobacter* are gram-negative, motile, S- or spiral-shaped bacilli ranging from 0.2 to 0.5 μm wide by 0.3 to 0.8 μm long. These organisms cause abortion in cattle and sheep and diarrheal disease in humans, including "traveler's diarrhea" (Table 18–4). The first studies of *Campylobacter* involved their role in causing veterinary disease in domestic animals. Since the beginning of this century, it was recognized that these microorganisms could cause abortion in cattle. Two forms of this disease were latter distinguished. One form of abortion occurred in cows that were members of an otherwise healthy herd. The other form of this disease occurred in cows from herds with greatly reduced fertility. It was not until 1959 that it became clear that these two very similar diseases were caused by different microorganisms. Only in the early 1970s following improved techniques of bacterial culture did

Table 18–2 ■ *Wolinella*	
Characteristics	Gram-negative anaerobe
	Motile by means of polar flagella
	Three colony types
	Hexagonal subunits on the outer cell membrane
Major species	*W. recta*
	W. succinogenes
	W. curva
Growth	Anaerobic at 37° C
Disease	Associated with adult periodontitis (*W. recta*)
Pathogenesis	Unknown

Table 18–3 ■ Predominant bacterial species in subgingival plaque from periodontitis patients with non–insulin dependent diabetes mellitus

Bacterial Species	Bacterial Isolates No. (%)	Positive Sites No. (%)	Positive Patients No. (%)	Range—% Total Viable Count
Bacteroides intermedius	67 (15.9)	9 (56.3)	7 (88)	66.7
Wolinella recta	56 (13.3)	8 (50.0)	5 (67)	66.7
Bacteroides gingivalis	55 (13.0)	9 (56.3)	6 (75)	73.3
Streptococcus sanguis	33 (7.8)	12 (75)	7 (88)	40.0
Actinomyces naeslundii	29 (6.9)	11 (68.8)	7 (88)	25.0
Capnocytophage species	17 (4.0)	7 (43.8)	5 (67)	15.6
Actinomyces odontolyticus	14 (3.3)	4 (25)	2 (25)	28.1
Fusobacterium nucleatum	12 (2.8)	6 (37.5)	4 (50)	18.8
Veillonella dispar	10 (2.4)	5 (31.3)	4 (50)	16.7
Actinomyces viscosus	9 (2.1)	6 (37.5)	4 (50)	9.1
Fusobacterium species	8 (1.9)	4 (25)	3 (38)	13.3
Eikenella corrodens	7 (1.7)	3 (18.8)	3 (38)	20.0
Haemophilus actinomycetemcomitans	7 (1.7)	1 (6.3)	1 (13)	23.3
Propionibacterium species	7 (1.7)	6 (37.5)	5 (67)	10.0
Gram negative anaerobic rods	7 (1.7)	3 (18.8)	2 (11)	15.1
Eubacterium species	6 (1.4)	5 (31.3)	3 (38)	6.7
Neisseria species	6 (1.4)	3 (18.8)	3 (38)	12.5
Peptostreptococcus anaerobius	5 (1.2)	1 (6.3)	1 (12)	16.7
Arachnia propionica	4 (0.9)	2 (12.5)	2 (25)	6.7
Bacteroides loeschii	4 (0.9)	2 (12.5)	1 (12)	10.0
Actinomyces meyerii	3 (0.7)	1 (6.3)	1 (12)	10.0
Selenomonas sputigena	3 (0.7)	2 (12.5)	2 (25)	6.7
Campylobacter concisus	2 (0.5)	1 (6.3)	1 (12)	12.5
Haemophilus aphrophilus	2 (0.5)	2 (12.5)	1 (12)	6.3
Staphylococcus epidermidis	2 (0.5)	2 (12.5)	2 (25)	6.3
Actinomyces israelii	1 (0.2)	1 (6.3)	1 (12)	3.1
Bacteroides buccae	1 (0.2)	1 (6.3)	1 (12)	3.3
Bacteroides corporis	1 (0.2)	1 (6.3)	1 (12)	3.3
Bacteroides denticola	1 (0.2)	1 (6.3)	1 (12)	3.3
Bacterionema matruchotii	1 (0.2)	1 (6.3)	1 (12)	3.3
Fusobacterium periodonticum	1 (0.2)	1 (6.3)	1 (12)	3.3
Veillonella parvula	1 (0.2)	1 (6.3)	1 (12)	3.3

(From Zambon, J. J., Reynolds, H., Fisher, J., Shlossman, M., Dunford, R., and Genco, R. J.: Microbiological and immunological studies of adult periodontitis in patients with non-insulin dependent diabetes mellitus. J Periodontol 51:23, 1988, with permission.)

the importance of *Campylobacter* in human disease become apparent.

Campylobacter species range in oxygen sensitivity from those that are microaerophilic to those that are strict anaerobes. The genus *Campylobacter* together with the genus *Spirillum* compose the bacterial family *Spirillaceae*. The *Campylobacter* species can be distinguished from the *Spirillum* by their inability to accumulate intracellular granules of polyhydroxybutyric acid (PHB), by a mol% G + C content of 29 to 38 percent, and by the presence of a single flagellum on one or both ends. This flagellum enables the *Campylobacter* species to move with a characteristic darting and corkscrew motion similar to the movement of *Wolinella*. The *Spirillum*, by contrast, can accumulate intracellular PHB, have a mol% G + C of 38 to 65 percent, and have tufts of flagella at the poles. The *Campylobacter* species are oxidase-positive but neither

ferment nor oxidize carbohydrates. A key feature that is used in the taxonomy of *Campylobacter* is the catalase reaction. The genus *Campylobacter* is divided into two major

Table 18–4 ■ *Campylobacter*

Characteristics	Gram-negative, motile, S- or spiral-shaped bacilli Microaerophilic to anaerobic Catalase-positive and -negative species
Major species and diseases	*C. fetus* subsp. *fetus*—sporadic abortion in cattle and sheep *C. fetus* subsp. *venerealis*—enzootic sterility and abortion in cattle *C. jejuni*—human gastroenteritis, sporadic abortion in sheep *C. coli*—human gastroenteritis
Prevention	Thorough cooking of meat products
Treatment	Self-limiting, antibiotics of limited use

groups based on this test: the catalase-positive species and the catalase-negative species (Table 18–5). The catalase-positive species can also be distinguished from the catalase-negative species in that they grow best in a higher oxygen environment and they do not produce hydrogen sulfide or reduce nitrite (Table 18–6). Another key test is hippurate hydrolysis; this test can be used to distinguish *C. jejuni* from *C. coli*.

Among the catalase-positive *Campylobacter* species is *C. fetus*, which causes enzootic sterility and abortion in cattle. Enzootic sterility, also known as venereal bovine campylobacteriosis, is the result of transmission of the microorganism from the prepuce of an infected bull to the vagina of a cow following sexual intercourse. In the cow, the organism multiplies and produces inflammation of the endometrium. Any fetus present will suffer owing to this inflammation and is usually aborted. The term "enzootic sterility" follows from the fact that a single bull may spread this type of infection to an entire herd of cows. *C. fetus* subsp. *venerealis* serotype A and *C. fetus* subsp. *fetus* serotype B cause enzootic sterility. *C. fetus* subsp. *fetus* serotype A causes sporadic abortion. Here, the organism may be present as a commensal in the gallbladder or gut of the cow and may spread to the developing placenta where it can cause anoxia and spontaneous abortion late in the course of the pregnancy.

The important human pathogens among the *Campylobacter* include *C. coli*, *C. fetus* subsp. *fetus*, and *C. jejuni*, all of which can cause diarrheal disease. *C. fetus* and subsp. *fetus* can also cause septicemia, cardiac disease, meningitis, arthritis, and localized suppuration. It usually affects patients who are already debilitated as a result of another underlying disease. *C. fetus* subsp. *fetus* is susceptible to several antibiotics including tetracycline, aminoglycosides, and erythromycin. The organism is found in domestic animals—especially pigs—and is found as a commensal in the gastrointestinal tract of sheep, in which it can cause abortion.

C. jejuni infection in humans, including "traveler's diarrhea," usually starts with a prodromal period of 24 to 48 hours characterized by a high fever, sometimes with delirium. Over the next 2 to 3 days, the patient

Table 18–5 ■ *Campylobacter* species

Species	Disease
Catalase-Positive	
C. fetus subsp. *fetus*	Sporadic abortion in cattle and sheep
C. fetus subsp. *venerealis*	Enzootic sterility and abortion in cattle
C. jejuni	Human gastroenteritis, sporadic abortion in sheep
C. coli	Human gastroenteritis
NARTC group	? Isolated from seagulls
C. fecalis	? Isolated from birds and cattle
Catalase-Negative	
C. sputorum subsp. *sputorum*	Human oral isolate
C. sputorum subsp. *bubulus*	Genital tract of cattle and sheep
C. sputorum subsp. *mucosalis*	Gastrointestinal disease in pigs
C. concisus	Human oral isolate

experiences periumbilical pain, abdominal cramps, and produces profuse, watery, slimy stools, sometimes with blood. Microscopic examination of feces can demonstrate *Campylobacter* and polymorphonuclear leukocytes. Antibiotic therapy is usually not indicated, since the disease rarely lasts longer than 1 week.

C. jejuni is also associated with diarrheal disease in domestic animals, although it is usually present together with other pathogens. These diarrheal diseases include winter diarrhea or winter dysentery in calves and diarrheal disease in pigs. Significant proportions of domestic animals are infected with *C. jejuni*, including up to as many as 92 percent of chickens and 59 percent of pigs.

Other catalase-positive *Campylobacter* species include the nalidixic acid–resistant thermophilic *Campylobacter*, known as the NARTC group, which has been isolated from seagulls and children with diarrheal disease, and *C. fecalis*, which has been isolated from birds and cattle. The pathogenicity of these two species is still under investigation.

Among the catalase-negative *Campylobacter* species is *C. sputorum* subspecies *sputorum*, which is found as a commensal in the human oral cavity. The pathogenic potential of this species is unknown. *C. concisus* is also a catalase-negative *Campylobacter* found in the human oral cavity; it also has an unknown pathogenic potential. *C. sputorum* subspecies

Table 18–6 ■ Differentiating catalase-positive from catalase-negative *Campylobacter*

	Growth in O_2	Nitrite Reduction	H_2S Production
Catalase-positive	Higher optimal O_2 tension	Negative	Negative
Catalase-negative	Lower optimal O_2 tension	Positive	Positive

mucosalis is found in pigs and is associated with porcine gastrointestinal diseases, including ileitis and hemorrhagic enteropathy. *C. sputorum* subspecies *bubulus* can be isolated from the genital tract of cattle or sheep.

REFERENCES

Butzler, J. P. (ed.): Campylobacter infection in man and animals. CRC Press, Orlando, FL, 1982.

Lai, C.-H., Listgarten, M. A., Tanner, A. C. R., and Socransky, S. S.: Ultrastructures of *Bacteroides gracilis*, *Campylobacter concisus*, *Wolinella recta*, and *Eikenella corrodens*, all from humans with periodontal disease. Int J Syst Bacteriol 31:465, 1981.

Tanner, A. C. R., Badger, S., Lai, C.-H., Listgarten, M. A., Visconti, R. A., and Socransky, S. S.: *Wolinella* gen. nov. *Wolinella succinogenes* (*Vibrio succinogenes*) Wolin et al. comb. nov., and description of *Bacteroides gracilis* sp. nov., *Wolinella recta* sp. nov., *Campylobacter concisus* sp. nov., and *Eikenella corrodens*, all from humans with periodontal disease. Int J Syst Bacteriol 31:432, 1981.

chapter 19

The spirochetes

Walter J. Loesche, D.M.D., Ph.D.

CHAPTER OUTLINE

- ORAL SPIROCHETES
- MORPHOLOGY AND TAXONOMY
- ACQUISITION OF SPIROCHETES
- ISOLATION AND CHARACTERIZATION
- ASSOCIATION STUDIES
- LONGITUDINAL STUDIES

- RESPONSE TO TREATMENT
- VIRULENCE MECHANISMS
- DIAGNOSTIC IMPLICATIONS OF SPIROCHETES
- OTHER SPIROCHETES
- SUMMARY

Oral Spirochetes

Many bacterial species live in the dental plaque, but the most recognizable of these organisms are the **spirochetes**. The spirochetes are long, thin, corkscrew-like gram-negative anaerobic bacteria whose characteristic motility and morphology can readily be discerned by darkfield and/or phase contrast microscopic examination of subgingival plaque. Spirochetes are observed mainly in plaques removed from diseased periodontal sites, and this has caused some investigators to suggest or claim that these organisms are periodontopathogens. Others have suggested that the pre-eminence of spirochetes is secondary to some other event and that the spirochetes are opportunistic organisms thriving on the nutrients that are relatively abundant in a periodontally inflamed site. In either case, the increase of spirochetes in plaque is not a favorable sign, and efforts should be made to reduce and/or eliminate them from the subgingival plaques.

Morphology and Taxonomy

Spirochetes are unique bacteria in that they have internal flagella-like structures called **axial filaments**, which are located between an outer osmotically labile envelope and an inner rigid protoplasmic cylinder (Fig. 19–1). A variable number of axial fibers are inserted at each end of the cylinder and then flow back along the cylinder for about two thirds of its length. Listgarten and Socransky have suggested that the number of fibrils can be used to classify the spirochetes. In Figure 19–1, a 1-2-1 spirochete is shown, a designation that is based upon the insertion of one axial filament at each end of the spirochete and the overlap of these two filaments in the middle section. A classification scheme based upon ultrastructure is shown in Table 19–1. Small spirochetes have 1-2-1 or 2-4-2 fibril patterns, and their protoplasmic cylinder has a diameter of 100 to 250 nm. Some of these spirochetes have been cultivated and, upon

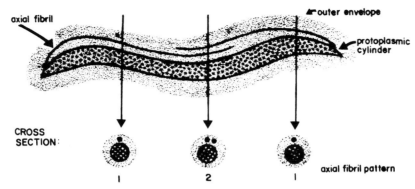

Figure 19–1 ■ Schematic diagram of a 1-2-1 small oral spirochete. Note that one axial fibril inserts at each end of the protoplasmic cylinder and that they overlap in the center. The axial fibrils are inside the outer envelope, so they are not true flagella. (From Loesche, W.J.: Dental Caries: A Treatable Infection. University of Michigan School of Dentistry, 1987. Used by permission.)

the basis of biochemical and physiologic criteria, can be divided into three species: *Treponema denticola, T. pectinovorum,* and *T. socranskii.*

The intermediate-sized spirochetes have a protoplasmic cylinder that is 200 to 500 nm in diameter and have from 3 to 20 axial fibrils inserted at each end. These spirochetes have rarely been cultured and may contain several species, including the cultivable organism known as *T. vincentii.* Microscopic evidence implicates these spirochetes in acute necrotizing ulcerative gingivitis (ANUG). Undoubtedly, they include the *Treponema* that Vincent originally described in ANUG, which was subsequently referred to as *Borrelia vincentii.* The large spirochetes have a protoplasmic cylinder with diameters in excess of 50 nm and at least 12 axial fibers. They have also never been cultured. Hence, when the term "oral spirochetes" is used it should be understood that this is a general morphologic description and that, within this grouping, morphologically and biochemically distinct species exist. This complicates matters when trying to associate spirochetes with ANUG or other forms of periodontal disease, and there is no way to determine whether any one type is particularly periodontopathic.

Acquisition of Spirochetes

Definitive information on the acquisition of the oral spirochetes is lacking, forcing one to sketch in outline form what is known or presumed to be known, or both. The human oral spirochetes appear to be distinct from human genital and intestinal spirochetes, from animal species, from overtly pathogenic species, and from free-living forms. This implies that the oral spirochetes are acquired from other humans via oral contact. Spirochetes have been detected by darkfield microscopy in the dental plaque of about 50 percent of the 3- to 5-year-old children and in about 50 percent of the 6- to 12-year-old children whom we have examined. However, their numbers were less than 0.5 percent of the flora and they were uncultivable. Almost all 6- to 12-year-old Dutch and Tanzanian children examined had detectable spirochetes in their plaques, and their numbers and proportions were greater when the plaques were removed from sites of gingival bleeding.

These data suggest that most if not all individuals acquire some type of spirochete in their early life. As the oral spirochetes comprise at least four species (Table 19–1)

Table 19–1 ■ Taxonomic characteristics of oral spirochetes

Species	Size	No. of Axial Fibrils	Carbohydrate Fermentation	% G+C
T. denticola	small	2-4-2, 5-10-5	No	37–38
T. vincentii	Intermediate	5-10-5	No	44
T. socranskii	Small	1-2-1	Yes	51
T. pectinovorum.	Small	2-4-2	Pectin	39
T. oralis	Small	1-2-1	No	?
T. macrodentium	Small	1-2-1	Yes	?

and undoubtedly more, one assumes from the above frequency data that the acquisition of any one of these spirochetes is a likely event once the teeth erupt. Once acquired, the spirochetes show a predilection for the subgingival plaque presumably because in this ecosystem these motile organisms are not at as great a risk of being swept away by the saliva and masticatory forces. Also, the lower oxygen tension present in these plaques, combined with the availability of preformed nutrients derived from the host and cohabitating plaque bacteria, enable them to grow and persist.

Under conditions of good oral hygiene, the spirochetes remain in low proportions and are often undetectable in plaque smears. However, if oral hygiene is suspended, as during participation in the experimental gingivitis model, spirochetes invariably become detectable after 15 to 21 days. The universality of this emergence of the spirochetes reflects the growth of the indigenous spirochetes in response to increased nutrient availability, secondarily to gingival inflammation, rather than to de novo colonization from the outside.

These data from children and from the experimental gingivitis model form the basis for the assumption that spirochetes are ubiquitous to the subgingival plaque and are normally members of our supplemental flora. They contribute to gingival pathology only when their numbers increase beyond a certain threshold, and in this sense, periodontal disease can be considered an endogenous infection.

Isolation and Characterization

The spirochetes are notoriously difficult to isolate and most oral species—especially the intermediate and large size spirochetes—have probably never been cultivated. In many instances, this can be attributed to the failure of the isolating medium to contain the specific nutrients that these organisms require. A case in point is the requirement for pectin or its constituents galacturonic and glucuronic acids by the recently described species *T. pectinovorum*. If these unusual substrates were not present in the isolation medium, then this species would not have been isolated. This then requires the investigator to know a priori what the nutrient requirements of these unknown species are. In the absence of this information, most investigators use complex media that are supplemented with biologic fluids such as serum, rumen fluid, or ascitic fluid. This approach has led to the isolation of *T. denticola* and *T. vincentii*, which grow well on most commercially available media supplemented with rabbit serum, whereas *T. pectinovorum*'s and *T. socranskii*'s requirement for rumen fluid can be replaced by volatile short chain fatty acids.

Spirochetes are delicate organisms relative to the other bacterial types that are found in dental plaque. This affects their isolation, as procedures used to disrupt the plaque so as to facilitate both colony formation from single cells, and to maximize the number of colonies usually lyse the spirochetes. This was demonstrated by experiments in which subgingival plaques were gently disrupted by mechanical mixing, in order to obtain a microscopic count, and then were subjected to vigorous disruption by either sonification or by homogenization (Table 19–2). Spirochetes averaged about 55 percent of the microscopic count but only accounted for about 0.5 per cent of the viable count. *T. denticola* was the most common spirochetal isolate, and as this organism can grow readily on the media and in the anaerobic environment employed, these data indicate that its failure to be cultured reflected that it was destroyed by

---

Table 19–2 ■ Effect of dispersal procedures on recovery of spirochetes from subgingival plaque samples (n = 15)

Dispersal Procedure	Morphotype			
	Small	Intermediate	Large	Total
	Spirochetes as % of microscopic count			
Gentle mechanical	31%	15%	8%	54%
	Spirochetes as % of viable count			
Harsh mechanical	0.8%*	No growth	No growth	0.8
Homogenization	0.9%	No growth	No growth	0.9
Sonification	0.1%	No growth	No growth	0.1

*91% of isolates were *T. denticola*; 5% were *T. socranskii*, and 4% were unspeciated.

the routine dispersal procedures that are normally used in cultural studies.

Thus, harsh dispersal procedures and exacting nutrient requirements, and **not** anaerobiosis, are the main obstacles toward the isolation and subsequent characterization of the oral spirochetes. Until investigators can reliably identify and quantitate which spirochetes are indeed present in the plaque, it will be difficult to implicate any specific spirochetal species, or for that matter any other bacterial species, as periodontopathic. This caution is usually ignored as investigators seek to show that organisms such as *Actinobacillus actinomycetemcomitans* and *Bacteroides gingivalis,* which are often present in very low numbers relative to the spirochetes, are exclusively periodontopathic.

Association Studies

These problems related to spirochetal isolation and characterization have to be kept in mind when reviewing the extensive literature associating microscopic counts of spirochetes with various forms of periodontal disease. Spirochetes either are not detectable or, when detectable, are present in low proportions in plaques taken from healthy tooth sites. However, they most likely are always present in these nondiseased plaques, given the universality of their detection in the 3- to 4-week-old plaques formed when periodontally healthy individuals refrain from oral hygiene procedures while participating in the experimental gingivitis model.

Studies in 6- to 12-year-old children show a relationship between bleeding and increased proportions of spirochetes (Table 19–3). When the gingivitis is long-standing, the proportions of spirochetes increase still further to account for 8 to 20 percent of the plaque organisms. If the gingivitis is acute, as in ANUG, or of a severe generalized nature, the spirochetes can account for over 30 percent of the plaque flora.

The severe gingivitis condition was noted among Africans living in an endemically high fluoride area, raising the possibility that the overgrowth of spirochetes was not necessarily associated with extensive periodontal attachment and bone loss. Periodontitis could reflect that the spirochetes that had overgrown did not contain the same periodontopathic species that presumably were present in those plaques associated with periodontitis; also there could be host factors, such as the high fluoride consumption, which made the alveolar bone in these individuals less susceptible to resorption. These exceptional data point out the need to identify which of the various spirochetal species are present within the spirochetal grouping. This will soon be possible with the cultivable small spirochetes, as monoclonal antibodies, and DNA probes, to *T. denticola, T. socranskii, T. pectinovorum,* and *T. vincentii* are being developed.

Numerous investigators have noted elevated levels and proportions of spirochetes in adult periodontitis (AP) and early onset periodontitis (EOP). Table 19–4 lists several studies that showed spirochetes to average 37 percent of the flora in AP (range 21 to 56 percent). Only in local juvenile periodontitis are spirochetes not conspicuously associated with periodontal morbidity. These findings in toto would seem to make the spirochetes pathognomonic of periodontal disease.

Longitudinal Studies

The development of periodontal disease from gingivitis to periodontitis has not been documented. However, in recent years, two clinical situations or models have been de-

Table 19–3 ■ Prevalence of spirochetes in the subgingival plaque of 6- to 12-year-old Dutch and Tanzanian children

	% Spirochetes				Isolation Frequency
	Small	*Medium*	*Large*	*Total*	
Dutch					
Bleeding (77)*	1.5	1.20	0.006	2.6	66%
Nonbleeding (67)	0.1	0.06	0.000	0.2	19
Tanzanian					
Bleeding (69)	6.5 ↕	3.1 ↕	0.06	9.7 ↕	100%
Nonbleeding (71)	2.5	1.4	0.07	3.8	93

*Number of sites.
↕ Values connected by arrows are significantly different.
(Adapted from Mikx et al.)

Table 19–4 ■ Reported studies that associate spirochetes with periodontal disease

% Spirochetes in Plaque

Healthy Gingiva	Gingivitis	Periodontitis	
0.2%*	2%*	21%	38%*
0.6	3	23	38
0.8	8	30	44
1.8	10	32	45
2.0	18	34	49
4.0	30	34	50
	36	35	52
	36	38	56
n = 6	n = 8	n = 16	
ave. 1.6%	ave. 17.8%	ave. 37%	

*Each percentage value is taken from a published study.

scribed that monitor the further loss of attachment about periodontally involved teeth. In one study, 20 patients previously treated for moderate to advanced periodontitis were not given any further treatment during recall visits. During a 1-year-period, 7 patients had 2 or more teeth which lost 3 mm or more of attachment, whereas 6 patients exhibited no teeth with 3 mm attachment loss. The patients with the attachment loss had significantly higher proportions of spirochetes in pooled plaques than did patients with no attachment loss. This attachment loss was also correlated with baseline proportions of spirochetes but could not be correlated with plaque or gingivitis scores, probing depth or gingival recession. This suggested that plaque proportions of spirochetes were predictors of subsequent tissue loss.

Response to Treatment

If spirochetes are of etiologic significance in periodontal disease, then their demise in the subgingival plaque should coincide with the restoration of periodontal health. Many studies show that mechanical debridement with and without antimicrobial agents such as metronidazole, chlorhexidine, or tetracycline result in a decrease in spirochetes and a concurrent improvement in periodontal health as measured by reduced probing depth or increased apparent attachment, or both.

The proportions of spirochetes remaining after these treatments may be a sensitive indicator of the efficacy of treatment. In double blind studies involving systemic metro-

nidazole or placebo treatment (250 mg tablets taken 3 times a day for 1 week) superimposed upon rigorous mechanical debridement, the levels and proportions of spirochetes were reduced in both groups but significantly more so in the metronidazole groups (Table 19–5). This bacteriologic difference was manifested by a difference in the subsequent treatment needs of the two groups of patients. Thus, the clinician who examined the patients, without knowing which group they were in, initially estimated that the metronidazole patients had an average of 19 teeth and the placebo group 17 teeth that would require either periodontal or oral surgery. However, upon completion of the usage of the antimicrobial agents, he re-examined the patients, again not knowing which treatment group they were in, and found that those patients in the metronidazole group had 8 fewer teeth that required periodontal surgery, whereas those in the placebo group had 3 fewer teeth. This difference between groups was significant and was reflected only by the spirochetal parameters of the more than 30 bacteriologic parameters that were monitored.

These data indicate that the spirochetal levels and/or proportions are sensitive indicators of treatment efficacy.

Virulence Mechanisms

If spirochetal overgrowth is synonymous with the presence of clinical inflammation, then it is likely that these organisms are active contributors to this inflammation. Data

Table 19–5 ■ Effect of debridement of root surfaces with and without systemic metronidazole for one week upon proportions of spirochetes and periodontal surgical needs

	Metronidazole Plus Mechanical (17)*		Placebo Plus Mechanical (20)*	
	Before	After	Before	After
% Spirochetes	52%	‡ ⟵⟶ 22%§	57%	42§
No. of teeth needing surgery†	19	‡ ⟵⟶ 11	17	14

*Number of patients in each group.
†Surgery includes both periodontal surgery and tooth extraction because of periodontal disease.
‡Values connected by arrow are significantly different.
§Difference between metronidazole and placebo groups is significant.

on how this is accomplished are minimal, because of the difficulty in isolating and growing many of these organisms. Spirochetes contain endotoxin and therefore would contribute to those toxic and pharmacologic effects attributed to the total endotoxin load found in the subgingival plaque. More importantly, however, the small size of the spirochetes and their motility enable some of them to invade the periodontal tissue and release their endotoxin and other toxic components directly adjacent to fibroblasts, epithelial cells, and other tissue components.

The availability of cultivable species has permitted in vitro studies of virulence mechanisms. A surprising finding was that *T. denticola, T. socranskii,* and possibly *T. vincentii* are not immunologically reactive in the periodontal patient. Thus, there was no correlation between the number of spirochetes in the plaque sample (despite the fact that high numbers of spirochetes came from patients and low numbers came from healthy subjects), and either the titers of antibodies to *T. denticola* or *T. vincentii* or the lymphocyte blastogenic response of the sera. In another study, in those individuals with the most severe periodontal involvement, the serologic response to *T. denticola* and *T. socranskii* was reduced compared with healthy controls and to individuals with less periodontal morbidity.

These studies raise the possibility that high antigen loads of these spirochetes may lead to some type of immune suppression, which would enable the spirochetes to escape the normal host defense mechanisms and thereby remain in high numbers in the plaque. This suppression concept was verified in vitro in regard to lymphocyte response to various antigens and mitogens. Thus, sonicates of some strains of *T. denticola,* when preincubated with human lymphocytes, caused a dose-dependent inhibition of responsiveness to ConA, PHA, PWM, and SKSD. This inhibitory effect, seen only with *T. denticola* and not with *T. vincentii,* was dependent on the presence of monocytes and was reversed by the addition of both indomethacin and catalase to the mixture.

T. denticola and *T. vincentii* also inhibit polymorphonuclear leukocyte (PMN) function in vitro. Thus, the PMNs can readily phagocytize these spirochetes but were unable to degrade them. This was associated with a failure of the lysosomal granules to degranulate and suggested that the spirochetes may limit the fusion of the lysosomes to the phagosomes. If this is the case, then these spirochetes could evade the host protective effects of the PMNs and persist in the plaques. These studies indicate that the cultivable spirochetes possess mechanisms by which they can evade the normal host immunologic and phagocytic surveillance. These mechanisms could account then for their high levels and proportions in subgingival plaques removed from diseased sites.

Diagnostic Implications of Spirochetes

The association and response to treatment studies indicate that subgingival plaque levels and/or proportions of spirochetes could be used clinically to identify those sites or individuals, or both, requiring periodontal treatment. This information can be routinely obtained by the use of phase or darkfield microscopy using a simple qualitative enumeration system. However, if other periodontopathic organisms are more involved in the plaque infection than the spirochetes, these other organisms would not be detected by the microscopic approach and accordingly some false-negative results would be recorded. Thus, a more broad-base diagnostic procedure would be preferred.

The taxonomic screening of periodontopathic organisms with various enzyme assays have shown that *T. denticola, B. gingivalis, B. forsythus,* and an unspeciated *Capnocytophaga* possess a trypsin-like enzyme that can be detected by the hydrolysis of benzoyl-DL-arginine-2-naphthylamide (BANA). This BANA hydrolytic enzyme could also be detected in subgingival plaque samples and was statistically related to the plaque levels and proportions of spirochetes and with probing depth. Thus, a BANA-positive plaque was indicative of subgingival plaques containing more than 30 percent spirochetes that were removed from sites with probing depths of 7 mm or more. The other BANA-positive species accounted for only 10 percent of the BANA-positive reactions, indicating that the plaque BANA test was essentially a *T. denticola* reaction.

Seventy-one percent of the plaques removed from untreated periodontal patients were BANA positive, averaged 40 percent spirochetes, and came from sites that had average probing depths of 7 mm. The BANA-negative plaques in these patients averaged 12 percent spirochetes and came from sites that had average probing depths of 5.4 mm. In contrast, only 8 per cent of the plaques removed from treated patients seen at recall visits were BANA positive, and these plaques had significantly higher proportions of spirochetes and came from deeper pockets than the BANA-positive plaques.

These data indicate that the ability of subgingival plaque to hydrolyze BANA is a reliable marker for the presence of high proportions of spirochetes and possibly could be used clinically to identify those sites or individuals, or both, that might require either initial treatment or retreatment to reduce this spirochetal overgrowth. If so, BANA hydrolysis has the potential to be an objective indicator of periodontal disease activity and could be used in combination with clinical criteria both to initiate therapy and as a means to monitor the efficacy of treatment.

Other Spirochetes

OTHER INFECTIONS

Spirochetes are also found on the intestinal and to a lesser extent on the genital urinary surfaces of humans. Most of these spirochetes are presumed to be nonpathogenic, but notable exceptions occur, such as *T. pallidum* being the etiologic agent of **syphilis,** *T. pertenue* being the etiologic agent of the childhood infection known as **yaws,** and *T. carateum* being the etiologic agent of **pinta.**

There are other types of spirochetes, such as the very thin aerobic species classified in the genus *Leptospira,* and the larger anaerobic species classified in the genus *Borrelia.* Pathogenic leptospira reside in domestic and wild animals, where they can cause life-threatening infections that are a major concern to the meat and dairy industry. Humans can become accidentally infected with leptospira

when they come into contact with soil or water that has been contaminated with urine from the infected animal. Rarely does the individual develop a fatal infection, but on occasion a severe icteric infection (jaundice), known as **Weil's disease,** occurs.

Human infections due to *Borrelia* species are more common than those due to leptospira and invariably involve transmission by infected lice or ticks. Many of these infections manifest as febrile diseases characterized by a remittent fever and are known as **relapsing fevers.** The louse-borne infection occurs under conditions of poor personal hygiene and sanitation, and for this reason it can reach epidemic proportions in communities devastated by wars or natural disaster. The tick-borne infection occurs only in individuals exposed to infected ticks, and these infections are called **endemic relapsing fever.** Recently, a new type of tick-borne infection was described in residents of Lyme, Connecticut, who exhibited skin and joint lesions and involvement of the heart and nervous system. This complex of symptoms has been called **Lyme disease,** and the high number of reported cases since its initial description has made Lyme disease an important public health problem.

The salient features of these other spirochetal infections are given in Table 19–6. Syphilis, the most important of these nonoral spirochetal infections, will be briefly described subsequently.

SYPHILIS

Syphilis invoked as much dread and censure in the 19th and early 20th century as AIDS does in the 1980s. The advent of effective chemotherapeutic agents and an apparent decreased virulence of *T. pallidum* have made syphilis a considerably less fearsome

Table 19–6 ■ Aspects of various human spirochetal infections

	Leptospira	Borrelia		Treponema		
Disease	Weil's disease	Relapsing fever	Lyme disease	Syphilis	Yaws	Pinta
Agent	*L. interrogans* serotype *icterohaemorrhagiae*	*B. recurrentis*	*B. burgdorferi*	*T. pallidum*	*T. pertenue*	*T. carateum*
Age group	All	All	All	Adults	Children	Children
Spread	Contact with contaminated animal urine	Louse or tick bite	Tick bite	Venereal	Skin	Skin
Cultivable	Yes	Yes	Yes	No	No	No
Treatment	Penicillin Tetracycline	Tetracycline	Tetracycline	Penicillin	Penicillin	Penicillin

disease today. Syphilis was the target disease for Paul Ehrlich's magic bullet, and the conceptual and therapeutic breakthrough of his arsenic compound, arsphenamine, ushered in the modern age of antimicrobial chemotherapy. Penicillin has long since replaced arsphenamine as the drug of choice, and the remarkable effectiveness of this agent against *T. pallidum* has led to the general easing of concern over syphilis as a major health concern. Yet syphilitic infections still occur with a greater frequency than is necessary, given today's knowledge of venereal disease control, and the possibility that *T. pallidum* will develop clinical resistance to penicillin cannot be ignored.

Syphilis is transmitted from person to person usually by sexual intercourse, but the lesions of secondary syphilis, which would include oral lesions, are also infectious. Spirochetes can be transferred across the placenta to the fetus, but fortunately congenital syphilis can be prevented by aggressive treatment of the mother with penicillin in the early stages of pregnancy, and still later by treating the newborn. Such treatments have made a diagnostic rarity of **Hutchinson's triad** observed in congenital syphilis, which included tooth deformities (notched incisors, moon molars), interstitial keratitis, and nerve deafness.

Syphilis, when it was most prevalent, was known as the "the great imitator," because the diverse array of lesions that it caused in many organ systems often resembled the symptoms of other diseases. The clinical course of untreated syphilis has a primary, secondary, and often a fatal tertiary phase. The **primary phase** reflected the erythema and induration that followed the multiplication of the spirochetes at the entry site. The hard chancre that forms is highly contagious and should cause the individual to seek prompt medical care. If untreated, the lesion heals leaving remnants of scar tissue. After an asymptomatic period of 2 to 24 weeks the **secondary stage** begins with a high fever and culminates with a mucocutaneous rash that spreads from the palms and soles to include almost all surface areas of the body and many internal organs. White mucoid patches of moist papules or condylomata occur on the mucous membranes of the mouth, vagina, and anus. These lesions are also highly contagious and care should be exercised when examining them.

Within several weeks the host mounts an effective immune response and the lesions heal, although in about 25 percent of patients there may be several recurrences of the rash. After clinical resolution *T. pallidum* seems to disappear from the skin and mucous membranes but can still be detected in the spleen and lymph nodes. Tertiary syphilis occurs from 5 to 30 years later, when cardiovascular (80 percent of cases) and neurologic (20 percent of cases) symptoms occur, which can be fatal.

Most syphilitic infections do not progress through the three stages. The natural history of the infection was followed for 30 to 50 years in 1000 untreated Norwegian patients in the early part of this century. Seventy-five percent of the subjects did not progress to secondary syphilis, and only 13 percent developed tertiary syphilis. This indicates that the host can mount a protective immune response that can thwart the progression of the infection in the majority of infected individuals who are untreated. This protection also extends to prevent new instances of primary syphilis. Thus, individuals who have once been infected appear to be resistant to subsequent new infections. However, in the modern era this protective immunity rarely develops, as most individuals with primary syphilis are promptly treated prior to the mounting of a protective immune response.

This immunity is due to antigens shared with the other pathogenic treponemes, such as *T. pertenue* and *T. carateum*, as children with yaws and pinta infections rarely develop syphilis as adults. This was dramatically demonstrated by a public health program, which was successful in treating yaws in children, but led eventually to an outbreak of syphilis in these children when they became older and sexually active. Apparently the immune response to *T. pertenue* included antibodies that recognized *T. pallidum*, and thus the yaws infection served as a vaccine against syphilis.

These findings indicate that a vaccine against *T. pallidum* would be protective. Indeed, prior to the demonstration of the efficacy of penicillin in syphilis, the pursuit of a vaccine against *T. pallidum* was of the highest medical priority. The main problem in vaccine development was and remains to this day the inability to identify, isolate, and purify those antigens that conferred immunity. As noted earlier, the discovery of penicillin reduced the importance of a vaccine, and medical science has since moved on to other matters. Syphilis, however, remains endemic in the United States, with approximately 10 cases per 100,000 individuals reported annually, for a total of about 23,000 cases per year.

The inability to grow *T. pallidum* on artificial media means that very little is known about its metabolism, physiology, genetics, and pathogenicity. Accordingly, very few researchers have chosen to work on spirochetes as a group, and this avoidance has carried over somewhat to the oral spirochetes.

Summary

The spirochetal accumulation in subgingival plaques appears to be a function of the clinical severity of periodontal disease. It is not known how many different spirochetal species colonize the plaque, but based on size alone, there are small, intermediate, and large spirochetes. Four species of small spirochetes are cultivable, and of these *T. denticola* has been shown to possess factors or mechanisms that suppress lymphocyte blastogenesis and inhibit fibroblast and PMN function. This species also contains a BANA hydrolytic enzyme, which can be detected directly in plaque samples, and such detection may be useful for the diagnosis of periodontal disease activity.

REFERENCES

Africa, C. W., Parker, J. R., and Reddy, J.: Bacteriological studies of subgingival plaque in a periodontitis-resistant population. I. Darkfield microscopic studies. J. Periodont. Res. 20:106, 1985.

Boehringer, H., Berthold, P. H., and Taichman, N. S.: Studies on the interaction of human neutrophils with plaque spirochetes. J. Periodont. Res. 21:195, 1986.

Dunham, S. L., Goodson, J. M., Hogan, P. E., and Socransky, S. S.: Failure of darkfield microbiologic parameters to predict periodontal disease activity at periodontal sites. J. Dent. Res. 64:1657, 1985.

Keyes, P. H., and Rams, R. E.: A rationale for the management of periodontal diseases: rapid identification of microbial "therapeutic targets" with phase-control microscopy. J. Am. Dent. Assoc. 106:803, 1983.

Listgarten, M. A.: Subgingival microbiological differences between periodontally healthy sites and diseased sites prior to and after treatment. Int. J. Periodont. Restor. Dent. 4:27, 1984.

Listgarten, M. A., and Socransky, S. S.: Electron microscopy as an aid in the taxonomic differentiation of oral spirochetes. Arch. Oral Biol. 10:127, 1965.

Loe, H.: Human research model for the production and prevention of gingivitis. J. Dent. Res. 50:256, 1971.

Loesche, W. J.: Dental Caries: A Treatable Infection. Charles C Thomas, Springfield, IL, 1982.

Loesche, W. J.: The identification of bacteria associated with periodontal disease and dental caries in vitro and in vivo by enzymatic methods. Oral Microbiol. Oral Immun. 1:19, 1986.

Loesche, W. J., and Laughon, B.: Role of spirochetes in periodontal disease. In Genco, R. J., and Morgenhagen, S. E. (eds.): Host-Parasite Interactions in Periodontal Disease. American Society for Microbiology, Washington, DC, 1982, pp. 62–75.

Loesche, W. J., Syed, S. A., Laughon, B., and Stoll, J.: The bacteriology of acute necrotizing ulcerative gingivitis. J. Periodontol. 53:223, 1982.

Loesche, W. J., Syed, S. A., Schmidt, E., and Morrison, E. C.: Bacterial profiles of subgingival plaques in periodontitis. J. Periodontol. 56:447, 1985.

Loesche, W. J., Syed, S. A., and Stoll, J.: Trypsin-like activity in subgingival plaque: a diagnostic marker for spirochetes and periodontal disease? J. Periodontol. 58:266, 1987.

Mangan, D. F., Laughon, B. E., Bower, B., and Lopatin, D. E.: In vitro lymphocyte blastogenic responses and titers of humoral antibodies from periodontitis patients to oral spirochete isolates. Infect. Immun. 37:445, 1982.

Mikx, F. H., Matee, M. I., and Schaeken, M. J.: The prevalence of spirochetes in the subgingival microbiota of Tanzanian and Dutch children. J. Clin. Periodontol. 13:289, 1986.

Saglie, F., Carranza, F., Newman, M., Ching, L., and Lewin, K.: Identification tissue-invading bacteria in human periodontal disease. J. Periodont. Res. 17:452, 1982.

Shenker, B. J., Listgarten, M. A., and Taichman, N. S.: Suppression of human lymphocyte responses by oral spirochetes: a monocyte-dependent phenomenon. J. Immunol. 132:2039, 1984.

Slots, J., and Genco, R. J.: Black-pigmented Bacteroides species, Capnocytophaga species, and Actinobacillus actinomycetemcomitans in human periodontal disease: virulence factors in colonization, survival and tissue destruction. J. Dent. Res. 63:412, 1984.

Smibert, R. M., and Burmeister, J. A.: Treponema pectinovorum sp. nov. isolated from humans with periodontitis. Int. J. Syst. Bacteriol. 33:852, 1983.

Tew, J. G., Smibert, R. M., Scott, E. A., Burmeister, J. A., and Ranney, R. R.: Serum antibodies in young adult humans reactive with periodontitis associated treponemes. J. Periodont. Res. 20:580, 1985.

chapter 20

Mycoplasmas, chlamydiae, and rickettsiae

Joseph J. Zambon, D.D.S., Ph.D.

CHAPTER OUTLINE

- MYCOPLASMAS
- CHLAMYDIAE

- RICKETTSIAE

Mycoplasmas

The mycoplasmas are a group of 70 species of which approximately 11 are human pathogens (Table 20–1). They are very small, generally microaerophilic or anaerobic microorganisms, although one species, *Mycoplasma pneumoniae*, is an aerobe (Table 20–2). The mycoplasmas are, in fact, the smallest free-living organisms known to exist. One genus of mycoplasma, the ureaplasmas, are even referred to as *T (tiny) strains*. The mycoplasmas are pleomorphic. Cells from a single pure culture may exhibit coccoid, star-shaped, or filamentous forms. Mycoplasma cells lack a peptidoglycan cell wall and are composed of a cell membrane, ribosomes, and nucleoid, but they lack any internal membranous structures. This lack of structural rigidity may explain why the mycoplasmas have a highly pleomorphic cell morphology. The cells are very small, and coccoid, ranging from 0.3 to 0.8 μm. The mycoplasmas, like viruses chlamydiae and rickettsiae, are able to pass through a 450-nm pore size filter. However, unlike these other microorganisms, the mycoplasmas can be cultured on artificial media. The mycoplasmas do not react to Gram stain; they do stain with Giemsa, although poorly. The cells possess a *terminal structure*, which permits the mycoplasma to attach to host eukaryotic cells and which may be responsible for the gliding motility these organisms exhibit. Reproduction is by binary fission, although budding is evident in some species. The mycoplasma are distinguished from bacteria not only by their small size but also by their slow growth rate. The mean generation time is as long as 1 to 2 weeks. They can also be distinguished from bacteria in that they have 43 to 48 percent guanine plus cytosine in ribosomal RNA as compared with 50 to 54 percent seen in bacteria. These data suggest that mycoplasmas have a different evolutionary path than bacteria. Mycoplasmas have unique nutritional requirements, especially in their need for lipids and cholesterol, which are used in the mycoplasma cell membrane. One group, the *Acholeplasma*, does not, as the name implies, require cholesterol in its growth medium. Since the mycoplasmas do not possess a cell wall, antibiotics that inhibit cell wall synthesis do not affect the growth

Table 20–1 ■ Taxonomy of the Mycoplasmas

Class	Order	Family	Genus	Characteristics
Mollicutes	Mycoplasmatales	Mycoplasmataceae	Mycoplasma Ureaplasma	Requires urea for growth
		Acholeplasmataceae	Acholeplasma	Does not require exogenous cholesterol
				A. laidlawii unusual in its rapid growth—18–24 hours
		Spiroplasmataceae	Spiroplasma Anaeroplasma	

of these microorganisms as they do that of bacteria.

The colony morphology of the mycoplasmas is also unusual. These microorganisms produce tiny colonies from 10 to 600 μm in diameter, which can be seen only with a magnifying glass or under low power on a microscope. The colonies exhibit a "fried egg" appearance as a result of the colony center growing down into the agar. The mycoplasma grow only on complex media containing peptones, yeast extract, and serum. The same medium that supports the growth of mycoplasma may also allow for the growth of cell wall–deficient bacteria known as *L-forms*. Penicillin is often added to the isolation medium to inhibit bacterial growth. *Mycoplasma* species may be identified by inhibition of growth in proximity to a disk containing specific antisera—similar to an antibiotic susceptibility test.

Table 20–2 ■ Mycoplasma

Features	Small coccoid cells (0.3–0.5 μm), nonmotile, non–Gram-staining
	Pleuropneumonia-like organisms (PPLO)
	Generally microaerophilic or anaerobic
Species	M. pneumoniae—aerobic, causes primary atypical pneumonia
	M. hominis—cervix
	M. salivarium—in gingival crevice
	M. orale
	M. buccale ⎫ oral species
	M. faucium ⎭
	Ureaplasma urealyticum (T- strain mycoplasma)—nongonococcal urethritis
	Acholeplasma laidlawii—found in burns
Diseases	Primary atypical pneumonia
	Nongonococcal urethritis
Diagnosis	Culture on specific media
	Immunofluorescence microscopy
	Increase in serum antibody titer
Treatment	Tetracycline and erythromycin

MYCOPLASMA PNEUMONIAE

In the first half of this century, it became apparent that significant numbers of cases of pneumonia were culture-negative; that is, a specific bacterium could not be identified in certain patients, mainly children and young adults. These cases of culture-negative pneumonia could also be distinguished on clinical criteria. The patients developed cough, fever, and headache but the disease was usually self-limited. This type of pneumonia came to be known as primary atypical pneumonia. Studies by Eaton, however, suggested that there was a microbial origin to primary atypical pneumonia. He was able to take patient material, inoculate it into eggs, blindly passage the infectious agent, and then use it to produce pneumonia in rats and hamsters. In 1962, Chanock, Hayflick, and Barile developed a medium and were able to culture the agent responsible for primary atypical pneumonia, which was a mycoplasma, *M. pneumoniae*. This microorganism cannot penetrate epithelial cells but it is able to adhere to these cells in the respiratory tract by means of neuraminic acid receptors on the epithelial cell surface. Following attachment, the cilia on the epithelial cell cease movement (ciliostasis), are lost, and the cells die. This is thought to occur as a result of hydrogen peroxide production by *M. pneumoniae*.

Mycoplasma may also damage host tissues by means of hypersensitivity reactions. The major mycoplasmic antigens are cell membrane proteins and glycolipids, which may induce cross-reacting antibodies. In *M. pneumoniae*, for example, the major antigen is a glucose- and galactose-containing glycolipid, which induces antibodies that can cross-react with certain host tissues such as human brain. Patients with an initial mycoplasma infection can develop these cross-reactive antibodies. During a second mycoplasma infection, the antibody response may then damage host tissues as well as the microorganism.

M. pneumoniae generally causes only a mild upper respiratory infection but may cause primary atypical pneumoniae. The peak incidence for this disease is in children 5 to 15 years of age, and the microorganism is responsible for up to half of all cases of pneumonia in children and young adults.

OTHER MYCOPLASMAS

Other mycoplasmas such as *M. hominis* and *M. orale* may exist as commensals on human mucous membranes. Certain mycoplasmas such as *Ureaplasma urealyticum* exist on the mucous membranes of the urogenital tract. *U. urealyticum* has been implicated in the etiology of nongonococcal urethritis and pelvic inflammatory disease. Mycoplasmas are also frequently found as contaminants in animal cell cultures.

DIAGNOSIS AND TREATMENT

Mycoplasma infection can be diagnosed by culture of the microorganism on one of several special media, by the immunofluorescent detection of the organism from culture of patient specimens, and by increased serum antibody titers to mycoplasma antigens. Once cultured, the mycoplasma can also be speciated by immunofluorescence using species-specific antisera. Speciation can also be performed by growth inhibition and by metabolic inhibition. In these latter assays, the mycoplasma is grown on media on which a disk that contains species-specific antisera has been placed. If the unknown mycoplasma is the same species as the species-specific antisera, then growth will be inhibited much like in an antibiotic sensitivity test. Metabolic inhibition makes use of changes in, for example, sugar fermentation as a means of assessing the effect of the species-specific antisera.

Chlamydiae

The chlamydiae are an unusual group of human and animal microbial pathogens that are a leading cause of *human blindness* and *venereal disease* (Table 20–3). They are nonmotile, gram-negative microorganisms similar to the rickettsiae in being obligate *intra-*

Table 20–3 ■ Chlamydiae	
Features	Small (<1 μm), nonmotile, Gram-negative, obligate intracellular parasite
	Two stage life cycle:
	elementary body—infectious stage
	reticular body—intracellular stage
	Forms intracellular inclusions visible by light microscopy
Species	*C. trachomatis* causes
	1. Trachoma—leading cause of human blindness
	2. Inclusion conjunctivitis
	a. "Swimming pool" conjunctivitis in adults
	b. Inclusion blenorrhea in infants
	3. Sexually transmitted disease—infertility
	4. Lymphogranuloma venereum—Frei test
	C. psittaci causes
	1. Psittacosis

cellular parasites. The chlamydiae can be differentiated from viruses in having both DNA and RNA and in being susceptible to broad-spectrum antibiotics such as tetracycline. They have a limited metabolic capacity and use ATP produced by the host cell. They are smaller than other bacteria (less than 1 μm) and have an unusual two-stage life cycle. One stage, the *elementary body* (0.3 nm), is adapted for extracellular survival and the other stage, the *reticular body,* is adapted for intracellular growth and multiplication by means of cytoplasmic vesicles known as *inclusions.* The elementary body is phagocytosed by susceptible cells and forms a phagosome. Subsequent fusion with cellular lysosomes and formation of a phagolysosome is prevented. The elementary body in the cellular inclusion is then transformed into a reticular body, which is longer (1 nm) and richer in RNA. After about 8 hours, they divide by binary fission and are re-formed into elementary bodies. After an additional 18 to 24 hours, these elementary bodies are released during lysis of the infected host cell and can go on to infect other host cells. There are two main species, *Chlamydia trachomatis* and *C. psittaci.* Each microorganism exhibits heat-labile cell surface protein antigens that are species-specific, as well as heat-stable lipopolysaccharide antigens that are group-specific. The serotype antigens of *C. trachomatis* are proteins of 30,000 kilodalton.

CHLAMYDIA TRACHOMATIS

C. trachomatis causes disease primarily in humans, including both trachoma, the leading cause of human blindness, and inclusion conjunctivitis. Trachoma is caused by *C. trachomatis* serotypes A, B, Ba and C. *C. trachomatis* also causes sexually transmitted diseases such as lymphogranuloma venereum (LGV), which is due to serotypes L1, L2, and L3, and nongonococcal urethritis and epididymitis, from serotypes D through K. Humans are the only known reservoir of *C. trachomatis*.

The elementary body is that stage of the chlamydial life cycle in which the microorganism is transmissible between hosts. The elementary body has a rigid, impermeable cell envelope that contains a hemagglutinin. It is transmitted by person-to-person contact and is a problem especially in Third World countries where sanitation and personal hygiene may be poor. The elementary body can attach to human epithelial cells as in the conjunctiva and is taken up by the cell into a phagosome. Once in the cytoplasm of the host cell, the phagosome is resistant to degradation by hydrolytic enzymes and the elementary body undergoes a metamorphic change to form the reticular body. This metamorphosis includes lengthening to 1000 nm, a decrease in the rigidity and permeability of the cell envelope, and loss of the hemagglutinin. The reticular body is a noninfectious form that multiplies intracellularly 1 to 2 days after infection. It prevents DNA and protein synthesis by the host and destroys the host cell.

Clinically, the pathogenesis of *C. trachomatis* in trachoma is characterized by inflammation of the conjunctiva with follicle formation. The cornea becomes vascularized, injected, and, as a result, partial or complete blindness develops. Scarring may cause inversion of the eyelids and scarring of the cornea by the eyelashes. Alterations in the lacrimal glands can lead the way to secondary bacterial infections by other microorganisms. *C. trachomatis* infection results in a short-lived humoral immunity. IgG and secretory IgA are found in the eye secretions. Most *C. trachomatis* infections resolve spontaneously without severe complications such as blindness. However, approximately 10 percent of infected persons will become partially or completely blind. Since the disease is epidemic in some countries, trachoma is a leading cause of blindness.

The diagnosis of trachoma is based on clinical signs including conjunctival follicles, scars and corneal infiltration, and vascularization. The microorganism can be recovered from the conjunctiva and isolated by culture in a eukaryotic cell line. Cytoplasmic inclusion bodies can be seen by fluorescent antibody tests. Antibodies in serum or eye secretions can also be detected by serologic tests. Antibiotic therapy by means of orally administered tetracycline and ophthalmic ointment is effective in eliminating the infection.

A variant of trachoma is known as inclusion conjunctivitis or "swimming pool conjunctivitis." This disease occurs in adults and is similar to another variant of trachoma that occurs in infants known as inclusion blenorrhea. Clinically, both of these diseases exhibit conjunctival inflammation, but the diseases are self-limiting and do not generally cause blindness. Inclusion conjunctivitis is caused by ocular infection with genitourinary strains of *C. trachomatis* transmitted either by genital-to-hand-to-eye contact, sometimes through towels, or through genitourinary chlamydial contamination of improperly chlorinated swimming pools.

C. trachomatis, particularly serotypes D and K, can cause sexually transmitted genitourinary tract infections including nongonococcal urethritis and epididymitis in men and pelvic inflammatory disease in women. *C. trachomatis* is therefore a major cause of sexually transmitted disease and resulting *infertility*. Another form of *C. trachomatis*–related sexually transmitted disease is *lymphogranuloma venereum*. This is clinically apparent as herpetiform veiscles on the genitals with the development of enlarged and even suppurative regional lymph nodes referred to as *venereal buboes*. This disease can be detected by means of the *Frei test* in which heat-killed *C. trachomatis* is injected as a skin test and produces a delayed hypersensitivity reaction in infected individuals.

CHLAMYDIA PSITTACI

C. psittaci affects mainly domestic fowl and birds, causing a disease known as psittacosis. This disease can kill large numbers of infected birds. In humans, this microorganism causes only slight respiratory disease although severe cases of human pneumonia due to *C. psittaci* have been reported. Human disease is almost always related to contact with infected birds.

In birds, *C. psittaci* produces a widely disseminated infection throughout the animal, and the microorganism is eventually shed through secretions and feces. In certain species, *C. psittaci* can be transmitted through eggs to infect the next generation. Dust contaminated with bird feces can be inhaled to cause human disease. The diagnosis of ornithosis is made by culture of *C. psittaci* or by immunofluorescence.

DIAGNOSIS

Chlamydial infection can be detected by culture of appropriate clinical specimens or by serologic techniques. Chlamydiae can be cultured in egg yolk sacs or in the brain, liver, or spleen of mice; however, the most widely used method is by culture in eukaryotic cells such as the McCoy cell line. The clinical specimen to be tested is inoculated into cycloheximide-treated McCoy cells, incubated for 48 to 72 hours, stained with iodine or Giemsa, and examined by light microscopy for the development of the glycogen-rich inclusion bodies. Staining with fluorescent antibody enables detection after only 24 hours.

Rickettsiae

The rickettsiae are a group of intracellular parasites that are transmitted to humans through the bites of arthropod vectors including insects such as lice or arachnids such as ticks (Table 20–4). Once these microorganisms gain access to the vasculature, they infect endothelial cells, resulting in hyperplasia and focal obstruction. The resulting clinical diseases are characterized by a typical clinical course including fever, headache, and skin rash. The type and distribution of skin

---

Table 20–4 ■ Rickettsiae

Rickettsia	Obligate intracellular parasites
	Requires an extracellular energy source
Species	*Rickettsia prowazekii*
	Causes
	Primary louse-borne typhus
	Recrudescent typhus (Brill-Zinsser disease)
	Features
	Rash develops from trunk to arms and legs
	Rickettsia rickettsii
	Causes
	Spotted fever, tick-borne
	Features
	Intracytoplasmic and intranuclear parasite
	Rash from arms and legs to trunk

---

rash is, itself, clinically useful in diagnosing rickettsial disease as well as in distinguishing different types of rickettsial disease. One type of rickettsial disease, Q fever, results from inhalation of contaminated aerosols.

The rickettsiae are distinguished from bacteria by a number of important criteria:

1. The rickettsiae are obligate intracellular parasites and they exist within intracellular vesicles that are resistant to lysosomal degradation. Bacteria, by contrast, can exist as intracellular parasites but they can also survive extracellularly. In contrast to other intracellular parasites, the rickettsiae can parasitize even nonphagocytic cells.

2. The rickettsiae require an outside energy source. ATP, NAD, and CoA can diffuse from the cytoplasm of the host cell into the rickettsiae to serve as an energy source.

3. They are smaller than bacterial cells, generally 0.3 to 0.5 nm in diameter, and they approximate the size of eukaryotic intracellular organelles such as mitochondria. They have a cell wall with lipopolysaccharide and peptidoglycan and a plasma membrane.

CLASSIFICATION OF RICKETTSIAL DISEASE

Typhus Group

This group of rickettsial diseases includes: (1) primary louse-borne typhus, (2) Brill-Zinsser disease, and (3) murine typhus.

Primary louse-borne typhus is caused by *R. prowazekii*. This organism lives only in humans and in the human louse *Pediculus humanus*. The transmission cycle is, therefore, louse-to-human-to-louse-to-human. Humans, however, are the reservoir for this organism since *R. prowazekii* infection is fatal to lice. Lice become infected by feeding on contaminated human blood. The organism multiplies in the insect's gastrointestinal tract and contaminates the feces. When the insect subsequently bites a human, it defecates on the skin and the contaminated feces are inoculated into the underlying tissues by scratching.

About 2 weeks after being bitten, the person will experience headache, rash, fever, and chills. The organism then multiplies in the endothelial cells lining the small blood vessels and causes hyperplasia and focal obstruction of these vessels. This vascular obstruction is responsible for the signs and symptoms of the disease. Thrombosis and obstruction of small vessels in the skin result in a rash, while thrombosis and obstruction of small vessels in the meninges cause headache and stupor.

The rash is clinically characteristic. It develops about 1 week after infection and it starts on the thorax and spreads to the arms and legs but does not involve the palms of the hands or the soles of the feet. The rash also changes from a maculopapular lesion to petechial hemorrhages.

Recrudescent typhus (Brill-Zinsser disease) represents a second subsequent episode of typhus in persons who previously have had primary louse-borne typhus. After the primary course of typhus, the patient recovers but the microorganism enters a latent stage. The patient may then undergo repeated bouts of typhus if, in response to stress or decreased host immunity, or both, *R. prowazekii* leaves the latent stage and multiplies in host cells. Similar to repeated episodes of other infectious diseases, recrudescent typhus is of shorter duration and is milder, and it produces an immediate secondary (IgG) immune response. No vector is involved in recrudescent typhus, since the original infection may have occurred years or decades before. The patients may or may not develop a rash.

Murine typhus is, as the name suggests, spread by rats and the rat flea (*Xenopsylla cheopis,* the same organism that spreads *Yersinia pestis* to cause bubonic plague). The rat flea is infected with *R. mooseri* by feeding on an infected rat. The flea can then spread the microorganism from rat-to-rat or from rat-to-human through contaminated feces, the same as in primary louse-borne typhus. It also produces a similar but less virulent human disease in areas where rats are found in high numbers, such as coastal areas. This human disease is called Toulon fever in France, Moscow typhus in Russia, and red fever in the Congo.

The spotted fevers, the best known of which is Rocky Mountain spotted fever, are caused by *R. rickettsia*. This microorganism is spread by ticks—primarily the wood tick in the Western United States and the dog tick in the Eastern United States. Other rickettsiae that are antigenically similar to *R. rickettsia* produce Marseilles fever, Siberian tick typhus, and Queensland tick typhus. *R. rickettsia* differs from other rickettsiae in that it can be found in the nucleus of host eukaryotic cells as well as in the cytoplasm. The resulting disease is also different from that caused by the typhus group in that the rash starts on the arms and legs, including the palms of the hands and the soles of the feet, and proceeds to include the thorax. Like typhus, the primary lesion is intravascular thrombosis, which can be so severe as to cause disseminated intravascular coagulation. There is a 5 percent mortality from this disease, even with antibiotic treatment.

Ticks become infected with *R. rickettsia* but do not die of the infection as in primary louse-borne typhus. The organism can be passed on to the next generation of tick through transovarial infection. Eggs harboring *R. rickettsia* transform from larva to nymphs to adults. Ticks may also have *R. rickettsia* in saliva. When they bite humans, infected saliva is injected into the skin.

Scrub typhus (tsutsugamushi disease) is a disease seen in Japan, Southeast Asia, and the South Pacific islands and is spread by trombiculid mites infected with *R. tsutsugamushi*. The mites spread the microorganism by biting both rodents and humans. The organism is then spread to a subsequent generation of mites through infected eggs. The site of the bite in humans develops into a black, ulcerated scar and produces regional and later generalized lymphadenopathy, which is distinct from other rickettsial diseases. Like the other rickettsial diseases, the patient develops fever, headache, and rash 1 to 2 weeks after the bite.

Q Fever

Q fever is a completely different type of rickettsial disease. It does not occur only by means of an insect or arachnid bite, but is also spread by inhalation of infected aerosols. The primary site of human infection is the lung as opposed to the vasculature. The infectious agent is also in a different genus from the other rickettsial diseases. *Coxiella burnetii,* named after its discoverers, Cox in the United States and Burnett in Australia, causes Q fever. It is differentiated from the other rickettsiae in being stable outside the eukaryotic host cells and also in being antigenically distinct from them. *C. burnetii* can infect a variety of ticks worldwide. The ticks, in turn, bite domestic animals, which then harbor *C. burnetii* in a latent stage (similar to that of recrudescent typhus). When a period of stress occurs such as during parturition the organism multiplies. It then becomes present in high numbers in chorionic fluid, placental tissues, feces, and urine. People who develop Q fever are, therefore, those who come in contact with infected animals or animal tissues. These people include livestock tenders, slaughterhouse workers, textile workers (contaminated wool) and laboratorians. The microorganism can also be spread through infected dust or aerosols that are inhaled. Clinical symptoms include headache, fever, and pneumonia.

LABORATORY DIAGNOSIS OF RICKETTSIAL DISEASE

Serologic tests provide the primary means for the laboratory diagnosis of rickettsial disease; however, many times the patient will have developed severe symptoms before an antibody response has developed. Therefore, clinicians must many times rely on patient history and clinical signs and symptoms, especially the characteristic skin rash, in order to diagnose the rickettsial diseases. Serologic tests generally detect patient antibodies to one of two types of rickettsial antigens—the soluble group antigens, which are shared by most of the rickettsia, and the insoluble, type-specific antigens, which are unique to each species. The serologic assays used to detect patient antibodies include complement fixation to measure common antigens, immunofluorescence, and the *Weil-Felix reaction*. This latter test is based on the presence of cross-reactive polysaccharide antigens shared by the rickettsia and certain species of *Proteus*. The test is performed by mixing a drop of the patient's blood with each of three *Proteus* strains. The presence of antibody to the rickettsiae can be detected by bacterial cell agglutination, which appears after approximately 5 minutes.

Certain rickettsial diseases produce other laboratory results, which can be useful in diagnosis. Patients with Rocky Mountain spotted fever, for example, will often exhibit leukopenia and thrombocytopenia.

TREATMENT AND PREVENTION

The rickettsial diseases generally respond to systemic antibiotics, particularly those antibiotics that can eliminate intracellular parasites. These include chloramphenicol and the tetracyclines.

There are two main approaches to the prevention of rickettsial disease. These are immunization with appropriate vaccines and elimination of the rickettsial vector. Vaccines have been used to prevent primary louse-borne typhus but have only ameliorated the course of the disease rather than providing complete protection. Rickettsial diseases have been better prevented by elimination of the vector. Primary louse-borne typhus and subsequent recrudescent typhus have been controlled through the use of DDT to eliminate the human lice. Murine typhus is controlled by killing rat fleas and by the elimination of rodent populations.

REFERENCES

Mycoplasma

Chanock, R. M., Hayflick, L., and Barile, M. F.: Growth in artificial media of an agent associated with atypical pneumonia and its identification as a PPLO. Proc Nat Acad Sci (USA) 48:41, 1962.
Razin, S.: The mycoplasma. Microbial Reviews 42:414, 1978.
Tully, J. G., and Whitcomb, R. F. (eds.): The Mycoplasma. Academic Press, New York, 1979.

Chlamydiae

Schachter, J.: Chlamydial infections. N Engl J Med 298:428; 490; 540; 1978.
Schachter, J., and Caldwell, H. D.: Chlamydiae. Ann Rev Microbiol 34:285, 1980.

Rickettsiae

Ormsbee, R. A.: Rickettsiae (as organisms). Ann Rev Microbiol 23:275, 1969.
Weiss, E.: The biology of the rickettsiae. Ann Rev Microbiol 36:345, 1982.

Legionella

Joan Otomo-Corgel, D.D.S., M.P.H.

In July 1976, the Pennsylvania American Legion was having its 50th Annual Convention. A mysterious illness that took 29 lives shrouded the event. Approximately 6 months later, a gram-negative bacterium was isolated by techniques used for the isolation of rickettsial agents. Survivors demonstrated antibodies against the isolate. The first description of the legionnaires' disease bacterium had just been introduced.

Earlier outbreaks were later retrospectively linked to the same etiologic organism: 81 patients became ill and 14 died in 1965 at St. Elizabeth Hospital, Washington, D.C.; 144 cases related to air conditioning in a health department building occurred in Pontiac, Michigan, and two deaths from pneumonia were associated with an Oddfellows Convention in Philadelphia in 1974. Recognition of legionnaires' disease bacterium (**LDB**, or *Legionella pneumophila*) brought to light a sporadic epidemic that is increasing in frequency. While it is broadly referred to as legionnaires' disease or legionellosis, a number of species within the genus *Legionella* (i.e., *L. wadsworthii, L. gormanii,* or *L. micdadei*) are linked to disease.

Clinical-Epidemiologic Patterns

There are three distinct clinical-epidemiologic patterns.

1. **Pontiac fever** or **nonpneumonic legionnaires' disease** is devoid of mortality and pneumonia. It has a 5- to 66-hour incubation period, followed by flulike symptoms of abrupt-onset fever, chills, headache, and myalgia. Neurologic and gastrointestinal symptoms are similar to those of other legionnaires' outbreaks. In the Pontiac outbreak, the suspected source of *Legionella* was the air-conditioning system. Once the evaporator condenser was cleansed and relocated, the outbreak was suppressed.

2. **Pneumonic legionnaires' disease,** exemplified by the 1976 Philadelphia outbreak, has an incubation period of 2 to 10 days and a low attack rate. The clinical course begins with malaise, myalgia, headache with ensuing fever, pneumonia, and sometimes death. Central nervous system symptoms of slurred speech, clumsiness, ataxia, and confusion occur early. Lower respiratory symptoms (dyspnea and nonproductive cough) are

present in 4 to 7 days without previous upper respiratory symptoms. In half of the cases, coughs became productive. Once respiratory symptoms predominate, progression to pneumonia occurs. Diarrhea, vomiting, abdominal pain, abnormalities in serum electrolytes, leukocytosis, and renal abnormalities have also been noted.

3. The third form of legionnaires' disease has been described as **nosocomial**. Attack rates are low, but fatality rates are high. An outbreak occurred in 1978 at the Veterans Administration Medical Center, West Los Angeles, Wadsworth Division, where 75 people contracted the disease and 25 percent died. The clinical course was similar to the pneumonic form, but renal disease was absent and pneumonia progression was different. *Legionella pneumophila* was isolated from the water supply and treated primarily by hyperchlorination.

Epidemiology

The sex distribution in legionnaires' disease is 2 to 3:1 males to females. The average age of a patient is 60 years; however, there is a broad age range. It is also apparently more benign in children. A majority of patients have one or more predisposing underlying conditions including immunosuppression, malignancy, heart disease, and chronic renal failure.

Laboratory Diagnosis

Laboratory diagnosis is based on cultural isolation, identification in clinical specimens by direct immunofluorescence, elevated antibody titers in convalescent sera, and identification of bacterial antigens in body fluids. Newer tests for antibody determination include an indirect enzyme-linked immunosorbent assay (ELISA) using six serogroups of whole *L. pneumophila* and a microagglutination assay, which are both rapid and sensitive. *Legionella* antigens can also be detected by ELISA. At present, DNA probes are being investigated for identifying species of *Legionella*.

Microbiology

The initial classification of *Legionella* was family *Legionellaceae*, genus *Legionella*, and

Table 21–1 ■ *Species of Legionella*

Legionella pneumophila
Legionella gormanii
Legionella dumoffii
Legionella bozemanii
Legionella jordanis
Legionella micdadei
Legionella longbeachae
Legionella wadsworthii
Legionella oakridgensis
LLO (*Legionella*-like organisms)

Note: The above are similar in physiologic characteristics but differ in DNA homology and major cell surface antigens.

single species *pneumophila*. There are now at least eight *pneumophila* serogroups and 10 *Legionella* species, with more species being named (Table 21–1). The genus identification is based on ability to grow on charcoal-yeast agar or other media containing cysteine and iron salts. Species identification is done serologically and, more recently, by DNA relatedness. Species designation may then be supported by antigen analysis and cell wall fatty acid profiles supported by gas-liquid chromatography. The bacterial cell wall is composed of diaminopimelic acid, typical of gram-negative bacilli, but with an unusually high cross-linkage of 80 to 90 percent.

Pathogenesis

L. pneumophila is an opportunistic facultative organism with a number of serotypes indicating antigenic diversity in humans. The mode of infection is thought to be via inhalation or ingestion. Small particles (less than 5 μm) are necessary to ensure respiratory bronchiole penetration. Potable water ingestion with entry into the lymphatics and lung dissemination may also occur. Mortality ranges from 10 to 20 percent of untreated cases. **Legionellosis** is an acute fibropurulent pneumonia affecting the sinus with leakage of the edema and fibrin from damaged capillaries affecting gaseous exchange leading to hypoxia. The bacterium causes cellular damage besides lung infiltration and consolidation. Histologically, there are intra-alveolar macrophages and monocytes. There is either direct tissue invasion or systemic-toxic effects of the bacterium (pyrexia or gram-negative septicemia) on extrapulmonary organs: renal, hepatic, gastrointestinal, and neurologic. Inflammation and tissue injury can occur in the absence of organisms, suggesting production of an "endotoxin-like polysaccharide substance."

Immunology

There is no agreement on the chemical structure of serogroup-specific and species-specific antigens, but antigenic activity of serogroup-specific antigens of *L. pneumophila* resides in the polysaccharide portion of the antigen. The antigen has a molecular weight of approximately 4×10^4 and consists of less than 10 percent carbohydrate, 15 percent protein, 1.1 percent phosphate, and a lipid. There is a similarity between serogroup antigens of *L. pneumophila* (cell-like surface location, high molecular weight, and chemical composition) and the lipopolysaccharide endotoxin classically associated with other gram-negative bacteria. *L. pneumophila* produces compounds similar to classic endotoxin in biologic activity and chemical structure, but further study is required to implicate serotype-specific antigens to endotoxin activity. Skin testing for antigens specific to legionellosis is also being developed.

Legionella pneumophila may multiply intracellularly in human mononuclear phagosomes (facultative, intracellular parasite), thus belonging to a special group of pathogens that can evade host defenses by parasitizing mononuclear phagocytes. Humans are probably incidental hosts for legionnaires' disease bacteria, which developed a capacity for intracellular survival in amoebae and mononuclear phagocytes. In vitro antibody studies suggest that humoral immunity may not be effective against *L. pneumophila* and that a vaccine that elicits only antibody protection also may be ineffective. The organism inhibits phagosome-lysosome fusion, which is important to its survival in mononuclear phagocytes (comparable to *M. tuberculosis* and *T. gondii*). In contrast to humoral defense, cell-mediated immunity seems to play a major role. Patients with legionnaires' disease develop a mononuclear response to *L. pneumophila* antigens with proliferation and generation of monocyte-activating cytokinins. Mononuclear phagocytes activated by the cytokinins inhibit intracellular multiplication of *L. pneumophila*. Monocytes and PMNs phagocytose a limited portion of an inoculum of antibody and complement-coated bacteria.

Treatment

Owing to the ubiquity of the organism, eradication is not feasible and control in water is difficult. Hyperchlorination is effective in nosocomial legionellosis from potable water. Low hot water temperatures, water stagnation, and faucet obstructions (rubber washers) act as reservoirs for bacterial growth. Cooling towers provide an environment for amplification of *L. pneumophila* due to thermal enhancement. Legionnaires' disease bacteria are not active at 45°C and are relatively inactive at 75°C. Therefore, current recommendations for hospitals are chlorination at or raising temperatures of hot water systems to above 63°C.

In clinical treatment, erythromycin and tetracycline decrease mortality and provide clinical improvement. Differences exist, however, between clinical response to antibiotic therapy and in vitro susceptibility studies. Based on data from epidemics, antibiotics are indicated for suspected or diagnosed legionellosis (Table 21–2). Erythromycin and rifampin inhibit *L. pneumophila* intracellular multiplication but do not kill intracellular bacteria even at high concentrations. Once the antibiotic is stopped, multiplication in monocytes resumes. Therefore, antibiotics provide an opportunity for the host to mount an immune defense against the unique bacterium. A combination of erythromycin and rifampin may be best because erythromycin does not prevent widespread lung lesions, but rifampin penetrates well into the macrophage to reach the legionnaires' disease bacteria and confines the lung lesions.

Supportive care for the patients with legionnaires' disease must be maintained. Because of the pyrexia, lung infiltration, fibrosis, and septicemia associated with this disease, attention should be placed on prevention of hypotension, renal failure, and respiratory failure. Maintenance of fluid-electrolyte and acid-base balance is also important. Secondary infection is also a potential complicating factor.

DENTAL TREATMENT CONSIDERATIONS

There are no clinical guidelines for treating patients with a history of or active legionnaires' disease in the dental environment. There is a paucity of information relating to transmission of legionnaires' disease bacteria infections. Dental personnel should be aware of clinical signs and symptoms and suspect patients with pneumonia of unknown etiology. Elective dental treatment should not be performed on a legionnaires' disease patient.

Table 21-2 ■ Antimicrobial therapy for *Legionella* disease

Antimicrobial	Dose	Route	Duration	Miscellaneous
Erythromycin gluceptate or erythromycin lactobionate	25–50 mg/kg not to exceed 4 g/day	IV	3 wk	Dilute 0.5–1 g in 250 ml 5% dextrose or 0.9% sodium chloride solution for continuous 6 hr infusion.
Tetracycline	250–500 mg q6h not to exceed 2 g/day	IV	2 wk	In children >8 yrs 15 mg/kg q12h. When clinical improvement is noted, 500 mg qid oral.
Doxycycline	100 mg q12h	IV	2 wk	For patients with renal insufficiency.
Rifampin	10–20 mg/kg not to exceed 600 mg/day	Oral dose + erythromycin or tetracycline on empty stomach		For critically ill. Increases hepatic enzymes.
Imipenem Imipenem + cilastatin	500 mg each tid	Oral dose	Minimum 5 days	New carbapenem β-lactam antibiotic. Studied by Farrell et al. and Beasley et al. in 1985.

If it is an emergency, the physician should be consulted and infection control procedures should be followed closely:

Barrier technique
Minimal use of air or water syringes
Strict septic technique
Slow-speed handpiece only
In-hospital treatment only (isolation)

The patient should not be placed in a fully reclining position, if this is uncomfortable. Stress reduction protocols should be employed.

In patients who have recovered from legionellosis, there are no contraindications to routine dental therapy. The dentist should be aware of patients with possible lung fibrosis, permanent cerebellum dysfunction, cranial nerve palsies, seizures, renal dysfunction, peripheral neuropathy, and even endocarditis. The disease is not spread from person to person but from water sources to immunosusceptible hosts. Relapse of the infection is infrequent.

The incidence of legionnaires' disease is increasing. It is epidemic and sporadic, but bacterial identification is rapid. Identification of reservoirs and mechanisms of aerosolization, transmission, and bacterial virulence are better understood but need greater focus. Prophylaxis is of paramount importance, especially in hospitals, where the immunocompromised patient is a prime target. Extrathoracic manifestation of legionellosis is poorly understood, and protective immunity from prior infection with bacteria of a different serogroup is unknown. Great strides have been made since 1976, but further knowledge is necessary before a solution to the problem will be found. Along with improvements in diagnosis and treatment, the management of dental patients will become clearer.

REFERENCES

Barka, N., et al.: ELISA using whole *Legionella pneumophila* as an antigen. Comparison between monovalent and polyvalent antigens for the serodiagnosis of human legionellosis. J. Immunol. Methods 93:77, 1986.

Beasley, C.R.: Treatment of pneumonia with imipenem/cilastatin. N. Z. Med. J. 98:494, 1985.

Beaty, H.N.: Clinical features of legionellosis. Legionella Proceedings of the International Symposium, American Society for Microbiology, Washington, D.C., pp 6–10, 1984.

Blackmon, J.A., et al.: Legionellosis. Am. J. Pathol. 103:429, 1981.

Brenner, D.J., et al.: Classification of Legionnaires' disease bacterium: *Legionella pneumophila*, genus novum, species nova of the family *Legionellaceae*, familia nova. Ann. Int. Med. 90:656, 1979.

Broome, C.V., and Fraser, D.W.: Epidemiologic aspects of legionellosis. Epidemiol. Rev., 1:1, 1979.

Centers for Disease Control: Respiratory infection—Pennsylvania. MMWR 25:244, 1976.

Farrell, I.D., et al.: The activity of imipenem on *Legionella pneumophila*, with a note on the treatment of two cases. J. Antimicrob. Chemother. 16:61, 1985.

Flesher, A.R.: Isolation of a serogroup 1-specific antigen from *Legionella pneumophila*. J. Infect. Dis. 145:224, 1982.

Fliermans, C.B.: Measure of *Legionella pneumophila* activity *in situ*. Curr. Microbiol. 6:89–94, 1981.

Fraser, D.W., et al.: Legionnaires' disease: description of an epidemic of pneumonia. N. Engl. J. Med. 297:1189, 1977.

Glavin, F.L.: Ultrastructure of lung in Legionnaires'

disease. Observation of three biopsies done during the Vermont epidemic. Ann. Intern. Med. 90:555, 1979.

Glick, T.H., et al.: Pontiac Fever. An epidemic of unknown etiology in a health department. I. Clinical and epidemiological aspects. Am. J. Epidemiol. 107:149, 1978.

Haley, C.E.: Nosocomial Legionnaires' disease. A continuing common-source epidemic at Wadsworth Medical Center. Ann. Intern. Med. 90:583, 1979.

Horwitz, M.A.: Interactions between *Legionella pneumophila* and human mononuclear phagocytes. Legionella, American Society for Microbiology, Washington, D.C., 159–166, 1984.

Horwitz, M.A., and Silverstein, S.C.: The Legionnaires' disease bacterium multiplies intracellularly in human monocytes. J. Clin. Invest. 66:441, 1980.

Johnson, W., et al.: Serospecificity and opsonic activity of antisera to *Legionella pneumophila*. Infect. Immun. 26:698, 1979.

Kirby, B.D., et al.: Legionnaires' disease: Report of sixty-five nosocomial acquired cases and review of the literature. Medicine 59:188, 1980.

Lattimer, G.L., and Ormsbee, R.A.: Legionnaires' Disease. Marcel Dekker, New York, 1981.

McDade, J.E., et al.: Legionnaires' disease. Isolation of a bacterium and demonstration of its role in other respiratory diseases. N. Engl. J. Med. 297:1197, 1977.

Meyer, R.D.: Legionella infections: a review of five years of research. Rev. Infect. Dis. 5:258, 1983.

Muder, R.R., et al.: Pneumonia due to the Pittsburgh pneumonia agent: new clinical perspective with a review of the literature. Medicine 62:120, 1983.

Shands, K.N., et al.: Potable water as a source of Legionnaires' disease. JAMA 253:1412, 1985.

Tang, P.W., and Toma, S.: Broad-spectrum enzyme-linked immuno-absorbent assay for detection of Legionella-soluble antigens. J. Clin. Microbiol. 24:556, 1986.

Thacker, S.B., et al.: An outbreak in 1965 of severe respiratory illness caused by the Legionnaires' disease bacterium. J. Infect. Dis. 138:512, 1978.

Tsai, T.F., et al.: Legionnaires' Disease: Clinical features of the epidemic in Philadelphia. Ann. Intern. Med. 90:509, 1979.

U.S. Dept. of Health, Education and Welfare, Centers for Disease Control: Epidemiology of Legionnaires' Disease. Baine, W.B. 1980.

Wong, K.H.: Endotoxicity of the Legionnaires' disease bacterium. Ann. Intern. Med. 90:624, 1979.

section III

Virology and parasitology

III

chapter 22

Virology

No-Hee Park, D.M.D., Ph.D.

CHAPTER OUTLINE

- GENERAL STRUCTURE OF VIRUSES
- CLASSIFICATION OF ANIMAL VIRUSES
- VIRUS REPLICATION
- DIAGNOSIS OF VIRAL DISEASES
- EFFECT OF VIRUSES ON HOST CELL
- HOST RESPONSE TO VIRAL INFECTIONS
- HERPESVIRUSES
- HEPATITIS VIRUSES
- ONCOGENIC VIRUSES
- AIDS AND HUMAN IMMUNODEFICIENCY VIRUS
- ANTIVIRAL THERAPY
- VACCINES

General Structure of Viruses

Over the past two decades, significant advances have occurred in our understanding of the nature of viruses as well as the pathogenesis and treatment of human viral infections. Viruses are a major cause of disease in humans, being responsible for illnesses ranging in severity from the common cold to fatal encephalitis. In order to establish the etiologic diagnosis and effective prophylactic and therapeutic measures of a viral disease, it is essential to understand the detailed mechanism and pattern of that virus' dissemination within the population, its mode of entry into and spread within the hosts, the nature of its interaction with host cells, and its mode of replication within individual host cells. All of these parameters are closely related to virus structure and composition. The main structural components of a virion are nucleic acid, capsid, and viral envelope (Figs. 22–1 and 22–2).

NUCLEIC ACIDS

Viruses contain either single or double strands of nucleic acid, either DNA or RNA, which contain the genetic information and direct the cell to construct a series of proteins. The size of nucleic acid differs among viruses and determines the complexity of virions. The nucleic acid genome can be double-stranded (ds) circular or linear DNA, single-stranded (ss) linear DNA, ds or ss broken linear RNA, ss intact linear RNA, or ss broken circular RNA.

CAPSID

Proteins are indispensable components of all virions together with nucleic acids. The protein coat that surrounds the nucleic acid genome of all viruses is called the capsid. Nucleocapsid is the name for the complex of the capsid and the nucleic acid. In a virion lacking an envelope, the capsid provides the

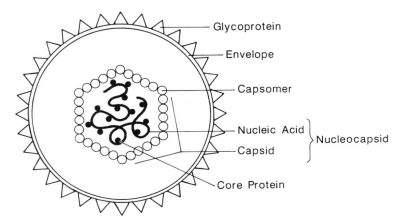

Figure 22–1 ■ A schematic representation of an enveloped virion. The viral nucleic acid, either RNA or DNA, is enclosed by protein molecules forming the capsid. The capsid is enclosed in an envelope to whose outer surface viral specific glycoproteins are attached.

only protection for the nucleic acid. The capsid also determines the host range and is responsible for the initiation of infection. Most viral capsids exhibit one or two types of symmetry: icosahedral (cubic) or helical (certain complex viruses, such as the poxviruses and T-even bacteriophages exhibit bilateral symmetry). The capsids are composed of subunits called capsomeres, which may be made up of more than one polypeptide molecule. In addition to capsid proteins, some viruses contain a variety of virion enzymes of which discovery has aided greatly in providing an understanding of the life cycles of viruses. Some of the enzymes present may be of host cell origin, serving no apparent useful function for the virus. The presence of some virus-coded enzymes is, however, essential for the viral infectivity. One of the most important enzymes found in some virions is **transcriptase**. Four different transcriptases (or polymerases) have so far been found in the virion: DNA-dependent RNA polymerase in poxvirus, RNA-dependent RNA polymerase in all negative-stranded RNA viruses, RNA transcriptase in viruses with ds RNA genomes, and RNA-dependent DNA polymerase (or reverse transcriptase).

ENVELOPE

Many viruses have a lipid envelope surrounding their nucleocapsid. The envelopes are derived from host cell membranes, that is, nuclear membrane, endoplasmic reticulum, Golgi apparatus, plasma membrane, or vacuolar membrane. Therefore, the viral envelopes are structurally similar to cellular membranes—a lipid bilayer with protein molecules embedded in it and, frequently, with glycoprotein spikes protruding on the outer

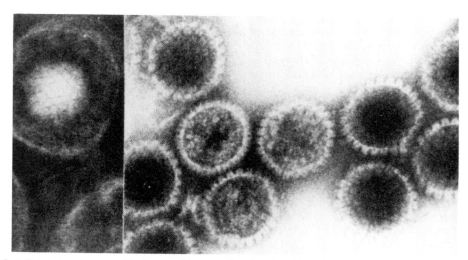

Figure 22–2 ■ Electron micrographic figure of herpes simplex virus type 1, enveloped *(left)* and naked capsids *(right)*. Magnification × 189,000. (From Fields, B. N., and Knipe, D. M.: In Fields, B. N., et al. (eds): Fields' Virology. Raven Press, New York, 1985, p. 12, with permission.)

surface. The envelope represents the outermost barrier of the virion. It contributes to the resistance of the virus to various physical and chemical agents, and it also determines the host range of the virus.

Classification of Animal Viruses

Animal viruses have been classified by various criteria. The potential bases for classification are host (tissue and cell trophism), pathology and symptomatology, epidemiology, virion morphology, nucleic acids, and immunologic properties. In general, viruses are classified according to the characteristics of the virion itself, using a combination of criteria. In practice, however, more or less weight is given to certain properties, depending upon the needs and the point of view of the classifier.

The nomenclature used for animal viruses consisted of giving the name of the disease produced in the major host followed by the word "virus." However, one faces the problem of the choice of criteria: the nature of the major hosts, the type of disease produced, the properties of virions, or the feature of the reproductive cycle. Therefore, a good system for viral classification has been sought, and the International Committee on Nomenclature of Viruses has proposed a dual system of nomenclature consisting of generic names ending in "-virus" for individual virus groups and of eight-digit cryptograms purported to describe each virus according to a conventional key.

In general, the animal viruses are divided into two groups according to properties of the genetic nucleic acids: RNA viruses and DNA viruses. RNA viruses that cause diseases in humans include picornavirus, togavirus, paramyxovirus, orthomyxovirus, rhabdovirus, reovirus, and retrovirus. DNA viruses are parvoviruses, papovavirus, adenovirus, herpesvirus, and poxvirus (Table 22–1).

RNA VIRUSES

Human RNA viruses are classified as follows (Table 22–2).

1. *Picornaviruses:* Picornavirus is small (27 nm in diameter) and naked, contains single-stranded RNA of 2.7×10^6 daltons, and exhibits icosahedral symmetry. This virus group includes poliovirus, coxsackievirus, rhinovirus, and the foot and mouth disease virus of cattle (Table 22–1). Coxsackievirus causes a variety of symptoms, especially myositis. There are three serotypes of poliovirus that can cause paralysis. More than 100 serotypes of rhinoviruses are identified, and the rhinoviruses are the most important agents of the "common cold" in humans.

2. *Togaviruses:* Togavirus is an enveloped virus, and its capsid is icosahedral with a diameter of 50 to 70 nm. It has single-stranded infectious RNA of 4×10^6 daltons. Togavirus was formerly known as "arbovirus" and infects animals, birds, insects, and humans. Two subgroups of togavirus are known. Type A (alphaviruses) is mosquito-borne and includes 20 viruses that show

| Table 22–1 ■ Classification of animal viruses and their characteristics |

Class	Nucleic Acid	Capsid	Envelope	Polarity	Infectivity of Naked Nucleic Acid
Poxvirus	ds DNA	Complex	+		
Herpesvirus	ds DNA	Icosahedron	+		+
Adenovirus	ds DNA	Icosahedron	0		+
Papovavirus	ds DNA	Icosahedron	0		+
Parvovirus	ss DNA	Icosahedron	0	+, −	+
Reovirus	ds DNA	Icosahedron	0		−
Orthomyxovirus	ss RNA	Helix	+	−	−
Paramyxovirus	ss RNA	Helix	+	−	−
Rhabdovirus	ss RNA	Helix	+	−	−
Coronavirus	ss RNA	Helix	+	+	+
Oncornavirus	ss RNA	Helix	+	+	−
Picornavirus	ss RNA	Icosahedron	0	+	+
Togavirus	ss RNA	Icosahedron	+	+	+
Hepatitis B	ds DNA	Icosahedron	+		+
Hepatitis A	ds RNA	Icosahedron	+		−

ss DNA = single-strand DNA.
ds DNA = double-strand DNA.
ss RNA = single-strand RNA.
ds RNA = double strand RNA.

Table 22–2 ■ Examples of human RNA viruses

Class	Name of Virus	Major Clinical Diseases
I. Picornaviruses	Poliovirus	Poliomyelitis
	Coxsackievirus A	Herpangina, aseptic meningitis, paralysis, common cold syndrome
	Coxsackievirus B	Pleurodynia, aseptic meningitis
	ECHO viruses	Paralysis, diarrhea, aseptic meningitis
	Human enterovirus 72 (hepatitis A virus)	Infectious hepatitis, jaundice
	Rhinoviruses	Common cold, bronchitis
II. Togaviruses	Rubella virus	Rubella
	Yellow fever virus	Yellow fever
III. Orthomyxoviruses	Influenza virus A, B, C	Influenza
IV. Paramyxoviruses	Measles virus	Measles
	SSPE (subacute sclerosing panencephalitis)	Chronic degeneration of CNS
	Mumps virus	Mumps
	Parainfluenza viruses	Respiratory tract infection
	Sendai virus	Croup, common cold syndrome
V. Rhabdoviruses	Rabies virus	Encephalitis, almost invariably fatal
	Vesicular stomatitis virus	Mostly occurs in cattle
VI. Reoviruses	Reovirus types 1, 2, 3	Not known
	Rotavirus	Diarrhea in infants

serologic cross-reactivity. Alphaviruses cause encephalitis in humans and other mammals and can be fatal. Type B (flaviviruses) is either mosquito-borne or tick-borne and includes several dozen cross-reacting species. Flaviviruses also cause encephalitis and other serious systemic illnesses.

3. *Paramyxoviruses:* Members of the paramyxovirus family are enveloped, and the overall particle shapes are pleomorphic with a diameter of approximately 150 nm. These viruses contain single-stranded "negative-strand" RNA of 7×10^6 daltons. Of the paramyxoviruses, mumps virus and the Newcastle disease virus of chickens contain neuraminidase and hemagglutinin in single protein and are infectious for many tissues. Measles virus and respiratory syncytial virus of humans do not contain neuraminidase, but have hemagglutinin.

4. *Orthomyxoviruses:* Members of the orthomyxovirus family are enveloped, have pleomorphic shapes, and are 80 to 120 nm in diameter. They contain a helical nucleocapsid with a diameter 6 to 9 nm. The RNA is segmented and single stranded, with a molecular weight of 2.4×10^6 daltons. Examples of orthomyxoviruses are influenza viruses A, B, and C. These viruses contain neuraminidase and hemagglutinin in separate proteins. The A strain is the most important for human disease and undergoes constant antigenic variation.

5. *Rhabdoviruses:* Rhabdoviruses are enveloped, bullet-shaped virions 70×175 nm in size, and contain helical nucleocapsids with single-stranded negative-strand RNA of 4×10^6 daltons and virion mRNA polymerase. Vesicular stomatitis virus and rabies virus belong to the rhabdovirus family.

6. *Reoviruses:* Viruses within the family of reoviruses are naked, icosahedral, and double-shelled virions. The virion contains 10 or more double-stranded RNA molecules ranging from 0.4 to 2.8×10^6 daltons and virion transcriptase. Reovirus types 1, 2, and 3, human rotavirus types 1 and 2, and Colorado tick fever virus belong to the reoviruses. Reovirus type 1 may cause diarrhea in children, and rotaviruses cause acute diarrhea in infants of many species.

7. *Retroviruses:* Members of the retrovirus family are enveloped and roundish particles about 100 nm in diameter with a helical nucleocapsid containing 6×10^6 daltons of RNA consisting of two identical molecules 3×10^6 each. They also contain reverse transcriptase and multiply by integration into DNA of the host and may cause leukemia, sarcoma, and other various malignancies.

DNA VIRUSES

Human DNA viruses are classified as follows (Table 22–3).

1. *Parvoviruses:* Parvoviruses are naked virions with a diameter of 18 to 26 nm and include an icosahedral nucleocapsid with 32 capsomeres. Virions contain single-stranded DNA of 1.2 to 1.8×10^6 daltons. Both defective and infectious types of parvoviruses ex-

Table 22–3 ■ Examples of human DNA viruses

Class	Names of Virus	Major Clinical Diseases
I. Parvoviruses	Adeno-associated virus	No known symptoms
II. Papovaviruses	Human papilloma viruses	Plantar warts
	Human polyoma virus	Isolated from brains of patients with progressive multifocal leukoencephalopathy
III. Adenoviruses	Adenovirus A	No known pathogenicity
	Adenovirus B and E	Acute respiratory disease
	Adenovirus C	Mild infections of respiratory tract, latent infection in lymphoid tissue
	Adenovirus D	Epidemic keratoconjunctivitis
IV. Herpesviruses	Herpes simplex virus type 1	Primary herpes stomatitis, recurrent herpes labialis, upper respiratory infections, herpes keratitis and genitalis, fetal encephalitis
	Herpes simplex virus type 2	Mainly herpes genitalis, rarely keratitis and stomatitis, recurrent herpes labialis, fatal encephalitis and meningitis
	Varicella zoster virus	Chickenpox in children, shingles, fatal encephalitis, keratitis
	Cytomegalovirus	Jaundice, hepatosplenomegaly, brain damage, birth defect, mononucleosis, death
	Epstein-Barr virus	Burkitt's lymphoma, nasopharyngeal carcinoma, infectious mononucleosis
V. Poxviruses	Variola virus (major)	Smallpox
	Variola virus (minor)	Alastrim
	Monkeypox virus	Smallpox-like disease
	Vaccinia virus	Vesicular eruption of the skin
VI. Hepatitis B virus	Hepatitis B virus	Hepatitis B (serum hepatitis)

ist: minute virus of mice (nondefective) and adeno-associated virus (AAV; defective).

2. *Papoviruses:* Members of the papovavirus family are naked virions with icosahedral capsids 45 to 55 nm in diameter. They contain closed circular double-stranded DNA from 3 to 5×10^6 daltons. The members are polyoma virus of mice, simian virus 40 (SV 40), Shope papilloma virus, and human wart virus. These viruses can cause cell transformation and tumors in animals.

3. *Adenoviruses:* The members of the adenovirus family are naked DNA viruses 80 to 90 nm in size. They are 20 to 30×10^6 daltons in molecular weight and can transform cells. Human adenovirus types 1 and 2 belong to this family. Some adenovirus types can cause respiratory illness and conjunctivitis in humans.

4. *Herpesviruses:* The herpesviruses are enveloped and contain icosahedral 100 nm nucleocapsids with double-stranded linear DNA of 100×10^6 daltons. They grow in the nucleus, bud through the nuclear membrane, and cause latent infections. Herpes simplex virus types 1 and 2, Epstein-Barr virus, varicella zoster virus, and cytomegalovirus are herpesviruses that cause diseases in humans. Pseudorabies virus causes "mad itch" in swine and cattle, and Lucke virus causes frog adenocarcinoma.

5. *Poxviruses:* Poxviruses are enveloped, complex brick-shaped virions (300 × 200 × 100 nm) with double-stranded linear DNA of 160×10^6 daltons in molecular weight. The virions contain many enzymes and at least 30 proteins including virion RNA polymerase. Poxviruses include human variola virus, human vaccinia virus, mammalian poxviruses for many species, and myxoma-fibroma virus. Human variola virus causes smallpox and human vaccinia virus can provide immunity to smallpox.

Virus Replication

Viruses have a unique mode of reproduction that differentiates them from the more complex cellular microorganisms. The mechanism by which virions replicate within the cells can be divided into a number of distinct steps. The steps in the replication of a typical animal virus are as follows (Figs. 22–3 and 22–4):

1. Attachment (adsorption)
2. Penetration
3. Uncoating of the viral nucleic acid
4. Transport of virion, core, or virion nucleic acid to site of replication
5. Synthesis of viral messenger RNA (mRNA)
6. Synthesis of viral proteins
7. Replication of the virion nucleic acid

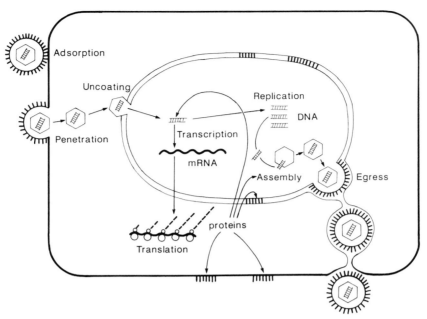

Figure 22–3 ■ Replicative cycle of adenovirus (DNA virus).

8. Assembly (maturation) of virions
9. Egress of virions from the cell

It is, however, important to recognize that in the case of animal viruses, the susceptible cells are always part of a complex multicellular organism. The virus infects a susceptible host, replicates (or at least persists) within it, exists at some time prior to the host's demise, and then infects another susceptible host. Viral multiplication in cells accompanies gen-

eral cytopathic changes including rounding of cells and the appearance of large intranuclear eosinophilic inclusion bodies (Fig. 22–5).

ATTACHMENT (ADSORPTION)

Physical contact of the infecting virion with the host cell is the first requirement of repli-

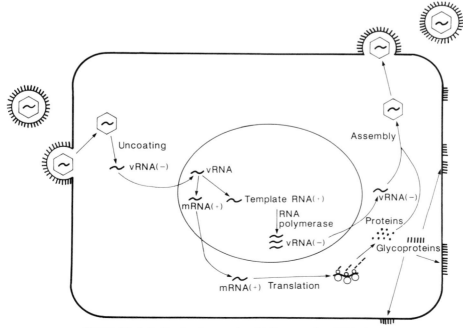

Figure 22–4 ■ Replicative cycle of influenza virus (RNA virus).

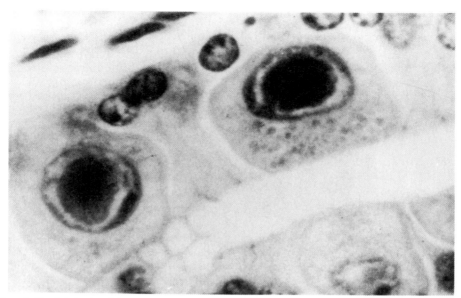

Figure 22–5 ■ Epithelial duct cell from a human submaxillary gland infected with human cytomegalovirus, showing typical eosinophilic nuclear and basophilic cytoplasmic inclusions. Magnification × 1500. (From Nelson J. S. N. and Wyatt J. P. W.: Medicine 38:223, 1959, with permission.)

cation. Brownian movement of virions may cause them to randomly collide with cell surface, where they bind electrostatically. Infection and viral diseases are determined to a considerable degree by the ability of viruses to bind to cells of a particular animal species. Tropism appears to be due to localization of viruses of different cells determined by the presence of receptors. Receptors are virus-specific; even closely related viruses do not share the same receptors. However, rarely, unrelated viruses may share common receptors. The viral receptors have not been characterized, but it is thought that they may be glycoprotein.

PENETRATION

The virion attached to the surface of cell enters the cell by penetration. Penetration and internalization of absorbed virions can occur by three mechanisms.

1. *Pinocytosis or viropexis:* Pinocytosis, which is akin to phagocytosis, is the most common mode of penetration of animal viruses. Both naked and enveloped virions enter the cell by this mechanism.

2. *Direct entry:* In some instances the virion appears to cross the cell membrane by direct entry without gradual engulfment. The actual mechanism is unknown. Only naked virions are taken up by this mode of entry.

3. *Fusion of viral envelope with cellular plasma membrane:* The viral membrane fuses with the host cell plasma membrane, and the nucleocapsid is introduced into the cellular cytoplasm. Most enveloped virions appear to enter the cells by this mechanism.

UNCOATING

Uncoating is defined as the release of nucleic acid from the nucleocapsid after it has entered the host cell. Although there is no evidence that the uncoating process results from the cellular enzymatic removal of viral capsid proteins, the conformation of capsid proteins may be changed following the viral attachment to cell receptors. These changes in capsid protein conformation may then trigger the release of the nucleic acid. The cytoplasmic locations where the uncoating takes place may differ among viruses. In simple plus-stranded RNA viruses (i.e., picornavirus and togavirus), uncoating occurs immediately after engulfment near the cellular plasma membrane. The uncoating of adenoviruses and herpesviruses appears to take place mainly in the vicinity of nuclear pores, the viral DNA thus gaining access into the nucleus.

TRANSPORT TO SITE OF REPLICATION

Following penetration and uncoating, the virion must be transported to a site where the subsequent steps in the replication can take place. For example, adenovirus virions which are taken up by either endocytosis or direct transport across the cell membrane are rapidly moved to the vicinity of nuclear pores. This transport takes place in the cytoplasmic matrix, probably along the network of microtubules. Adenovirus DNA then enters the nucleus through the nuclear pore, while the empty capsid stays outside the nucleus.

SYNTHESIS OF VIRAL mRNA

At the site of replication, the viral genome transcribes viral mRNA. Animal viruses can be divided into six classes according to the mode of duplication of genetic material and a characteristic pattern of genetic information as follows:

Class I: double-stranded DNA viruses (poxvirus, herpesvirus, adenovirus, and papovavirus)

Class II: single-stranded DNA viruses (parvovirus)

Class III: double-stranded RNA viruses (reovirus)

Class IV: plus-stranded RNA viruses (picorna and togavirus)

Class V: minus-stranded RNA viruses (orthomyxovirus, paramyxovirus, and rhabdovirus)

Class VI: RNA viruses with DNA intermediate (retrovirus)

Only the RNA genome of class IV viruses can act as mRNA. In all other classes of viruses, mRNA must be newly synthesized from the viral genome. For the synthesis of mRNA, viral encoded enzymes are required if the host cell cannot provide the appropriate enzyme. Pox-, orthomyxo-, paramyxo-, rhabdo-, reo-, and retroviruses contain the virion-associated polymerases for the transcription.

The synthesized mRNA is spliced after its synthesis. A spliced RNA is defined as a covalently continuous RNA molecule composed of sequences that are encoded in separate regions of a DNA genome. The RNA sequence that is colinear with a DNA sequence is referred to as a colinear transcript. Thus, the spliced RNA is composed of two or more colinear transcripts. The splicing of mRNA has been shown to occur in SV40 and adenovirus.

SYNTHESIS OF VIRAL PROTEINS

The major function of viral mRNA is as a template for the synthesis of viral proteins. Viral proteins are usually referred to as structural and nonstructural proteins. Structural proteins are found on purified virions, and nonstructural proteins are found in infected cells but not as virion proteins or precursors to virion proteins. Some DNA viral genes are expressed during the early phase of replication while other genes are expressed during the late phase. In general, enzymes needed for nucleic acid replication and proteins that inhibit the host cell's macromolecular synthesis are early proteins. The capsid proteins and envelope proteins are synthesized during the late phase of replication. Viral proteins are synthesized in the cytoplasm, utilizing cellular protein-synthesizing machinery.

REPLICATION OF VIRION NUCLEIC ACID

Viral nucleic acids are synthesized in the nucleus or in the cytoplasm. In general, DNA replication takes place in the nucleus (except for poxvirus) and RNA replication in the cytoplasm. Viral infected cells show inclusion bodies, which are structures in the nucleus or cytoplasm of cells infected with viruses when observed under microscope. The location or staining characteristics of inclusion bodies sometimes differ among viruses. For instance, poxvirus inclusion bodies are found in the cytoplasm, while herpesvirus inclusion bodies are found in the nucleus. The rabies inclusion bodies called Negri bodies are found in the cytoplasm and the measle inclusion bodies occur in both cytoplasm and nucleus. Both herpesvirus and adenovirus inclusion bodies occur in the nucleus, but the former is eosinophilic while the latter is basophilic.

ASSEMBLY AND MATURATION

Assembly refers to the formation of the capsid around the viral genome or encapsidation of the viral nucleic acid. Maturation refers to the genesis of progeny virions. Assembly and maturation are the same events for naked virions, but the nucleocapsid of an enveloped virion must obtain an envelope for maturation. After the synthesis of individual components of the virion, they are transported to the site of nucleocapsid assembly. The nucleocapsid assembly of most DNA viruses takes place in the nucleus, whereas the final assembly of RNA-containing nucleocapsids occurs in the cytoplasm. Little is known about the regulation of intracellular transport of the newly synthesized viral proteins. In general, the assembly of viral components is an autocatalytic process that does not require the mediation of enzymes.

RELEASE AND ENVELOPMENT

After the assembly and maturation processes, the nucleocapsids of naked viruses accumulate in the cells, and then most are released simultaneously in a relatively short period of time. In contrast, the enveloped viruses are released one by one as they mature. During the late phase of replication, the enveloped viral nucleic acids express glycoproteins, which are inserted into the cell membrane. The assembled nucleocapsid moves toward the area of the cell membrane containing viral glycoproteins. These regions loop out (reverse phagocytosis) and by doing so include the nucleocapsids. The loop is eventually pinched off from the membrane and an enveloped virion is released from the cell. Replication of enveloped viruses often is not cytocidal, so that the host cell may survive for a while and continuously produce progeny virus.

Diagnosis of Viral Diseases

Viruses are detected, identified, and quantitated by various methods. Specific diagnosis of virus infection is important for the practicing physician by delineating an etiologic agent for the observed illness.

DETERMINATION OF VIRAL ANTIBODIES

Although a certain virus is isolated from a patient, it does not always prove an etiologic relationship to the illness. Therefore, the patient's sera must be thoroughly examined for antibody determination during the acute and convalescent period of illness. An acute-phase serum is obtained when the patient is first seen, hopefully within 7 days after the onset of disease, and the convalescent specimen is drawn 2 to 3 weeks later. The serum must be kept in a refrigerator or freezer.

When the specimens are received by the laboratory, the antibody levels of the viruses are measured by a neutralization method, a hemagglutination inhibition (HI) test, or a complement fixation (CF) test. In viral infection, the antibody titer is risen by fourfold or greater when serial twofold dilutions of serum are employed in these test procedures.

1. *Neutralization test:* Since neutralizing antibodies are highly specific for virus type, this test is an extremely accurate and sensitive method for the determination of specific viral antibodies. Neutralizing antibodies appear early in the course of illness and persist for a long period of time thereafter. The patient serum is incubated with the suspected virus and is then placed into the appropriate cell culture system. The presence of neutralizing antibodies will prevent the cytopathic effect of suspected virus.

2. *Hemagglutination inhibition (HI) test:* This test is limited for the determination of viruses that possess hemagglutinin, including influenza, mumps, measles, the parainfluenzae, rubella, variola, arboviruses, reoviruses, some adenoviruses, and some echoviruses. These viruses cause certain types of red cells to clump together, or hemagglutinate. If antibody is added to the virus, hemagglutination is inhibited. In the HI test, each dilution is mixed with virus, and the mixtures are added to red blood cells to ascertain the highest dilution that prevents hemagglutination. This test is very sensitive and type-specific.

3. *Complement fixation (CF) test:* This test is a rapid and efficient method of screening a number of viral antibodies. In general, antibodies detected are group-specific, but not type-specific. For example, herpes simplex virus antibodies are distinguished from the adenovirus antibodies, but antibodies to herpes simplex virus type 1 cannot be distinguished from antibodies to herpes simplex virus type 2. Complement fixation antibodies disappear earlier than neutralizing antibodies.

DETERMINATION OF VIRAL ANTIGEN

Recently, new methods such as ELISA (enzyme-linked immunoabsorbent assays), RIA (radioimmunoassays), immunoprecipitation, and immunoelectrophoresis have begun to be applied for the determination of viral antigen in clinical specimens. The introduction of monoclonal antibodies tremendously increases the sensitivity and specificity of viral antigen determination.

1. *ELISA:* This assay is an extremely sensitive technique, in which viral antigen is immobilized on some surface, such as the wells of plastic microtiter plate or metal beads, and the test serum is added to allow the formation of antigen-antibody complex. Then antiglobulin coupled with alkaline phosphatase or peroxidase attaches to the bound antigen-antibody complex. Following extensive washing, substrate (e.g., p-nitrophenyl phosphate) is added to induce visible color change, which can be determined with spectrophotometry. This technique is more than 100 times more sensitive than the complement fixation test.

2. *Immunofluorescence:* This technique has been used for the rapid determination of viral infections such as respiratory tract infections and vesicular exanthem. The cells obtained from the viral lesions are examined by indirect immunofluorescence for the presence of viruses.

3. *Determination of viral nucleic acids and proteins:* After immobilizing viral DNA, RNA, or proteins in nitrocellulose paper, the nucleic acids or proteins can be detected with enzyme or radiolabeled probe. This method is extremely sensitive and is the backbone of molecular biology research.

CELL CULTURES AND QUANTITATION OF VIRUS

Laboratory specimens can be cultured into monolayer cells to isolate viruses. Most viruses replicate, damage, and eventually kill the infected cells, which is called the cytopathic effect (CPE) of virus and can be readily examined under light microscope (Fig. 22–6). Numerous types of CPE can occur including rounding of cells, cell swelling, and fusion of several cells into a syncytium. Adenovirus CPE are grape-like clusters of rounded, refractile cells that have intranuclear inclusions when stained with hematoxylin and eosin. The amount of infectious virus is determined in many different ways, such as plaque formation assay, pock formation assay, focus formation assay, and the serial dilution endpoint method.

Plaque Formation Assay

This is the fundamental assay technique for the determination of viral infectivity, and it is also of great value in viral diagnosis. It is highly reproducible, accurate, and extremely simple. When virions infect the monolayer cells, progeny viruses are produced, released, and then infect adjoining cells. This process will eventually allow one to see the

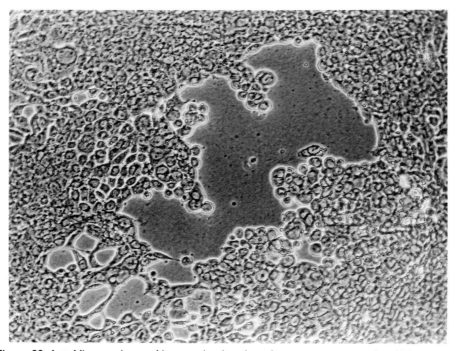

Figure 22–6 ■ Microanatomy of herpes simplex virus plaque on green monkey kidney cells.

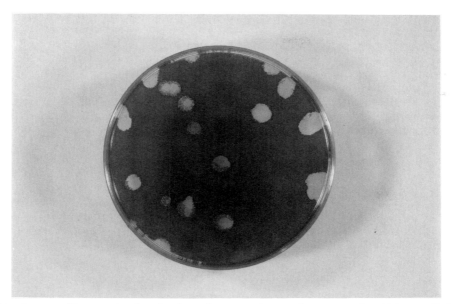

Figure 22–7 ■ Plaques of herpes simplex virus type 1 on monolayers of green monkey kidney cells, 3 days after inoculation. The monolayers were stained with crystal violet.

infected area with the naked eye. These infected areas are called "plaques." To ensure that progeny virus particles liberated into the medium do not diffuse away and initiate separate plaques, agar or specific antiserum is incorporated into the culture medium. This assay technique is most widely used in virology laboratory for the titration of viruses and the units are expressed as plaque forming units per milliliter (PFU/ml) (Fig. 22–7).

Pock Formation Assay

When the chorionic epithelium of the chorioallantoic membrane of a chick embryo is infected by certain viruses, macroscopically recognizable foci (pocks) appear. The pocks appear after 36 to 72 hours as opaque white or red areas caused by cell disintegration, migration, and proliferation on the transparent chorioallantoic membrane. This assay is readily available, and numerous viruses such as herpes simplex virus and poxvirus produce the pocks.

Focus Formation Assay

Instead of producing plaques, many tumor viruses change the morphology of the infected cells and allow these cells to grow faster than uninfected cells. The transformed cells develop into foci that gradually become large enough to be observable by the naked eye.

Serial Dilution End-Point Method

Serial dilutions of virus are inoculated into monolayer cells and cultured in the cells until the CPE of virus is observable. The highest dilution of virus with the induction of the CPE becomes the titer of the virus. This method of viral titration is extremely accurate and also is useful in titrating virus in laboratory animals.

Effect of Viruses on Host Cells

The effect of viruses on cells can be very diverse causing lytic infections, persistent infections (chronic, slow, and latent infections), transformations, and induction of interferon.

LYTIC INFECTION

Lytic cytopathic effects of viruses are easily observed during the course of productive viral infection in tissue culture. Microscopically, the shape of cells is changed (e.g., cell rounding or cell fusion). The mechanism of morphologic cellular alterations by viral infections is not completely known. Many different events may contribute to the development of cytopathic changes and cell death.

1. An inhibition of host cell DNA, RNA,

and protein synthesis may occur during the lytic infection.

2. Some virion proteins may exert toxic effects on the host cell.

3. Activation of lysosomal enzymes may occur in cells infected with some viruses.

4. The normal ionic environment inside cells may be altered with increased intracellular Na concentration because of the inhibition of Na^+-K^+ pump by the lytic viral infection.

PERSISTENT INFECTIONS

Following infection some viruses persist in some cells for long periods of time or for life. There are three forms of persistent infections: chronic infections, latent infections, and slow viral infections. In chronic infections, viral infections are easily detectable. The individual is considered a carrier of the viral disease. In latent infections the virus goes into hiding after the primary infection and later is activated by certain factors leading to recurrent viral diseases. For example, herpes simplex virus induces primary herpes stomatitis or nonsymptomatic primary infectious diseases followed by the establishment of latent infection in autonomic or sensory neuronal ganglia. This latent herpes simplex virus is reactivated, leading to recurrent herpes labialis. One of the best examples of slow viral infections is systemic sclerosing panencephalitis (SSPE). SSPE is a disease of children and adolescents that occurs some years after recovery from measles.

TRANSFORMATION

Some viral infections may convert normal cells into transformed or tumorigenic cells. Cell transformation is characterized by a hereditary change from the normal phenotype to the transformed phenotype. Both DNA (papovaviruses, adenoviruses, and herpesviruses) and RNA (retroviruses) viruses cause malignant transformation of cells in culture and produce tumors on injection into some animals. Transformation by most DNA viruses occurs in the absence of virus multiplication.

INDUCTION OF INTERFERON

Viral infections induce the biosynthesis of interferon, which is a glycoprotein. Inter-

feron is synthesized in the viral infected cells and produces antiviral activity in secondary cells by inducing synthesis of new proteins, which makes these cells resistant to viral infection. A detailed mechanism of action of interferon in its antiviral activity will be discussed later.

Host Response to Viral Infections

Upon viral infection, the host responds immunologically with antibody and cell-mediated immune responses and nonimmunologically.

ANTIBODIES

Antibodies are classic markers of immunity to viruses and play an important role in the control of viral infections. IgA antibodies at the portals of entry (i.e., respiratory, alimentary, and urogenital mucosal surfaces) are important in resistance to reinfection but probably also play a role in resistance and recovery from primary infections. Both IgM and IgG antibodies are responsible for virus neutralization in serum, while IgA antibodies neutralize viruses on mucosal surfaces. IgM antibodies, as larger molecules, do not enter extravascular tissue spaces to any great extent and are not transmitted to the fetus. IgM antibodies appear earlier than IgG antibodies during primary infections by 1 or 2 days, and thus could be of critical importance in resistance in viral infection. IgE antibodies are present in serum at low concentration. IgE antibodies are known to bind to mast cells via specific receptors. When antigen reacts with the cell-bound IgE, inflammatory mediators are released from the mast cell. However, little is known regarding the response of IgE to viral infections.

CELL-MEDIATED IMMUNITY

Cell-mediated effector mechanisms against viruses are natural killer (NK) cells, antibody-dependent cell-mediated cytotoxicity, delayed-hypersensitivity, and virus-specific cytotoxic T lymphocytes. Human peripheral blood lymphocytes produce a spontaneous lysis of virus-infected cells, and the cells responsible for the lysis are called natural killer (NK) cells. This lysis does not show conventional immunologic specificity and is a natural cytotoxicity. The cytotoxic activity of NK cells is enhanced by interferon and interleukin-2 (IL-2). Among the peripheral blood lymphocytes, K (killer) cells lyse the cells bearing IgG antibody on the surface. This phenomenon is called antibody-dependent cell-mediated cytotoxicity (ADCC). Delayed hypersensitivity is an inflammatory reaction in tissues characterized by infiltration with activated macrophages at the site where antigen is present. The sensitized T cells produce numerous mediators responsible for the activation of macrophages. Delayed hypersensitivity plays an important role in host resistance to viral infections. In many viral infections, virus-specific T cells appear to be of critical significance in recovery from infection. For instance, patients with thymic aplasia are unable to limit poxvirus infections and develop measles giant cell pneumonia without a rash. Virus-specific cytotoxic T cells have been demonstrated in both acute and persistent infections in humans.

NONIMMUNOLOGIC FACTORS

Fever, interferon, and genetic factors are nonimmunologic factors which convey resistance to viral infection. The role of interferon will be discussed in the section on antiviral therapy. Fever may play an important role in host resistance because (1) elevated body temperature can produce a decrease in viral replication in target tissue, (2) elevated body temperature can prevent otherwise fatal herpes simplex viral infection in puppies, and (3) certain viral strains grow slowly and poorly in tissue cultures at high temperature.

Herpesviruses

Herpesviruses are the most ubiquitous communicable infectious viruses in humans. Herpes virion is enveloped, has double-stranded DNA and icosahedral nucleocapsid, replicates in the cell nucleus, and acquires its envelope from the inner nuclear membrane. The size of naked virion is approximately 110 nm and, with envelopes, 180 to 250 nm. Infection with herpesviruses can be either productive or nonproductive, which can result in acute infection or latent and recurrent infection. Some human herpesviruses are oncogenic. There are four known human herpesviruses: herpes simplex virus (HSV) types

I and II, cytomegalovirus (CMV), Epstein-Barr virus (EBV), and varicella-zoster virus (VZV).

HERPES SIMPLEX VIRUS (HSV)

HSV virion consists of four major architectural and structural components: core (DNA), capsid, teguments (fibrillar substance), and envelope. HSV DNA is double stranded and its molecular weight is approximately 100 million daltons. The DNA consists of two unique regions flanked by inverted repeat sequences. Type 1 HSV (HSV-1) and type 2 HSV (HSV-2) share many common antigens and are about 50 percent genetically homologous. Three classes of viral proteins—alpha (immediate early), beta (early), and gamma (late) proteins—are translated in a cascade manner during HSV replication. Alpha proteins are necessary for the synthesis of beta proteins. Beta proteins in turn are needed for the production of gamma proteins. DNA replication is done in a semiconservative manner (Fig. 22–8).

Pathogenesis and Clinical Diseases Caused by HSV

HSV commonly attacks mucosa, skin, eyes, and the nervous system. In immunocompromised persons and neonates, HSV also involves the liver and lungs. Primary infection may or may not be clinically evident: from 88 to 99 percent of primary oral infections with HSV are asymptomatic. After the primary infection, the virus ascends sensory or autonomic nerves at the site of the primary infection and persists in neuronal ganglia that innervate the site as latent HSV (Fig. 22–9). In response to various stimuli such as exposure to ultraviolet light, trauma, fever, hormonal imbalance, stress, steroids, and cancer chemotherapy, the latent virus is reactivated, grows in the neuron, travels back down the nerves, and causes recurrent viral lesions in the initially infected area. Antibodies and cell-mediated responses may not affect the frequency of recurrences, but do limit subsequent infections to local extension or viremic spread.

HSV is the most ubiquitous communicable infectious virus in humans and causes a wide variety of chronically recurring diseases:

1. Recurrent herpes labialis, usually due to HSV-1, afflicts approximately one third of the world's population with one half of them

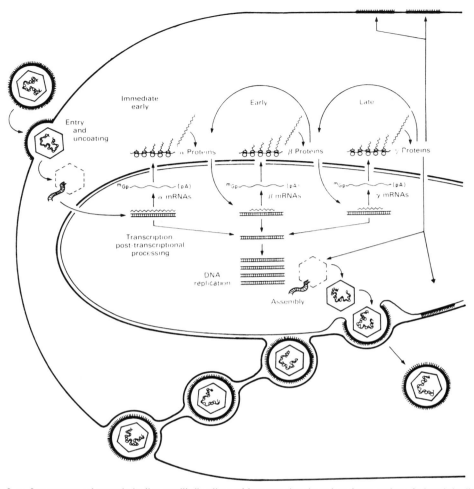

Figure 22–8 ■ Sequence of events in the multiplication of herpes simplex virus from entry of virus into the cell by fusion of the virion envelope with the cell plasma membrane to assembly of virions and their exit from the cell through the endoplasmic reticulum. (From Davis, B. D. et al. (eds): Microbiology. Harper and Row, Philadelphia, 1980, p. 1065, with permission.)

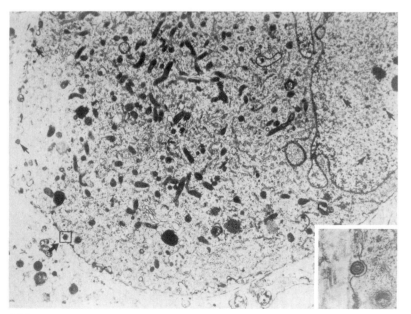

Figure 22–9 ■ Electron microgram of a sectioned trigeminal ganglion from a mouse sacrificed 30 days after oral HSV-1 inoculation. The ganglion was cultured in vitro for 4 days to reactivate latent HSV-1. Typical; HSV particles are seen within nucleus and outside of the cellular membrane (arrows). Magnification × 15,700. Complete herpes virion is in inset (Magnification × 47,000). (From Park, N. H., et al: Oral Surg 53:256, 1982, with permission.)

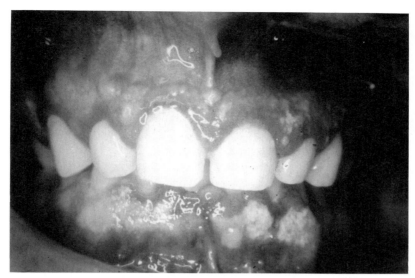

Figure 22–10 ■ Primary herpes gingivostomatitis. Note the gingival vesicles at the attached gingiva. (Courtesy of G. Shklar.)

suffering multiple attacks annually (Figs. 22–10 and 22–11).

2. Herpes genitalis, caused by both HSV-1 and HSV-2 although predominated by HSV-2, is the most common genital disease in women, and second only to syphilis as the genital lesion in men. At least 100,000 cases of herpes genitalis are reported each year in the United States.

3. Ocular HSV infection, due primarily to HSV-1 but occasionally to HSV-2, is the leading cause of blindness due to corneal infection in the United States. Approximately 500,000 cases of primary or recurrent ocular

herpetic diseases are reported annually in the United States (Fig. 22–12).

4. Herpes encephalitis is the most common acute sporadic viral disease of the brain in the United States. It is a devastating process, with mortality in excess of 50 per cent and severe complications in over 80 percent. HSV-1 is the usual culprit in adults and HSV-2 in neonates. HSV-1 appears to spread directly by neural routes and HSV-2 by hematogenous routes.

5. The primary HSV attack in neonates and immunologically compromised patients such as those with leukemia, organ-trans-

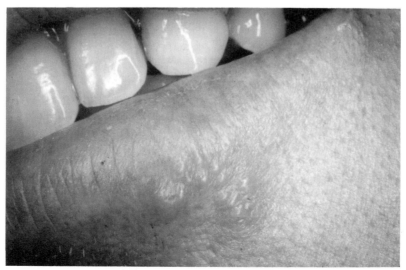

Figure 22–11 ■ Recurrent herpes labialis (RHL). RHL usually occurs at the mucocutaneous junctions and results from the reactivation of latent virus. (Courtesy of L. Gangarosa.)

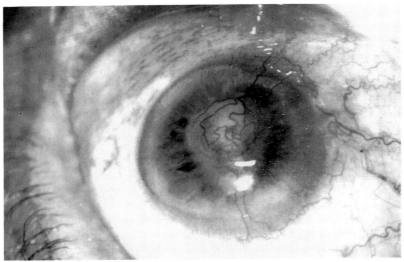

Figure 22–12 ■ Herpetic keratitis caused by HSV-1. There is a growth of capillaries into the cornea (conjunctival injection) and haziness of stoma. (Courtesy of D. Pavan-Langston.)

plant recipients, and patients with acquired immunodeficiency syndrome (AIDS) is associated with a high degree of mortality and morbidity.

Latency and Recurrence of HSV Infections

Between the episodes of disease, HSV remains in the regional sensory ganglia as latent HSV. Mostly HSV-1 remains in the trigeminal ganglia and HSV-2 remains in the sacral ganglia. Latent virus in the ganglionic cells may exist as nonreplicating, truly latent entities. Therefore, demonstration of the presence of the virus in the ganglia requires organ culture of ganglionic tissue. The presence of viral DNA, virus specific RNA, and some viral proteins, however, is demonstrated in latently infected ganglia. Although the detailed aspects of recurrent HSV infection are relatively unknown, the ganglionic latent HSV serves as the source of virus in the recurrent disease. Recurrent disease can be induced by various stimuli, including fever, menstruation, exposure to sunlight, and emotional stress (Fig. 22–11).

Laboratory Diagnosis of HSV Infections

The quickest and most economic test for the diagnosis of HSV infection is to demonstrate multinuclear giant cells, containing intranuclear eosinophilic inclusion bodies, in scrapings from the base of vesicles. However, this procedure does not distinguish HSV infection from infections caused by cytomegalovirus or varicella zoster virus. Virions can be determined by an electron microscopic examination, and specific HSV antigens can be detected in cells from the lesion by immunofluorescence. Virus can also be isolated by inoculating vesicular fluid or scrapings into susceptible culture cells. Finally, a rise in HSV antibody can be determined by serologic tests from serum obtained early in the primary disease and again 14 to 21 days after onset (paired sera).

CYTOMEGALOVIRUS (CMV)

CMV is antigenetically distinct from other herpesviruses and has a very narrow host range, being nearly species-specific. In vitro, CMV grows more readily in fibroblasts than in epithelial or lymphoid cells. Replication of CMV is slow and inefficient. CMV causes latent infections in epithelial cells of kidney, salivary glands, and certain leukocytes.

Pathogenesis

Transmission of CMV occurs via various routes—through congenital infection, close sexual or oral contact, and blood transfusion or organ transplantation. The latent CMV can be reactivated during periods of immunosuppression. Primary infection is usually subclinical but in fetuses or immunocompromised individuals can cause severe disease. Like HSV, serum antibody is unimportant in preventing reactivation or limiting spread of infection, but cell-mediated immunity may be critical in the latter. CMV also suppresses the cell-mediated immunity of the host, and by so doing may increase the susceptibility of transplant recipients or patients with AIDS to infectious and neoplastic complications, i.e., *Pneumocystis carinii* pneumonia and Kaposi's sarcoma.

Clinical Diseases Associated With CMV

CMV also causes numerous clinical diseases:

1. Congenital CMV infection causes cytomegalic inclusion disease. One out of every 100 neonates in the United States excretes CMV in urine. A small percentage (1 percent) exhibits severe CNS malformation, hepatosplenomegaly, petechiae, or chorioretinitis. Others will exhibit subtle abnormalities of hearing mentation that may not be appreciated for several years. The majority of infected infants are asymptomatic.

2. CMV mononucleosis results from primary infection by CMV in healthy young adults. This is characterized by prolonged fever, malaise, abnormal liver function, and peripheral blood mononucleosis.

3. Most renal transplant recipients excrete CMV after the transplantation. Many have subclinical syndromes often with leukopenia or pneumonia.

4. Kaposi's sarcoma, a vascular tumor that is observed in AIDS patients, renal transplant recipients, and young male homosexuals, may be associated with CMV.

Laboratory Diagnosis of CMV Infection

The most sensitive method to detect an infection is virus isolation in human embryonic fibroblast cultures. Characteristic cytomegalic cells with intranuclear and cytoplasmic inclusions can be identified from the urinary sediment or bronchial and gastric washings. Furthermore, CMV antibodies can be determined by immunofluorescence, indirect hemagglutination, and complement fixation.

EPSTEIN-BARR VIRUS (EBV)

EBV was discovered in 1964 by Epstein, Barr, and Achong in electronmicroscopic examination of lymphoblasts from a patient with Burkitt's lymphoma. EBV was suggested to be the causative agent of infectious mononucleosis in 1968. EBV is antigenically unrelated to other human herpesviruses. It only infects B cells in vitro and can also establish latent infections in B cells. EBV may persist in peripheral blood lymphocytes for years after infection. EBV may also infect certain epithelial cells of the white, hairy tongue in patients with AIDS or AIDS-related condition (ARC) or of the nasopharynx. Infected B cells may undergo blast transformation and go into long-term culture ("immortalization").

Pathogenesis

EBV infections are extremely common; over 90 per cent of adults have antibody to EBV. Infection is acquired primarily by oral-oral contact (mononucleosis has been called the "kissing disease") and less commonly through blood transfusion. EBV may be excreted into saliva during mononucleosis and for weeks thereafter. Primary infection in children is usually asymptomatic, but in young adults, it is often manifest as infectious mononucleosis.

Clinical Diseases Associated With EBV

EBV induces lymphoproliferative disorders:

1. Infectious mononucleosis is caused by EBV primary infection in young adults. The virus replicates in the oropharynx for long periods and the individual continues to be infectious. The incubation period of infectious mononucleosis is 4 to 7 weeks and the characteristic clinical picture consists of fever, pharyngitis, and cervical lymphadenopathy, accompanied by splenomegaly, swollen eyes, and palatal petechiae. Differentiation from CMV and other causes of mononucleosis can be made by the determination of heterophile antibody. Infectious mononucleosis may last for weeks but is usually benign and self-limiting.

2. Seroepidemiologic, molecular biologic, and animal studies have shown that certain cancers (e.g., Burkitt's lymphoma and nasopharyngeal carcinoma) are associated with EBV. EBV may also cause progressive B-cell lymphoproliferative disease in immunocompromised people and may be associated with primary cerebral lymphomas.

3. A number of neurologic syndromes (e.g., Guillain's syndrome, Bell's palsy, meningoencephalitis, and transverse myelitis) may be related to EBV.

4. Recently some studies have indicated that EBV virions are found in white, hairy tongues of patients with AIDS or healthy homosexuals.

Laboratory Diagnosis of EBV Infection

The practical laboratory diagnosis rests upon finding abnormal, large lymphocytes and heterophile antibodies. However, the specific diagnosis can be only made by determination of elevated antibody to early antigens and to the viral capsid proteins.

VARICELLA-ZOSTER VIRUS (VZV)

VZV is relatively unstable and has limited host range but replicates in a variety of human and monkey cells in vitro.

Pathogenesis

VZV enters the body through the respiratory route. After an incubation period of 2 weeks in which viremia and local replication occur, cutaneous vesicles develop. In a normal host, humoral and cell-mediated immune mechanisms limit the spread of the disease. However, dissemination may continue and visceral organs may become involved in an immunocompromised individual. During the primary infection, VZV migrates to the dorsal root ganglia along the sensory nerves and establishes latent infection in the ganglia. In zoster, the latent virus is reactivated and travels down sensory nerves to the skin, where clusters of vesicles occur.

Clinical Diseases Caused by VZV

The primary infection of VZV is called varicella, or chicken pox. Varicella may be preceded by a 1- to 2-day prodrome of fever, headache, malaise, and anorexia. The rash evolves rapidly in crops mainly on the trunk. Primary varicella is more severe in adults, in whom it is frequently accompanied by pneumonia. The infection is highly communicable, and occurs most commonly in winter and spring.

Recurrent infection of VZV is called shingles, or zoster. In contrast to varicella, zoster shows no epidemic or seasonal pattern and is caused by the reactivation of latent virus. It can occur at any age, but the incidence increases sharply in elderly individuals. The zoster eruption is characteristically unilateral. Patients with decreased immune function are more susceptible to developing zoster.

Laboratory Diagnosis of VZV Infection

The typical varicella giant cells and cells with characteristic inclusion bodies can be easily and rapidly detected in smears from the base of vesicles. In addition, virus can be detected by electron microscopic examination and culture.

Hepatitis Viruses

Since Voeght found that hepatitis was transmissible in 1942, the etiologic agents of hepatitis were subsequently found to be filterable and the disease transmitted in two ways—by the intestinal-oral route (infectious hepatitis) and by the injection of infected blood or its products (serum hepatitis). However, the differences in transmission are found not absolute, so that they have been renamed to hepatitis A virus (HAV) for infectious hepatitis and hepatitis B virus (HBV) for serum hepatitis. Furthermore, at least one other hepatitis virus not related to HAV or HBV has been recognized and called hepatitis C virus (or non-A non-B hepatitis virus). The hepatitis C virus is the major cause of hepatitis following transfusions in the United States (Table 22–4; Fig. 22–13).

HEPATITIS A VIRUS (HAV)

HAV virion is similar to picornaviruses and consists of a single-stranded RNA genome and three major polypeptides without envelope. A 27 nm viral particle is found in the stool of patients with viral hepatitis A.

The virus multiplies in the cytoplasm of infected cells and its growth is limited in cell culture. HAV enters the body mainly through the oral route and grows in the gastrointestinal tract. After systemic viremia, the virus spreads to the liver, spleen, and kidneys. By this time HAV virions are detected in the feces, duodenal contents, blood, and urine. HAV has an incubation period of 25 to 30 days from the time of exposure. Patients with the disease may be asymptomatic, with only abnormal liver function or seroconversion. Usually children and young adults are susceptible to HAV infection, especially in the autumn and winter. The danger of HAV dissemination from an infected individual is highest during the last stage of incubation. Since the viral shedding in feces is maximal prior to clinical disease, the virus is very contagious. Type A hepatitis may be prevented by passive immunization with pooled adult gamma-globulin. The gamma-globulin must be given no later than 2 weeks after the exposure.

Table 22–4 ■ Comparison of hepatitis viruses

Characteristics	HAV	HBV	HCV
Size	27 nm	42 nm Dane particle 22 nm surface antigen	Unknown
Nucleic acid	ss RNA	ds DNA	Unknown
Antigen	HA Ag (major antigen)	HBsAg (surface antigen) HBcAg (core antigen) HBeAg (core-related antigen)	Reportedly identified but not confirmed
Antibody	Anti-HA, IgG, IgM	Anti-HBs, anti-HBc, anti-HBe	Reportedly identified but not confirmed
Route of infection	Oral and parenteral	Oral, parenteral, and sexual or maternal-fetal contact	Mainly parenteral
Incubation period	15–45 days (mean 30)	45–150 days (mean 60–90)	15–160 days (mean 50)
Presence of virus in body fluid	Feces, blood, urine	Feces, blood, saliva	Blood
Severity	Mild	Often severe	Moderate
Prognosis	Generally good	Worse with age and debility	Moderate
Immune serum globulin (ISG) prophylaxis	Good	Partial	Unknown
Hepatitis B immune globulin prophylaxis	No	Yes	No
Carrier state	Rare	0.1–1.0%	Exists, but prevalence unknown

HAV = Hepatitis A virus.
HBC = Hepatitis B virus.
HCV = Hepatitis C virus (non-A, non-B hepatitis virus).

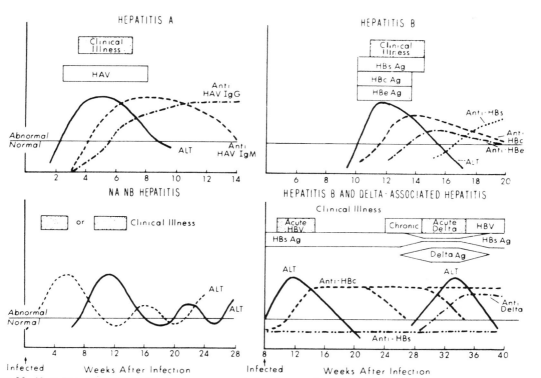

Figure 22–13 ■ The panels illustrate the sequence of development of clinical illness, liver function abnormalities, and hepatitis antigen and antibody for each of the four currently recognized forms of viral hepatitis. (From Jaklik, W. K. (ed.): Virology. Appleton-Century-Crofts, New York, 1985, p. 300, with permission.)

HEPATITIS B VIRUS (HBV)

Serum of patients with clinical hepatitis B contains three different structures: the Dane particle, spherical particle, and filamentous form. The Dane particle is 42 nm in diameter with an electrodense nucleocapsid 27 nm in diameter and is the least common in serum. Spherical particles are 22 nm in diameter and the most abundant. Filamentous particles are also plentiful in serum and are 22 nm in diameter and 50 to 230 nm in length. The Dane particle contains partially double-stranded circular DNA as the genome and two major antigens, the surface antigen (HBsAg) and the core antigen (HBcAg) (Figs. 22–14, 22–15, 22–16, 22–17). Spherical and filamentous particles in the serum only contain HBsAg. The HBcAg is found only in the core of Dane particles. High antibody titers to HBcAg are detected during the early phase of the disease, and these antibodies are consistently present in chronic carriers of HBsAg.

Although HBV mainly enters via the parenteral route, its primary site of replication is unknown. The disease caused by HBV varies from mild to a severe and prolonged disease. The incubation period also varies from a few weeks to 4 months. The clinical signs and symptoms of hepatitis B are similar to those of hepatitis A: jaundice, fever, headache, malaise, anorexia, abdominal pain, nausea, vomiting, serum-sickness like syndrome with arthralgia, skin rashes and arthritis, periarthritis, glomerulonephritis. Although 10 to 20 percent of adult patients and 35 percent of children show HBsAg for extended periods, less than half of them become chronic HBsAg carriers. More than half the chronic HBsAg carriers continuously manifest chronic liver disease. The risk of persistent infection is highest in infants and decreases with age. Infected males are two to three times more likely to become carriers than infected females. The probability of persistent infection is increased in high-risk groups including male homosexuals and persons with immune defects, on immunosuppressive therapy, or with chronic renal disease. Approximately 5 to 10 percent of persons infected with the disease will circulate the HBsAg for a prolonged period of time.

There are a number of tests for detection of HBV antigens, particularly HBsAg. These include radioimmunoassay, complement fixation, immune adherence, and enzyme immunoassays. Although there are sensitive immunologic blood tests for detection of viral carriers, blood transfusions are the major route of viral transmission. Therefore, individuals with a history of jaundice or with detectable HBsAg in the serum should be excluded from being blood donors. HBV is also associated with hepatocarcinoma. The

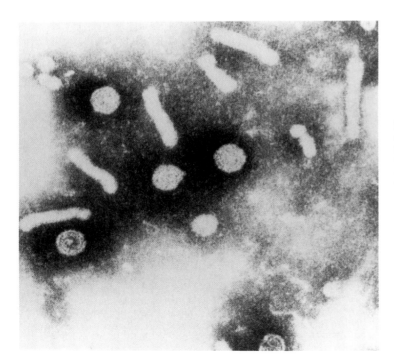

Figure 22–14 ■ Electron micrograph of negatively stained hepatitis B virus Dane particles, filaments, and 22 nm HBsAg particles present in the serum of a patient with active infection. Magnification × 150,000. (Courtesy of J. Gerin, Oak Ridge National Laboratory; from Davis, B. D. et al. (eds.): Microbiology, 3rd ed. Harper and Row, Philadelphia, 1980, p. 1221, with permission.)

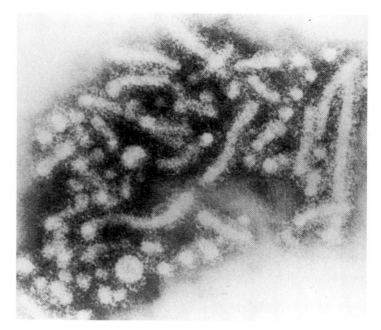

Figure 22–15 ■ Immunoelectron micrograph of Dane particles, filaments, and 22 nm HBsAg particles aggregated by serum from a late-convalescent patient. Magnification × 150,000. (Courtesy of J. Gerin, Oak Ridge National Laboratory; from Davis, B. D. et al. (eds.): Microbiology, 3rd ed. Harper and Row, Philadelphia, 1980, p. 1221, with permission.)

evidence is (1) a close correlation between the geographic distribution of HBV infection and hepatocarcinoma and (2) a high frequency of detection of HBsAg in patients with hepatocarcinoma.

Passive immunization with serum containing high antibody titers to HBs has marginal benefit in high-risk groups. However, inactivated hepatitis B vaccine was effective in a high-risk population of male homosexuals. This was prepared by purification and formalin inactivation of HBsAg collected from the serum of chronic carriers. Following two initial injections one month apart and a booster 6 months later, 96 percent of those vaccinated had acquired anti-HBs and experienced a reduced incidence of hepatitis B greater than 90 percent.

HEPATITIS C VIRUS (NON-A NON-B HEPATITIS VIRUS)

Hepatitis C virus was identified by prospective studies of patients with post-transfusion hepatitis without evidence of hepatitis A or B. The virions of hepatitis C virus are nonenveloped icosahedrons, about 27 nm in diameter, resembling picornaviruses in morphologic and physical characteristics. The hepatitis C virus antigens do not cross-react immunologically with antigens of HAV and HBV.

Recent studies indicate that over 90 percent of post-transfusion hepatitis cases are attributed to hepatitis C virus. Transmission by

means other than blood is still unknown since specific viral antigens have not yet been identified. The incubation period of this virus is 6 to 12 weeks. The clinical manifestations

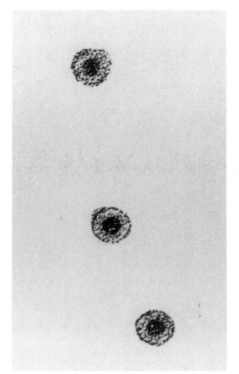

Figure 22–16 ■ Purified Dane particles stained with uranyl acetate to show the DNA core. Magnification × 200,000. (Courtesy of J. Gerin, Oak Ridge National Laboratory; from Davis, B. D. et al. (eds.): Microbiology, 3rd ed. Harper and Row, Philadelphia, 1980, p. 1221, with permission.)

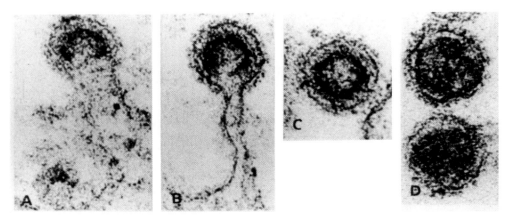

Figure 22–17 ■ Thin sections of type C particles from cells producing a mouse leukosis virus. *A* and *B,* Two phases of budding of the virions at the cell surface. *C,* Detached immature virion, with an electron-lucent nucleoid. *D,* Two mature particles with dense nucleoids. (Courtesy of L. Dmochowski; from Davis, B. D. et al. (eds.): Microbiology, 3rd ed. Harper and Row, 1980, p. 1284, with permission.)

of non-A non-B hepatitis are similar to those of hepatitis A or B. The most important finding in non-A non-B hepatitis research is a strong association between elevated alanine aminotransferase (ALT) levels in donor blood and appearance of non-A non-B hepatitis in the blood recipients. The higher the ALT level in the blood, the greater the risk of transmission of the disease.

HEPATITIS VIRUSES AND HEALTH CARE PROFESSIONALS

Hepatitis viral infection is one of the most serious occupational risks of health care professionals such as dentists, nurses, physicians, and laboratory technicians who have contact with patients and their blood. Hepatitis A outbreaks have occurred in hospitals, but the risk in health care professionals is mainly hepatitis B. The transmission of HBV is usually via blood, saliva, and semen of patients. Although chronically infected professionals can transmit the virus to their patients, the risk of patient transmission to health professionals appears much greater than the reverse. Hepatitis B markers are found in 20 to 40 percent of high risk health care worker groups, in contrast to only 5 percent in the members of general population. Asymptomatic HBsAg-positive carriers represent the greatest risk to health care personnel because there is no readily identifiable clinical feature such as jaundice. Therefore, patients with a past history of hepatitis or multiple blood transfusion, and those with parenteral drug abuse, chronic liver disease, chronic renal failure, leukemia, Hodgkin's

disease, and Down's syndrome must have routine HBsAg determinations because of the high frequency of the HBsAg carrier state in those groups. If positive, they must be treated as potentially infectious, and appropriate precautions must be taken.

In treating dental patients with a history of hepatitis B, dentists and assistants should adhere to aseptic techniques and wear masks and gloves. The handpieces should be either autoclaved or sterilized in a gas sterilizer following use. Usually cold sterilizing solutions are not effective. Nonautoclavable items must be gas sterilized and chairs should be covered with disposable head covers. Furthermore, disposable covers should be placed on the top of the mobile cabinets before and after use. Tray set-ups are advisable for instruments. Although dentists and auxiliaries with a history of hepatitis B have a moral, ethical, and legal obligation to protect their patients, there is insufficient evidence to prevent a health care professional from practicing because of positive antigen-screening tests. However, dentists and assistants must follow aseptic techniques to prevent transmission.

For the prevention and treatment of hepatitis A, immune serum globulin (ISG) containing anti-HAV is administered. When given before exposure or during the early incubation period, ISG is effective in aborting the development of clinical symptoms. For intimate contact with hepatitis A patients, administration of 0.02 ml/kg of ISG is recommended. For travelers to tropical and developing countries, ISG prophylaxis is recommended: 0.02 ml/kg for travel less than 3 months and 0.05 ml/kg every 4 to 6 months for longer travel. For postexposure prophylaxis against hepatitis B, high titer of hepatitis B immune globulin (HBIG) is recommended: 0.05 to 0.07 ml/kg as soon as possible after exposure. Preparations of purified HBsAg have shown to be effective in protecting laboratory animals from hepatitis B infection, but further investigation is needed for use in humans.

Oncogenic Viruses

Since Ellerman and Band in 1908 demonstrated the development of chicken leukemia by cell-free filtrates of other chickens, viruses have been suspected as causative agents of certain tumors in humans and other mammals. The oncogenic viruses are classified into DNA-containing viruses and RNA-containing viruses. DNA-containing oncogenic viruses include papovaviruses, adenoviruses, and herpesviruses. RNA-containing oncogenic viruses include C-type leukosis-sarcoma viruses and B-type (mammary tumor) virus.

PAPOVAVIRUSES (POLYOMA AND PAPILLOMAVIRUSES)

The virions of papovaviruses are naked icosahedrons with a diameter of 45 nm. They contain a circular, double-stranded DNA as genome and are resistant to heat and formalin. The outcome of infection by these viruses may be either productive or nonproductive. The productive infection leads to production of progeny viruses and the nonproductive infection can lead to abortive transformation of the cells. Cells transformed by papovaviruses express two viral proteins related to the transformation—tumor (T) antigen and tumor-specific transplantation antigen (TSTA). Both T and TST antigens are virus-encoded and appear early in the productive viral infection. These viral proteins are identical in cells of different species transformed by the same virus, but differ in transformed cells or tumors induced in the same species by the two different viruses. Neither of these proteins is a structural protein, or associated with the virion. After the adsorption, penetration, and uncoating, the papovaviral DNA enters the nucleus where it starts to transcribe an early mRNA to synthesize early proteins such as T antigen and TSTA. In a nonproductive infection, the viral DNA is then integrated into the cellular DNA

and continuously transcribes early regions of viral DNA to make early proteins. This transformed cell continuously replicates without production of progeny virus. In case of productive infection, late gene products (structural proteins) are produced after the early transcription and translation process. Then virion assembly and cell death follow within 48 hours after the virus infection.

In general, only a fraction of the viral genome is required for the induction of transformation of cells. Radiation treatment or chemical inactivation of viruses increases the oncogenic capacity of the viruses. In case of papovaviruses half of the viral genetic material is involved in the process of transformation. This amount of viral DNA is sufficient to code a single frame for only a few discrete proteins.

Among the papovaviruses, papillomaviruses are closely related with papillomas found in skin and mucous membranes. Papillomaviruses induce epithelial proliferation in animals and humans but cannot propagate in tissue culture. Human papillomavirus (HPV) is known to induce a variety of warts and papillomas in skin and mucous membrane including the oral cavity. In the oral cavity HPV induces verruca, condyloma accuminatum, squamous cell papilloma, and focal epithelial hyperplasia. So far, 25 different HPVs have been identified. Although some papillomas regress spontaneously, some remain for a long period of time and transform to malignant forms after the involvement of other environmental factors such as radiation or trauma.

RETROVIRUSES

Retroviruses are enveloped, ether sensitive, 110 nm in diameter, and contain single-stranded RNA as a genome. The 60 to 70S RNA genome is diploid having two identical molecules of 35S RNA held together near their 5' termini. The most peculiar characteristic of retroviruses is the presence of reverse transcriptase in the virions. Approximately 30 molecules of reverse transcriptase are present in one virion. This enzyme encoded by viral genome is capable of synthesizing complementary DNA (minus strand) from viral RNA and has an exonuclease activity (RNase H) that degrades the RNA strand in RNA-DNA hybrids from the 5' end of the RNA. Cellular tRNA participates in the synthesis of complementary DNA as a primer. The nucleoprotein core is central in viruses in C type morphology, whereas it is eccentric in viruses with B type morphology.

Replication Cycle

Less than 1 hour after viral infection, the complementary viral DNA (minus strand) synthesis begins in the cellular cytoplasm; then the synthesis of plus strand (complementary to the minus strand) begins to make linear double-stranded viral DNA. This linear DNA moves into the nucleus, circularizes, and then is incorporated into cellular DNA as proviral DNA. The linear, circular, and proviral forms of DNA contain a complete genome and are infectious. The replication cycle of retroviruses requires 10 to 12 hours under proper conditions. Cells survive by the productive infections of these viruses. Cells may be transformed or nontransformed with or without the production of progeny viruses (Fig. 22–18).

Transmission

Retroviruses are transmitted by horizontal transmission, congenital transmission, or vertical transmission. Feline leukemia viruses and sarcomaviruses can be transmitted by horizontal transmission, that is, can be acquired from the outside, as infectious agents can. Mammary tumor viruses and avian leukosis viruses are transmitted congenitally.

Vertical transmission is unique to endogenous retroviruses and consists of genetic transmission of proviral DNA in the same manner as any other chromosomal gene of the host.

Evidence for Involvement of Retroviruses in Human Cancers

Human T-cell leukemia, which is endemic to Southeast Japan and West India, is strongly associated with type 1 or 2 human T-cell leukemia virus (HTLV-I or HTLV-II). High antibody titer to HTLV-I or -II is found in all patients with T-cell leukemia, whereas they are absent in healthy individuals. HTLVs are C-type retroviruses. Their viral oncogene has not yet been identified.

AIDS and Human Immunodeficiency Virus (HIV)

Since the late 1970s a number of previously healthy male homosexuals have developed various opportunistic infectious diseases or neoplasms, such as Kaposi's sarcoma, complicating an underlying defect in the cellular immune mechanism. Since these diseases had almost never been seen in immunocompetent individuals, extensive effort has been

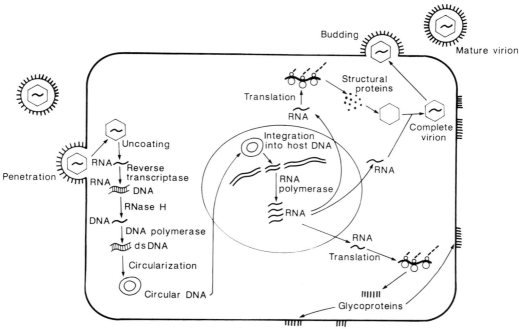

Figure 22–18 ■ Replicative cycle of retrovirus.

given to find the causes of them. Finally, the Centers for Disease Control (CDC) named this syndrome acquired immunodeficiency syndrome (AIDS). AIDS results from the quantitative deficiency of the T-helper cell population.

CLINICAL SIGNS AND SYMPTOMS OF AIDS

CDC defines AIDS as a disease that occurs by a defect in cell-mediated immune function. There is a great variation in the clinical course of AIDS. Many patients have no prodromal symptoms until they show cutaneous Kaposi's sarcoma, life-threatening *Pneumocystis carinii* pneumonia, or cryptococcal meningitis. Some patients, however, experience malaise, weakness, weight loss, oral candidiasis, oral hairy tongue leukoplakia, and diarrhea for several weeks or months before exhibiting the life-threatening opportunistic infectious diseases. Finally, in some patients, the prodromal malaise, fever, and weight loss may last several months or years before a specific opportunistic infection or Kaposi's sarcoma occurs. Some patients also show generalized lymphadenopathy for months or years. Opportunistic infectious diseases under the CDC definition include (1) pneumonia, meningitis, or encephalitis due to aspergillosis, candidiasis, cryptococcus, cytomegalovirus (CMV), herpes simplex virus (HSV), or nocardiosis; (2) esophagitis due to candida, HSV, or CMV; (3) extensive mucocutaneous HSV infections; (4) progressive multifocal leukoencephalopathy; (5) Kaposi's sarcoma; (6) lymphoma limited to the brain; (7) chronic enterocolitis; or (8) central nervous system infection due to coccidiomy-cosis, cryptococcosis, or histoplasmosis. Among these, the most common opportunistic infections in AIDS are *Pneumocystis carinii* pneumonia, disseminated CMV infection, disseminated *Mycobacterium avium-intracellulare*, candidal esophagitis, mucocutaneous HSV infection, cryptococcal meningitis, cerebral toxoplasmosis, and enteric cryptosporidiosis. The most common clinical manifestations in AIDS are fever of unknown origin, weight loss, fatigue, diffuse pneumonia, diarrhea, neurologic disorders, and retinitis (Figs. 22–19, 22–20, and 22–21).

EPIDEMIOLOGIC STUDIES

The CDC reported over 50,000 cases of AIDS in the United States as of the end of 1987. Among them, (1) 72.1 percent are homosexual and bisexual men; (2) 17 percent are heterosexual men or women involved in intravenous drug abuse; (3) 1.5 percent are patients who have had whole blood or blood component transfusion within the past 5 years; (4) 1 percent are heterosexual partners of AIDS patients or of persons at increased risk for AIDS; (5) 1.3 percent are infants and children born to parents who have AIDS, have hemophilia, or have had whole blood transfusion; and (6) 6.4 percent are people with no risk factors. So far, approximately half of the AIDS patients have died. According to the CDC report, certain populations are at increased risk of getting AIDS: promiscuous homosexual males, intravenous drug abusers, hemophiliacs, recent Haitian immigrants, heterosexual contacts of the aforementioned groups, newborns of high-risk mothers, and persons receiving whole blood or blood component transfusion.

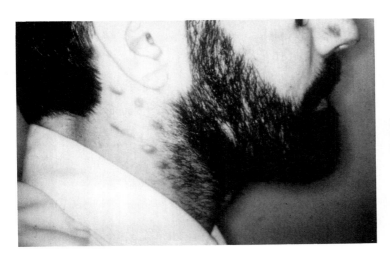

Figure 22–19 ■ Kaposi's sarcoma in the face and neck of an AIDS patient. (Courtesy of F. Lucartoto.)

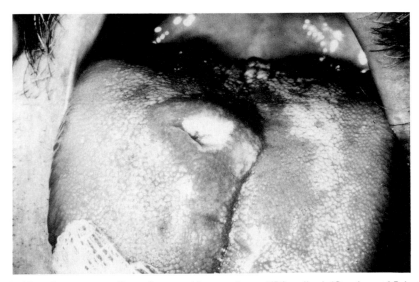

Figure 22–20 ■ Squamous cell carcinoma of tongue in an AIDS patient. (Courtesy of F. Lucartoto.)

Epidemiologic studies have indicated that a transmissible infectious agent must be involved in the development of AIDS. Since a number of viruses capable of suppressing body immune mechanisms, including HSV, CMV, Epstein-Barr virus, hepatitis B virus (HBV), and adenovirus, are frequently found in AIDS patients, these viruses were initially suspected as the causative agents. Recently human immunodeficiency virus (HIV) was isolated frequently in AIDS and pre-AIDS patients. Almost 100 percent of all AIDS sera showed antibody to HIV.

MODE OF TRANSMISSION OF HIV

HIV is transmitted mainly by sexual contact. Although most cases of AIDS are reported in homosexual men, there are documented cases of women acquiring the disease from bisexual men. In these cases, HIV or HIV-infected cells in semen may play a major role in the transmission of disease. Although the initial reports suggested the presence of HIV in the saliva of asymptomatic male homosexuals and AIDS patients, the number of viral particles found there may be very min-

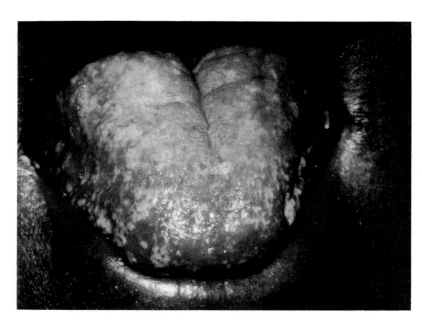

Figure 22–21 ■ Candida albicans of tongue in an AIDS patient. (Courtesy of F. Lucartoto.)

imal. Thus, the possibility of the transmission of HIV through saliva may be negligible.

PROPERTIES OF HIV

Like HTLV-I or -II, HIV is a human T-lymphotropic virus. However, in contrast to HTLV-I or -II, which lead to uncontrolled cell proliferation and leukemias and lymphomas, HIV kills the cells it infects. HIV contains the transactivating transcriptional (tat) gene, which expresses transactivating proteins, an absolutely necessary polypeptide for the replication of the virus (Fig. 22–22).

AIDS AND THE DENTIST

Although HIV is not transmissible through casual contact, occupational exposure of health care workers to HIV has been reported in clinical and laboratory workers. Since dentists and auxiliaries have regular contact with patients' blood and saliva, there is great concern among dental professionals. Further-

more, as of February 1986, the Centers for Disease Control reported that 26 out of 17,115 reported AIDS cases were in dental personnel. However, there is no evidence that health care or laboratory personnel are at significant risk of contracting AIDS as a consequence of their occupation. Precautions for avoiding AIDS closely resemble those recommended for hepatitis B. To minimize the transmission of infection from AIDS patients, dentists must follow recommended procedures:

1. Employment of strict aseptic techniques to exclude all microorganisms from hands, instruments, and treatment area.

2. Treatment of patients with an established barrier, e.g., latex or rubber gloves, gown, mask, and protective eye glasses.

3. Use of disposable materials when possible.

4. Cleansing of instruments in an ultrasonic cleaner for 3 minutes, rinsing three times in clean water, bagging in autoclave bags, and sterilizing in formaldehyde at 25 lbs for 25 minutes.

5. Sterilization of nonautoclavable items in

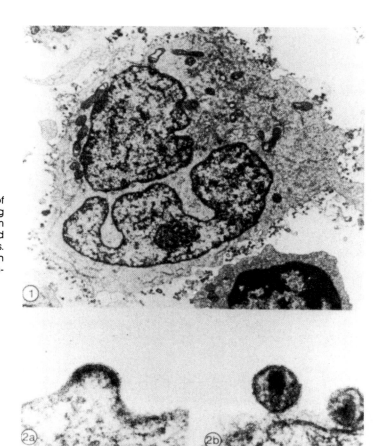

Figure 22–22 ■ Electron micrograph of HIV-infected cells *(1)*, showing the budding virus *(2a)* and mature virion *(2b)*. (From Sarngadharan, M. G., Markham, P. D., and Gallo, R. C.: Human T-cell leukemia viruses. In Fields, B. N., et al. (eds.): Virology. Raven Press, New York, 1985, p. 1360, with permission.)

glutaraldehyde or iodophor disinfectant for 7 hours.

6. Cleansing and disinfecting of the dental unit and chair by wiping with a 1:5 dilution of 5.25 percent sodium hypochlorite solution followed several minutes later with 70 percent alcohol containing 2 percent betadine solution.

7. Control of patient's blood and saliva. Use of rubber dam, high-speed evacuation during use of a high-speed air turbine handpiece and the judicious use of air/water syringe is recommended.

8. Use of resuscitation bags or disposable devices for mouth-to-mouth CPR must be available in dental office.

Antiviral Therapy

During the last two decades, a number of potent and selective antiviral agents have been introduced. Among the viruses, herpesviruses are particularly susceptible to chemotherapeutic agents. Since herpesviruses—especially herpes simplex virus (HSV)—are the most ubiquitous, communicable, and infectious viruses in humans and are the etiologic agents of a wide variety of chronically recurring diseases, herpesviruses are generally among the first to be studied when new antiviral agents are developed.

To date, only five antiviral agents have been approved for clinical use by the Food and Drug Administration: (1) amantadine HCl (1-adamantanamine hydrochloride, Symmetrel) for the prophylaxis and treatment of influenza A viral infections; (2) idox-uridine (5-iodo-2'-deoxyuridine, iododeoxy-uridine, IDU, Herpelex) for the topical treatment of herpes keratitis; (3) vidarabine (Ara-A, Vira-A) for the topical treatment of herpes keratitis and systemic treatment of herpes encephalitis; (4) trifluridine (5-trifluorothym-idine, Viroptic) for the topical treatment of herpes keratitis; and (5) acyclovir (9-[(2-hydroxyethoxy) methyl] guanine, ACV, Zovi-rax) for topical and systemic treatment of primary and recurrent herpes genitalis, mucocutaneous herpes infection and other herpes infections in immune compromised patients. All these drugs except amantadine HCl act on herpes infections (Table 22–5).

AMANTADINE HCl

Amantadine HCl interferes with the early interaction of influenza viruses with the cell membrane; it blocks the penetration and uncoating processes. Amantadine is approximately 60 percent effective as a prophylactic agent against influenza A strains. Side effects of amantadine include tremor, instability of motion, frank ataxia, inability to concentrate, insomnia, and slurred speech. Amantadine has been used more extensively as an agent in the treatment of Parkinson's disease than in the prophylaxis of influenza A (Fig. 22–23).

IDOXURIDINE

Idoxuridine is effective in the treatment of superficial herpes keratitis. Recurrences of

Table 22–5 ■ Comparison of antiviral agents

Name	Antiviral Spectrum	Mechanism of Action	Clinical Uses
Amantadine HCl	Influenza A virus	Blocking the penetration and uncoating process	Prophylaxis of influenza A infection
Idoxuridine	HSV-1 and HSV-2	Inhibition of DNA synthesis	Treatment of herpetic keratitis
Vidarabine	HSV-1 and HSV-2	Inhibition of DNA synthesis	Treatment of herpetic keratitis and encephalitis
Trifluridine	HSV-1 and HSV-2	Inhibition of DNA synthesis	Treatment of herpetic keratitis
Acyclovir	HSV-1 and HSV-2	Inhibition of DNA synthesis (selective to virus)	Treatment of herpes genitalis and encephalitis
Ganciclovir	HSV-1, HSV-2, CMV, and VZV	Inhibition of DNA synthesis (selective to virus)	Not approved by the FDA
Azidothymidine	HIV	Inhibition of viral cDNA synthesis	AIDS (acquired immunodeficiency syndrome)
Interferon	All viruses	Inhibition of viral protein synthesis	Certain systemic primary viral infections

HSV-1 = Herpex simplex virus type 1.
HSV-2 = Herpes simplex virus type 2.
CMV = Cytomegalovirus.
VZV = Varicella zoster virus.
HIV = Human immunodeficiency virus.
cDNA = Complementary DNA.

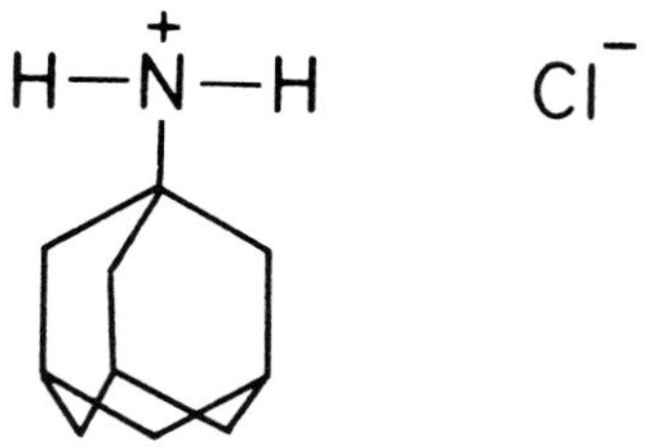

Figure 22–23 ■ Chemical structure of amantadine HCl.

Adenosine   Vidarabine

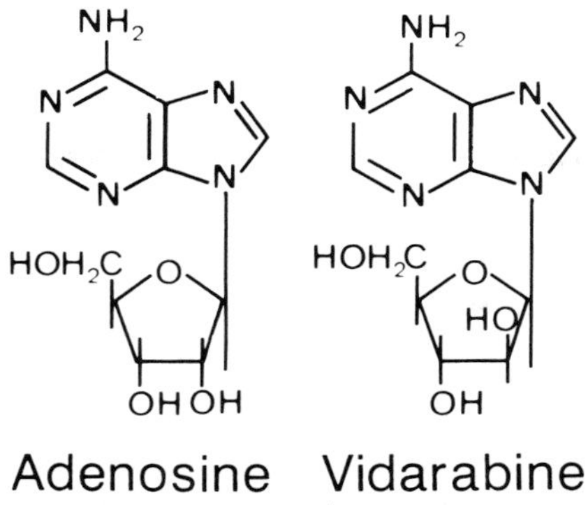

Figure 22–25 ■ Chemical structure of adenosine and vidarabine.

the disease and drug resistance are problems. The effectiveness of idoxuridine against recurrent herpes labialis and genitalis has not been established. Idoxuridine is a possible mutagenic, teratogenic, and carcinogenic substance. In cells, idoxuridine is metabolized to mono-, di-, and triphosphate forms. They competitively inhibit the activity of thymidine kinase, thymidylate kinase, and DNA polymerase. Thus, idoxuridine inhibits the synthesis of viral and cellular DNA. Furthermore, idoxuridine is incorporated into cellular and viral DNA, and makes defective DNA. Therefore, idoxuridine does not specifically attack the infected cells. Idoxuridine is known to increase the replication of retroviruses in transformed cells and to produce toxic effects in normal cells. Recently idoxuridine was found to activate the latently infected human immunodeficiency virus in vitro (Fig. 22–24).

VIDARABINE

Vidarabine has a broad spectrum of antiviral activity. It is active against herpes simplex virus, poxviruses, retroviruses, and rhabdoviruses. Vidarabine is metabolized in

cells to vidarabine mono-, di-, and triphosphate. Vidarabine diphosphate and triphosphate are responsible for the antiherpes activity by inhibiting the activity of viral and cellular ribonucleotide reductase and DNA polymerase. Thus, vidarabine does not show specific selectivity. It was first approved for the treatment of herpes keratitis. Subsequently, it was shown to improve the mortality and morbidity among patients with herpes encephalitis. Side effects of vidarabine are anorexia, nausea, vomiting, weight loss, weakness, and bone marrow depression (Fig. 22–25).

TRIFLURIDINE

Trifluridine is fluorinated thymidine derivative (Fig. 22–26) and a potent antiherpetic agent. It has an antiviral effect against DNA viruses such as herpes simplex virus types 1 and 2. Trifluridine is phosphorylated to become trifluridine monophosphate by thymi-

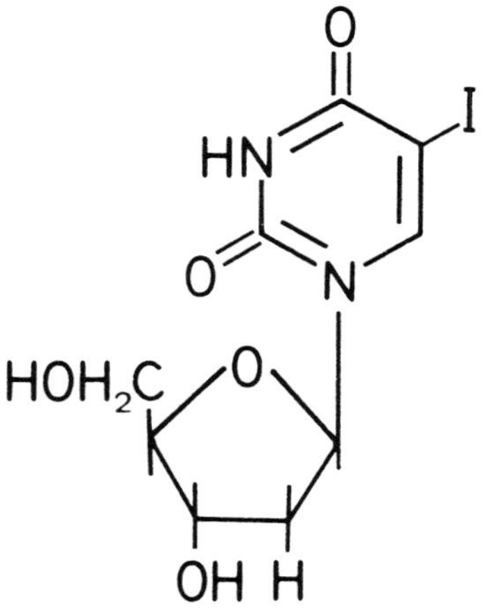

Figure 22–24 ■ Chemical structure of iododeoxyuridine.

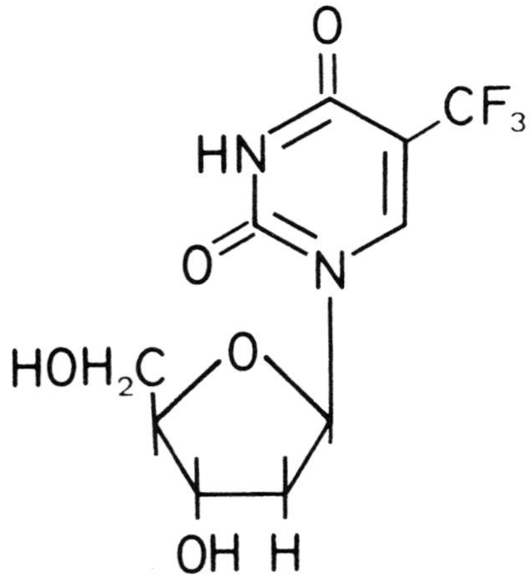

Figure 22–26 ■ Chemical structure of trifluorothymidine.

dine kinase. The monophosphate form is further phosphorylated to become di- and triphosphate forms. Trifluridine monophosphate and triphosphate inhibit the activities of thymidylate synthetase and DNA polymerase, respectively. Finally, the synthesis of viral DNA is inhibited by the agent. However, it is not selective and shows significant cytotoxic activity. This drug penetrates into human cornea and aqueous humor after topical instillation. It is marked for the control of superficial herpetic keratitis.

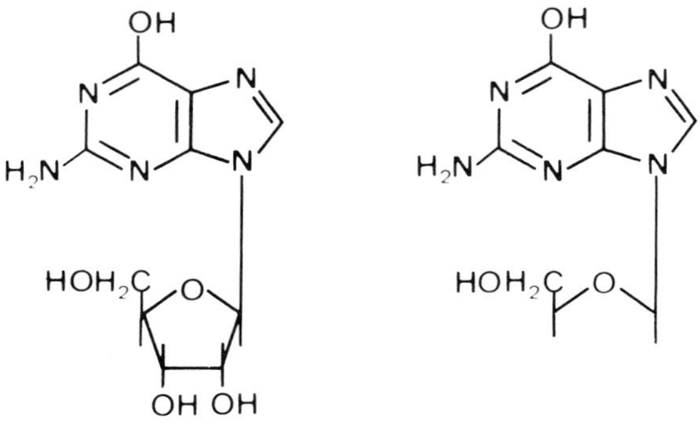

ACYCLOVIR

The major breakthrough in antiviral chemotherapy was the introduction of acyclovir. Acyclovir, an analogue of guanosine, was introduced as a potent and selective antiviral agent (Fig. 22–27). Acyclovir is phosphorylated to form acyclovir-monophosphate by herpesvirus-encoded thymidine kinase. Then acyclovir-diphosphate and -triphosphate are formed by cellular enzymes. Acyclovir-triphosphate inhibits the viral DNA polymerase and terminates the elongation of the viral DNA chain. Thus, it selectively affects only viral infected cells and leaves uninfected cells essentially untouched (Fig. 22–28). Acyclovir is highly effective in vitro against HSV-1, HSV-2, varicella zoster virus, and cytomegalovirus. Recently, intravenous and oral preparations have been released. The intravenous form is indicated for the treatment of primary and recurrent mucosal and cutaneous herpes simplex infections in immunocompromised

Guanosine   **Acyclovir**

Figure 22–27 ■ Chemical structure of guanosine and acyclovir.

patients. It is also used for severe initial episodes of herpes genitalis in patients who are not immunocompromised. Oral administration of acyclovir has recently been approved by FDA for the prevention of recurrent herpes genitalis. Up to 1000 mg of acyclovir per day could be given for a maximum of 6 months. However, the recurrent herpes disease rebounds when the drug administration is stopped.

GANCICLOVIR

More recently ganciclovir, also known as 9-(1,3-dihydroxy-2-propoxymethyl) guanine (DHPG), BW759U, BIOLF-62, and 2'nor-2'-deoxyguanosine, was introduced as a second generation of acyclovir. Ganciclovir is known to be more potent than acyclovir against

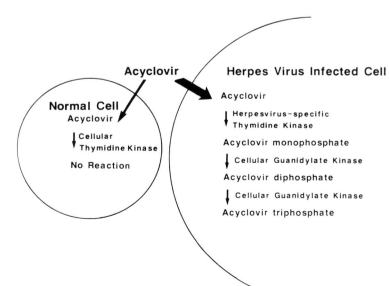

Figure 22–28 ■ Mechanism of action of acyclovir. Acyclovir is activated by herpesvirus thymidine kinase to be acyclovir monophosphate. Acyclovir monophosphate is further phosphorylated to be a triphosphate, which is responsible for the antiherpetic activity by inhibiting viral DNA polymerase and terminating the viral DNA chain elongation.

HSV-1 or HSV-2. Furthermore, ganciclovir has strong antiviral activity against cytomegalovirus, varicella zoster virus, and Epstein-Barr virus. Like acyclovir, ganciclovir is specific and activated by herpesviral thymidine kinase and inhibits the activity of DNA polymerase activity, thereby inhibiting the synthesis of viral DNA.

INTERFERONS

Interferons are glycoproteins secreted by virus-infected cells, which promote the establishment of an antiviral state in uninfected cells (Fig. 22–29). Although all cells in the body appear to be capable of synthesizing interferons, cells derived from the hematopoietic system (e.g., lymphocytes and macrophages) may contribute most of the total interferon synthesis in the body. All DNA or RNA viruses—single- or double-stranded, enveloped or not, with or without virion-associated polymerase, and replicating in the cytoplasm or nucleus—are sensitive to interferon, although differences in the degree of sensitivity exist.

Interferon induces two enzymes: an oligonucleotide polymerase, which synthesizes a series of oligonucleotide containing 2'5'-phosphodiester bonds from ATP (2'5'-oligo(A)polymerase), and a protein kinase, which phosphorylates the small subunit of initiation factor eIF-2. The product of 2'5'-oligo(A) polymerase pppA(2'p5'A)n is the activator of cellular endonucleases that restrict viral nucleic acids. Its activity depends on the continuous presence of pppA(2'p5')n with which it binds. Accumulation of viral RNA is also inhibited in interferon-treated cells and this may be the result of the action of endonucleases (Fig. 22–30). The average half-life of viral mRNA is approximately 12.7 hours in normal cells but only 4.8 hours in interferon-treated cells. The dsRNA-dependent protein kinase phosphorylates the alpha subunit of eIF-2 and subsequently inhibits the binding of initiator tRNA to 40S native ribosomal subunits. Interferon also blocks the proper formation of the viral mRNA cap by inhibiting the process of methylation. Interferon is a macromolecule and must be administered parenterally. It can cause increased pulse rate and temperature, decreased white blood cell counts, headache, and malaise.

Antiviral chemotherapeutic agents and interferons have different mechanisms of action and provide a different, rather than an alternative, way of dealing with a virus infection. For prophylaxis of infections or for early treatment, interferons may have advantages over narrow-spectrum antiviral agents. However, under other circumstances, a spe-

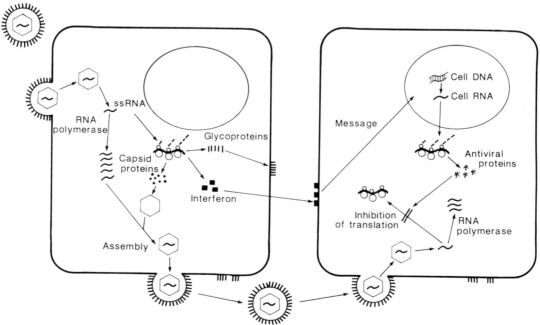

Figure 22–29 ■ Interrelationships of virus, interferon, and cells. Interferon is synthesized in the virus infected cells but shows antiviral activity in the second cell by inhibiting viral translation through the production of antiviral proteins.

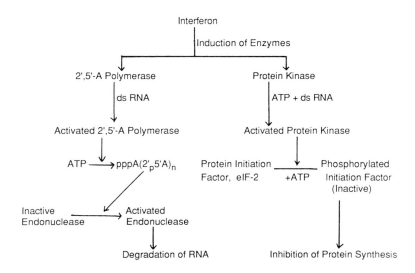

Figure 22–30 ■ Molecular mechanism of antiviral action of interferon.

cific antiviral agent may be preferable to interferons for convenience of administration, quicker onset of antiviral action, and lack of side effects.

ANTIVIRAL AGENTS FOR AIDS

Although AIDS was recognized as a new disease more than 4 years ago, the drug evaluation committee for the treatment of AIDS was only recently established at the National Institutes of Health. There are two difficult problems in developing anti-AIDS drugs; (1) HIV eventually becomes part of the cells it infects, which indicates that the virus cannot be removed from the body by antiviral chemotherapy; and (2) the HIV may infect the brain and establish a latent infection, which means antiviral drugs must cross the blood-brain barrier.

Recently, azidothymidine (3'-azido-3'-deoxythymidine, AZT), an analogue of thymidine, was approved by the FDA for treatment of AIDS (Fig. 22–31). AZT is phosphorylated by cellular enzymes to be AZT triphosphate, which is incorporated into DNA by the reverse transcriptase of HIV; the 3' substitution prevents further 5'- to 3'-phosphodiester linkages and terminates chain elongation of viral DNA. HIV reverse transcriptase is approximately 100 times more susceptible to inhibition by azidothymidine than the DNA polymerase of mammalian cells. Azidothymidine seems not only to block the replication of the virus but also to result in some regeneration of T-helper cells. Furthermore, AZT appears bioavailable when administered orally and penetrates the blood-brain barrier easily.

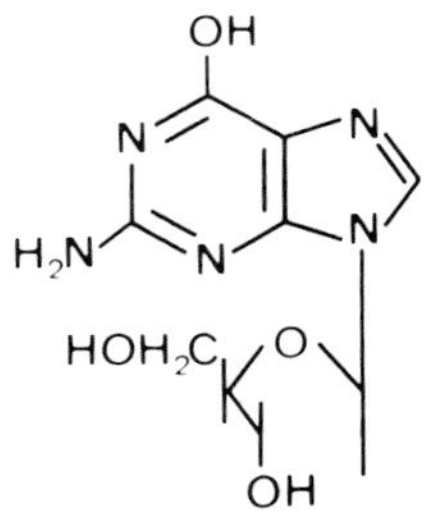

Ribavirin, an antiherpes and anti-influenza agent, also suppresses viral replication in laboratory tests and appears to do so in patients.

HPA-23 has been used in Europe extensively and is known as a reverse transcriptase inhibitor. The clinical trial of HPA-23 indicates the ineffectiveness of the drug. There is clearly a long way to go before an effective therapy for AIDS is developed.

Vaccines

The best way to prevent viral diseases is vaccination. Viral vaccination induces antibodies in serum and extracellular fluids, which provide the main protection against primary viral infections. There are two types of viral vaccines: inactivated viral vaccines and attenuated viral (living) vaccines (Table 22–6).

INACTIVATED VIRAL VACCINES

The essence of inactivated viral vaccines is complete inactivation of infectivity without

Figure 22–31 ■ Chemical structure of 5-azidothymidine.

Table 22–6 ▪ Viral diseases and currently available vaccines

| Diseases | Name of Virus | Vaccine | |
		Inactivated	Attenuated
Smallpox	Vaccinia virus		+
Yellow fever	Yellow fever virus		+
Poliomyelitis	Poliovirus	+	+
Measles	Rubeola virus		+
Influenza	Influenza virus	+	+
Mumps	Mumps virus	+	+
Rabies	Rabies virus	+	+
Adenovirus infections	Adenovirus	+	+ + +
Rubella	Rubella virus		+

+ = Currently available.

loss of antigenicity of viruses. Only a few substances and methods are used to inactivate the infectivity by disrupting the viral genomes without affecting the viral proteins, which are a source of antigenicity.

Ultraviolet Irradiation

Although ultraviolet (UV) irradiation can destroy the viral genomes without alteration of proteins, this method is not appropriate, because virus is frequently not completely inactivated by this manner. Furthermore, the UV inactivated virus such as herpes simplex virus can transform normal cells to be tumorigenic in vitro.

Photodynamic Inactivation

Photodynamic inactivation refers to the treatment of virus with numerous dyes such as neutral red dyes, which intercalate between viral nucleic acid bases; then the viruses are irradiated with white light to damage the nucleic acid without altering viral proteins. However, photodynamically inactivated virus can transform normal cells into tumorigenic ones.

Treatment With Formaldehyde

The best chemical to inactivate the function of viral genome without damaging the antigenicity of virus is formaldehyde. Formaldehyde reacts with nucleic acid bases containing amino group in its structure. Viruses containing single-strand nucleic acid are more readily inactivated by formaldehyde than ones with double-strand nucleic acid. Formaldehyde also reacts with viral capsid proteins and forms extensive crosslinkage, which prevents the access of formaldehyde to nucleic acid. Therefore, formaldehyde treatment can produce viral mutants with

altered capsid and intact nucleic acid, which show resistance to formaldehyde. All formaldehyde-inactivated vaccines must be carefully tested for infectivity before human use to ensure complete inactivation. Formalin-inactivated vaccines are available for the prevention of influenza, poliomyelitis, and rabies. These vaccines are prepared from virus that is grown in eggs (influenza virus types A and B), monkey kidney cell culture (poliovirus types 1, 2, and 3), or human diploid fibroblast cell culture (poliovirus, rabies) and then is inactivated in formaldehyde.

ATTENUATED VIRAL VACCINES

Since Jenner successfully demonstrated the prevention of smallpox infection in humans with live cowpox virus vaccine in 1798, numerous attenuated viral vaccines have been developed and used in clinic. These vaccines include the attenuated yellow fever virus, poliovirus, measles, mumps, and rubella virus vaccines. Since the attenuated virus can multiply in the human body, very small amounts of vaccines are needed for the effective induction of humoral and cellular immunity. The Sabin polio vaccine can be given orally to allow the virus to grow locally in the gastrointestinal tissue, which results in the massive production of secretory IgA in the infected local tissue. Since poliovirus is encountered by the fecal-oral route, the local IgA can neutralize the poliovirus in the gastrointestinal tissue and prevent systemic viremia.

VACCINES PRODUCED BY RECOMBINANT DNA TECHNOLOGY

Recent advances in molecular biology have led to the use of recombinant DNA techniques in the design of a new generation of vaccines. Many viral genomes are cloned and sequenced: as a result, amino acid sequences of proteins responsible for the production of neutralizing antibodies have become known. These known amino acid sequences of viral proteins will soon allow us to develop certain vaccines against influenza, paramyxovirus, hepatitis B, rotavirus, togavirus, and human immunodeficiency virus. Recently, a new type of recombinant DNA that contains vaccinia virus and herpes simplex virus glycoprotein D gene was introduced as a future vaccine to herpes simplex virus. This recombinant DNA was able to produce IgD against herpes simplex virus glycoprotein D in animals and protected them from the primary infections caused by herpes simplex virus types 1 and 2.

REFERENCES

Abramowicz, M.: Oral acyclovir for genital herpes simplex infection. Medical Letter 27:41, 1985.

Almeida, J.D., Howaltson, H.F., and Williams, M.: Morphology of varicella (chickenpox) virus. Virology 16:165, 1962.

Baltimore, D.: Expression of animal virus genomes. Bacteriol. Rev., 35:235, 1971.

Baker, L.F., Gerety, R.J., and Tabor, E.: The immunology of the hepatitis viruses. Adv. Med. 23:327, 1978.

Baringer, J.R., and Swoveland, A.J.: Recovery of herpes simplex virus from human trigeminal ganglions. N. Engl. J. Med. 288:648, 1973.

Ben-Porat, T., and Kaplan, A.S.: Studies on the biogenesis of herpesvirus envelope. Nature 235:165, 1972.

Beneson, A.S.: Smallpox. In Evan, A.S. (ed.): Viral Infections of Humans: Epidemiology and Control. New York, Plenum Press, 1976, p. 426.

Berk, A.J., and Sharp, P.A.: Spliced early mRNA of simian virus 40. Proc. Natl. Acad. Sci. 75:1274, 1978.

Bishop, J.M.: Retroviruses. Ann. Rev. Biochem. 47:35, 1978.

Buddingh, G.J., Schrum, D.I., Lanier, J.C., and Guidry, D.J.: Natural history of herpetic infections. Pediatrics 11:595, 1953.

Centers for Disease Control: Hepatitis Surveillance. U.S. Department of Health and Human Services, Public Health Service, Washington, D.C., Report 47, 1981.

Dale, D., and Avers, J.: AIDS: Reference guide for medical professionals. University of California, Los Angeles, 1984.

Epstein, M., Boav, Y., and Achong, B.: Studies with Burkitt's lymphoma. Wistar Inst. Symp. Monogr. 1:69, 1965.

Francis, D.P., Hadler, S.C., and Thompson, S.E.: The prevention of hepatitis B with vaccine: Report of CDC multicenter efficacy trial in homosexual men. Ann. Intern. Med. 97:362, 1982.

Fraenkel-Conrat, H., and Wagner, R.R. (eds.): Regulation and genetics—Genetics of animal viruses. Comp. Virol. Vol. 9, 1977.

Galasso, G.J., Merigan, T.C., and Buchanan, R.A.: Antiviral Agents and Viral Diseases of Man. Raven Press, New York, 1979, pp. 1–38.

Gerety, R.J. (ed.): Non-A, non-B hepatitis. New York, Academic Press, 1981.

Green, M.: Transformation and Oncogenesis: DNA Viruses. In Fields, B.N., Knipe, D.M., Chanock, R.M., Melnick, J.L., Roizman, B., and Shope, R.E. (eds.): Virology. Raven Press, New York, 1985, pp. 183–234.

Grob, P.J., and Jemelka, H.: Fecal SH (Australia) antigen in acute hepatitis. Lancet 1:206, 1971.

Henle, G., Henle, W., and Dieb, V.: Relation of Burkitt's tumor-associated herpes-type virus to infectious mononucleosis. Proc. Natl. Acad. Sci. USA 59:94, 1968.

Hiatt, H.H., Watson, D.J., and Wistein, J.A.: Origins of Human Cancer. Book B. Mechanisms of Carcinogenesis. Cold Spring Harbor Laboratory, Cold Spring Harbor, New York, 1977.

Hollinger, F.B., and Melnick, J.L.: Features of viral hepatitis. In Fields, B.N., Knipe, D.M., Chanock, R.M., Melnick, J.L., Roizman, B., and Shope, R.E. (eds.): Virology. Raven Press, New York, 1985, pp. 1417–1494.

Holmes, A.W., Wolfe, L., Deinhardt, F., and Conrad, M.E.: Transmission of human hepatitis to marmosets: further coded studies. J. Infect. Dis. 124:520, 1971.

Hutchinson, M.A., Hunter, T., and Eckhart, W.: Characterization of T antigens in polyoma-infected and transformed cell. Cell 15:65, 1978.

Jenson, A.B., Clifton, C.L. Jr., and Lancaster, W.D.: Papillomavirus Etiology of Oral Cavity Papillomas. In Hooks, J.J., and Jordan, G.W. (eds.): Viral Infections in Oral Medicine. Elsevier/North-Holland, New York, 1982, pp. 133–146.

Johnson, R.T.: Pathogenesis of viral infections. In Hooks, J.J., and Jordan, G.W. (eds.): Viral Infections in Oral Medicine. Elsevier/North-Holland, New York, 1982, pp. 3–12.

Joklik, W.K.: Interferons. In Fields, B.N., Knipe, D.M., Chanock, R.M., Melnick, J.L., Roizman, B., and Shope, R.E. (eds.): Virology. Raven Press, New York, 1985, pp. 281–308.

Kaplan, A.S. (ed.): The Herpesviruses. Academic Press, New York, 1973.

Lane, J.M., Miller, D., and Neff, J.M.: Smallpox and smallpox vaccination policy. Ann. Rev. Med. 22:251, 1971.

Long, W.K., and Francis, R.D.: Structure, replication, and classification of viruses. In McGhee, J.R., Michalek, S.M., and Cassell, G.H. (eds.): Dental Microbiology. Harper & Row, Philadelphia, 1982, pp. 549–575.

Lowy, D.R.: Transformation and Oncogenesis: Retroviruses. In Fields, B.N., Knipe, D.M., Chanock, R.M., Melnick, J.L., Roizman, B., and Shope, R.E. (eds.): Virology. Raven Press, New York, 1985, pp. 235–264.

Luria, S.E., Darnell, J.E. Jr., Baltimore, D., and Campbell, A. (eds.): General Virology, ed 3. John Wiley and Sons, New York, 1978.

Maynard, J.E.: Hepatitis A. Yale J. Biol. Med. 49:227, 1976.

McDougall, J.K., Crum, C.P., Fenoglio, C.M., Goldstein, L.C., and Galloway, D.A.: Herpesvirus-specific RNA and protein in carcinoma of the uterine cervix. Proc. Natl. Acad. Sci. U.S.A. 79:3853, 1982.

Melnick, J.L., Dreesman, G.R., and Hollinger, F.B.: Approaching the control of viral hepatitis type B. J. Infect. Dis. 133:210, 1976.

Nahmias, A.J., and Roizman, B.: Infection with Herpes Simplex virus 1 and 2. N. Engl. J. Med. 286:667; 719; 781, 1973.

Nathanson, N., and Cole, G. A.: Immunosuppression: A means to assess the role of immune response in acute virus infection. Fed. Proc. 30:1822, 1971.

National Institutes of Health: Workshop on the treatment of herpes simplex virus infection. J. Infect. Dis. 127:117, 1973.

Nichols, W.W.: Virus-induced chromosome abnormalities. Ann. Rev. Microbiol. 24:479, 1970.

Norman, C.: AIDS therapy: new push for clinical trials. Science 230:1355, 1985.

Overall, J.C.: Oral herpes simplex: pathogenesis, clinical and virologic course, approach to treatment. In Hooks, J.J., and Jordan, G.W. (eds.): Viral Infections in Oral Medicine. Elsevier/North Holland, New York, 1982, pp. 53–78.

Pagano, J.S.: Diseases and mechanisms of persistent DNA virus infection: Latency and cellular transformation. J. Infect. Dis. 132:209, 1975.

Park, N.-H., and Pavan-Langston, D.: Purines. In Came, P.E., and Caliguiri, L.A. (eds.): Chemotherapy of Viral Infections: Handbook of Experimental Pharmacology. Vol. 61. Springer-Verlag, Berlin, 1982, p. 117.

Park, N.-H.: Current aspects of anti-herpes research: problems, established work, and future goals. California Dental Association Journal, December 1984, pp. 167–169.

Park, N.-H., Pavan-Langston, D., and DeClercq, E.: Effect of acyclovir, bromovinyldeoxyuridine. vidarabine and L-lysine on latent ganglionic herpes simplex virus in vitro. Am. J. Med. 73:151, 1982.

Pavan-Langston, D.R.: Ocular viral diseases. In Galasso, G.J., Merigan, T.C., and Buchanan, R.A. (eds.): Antiviral Agents and Viral Diseases of Man. Raven Press, New York, 1979, pp. 253–304.

Pavan-Langston, D.R. (ed.): Ocular viral disease. Int. Ophthalmol. Clin. 15:171, 1975.

Rawls, W.E., Tompkins, W.A., and Melnick, J.L.: The association of herpesvirus type 2 carcinomas of the uterine cervix. Am. J. Epidemiol. 89:547, 1969.

Robinson, W.S., and Lutwick, L.I.: The virus of hepatitis, type B. N. Engl. J. Med. 295:1168; 1232, 1976.

Roizman, B. (ed.): The Herpesviruses. Plenum Publishing, New York, 1985.

Roizman, B., and Furlong, D.: Replication of herpesviruses. Comp. Virol. 3:229, 1974.

Sarngadharan, M.G., Markham, P.D., and Gallo, R.C.: Human T-cell leukemia viruses. In Fields, B.N., Knipe, D.M., Chanock, R.M., Melnick, J.L., Roizman, B., and Shope, R.E. (eds.): Virology. Raven Press, New York, 1985, pp. 1345–1372.

Shillitoe, E.J., Greenspan, D., Greenspan, J.S., and Silverman, S.: Antibody to early and late antigens of herpes simplex virus type 1 in patients with oral cancer. Cancer 54:266, 1984.

Smee, D.F., Martin, J.C., Verhyden, J.P.H., and Matthew, T.R.: Anti-herpesvirus activity of the acyclic nucleosides 9-(1,3-dihydroxy-2-propoxymethyl)-guanine. Antimicrob. Agents Chemother. 23:676, 1983.

Stevens, J.C., and Cook, M.L.: Latent herpes simplex virus in spinal ganglia of mice. Science 173:843, 1971.

Szmuness, W., Stevens, C.E., and Harley, E.J.: Hepatitis B vaccine—Demonstration of efficacy in a controlled clinical trial in a high risk population in the United States. N. Engl. J. Med. 303:8323, 1980.

Szmuness, W., Alter, H.J., and Maynard, J.E. (eds.): Viral Hepatitis. Franklin Institute Press, Philadelphia, 1981.

Tooze, J. (ed.): DNA tumor viruses—Molecular biology of tumor viruses. Cold Spring Harbor Laboratory, Cold Spring Harbor, New York, 1981.

Vilcek, J.: Fundamentals of virus structure and replication. In Galasso, G.J., Merigan, T.C., and Buchanan, R.A. (eds.): Antiviral Agents and Viral Diseases of Man. Raven Press, New York, 1979, pp. 1–38.

Wadsworth, T.H., Hayward, G.S., and Roizman, B.: Anatomy of herpes simplex virus DNA. V. Terminally repetitive sequences. J. Virol. 17:503, 1975.

Wellere, T.H.: The cytomegaloviruses: Ubiquitous agents with protean clinical manifestation. N. Engl. J. Med. 285:203, 1971.

Whitley, R.J., Ch'ien, L.T., Dolin, R., Galasso, G.L., Alford, C.A., and the Collaborative Study Group: Adenine arabinoside therapy of herpes zoster in the immunocompromised NIAID collaborative antiviral therapy. N. Engl. J. Med. 294:1193, 1976.

chapter 23

Oral mycology

Colin Franker, Ph.D.

CHAPTER OUTLINE

- THE FUNGAL CELL
- VEGETATIVE GROWTH IN FUNGI
- SEXUAL REPRODUCTION
- CLASSIFICATION OF FUNGI
- LABORATORY IDENTIFICATION OF FUNGI
- MYCOSES WITH OROFACIAL MANIFESTATIONS

Infections caused by fungi are called *mycoses*. Only a small minority of the 100,000 species are pathogenic in humans, and most of the frequently encountered mycoses are benign. While not as prevalent as bacterial and viral infections, the incidence of superficial as well as invasive mycoses has recently increased. Iatrogenic factors such as immunosuppressive treatments in transplant and oncotherapy, parenteral feeding, and widespread use of antibacterials have accounted for this increment. Most of the fungi associated with human disease are saprophytic members of soil microbial communities. Others exist either as commensals in the alimentary canal or as harmless residents of the skin and only infrequently assume the role of pathogens.

The Fungal Cell

Two major cell morphotypes can be distinguished for the majority of fungi of medical importance. Oval or spheroidal cell shapes are typical of *yeasts* or *blastospores* and range from 5 to 25 μM in diameter (Fig. 23–1). Tubular or filamentous cells are characteristic of *hyphae*, and a single hyphal cell may range from 5 to 50 μM in length and 2 to 5 μM in diameter (Fig. 23–2). Yeasts are usually seen as single cells or as clusters of two or three, with one of the cells distinctly larger than the others. Adjacent hyphal cells may or may not be compartmentalized by cross-wall–like structures called *septa*. A mass of septate hyphal cells constitutes a *mycelium*. A similar aggregate of hyphal cells lacking septa is referred to as a *pseudomycelium*. Both mycelia and pseudomycelia represent what is often meant by the term *mold*.

Many fungi can proliferate either as yeasts or as molds. This reversible transition is defined as *dimorphism*. Yeasts can be converted to filamentous hyphal cells by the outgrowth of a cylindrical *germ tube* (Fig. 23–3), and hyphal cells can differentiate during growth into nonfilamentous yeast-like cells. A variety of other cell morphotypes may also be differentiated from hyphal cells, and, as described later in the chapter, a number of these have specialized functions.

Vegetative Growth in Fungi

YEASTS

A process described as *budding* characterizes the reproduction of most pathogenic

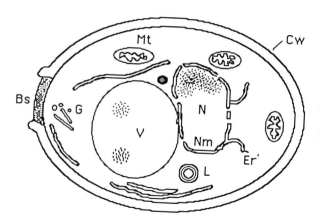

Figure 23–1 ■ Blastospore or yeast cell. Bs, Bud scar; Cw, Mannan-glucan cell wall; Er, endoplasmic reticulum; G, Golgi complex; L, lipid granule; Mt, mitochondria; N, nucleus; Nm, nuclear membrane; V, vacuole.

yeasts. Simple binary *fission* is another method employed by several species, but very few of these yeasts have been implicated in human diseases. As depicted in Figure 23–4, the budding process is initiated by a site-specific outgrowth in a region of the parent cell where curvature is maximal. The *bud initial* then increases in size until it is almost as large as the parental cell from which it was derived. A ring of chitin is then synthesized at the constriction between the mother cell and enlarging bud. After mitotic division and cytoplasmic partitioning of organelles such as mitochodria occurs, a primary septum is formed by the centripetal growth of the chitin ring separating the parent from progeny cells. Secondary septa compositionally similar to the cell wall are then synthesized on both sides of the primary septum. If the cells separate, the primary septum remains with the mother cell and can be identified on the surface as a *bud scar*. In instances in which there is no separation of cells, continuous rounds of budding may give rise to a cell chain or *pseudohypha.*

MYCELIAL GROWTH PATTERNS

Hyphal cells elongate by a process called *apical extension.* If the cells are partitioned by septa, de novo synthesis of cross-wall and nuclear division are coordinated with the growth of the apical tip. Hyphal cells can differentiate into *conidia* (sing. *conidium*) by a diversity of ontogenic processes, which result in the formation of a reproductive unit that in many instances is able to survive harsh environmental conditions. Conidiogenesis in fungi is a highly varied developmental sequence. Some hyphal cells, by a process analogous or identical to bud formation, can give rise to yeast-like *blastospores,* and in some mycelia this type of cell may become the numerically dominant morphotype. When some molds are growing on solid substrate, an elaborate variety of stalk-like conidiophoric structures can be observed. Growth on solid substrates can also elicit the differentiation of root-like structures called *haustoria,* which can anchor the mycelium to the underlying surface.

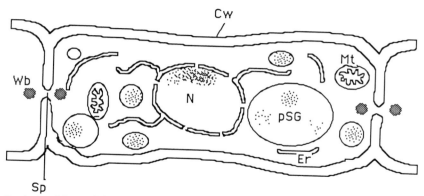

Figure 23–2 ■ Hyphal unit in septate mycelium. pSG, Polysaccharide granule; Sp, septal pore; Wb, Woronin body. See legend of Figure 23–1 for other symbols.

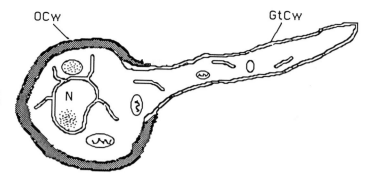

Figure 23–3 ■ Germ tube formation from blastospore. OCw, Old cell wall; GtCw, newly synthesized cell wall delimiting germ tube.

Sexual Reproduction

Gametic fusion, a process that defines eukaryotic sex, has only been observed in some of the fungi that have been identified as human pathogens. In the forms in which there is no apparent sexual component in the life cycle (*anamorphs*) genetic variation is sustained by mitotic recombinational mechanisms, that is, *parasexual reproduction*. The basic requirements for the more conventional pattern are fulfilled in a variety of ways. First, two compatible haploid nuclei are juxtaposed in the same cytoplasm (*plasmogamy*),

and this is followed by nuclear fusion (*karyogamy*) and a meiotic division sequence to yield four or more haploid progeny nuclei, which can be partitioned into cells that differentiate as *sexual* spores (Fig. 23–5). A number of complex variations of this fundamental sequence have evolved. In some forms there are discernible differences between gametes, while in others any somatic nucleus can assume the role of gamete. In some species gametic fusion can occur only between cells from distinct organisms (*thalli*), and in many of these kinds of situations specialized structures are available to promote interthallic

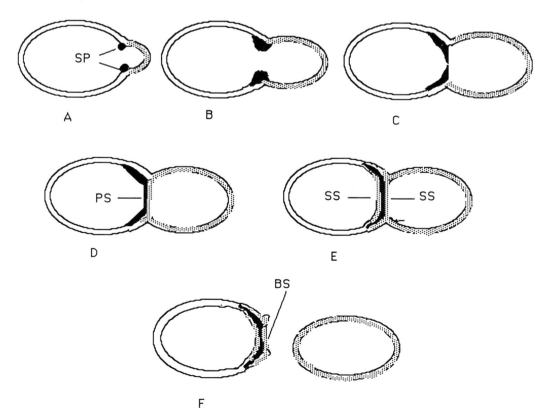

Figure 23–4 ■ Synthesis of chitin *(black areas)* and new cell wall *(shaded areas)* during cell division in budding yeasts. SP, Septal primordia; PS, primary septum; SS, secondary septum; BS, bud scar.

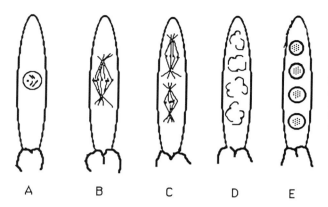

Figure 23–5 ■ Meiotic lineage of sexual spores in ascogenous hypha. *A,* Diploid nucleus in ascus mother cell; *B,* anaphase I; *C,* anaphase II; *D,* initiation of ascospore differentiation; *E,* mature ascus with four ascospores.

contact. Temporal phases of sexual cycles are also variable. In many fungi, karyogamy may not immediately follow plasmogamy, and in fact a multinucleate thallus may be produced consisting entirely of binucleate cells (*dikaryons*) and the dikaryophase may be the predominant state in the life cycle of the fungus. In other forms, the thallus may consist of diploid cells, as a result of an initial nuclear fusion but no ensuing postkaryogamic meiosis, and the diplophase is the temporally significant state of the organism.

Classification of Fungi

Fungal evolution has appeared to diverge along two distinct phyletic lines, the *Myxomycota,* which include the slime molds, and the *Eumycota,* the taxon that includes all human pathogens and opportunistic fungi. The *Eumycota* can be further resolved into subcategories that reflect basic structural and physiologic disparities that are useful in identification. The *Zygomycetes* represent the simplest forms of the *Eumycota* and are nonseptate filaments that are capable of differentiating into spore bearing sacs, or *sporangia* (Fig. 23–6). The latter house asexual spores, in contrast to the *zygospore,* which in this class of fungi is formed as the result of gametic fusion. The fungi classified as *Ascomycetes* also produce asexual and sexual spores, the former known as conidia and the latter designated *ascospores* because they are products of meiotic divisions that occur in *asci* (sing. *ascus*). Asci are in turn enclosed in complex fruiting body type structures known as *ascocarps* (Fig. 23–7). Another clinically significant group of fungi is the *Basidiomycetes* group, characterized by their septate hyphae and a structure specialized for the formation of sexual spores—the *basidium.*

Laboratory Identification of Fungi

Many mycotic infections are easily diagnosed because the etiologic agents can be readily observed in clinical specimens such as skin scrapings, hair, sputum, and/or biopsied tissue. Hyphal elements and yeast cells can be discerned with simple stains if the clinical material is pretreated with a dilute solution of potassium hydroxide that removes the alkali-soluble debris. Most pathogenic fungi also can be easily propagated on simple selective media, a feature that facilitates their identification. The yeast and mycelial phases of some dimorphic species can be observed by propagating the organism at 23°C and 37°C.

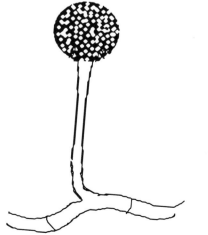

Figure 23–6 ■ Sporangium containing asexual spores in *Rhizopus.*

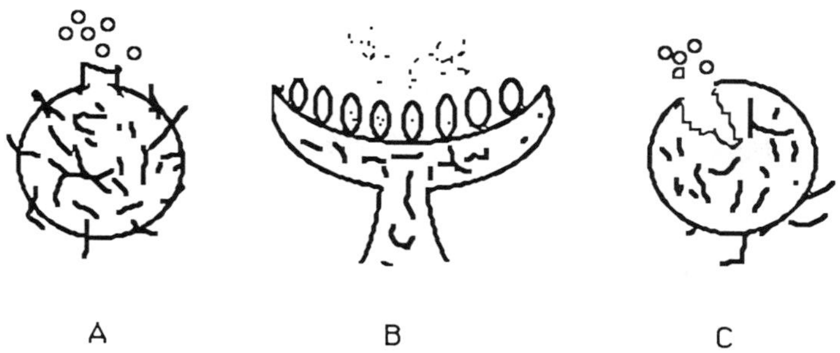

Figure 23–7 ■ Ascocarp types. *A*, Perithecium; *B*, Cleistothecium; *C*, Apothecium.

A   B   C

Mycoses with Orofacial Manifestations

Because some fungal pathogens exhibit distinct histotropisms, mycoses can be classified as *superficial, cutaneous, subcutaneous,* or *systemic.* The latter usually are initiated as pulmonary infections with subsequent dissemination to other sites, which in several instances may include the orofacial region of the body. The major features of the more commonly encountered clinical entities will be outlined here.

SUPERFICIAL OROFACIAL MYCOSES

A small number of fungi, some commensalistic members of the flora of the skin, can reach population densities that result in chronic but asymptomatic infections. These kinds of mycoses are referred to as superficial, and in most instances these elicit minimal host responses. The affected sites are commonly the outer layers of the stratum corneum and cuticular surfaces of hair shafts. One of the more prevalent examples is *pity-*

riasis versicolor, a condition that appears as a discolored area of the torso and/or upper limbs, and that is believed to be associated with local overgrowth of either or both of two lipophilic yeasts, *Malassezia furfur* and *M. ovalis* (Fig. 23–8). Occasionally, the face, eyelids, and ears may be involved. Depigmentation of the affected area may occur especially in tropical climates. Another superficial infection, in which bearded regions of the face can often be involved, is *white piedra*. This condition represents colonization of hair shafts by *Trichosporon beigelii* (Fig. 23–9) and is distinguishable from *black piedra*, which is a mycosis primarily of scalp hair with a different etiologic agent (*Piedraia hortae*). Very seldom is there discomfort with these infections and, except for their cosmetic impact, superficial mycoses represent minor clinical problems.

Orofacial Dermatophytoses

Keratinophilic fungi called *dermatophytes* are responsible for another clinical category of mycoses that also involve the skin, hair, and nails. This affinity for keratinized surfaces or structures, or both, reflects a conver-

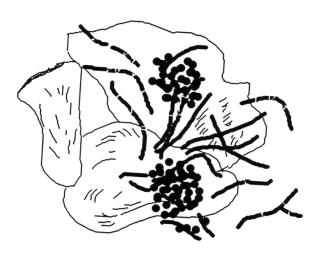

Figure 23–8 ■ Skin scales infected with short-branched mycelia and yeast cells of *Malassezia furfur.*

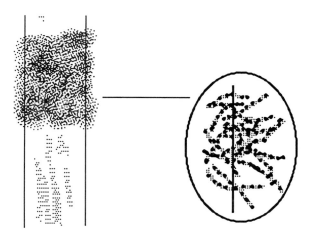

Figure 23–9 ■ Hair shaft infected with arthroconidia-enriched hyphae of *Trichosporon beigelli.*

gent specialization of species from three major genera, *Microsporum, Trichophyton,* and *Epidermophyton,* and includes the elaboration of enzymes that permit the use of epithelial and connective tissue as substrates (e.g., keratinases, elastases, and collagenases). The infections are also referred to as *tineas (ringworm)* and, as might be expected, the one most frequently encountered on orofacial surfaces is *tinea barbae,* ringworm of the beard. This dermatophytosis is usually associated with tissue colonization by *Trichophyton mentagrophytes* (Fig. 23–10). Deep pustular lesions, characteristic of the more severe form of the infection, are associated with *Trichophyton verrucosum.* Both of these dermatophytes can be identified by their morphologic and physiologic idiosyncrasies. *Microsporum canis* (Fig. 23–11), another significant dermatophyte, is often implicated in tineas of the eyebrow. Children appear to be more susceptible than adults to this form of dermatophytosis. Other dermatophytes, more frequently associated with tineas of other sites of the body, are capable of infecting orofacial tissue,

and these include *Trichophyton rubrum, Trichophyton concentricum,* and *Microsporum audounii.*

SUBCUTANEOUS MYCOSES IN OROFACIAL TISSUE

Subcutaneous mycosis usually is the sequela to implantation of fungus-contaminated material beneath the skin, as a result of a puncture wound or deep abrasion. Dissemination beyond the site of inoculation with these infections is rare and, if it does occur, is usually via lymphatic channels as opposed to more conventional hematogenous routes. Three major pathologic entities frequently involving subcutaneous orofacial sites have been documented—sporotrichosis, entomophthoromycosis conidiobolae, and rhinosporidiosis.

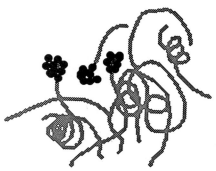

Figure 23–10 ■ Globose microconidia and coiled hyphae of *Trichophyton mentagrophytes.*

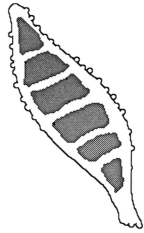

Figure 23–11 ■ Macroconidium of *Microsporum canis.*

Sporotrichosis

The etiologic agent for this mycosis is the dimorphic *Sporothrix schenckii* (Fig. 23–12), an organism usually associated with plants or plant-derived material, or both, such as timber or straw. Most of these orofacial infections result from being scratched by contaminated leaves, thorns, or twigs, and the primary signs of infection are the appearance of nodules that become discolored (pink-purple-black) and regional adenopathy. If the lesions break through the overlying skin and become necrotic, they assume the characteristic form of sporotrichotic chancres, which may remain without resolution for weeks or months. Secondary lesions may develop in adjacent areas connected by lymph channels, especially if the primary chancre is not treated. Most infections of the face and neck, however, are of the "fixed" type—that is, they are restricted to the site of inoculation—and these represent about 25 percent of human infections. Less frequent is involvement of mucous membranes (e.g., the mouth and pharynx), where the lesions may be ulcerative and painful and can be mistaken for aphthous ulcers, lichen planus, or other mycotic infections. All three kinds of infection can be chronic, with intermittent remissions. Spontaneous cure apparently does not occur. Successful treatment has been achieved by oral and/or topical administration of potassium iodide.

Entomophthoromycosis conidiobolae

The etiologic agent for this subcutaneous mycosis is a zygomycete, *Conidiobolus coronatus* (Fig. 23–13), which also infects arthropods but in humans exhibits a pronounced affinity for nasal submucosal tissue. The fun-

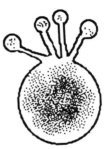

Figure 23–13 ■ Spore of *Conidiobolus coronatus* with papilla-like appendages.

gus is a soil saprophyte found in tropical and subtropical latitudes. Infection is thought to be initiated by implantation of contaminated insect parts or by abrasion with contaminated fingernails. Growth of the organism elicits a characteristic inflammatory reaction through which hyphal elements are ensheathed by large numbers of eosinophils (*Splendore-Hoeppli phenomenon*). Macroscopically a painless swelling develops around the inferior turbinates, which can expand to cause occlusion of the nares and severe disfigurement. Overlying tissue may become erythematous or acanthotic or both but remains intact. Except for recalcitrant cases, most infections respond to potassium iodide chemotherapy.

Rhinosporidiosis

Another mycosis with a decided bias for the submucosa of the nose is rhinosporidiosis. A minority of cases involve the palpebral conjunctiva and constitute the "ocular" form of the disease. The putative causal organism, *Rhinosporidium seeberi,* is thought to be a primitive *Phycomycete* and appears to be an obligate parasite, as it has not been propagated in vitro. The etiologic association is therefore predicated on consistent histologic observations. It is assumed that the infection is initiated by some traumatic event that breaches the mucosal surface. The infectious unit is thought to be a "spore" about 6 to 10 μm in diameter, which enlarges in size to become a 200 to 300 μm sporangium containing numerous endospores generated by successive mitoses (Fig. 23–14). The endospores are believed to escape from mature spherules through a pore-like rupture in the sporangial wall and to reinitiate the development cycle in adjacent tissue. Macroscopically a painless, vascularized, papillomatous mass develops as a reaction to the infection and in time can attain a size large enough to obstruct the nasal passage. Ocular lesions have similar

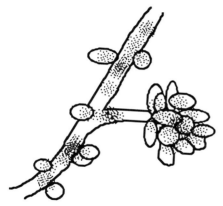

Figure 23–12 ■ Conidiophoric mycelium of *Sporothrix schenkii.*

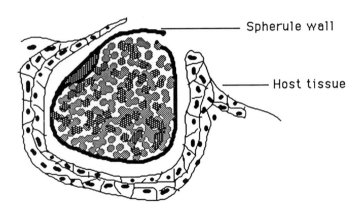

Figure 23–14 ■ Endospore-filled spherule (sporangium) of *Rhinosporidium seeberi.*

histologic lineages and, when sufficiently enlarged, may cause tearing, lid eversion, and secondary conjunctival infections. Nasal infection is noted for its high endemicity in India and Sri Lanka, and this may be attributable to exposure to fungus-containing bodies of water. The ocular form of the disease is more prevalent in arid regions where dust storms occur. Although only partly successful (there is a significant amount of recurrent infection), surgical removal of affected tissue remains the optimal method of control.

OROFACIAL COMPLICATIONS IN SYSTEMIC MYCOSES

The fungi responsible for systemic infections are usually classified as either "true pathogens" or "opportunistic," the former category including organisms that are inherently virulent and the latter comprising organisms that initiate disease in hosts with abrogated defense mechanisms. The group

with intrinsic pathogenicity is represented by four species: *Histoplasma capsulatum, Coccidioides immitis, Blastomyces dermatitidis,* and *Paracoccidioides brasiliensis.* The primary infection produced by these pathogens is usually pulmonary, but disseminated forms of the diseases with orofacial involvement are quite common. Species of the genera *Candida, Mucor,* and *Rhizopus* are most frequently implicated in the etiology of mycoses in patients who are immunocompromised or debilitated or both, and in several instances the primary infection occurs at oropharyngeal sites.

Histoplasmosis

The causal agent of this mycosis is an ascomycete with a well-documented teleomorphic (sexual) state (*Emmonsiella capsulata*), but it is the conidia from the anamorphic phase (*H. capsulatum*) that are the major vectors in the transmission of this disease. Conidiophoric mycelia (Fig. 23–15) of this organism flourish in nitrogen-enriched soil

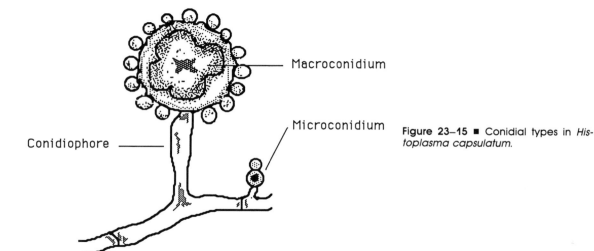

Figure 23–15 ■ Conidial types in *Histoplasma capsulatum.*

(especially with bird and bat droppings) and both micro- and macroconidia serve as infectious units because they can be easily aerosolized and inhaled. Inhaled conidia are phagocytosed by alveolar macrophages and proliferate as yeasts in host cells. This morphologic transition is also observed with some other fungal pathogens when translocated from a saprophytic environment to the cytoplasm of mammalian cells and is apparently temperature-dependent. In a substantial majority of instances infection elicits a benign, localized, inflammatory reaction that may be roentgenographically discernible because it calcifies upon healing. This type of finding and a positive histoplasmin skin test reaction are usually the only evidence of exposure to the fungus. This is particularly true in endemic areas. On the other hand, if large numbers of conidia are inhaled a more extensive and decidedly symptomatic course may ensue with fever and respiratory impairment (*acute pulmonary histoplasmosis*). The disease may become chronic and such situations enhance the possibility of dissemination via the reticuloendothelial system. Immunologic insufficiencies also predispose patients to disseminated histoplasmosis. Painful oropharyngeal ulcers appear in many individuals with the disseminated forms of the disease. As is the case with most systemic mycoses, amphotericin B administered intravenously in monitored amounts is effective, particularly when there is a potentially fatal fulminating infection in young children.

Coccidioidomycosis

Endemic in areas characterized by dry alkaline soils (e.g., the desert zones of the Southwest United States), *C. immitis* is a dimorphic fungus with an arthroconidium (Fig. 23–16) that is easily dispersed and small enough (3 to 6 μm) to be directly deposited onto alveolar surfaces. Postinhalation sequelae include phagocytosis by neutrophils as well as macrophages. The engulfed organism may then differentiate into a thick-walled spherule (30 to 60 μm) in which large numbers of endospores arise by successive cell divisions. The mature endospore (2 to 5 μm) is released by rupture of the spherule. In most individuals the infection is limited at this stage because endospores appear to be quite vulnerable to innate fungicidal mechanisms and the typical histologic response is a granuloma with empty spherules and nonviable endospores surrounded by eosinophilic material. Endospores that survive, however, can perpetuate the spherule-endospore cycle. Coccidioidin sensitivity, as revealed by intradermal injection of antigenic extracts, is often the only other indication of exposure to the organism in asymptomatic infections. More extensive involvement is characterized by fever, chest pain, and anorexia. In some individuals, symptomatic infection also elicits erythemas. Affected orofacial tissue indicates disseminated disease, and crusted granulomatous lesions on nose and face are the common manifestations of this advanced stage of the mycosis. Amphotericin B still prevails as the treatment of choice in severe cases.

Blastomycosis

All instances of blastomycosis begin as an alveolitis following inhalation of conidia from *B. dermatitidis* (Fig. 23–17), the anamorph phase of an ascomycete, *Ajellomyces dermatitidis*. The habitat of the conidiogenic morphotype is still not precisely known because it is difficult consistently to isolate the organism

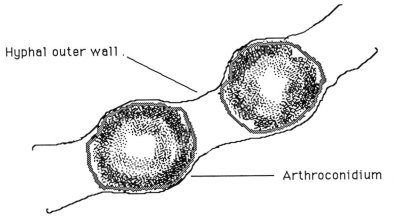

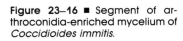

Figure 23–16 ■ Segment of arthroconidia-enriched mycelium of *Coccidioides immitis*.

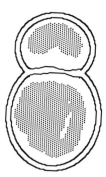

Figure 23–17 ■ Yeast cell of *Blastomyces dermatitidis* with broad-based bud.

from soil and fomites even in highly endemic areas. In vivo the predominant cell types are phagocytosed yeasts. Neutrophils appear to play a growth-promoting role in the course of the infection. The severity of pulmonary involvement can range from a small, well-healed fibrotic scar with mild symptoms to unresolved progressive blastomycosis entailing acute bronchopneumonia and pleuritis. The most common symptom of blastomycosis, however, is the skin lesion, which in turn reflects how easily the organism is disseminated to extrapulmonary sites. In fact, about half of the individuals with discernible symptoms have only cutaneous disease. Foci of organisms first appear in sucutaneous nodules, which become pustular and then ulcerate. The lips, tongue, and buccal mucosa, in addition to facial and nasal areas, are often affected, and in time the lesions evolve into characteristic verrucous granulomas. The latter may persist for months and contain yeast-type cells varying from 8 to 15 μm in diameter. Serologic assays for diagnostic purposes are still equivocal for *B. dermatitidis*, primarily because the organism shares antigens with other pathogenic fungi. Amphotericin B and hydroxystilbamine have been successfully used to treat blastomycoses.

Paracoccidioidomycosis

Until recently paracoccidioidomycosis was restricted to Latin America but, because of the large and recent influx of immigrants from endemic areas, this disease is now appearing in North America. The etiologic organism, *P. brasiliensis*, like other mycopathogens, is thermally dimorphic, with inhaled conidia producing a primary infection in the lungs and then phagocytosed yeast cells disseminating to form secondary infective foci in the mucosa of the mouth and nose. The

lesions in these areas initiate in submucosal lymph nodes and extend upward, developing into ulcerative granuloma. The formation of multiple buds (2 to 5 μm) from a single parent cell (15 to 40 μm) is typical of the yeast phase in this fungus (Fig. 23–18). A relatively reliable immunodiffusion assay is available for antigens of *P. brasiliensis* and is useful for prognosis. Paracoccidioidomycosis is now treated with ketoconazole, although amphotericin B has been very effective in the past.

OROFACIAL MYCOSES IN COMPROMISED INDIVIDUALS

Endocrinopathy and immunodeficiency constitute physiologic states that are conducive to serious and often life-threatening infections by fungi that either are part of the commensalistic human flora or are ubiquitous members of the human environment. Organisms with this potential have been designated as "opportunistic" pathogens, and two groups of fungi are frequently associated with orofacial infections in this context.

Candidiasis

Several "species" of the unnatural genus *Candida* are responsible for the spectrum of mycoses that can be included in this disease complex. The most frequently implicated representative is *C. albicans*, which has only been found in the anamorphic state and appears to be obligately associated with homeothermic animals. Candidiases attributable to *C. tropicalis*, *C. parapsilosis*, *C. pseudotropicalis*, and *C. stellatoidea* have been documented. Ordinarily harmless residents of mucous membranes, most *Candida* cells proliferate as

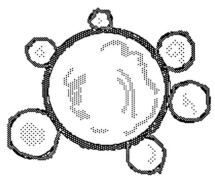

Figure 23–18 ■ Multiple bud formation in *Paracoccidioides brasiliensis*.

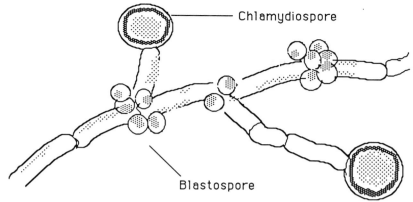

Figure 23–19 ■ Myceliation in *Candida albicans.*

budding yeasts (3 to 6 µM), and hyphae are rare. When the epithelium is breached by trauma or hormonally altered, however, invasion of submucosal tissue can occur, and in many instances there is significant conversion to hyphal growth (Fig. 23–19). In and around the mouth, two major kinds of infection are encountered. The most common of these, *thrush,* presents as a subepithelial invasion of lingual and buccal surfaces by the organism with the formation of a white opaque *pseudomembrane.* In infants the disease is often acquired from mothers with vaginal candidiasis. In older patients contributing circumstances are often intake of broad-spectrum antibiotics or immunosuppressive substances that reduce the level of commensalistic bacteria. Denture stomatitis is often accompanied by increments of oral populations of *Candida,* but a causal relationship has not been unequivocally established. Individuals with some T-cell aberrations are predisposed to *chronic mucocutaneous candidiasis,* characterized by widespread hyperplastic outgrowths that are particularly disfiguring when incurred on the face. Onset of the disease early in life suggests inherited defects in cell-mediated immunity. Thymomas are frequently associated with the condition in older patients. Hypothyroidism and hypovitaminoses have also been linked to susceptibility. An immunodiffusion assay of cytoplasmic antigens has been adopted as a useful serologic tool in candidiasis. Topical application of polyene as well as imidazole antifungal agents has been successful in treatment of thrush. A similar chemotherapeutic record does not exist for the chronic mucocutaneous form, but recent trials with the Lawrence transfer factor administration are promising.

Mucormycosis

Species of three major genera, *Rhizopus, Absidia,* and *Mucor,* can be responsible for severe and often fatal infections caused by the rapid proliferation and invasion of blood vessels with nonseptate hyphal cells from these types of fungi. Diabetics prone to episodes of ketoacidosis, burn patients, patients with leukemia, and malnourished or immunosuppressed individuals are at greatest risk. The form that involves the nose and palate—rhinocerebral mucormycosis—usually results from the inhalation of sporangiospores that germinate on the nasal epithelium. Mortality rates approach 90 percent. The particular susceptibility of patients with diabetes may be related to ability of many of the pathogens (especially *Rhizopus*) to elaborate ketoreductases and grow rapidly in the presence of high levels of glucose. Serologic parameters are of little value in mucormycosis. Intravenous administration of amphotericin B and debridement of infected tissue is currently indicated as a treatment regimen.

ADDITIONAL READING

General Mycology

Rippon, J. W.: Medical Mycology, ed. 2. W. B. Saunders, Philadelphia, 1982.

Speller, D. C. E.: Antifungal Chemotherapy. John Wiley, Chichester, 1980.

Warnock, D. W., and Richardson, M. D.: Fungal Infection in the Compromised Patient. John Wiley, Chichester, 1982.

Superficial Mycoses

Faergemann, J.: Tinea versicolor and *Pityrosporum orbiculare*: Mycological investigations, experimental infections, and epidemiological surveys. Acta Dermato-Venereol. (Suppl) 86:1, 1979.

Dermatophytoses

Ajello, L.: Natural history of the dermatophytes and related fungi. Mycopathologia 53:93, 1974.

Grappel, S. F., Bishop, C. T., and Bland, F.: Immunology of dermatophytes and dermatophytosis. Bacteriol. Rev. 38:222, 1974.

Rebell, G., and Taplin, D.: Dermatophytes. Their recognition and identification. University of Miami Press, Coral Gables, FL, 1974.

Subcutaneous Mycoses

Travassos, L. R., and Lloyd, K. O.: *Sporothrix schenkii* and related species of *Ceratocystis*. Microbiol. Rev. 44:683, 1980.

Vanbreuseghem, R.: Rhinosporidiose: klinischer Aspekt, Epidemiologic und ultrastrukturelle Studien von *Rhinosporidium seeberi*. Dermatol. Monatsschr. 162:512, 1976.

Systemic Mycoses

Domer, J. E., and Moser, S. A.: Histoplasmosis—a review. Rev. Med. Vet. Mycol. 15:159, 1980.

Lehrer, R. I., Howard, D. H., Sypherd, R. S., Edwards, J. E., Segal, G. P., and Winston, D. J.: Mucormycosis. Ann. Intern. Med. 93:93, 1980.

Odds, F. C.: *Candida* and Candidiasis. University Park Press, Baltimore, 1979.

San-Blas, G., and San-Blas, F.: *Paracoccidioides brasiliensis*: Cell wall structure and virulence. A review. Mycopathologia 62:77, 1977.

Stevens, D. A. (ed.): Coccidioidomycosis. A Text. Plenum, New York, 1980.

Tenenbaum, M. J., Greenspan, J., and Kerkering, T. M.: Blastomycosis. Crit. Rev. Microbiol. 9:139, 1982.

chapter 24

Parasitology

Philip T. LoVerde, Ph.D.

In a dental course in microbiology, the study of animal parasites is often omitted or its presentation justified as helping provide the student with a well-rounded education.

In this chapter the two organisms that inhabit the oral cavity, *Entamoeba gingivalis* and *Trichomonas tenax,* are presented. In fact, they are not parasites but commensals normally found in the gums and between the teeth in a low percentage of healthy individuals. Most often these two organisms are found associated with periodontal disease and caries and thus are an indication of poor oral hygiene.

Another group of organisms is presented in this chapter because it is associated with patients with acquired immune deficiency syndrome (AIDS) and its transmission to humans is through the oral ingestion of fecally contaminated material containing the infective stage of the parasite. In particular, transmission in homosexual males is due to oral-anal contact. An understanding of the biology and pathogenesis of these organisms will allow the dentist to evaluate accurately the risks of treating these patients. It is hoped that this will dispel some unfounded fears associated with treating AIDS patients or homosexual males.

Entamoeba gingivalis inhabits the oral cavity. This ameboid organism is a commensal and is cosmopolitan in distribution. Only the trophozoite stage has been described. Transmission is by direct contact (mouth to mouth). The trophozoite is 10 to 35 μm in diameter. The organism produces pseudopodia and behaves like a phagocyte. It contains a nucleus with a centrally located endosome. *E. gingivalis* is not a pathogen but is associated with periodontal disease, calculus around teeth, and carious teeth. Approximately 10 percent of people with healthy mouths harbor *E. gingivalis,* whereas more than 90 percent of people with oral disease harbor these organisms.

Trichomonas tenax inhabits the oral cavity. The flagellated organism (7 × 3 μm) is a commensal that appears to have a cosmopolitan distribution. The trophozoite is the only known stage (Fig. 24–1). Transmission is by direct contact (mouth to mouth). The trophozoite has four anterior free flagella of equal length, a relatively short undulating membrane, and a slender axostyle that protrudes

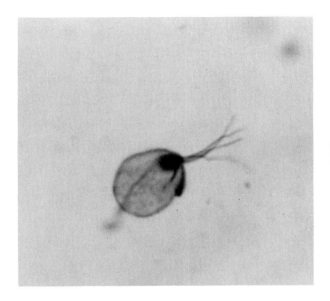

Figure 24–1 ■ Trophozoite of *Trichomonas tenax.* (Courtesy of D. D. Despommier.)

a distance beyond the posterior end of the body. The organism is associated with periodontal disease, calculus around teeth, and carious teeth. It is not pathogenic, but its presence indicates poor oral hygiene.

Entamoeba Histolytica

E. histolytica is the etiologic agent in amebiasis or amebic dysentery. This ameba is one of six species associated with humans. *E. histolytica* and *Dientamoeba fragilis* are pathogenic; the other four species are commensals. With the exception of *E. gingivalis*, which is found in the oral cavity, they all inhabit the intestine.

MORPHOLOGY AND LIFE CYCLE

E. histolytica has two stages in its life cycle: trophozoite and cyst (Fig. 24–2). Both stages are found in the feces; only trophozoites invade the tissues.

The trophozoite (the vegetative stage), which inhabits the large intestine and is capable of invading the tissues of the body, varies from 12 to 30 μm in diameter. It has a finely granular endoplasm that is sharply separated from the clear ectoplasm, and appears with a grayish tinge when observed under the microscope. Pseudopodia can be seen during movement. The single nucleus, which is used in distinguishing one species from the others, is spherical with an evenly distributed chromatin that is finely granular

around its periphery and contains a centrally located dense spherical chromatin body, the karyosome. The trophozoite is anaerobic and multiplies by binary fission. The cytoplasm contains food vacuoles that may contain host cells (e.g., red blood cells). The cyst stage, which is important in transmission, measures 5 to 20 μm in diameter. The mature cyst contains four nuclei, each identical in morphology to the nucleus of the trophozoite. As the cyst forms, the cytoplasm may contain chromatoid bodies that are diagnostically rod-shaped. Chromatoid bodies are not seen in the mature cyst. The mature cyst is the infective stage for humans. The cyst, which is passed in the feces, is surrounded by a protective covering that allows the parasite to resist dehydration, disinfectants, temperature changes, and gastric juices. The ingested cyst passes through the stomach and excysts in the small intestine. The quadrinucleated parasite undergoes nuclear division, giving rise to an eight-nucleated organism. The cytoplasm divides to produce eight uninucleate amebae. Intestinal stasis often enables the amebae to establish the site of infection in the cecal area of the colon. They begin to colonize the intestine by division. As stool containing parasites is passed down the intestine, the absorption of fluid triggers the trophozoite to expel its food vacuoles and undergo cyst formation. As an immature cyst, the nucleus, divides to give rise to a binucleate organism, the rod-shaped chromatoid bodies may appear. Each nucleus divides again, the chromatoid bodies disappear, the cyst wall forms, and the mature

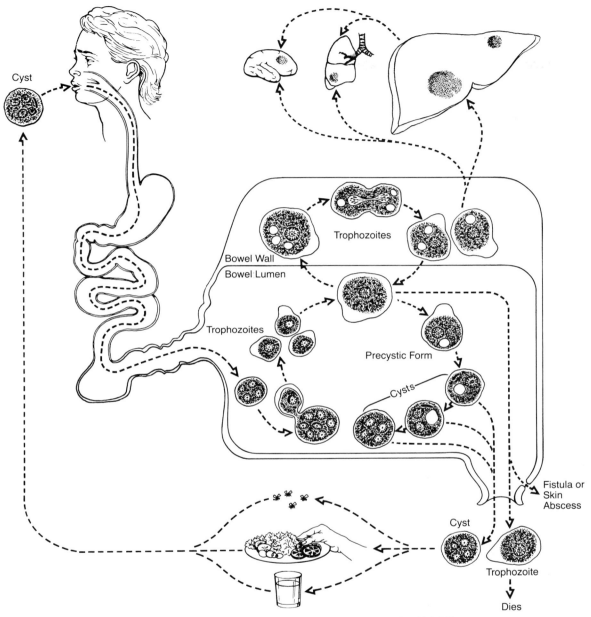

Figure 24–2 ■ Trophozoite and cyst stages of *Entamoeba histolytica.*

infective cyst is passed to the outside environment.

E. *histolytica* often behaves as a commensal inhabiting the lumen of the colon. The ability of E. *histolytica* to cause disease is, in part, determined by the environment of the gut. Individuals on a low-protein, high-carbohydrate diet have more amebae in the intestine. The species of bacteria present also influences pathogenicity, apparently by creating a reducing environment favorable for amebic growth.

PATHOGENESIS AND SYMPTOMATOLOGY

There are two forms of clinical manifestations: intestinal and extraintestinal (Fig. 24–2).

E. *histolytica* are able to quickly colonize the cecal and sigmoid-rectal areas of the intestine, where the colonic flow is slow. As they divide, the amebae release cytolytic enzymes that cause cell lysis. Cytolysis can also be caused by a cell contact–dependent mechanism. In either instance, release of cell juices induces amebic division. The progeny invade and advance the lesion as they divide. The first lesion appears as a button-hole ulceration (a small nodular elevation with a minute opening) in the intestinal mucosa. The increasing colony of amebae usually proceeds to the base of the more resistant muscularis and then spreads laterally to form a vase-shaped or crateriform ulceration. If this primary lesion is not complicated by accompanying bacteria, there is no host reaction (inflammation) to the invading amebae. Secondary bacterial invasion accounts for most of the clinical symptoms. The intestinal involvement can be localized or extensive and is classified as an ulcerative colitis. Destruction of tissue is followed by regenerative proliferation of connective tissue, which in cases of extensive damage may ultimately cause a fibrous thickening of the intestinal wall. From the submucosa, the amebae can extend into the mucularis and perforate the serosa, resulting in peritonitis. Amebae can extend to the diaphragm and enter the pleural cavity and lungs as well. Cutaneous amebiasis results from invasion of perianal tissue or genitalia. The cecal and sigmoid-rectal areas are those in which a majority of the lesions are found. In any lesion, E. histolytica inhabits only the perimeter of the necrotic tissue because the amebae feed only on living tissue.

When they occur, symptoms may be insidious, with vague abdominal discomfort or soft stools for a variable period and constipation alternating with mild diarrhea, or they may be abrupt with cramps, abdominal pain, diarrhea, and fever. There may be as many as 15 to 20 stools per day, resulting in dehydration. Stools are often bloody and contain mucus and sloughed tissue. The patient usually does not suffer the acute systemic intoxication seen in bacillary dysentery.

Extraintestinal amebiasis occurs when amebae invade mesenteric capillaries or venules and metastasize to other parts of the body, usually the liver. The amebae can be carried to any tissue or organ in the body (e.g., heart, lungs, kidneys, brain). The extraintestinal lesion, except in the case of cutaneous spread, is always secondary to intestinal involvement. The extraintestinal amebic lesion is caused by trophozoites that have lodged in a tissue and proceeded to colonize producing necrosis of surrounding host cells manifesting as a sterile abscess.

Patients with hepatic abscesses usually present with fever, an enlarged, tender liver, bulging in the right upper portion of the abdomen, and frequently pain in the right pleura radiating to the right shoulder.

DIAGNOSIS AND TREATMENT

Intestinal amebiasis must always be considered in any patient with protracted diarrhea and in all patients with dysentery. In cases of dysentery, it is important to differentiate bacterial from amebic etiologies because the latter may result in extraintestinal disease.

For intestinal amebiasis, one needs to demonstrate the parasite (trophozoite or cyst stage) in feces. A diagnosis cannot be reliably made on clinical evidence alone.

Identification of parasites in stool specimens requires fresh specimens to be examined by experienced personnel. Often multiple stool examinations are required to make a diagnosis. Purgatives (e.g., phosphate of soda) are used to obtain fresh samples. Typical stool from a patient with amebic dysentery will have exudates, mucus, blood, and cellular debris mixed with the feces. The amebae will most likely be found in the part of the stool containing the exudates, blood, and cellular debris.

Serologic tests such as indirect hemagglutination, ELISA, and countercurrent immunoelectrophoresis are helpful in diagnosis.

Diagnosis of extraintestinal amebiasis is made by a combination of serology and radiology, ultrasound, or radionuclide tests. Biopsy of the edge of the abscess may be helpful. Often patients with extraintestinal abscess show no history suggestive of amebic colitis, which makes the diagnosis more difficult.

The methods of treatment vary with the clinical type of amebiasis. No one treatment is ideal. Each drug carries with it certain contraindications. In severe amebic dysentery, the primary objective in treatment is to stop the dysentery and then to cure the infection. The drug of choice is metronidazole. Emetine hydrochloride and dehydroemetine are also given. With either of the latter two drugs, which arrest the dysentery, an amebicidal drug such as diiodohydroxyquin is also administered. With all treatments, antibiotics are also given to control symptoms due to bacterial invasion of the intestinal lesions. Several drugs, including diloxanide furoate and diiodohydroxyquin, provide good cure rates in nondysenteric intestinal amebiasis.

In the United States all asymptomatic patients should be treated. In endemic countries, usually only symptomatic patients are treated, partially because of the frequency of reinfection and the high incidence of infected patients who are asymptomatic.

For extraintestinal abscesses, metronidazole, emetine, or chloroquine, or a combination of the three, is recommended. Aspiration of the abscess may be necessary for cure.

EPIDEMIOLOGY AND CONTROL

E. histolytica has a worldwide distribution. Some 400 million people, approximately 10 percent of the world's population, are afflicted. In the United States there is a 4 percent incidence. Thirty-six million people have severe colitis or extraintestinal involvement. Approximately 75,000 people die each year. Infections are more prevalent and the intensity of infection more severe in tropical and subtropical climates than in temperate zones. People of all races and ages and of both sexes appear to be equally susceptible to infection. In the United States, the high-risk populations include (1) sexually active homosexual males, (2) residents of institutions, (3) travelers to endemic areas, (4) immigrants from endemic areas, (5) migrant workers, and (6) the lower socioeconomic class in the southern United States.

Transmission is fecal-oral. Therefore, food handlers, contaminated food (vegetables), and water with viable cysts and flies as mechanical vectors are common modes of transmission. Among homosexuals, anal-oral sex is the mode of transmission. In homosexuals, lesions occur in the oral cavity and on the genitalia owing to direct transmission of trophozoites. The cyst, however, is normally responsible for transmission.

Control of amebiasis results from improvements in sanitation and hygiene. In particular, the proper treatment of night soil is necessary to destroy cysts before it is used as fertilizer.

Giardia lamblia

Giardia lamblia is a flagellated parasite that has a cosmopolitan distribution. It is the most prevalent clinical infection caused by a protozoan in the United States today.

MORPHOLOGY AND LIFE CYCLE

G. lamblia has a trophozoite and cyst stage (Fig. 24–3). The trophozoite measures 9 to 20 μm in length by 7 to 15 μm in width and is 2 to 4 μm thick. The trophozoite appears pear-shaped, broadly rounded anteriorly, and tapered to a point posteriorly. On its ventral surface are two adhesive disks for attachment to epithelial surfaces. The parasite has four pairs of flagella that function in locomotion. In the center of the organism is a rod-shaped organelle, the parabasal body. In the area of each adhesive disk there is a nucleus containing a centrally located karyosome. The trophozoite appears bilaterally symmetrical. Multiplication of this anaerobic organism is by longitudinal binary fission.

The oval cyst, which is important in transmission, measures 9 to 12 μm long by 7 to 10 μm wide. The mature cyst contains four nuclei.

The cyst stage is ingested and excysts in the small intestine. Each cyst gives rise to two organisms that begin to multiply and colonize the upper two thirds of the small intestine. The trophozoites are not invasive. Instead they attach to the epithelial brush border by their powerful adhesive disks, and in a few days many millions pave the epithelium. As the intestine moves feces containing trophozoites into the large intestine, the parasite forms a cyst that is passed to the outside environment. The cyst is the infective form of the parasite and is seen in formed stools. Trophozoites are observed only in watery stools during diarrhea.

PATHOGENESIS AND SYMPTOMATOLOGY

G. lamblia infections are usually asymptomatic but occasionally cause protracted diarrhea or malabsorption. The parasites opposed to the brush border irritate the mucosa causing catarrhal inflammation. This can lead to diarrhea that can be mild to intensive and debilitating when the stools become watery and voluminous with 40 million parasites passed per day. Untreated, the diarrhea may last for months with exacerbations and remissions occurring. Symptoms consist of epigastric pain, abdominal cramps, flatulence, steatorrhea, and foul-smelling stools containing large amounts of mucus. There may be weight loss, dehydration, and fatigue. In

Giardiasis

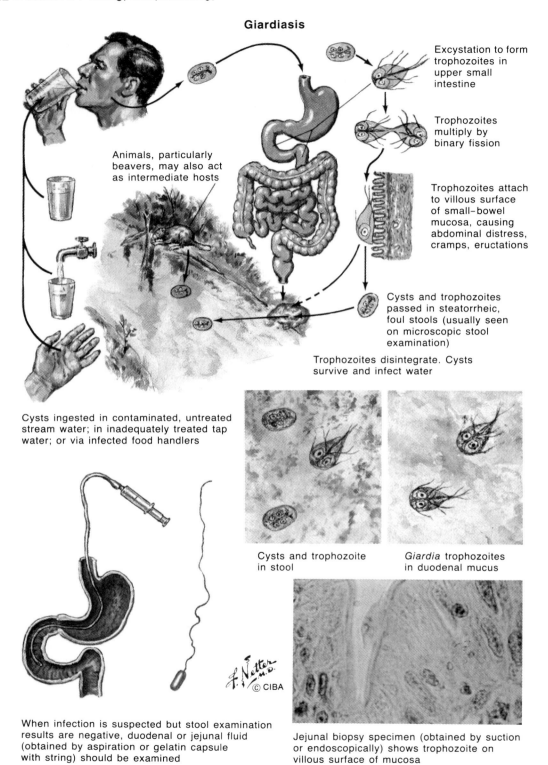

Excystation to form trophozoites in upper small intestine

Trophozoites multiply by binary fission

Trophozoites attach to villous surface of small-bowel mucosa, causing abdominal distress, cramps, eructations

Animals, particularly beavers, may also act as intermediate hosts

Cysts and trophozoites passed in steatorrheic, foul stools (usually seen on microscopic stool examination)

Trophozoites disintegrate. Cysts survive and infect water

Cysts ingested in contaminated, untreated stream water; in inadequately treated tap water; or via infected food handlers

Cysts and trophozoite in stool

Giardia trophozoites in duodenal mucus

When infection is suspected but stool examination results are negative, duodenal or jejunal fluid (obtained by aspiration or gelatin capsule with string) should be examined

Jejunal biopsy specimen (obtained by suction or endoscopically) shows trophozoite on villous surface of mucosa

Figure 24–3 ■ Trophozoite and cyst stages of *Giardia lamblia*. (Copyright 1984. CIBA Pharmaceutical Company, a division of CIBA-GEIGY. Reproduced with permission from Clinical Symposia—by Frank H Netter, M.D. All rights reserved.)

young children a malabsorption syndrome caused by atrophy of microvilli of the brush border and mechanical blockage of absorption of fats may result. Often vitamin A deficiency results. Clinically children are more seriously affected than adults; in adults infections are usually self-limiting. Secretory IgA appears to play an important role in pathogenesis. IgA-deficient patients develop more severe infections.

DIAGNOSIS AND TREATMENT

Diagnosis is based on demonstrating the parasite in stool samples—most often the cyst stage in formed stools, but sometimes the trophozoite stage in liquid stools. It often takes multiple stool examinations to make a diagnosis. Duodenal aspirates and a string test, a technique for sampling the duodenal mucosal surface, are also used in diagnosis. There are no routine serologic tests available. In the United States today one must consider giardiasis in any case of protracted diarrhea. Treatment is with quinacrine hydrochloride (Atabrine), with metronidazole, or with furazolidone. In severe cases supportive treatment is also recommended. All patients with *Giardia* infection, including asymptomatic carriers, should be treated.

EPIDEMIOLOGY AND CONTROL

Infection with *Giardia* results from ingestion of cysts. Reservoir hosts such as dogs, beavers, and muskrats are responsible for contaminating streams and watershed areas. Backpackers drinking from mountain streams often acquire infections. Inhabitants of towns where there was a break in the water purification systems have become infected. Sporadic epidemics have been reported in day care centers, nurseries, and institutions. In homosexual populations, giardiasis is very prevalent. Giardiasis is endemic in certain areas of the United States.

Control is very difficult because *G. lamblia* cysts are very resistant to chlorination. Boiling water for 2 to 5 minutes is recommended. Measures to prevent fecal-oral transmission apply.

Toxoplasma gondii

Toxoplasma gondii is an obligate intracellular parasite that has evolved a very complex life cycle. It is found in a large number of mammals including humans. The parasite is cosmopolitan in its host range and ubiquitous in its distribution.

MORPHOLOGY AND LIFE CYCLE

In humans, two forms of the parasite are found: the trophozoite (tachyzoite), usually seen during acute proliferative infection, and the pseudocyst (containing bradyzoites), found during chronic or latent infection (Fig. 24–4). Reproduction is by an asexual process of internal budding termed endodyogeny. The trophozoites measure 3 to 6 μm in length. They are crescent- or banana-shaped, with one end more pointed than the other. The cysts that occur in chronic infection are formed when the parasites multiply and produce a wall within a host cell; hence the term "pseudocyst."

Toxoplasma is a coccidian parasite of the cat family Felidae. The parasite has evolved a life cycle that includes transmission by (1) oocysts shed in cat feces, (2) pseudocysts ingested in improperly cooked meat, and (3) trophozoites involved in congenital transmission.

In the cat, the definitive host, the parasite infects the epithelial cells of the intestine. Here the parasite undergoes asexual reproduction (schizogony) and sexual reproduction (gametogony). The end result of sexual reproduction is the zygote, which protects itself with a resistant cell wall before elimination in the feces as an immature oocyst. Oocysts are approximately 9 μm in diameter. During primary infection, the cat sheds unsporulated oocysts for a period of 2 weeks. The freshly shed oocysts are not infective. However, after 3 to 4 days at 20 to 22°C the zygote contained within the oocysts divides into two sporocysts, and four sporozoites are contained within each sporocyst. These sporulated oocysts are infective. They are relatively resistant to a variety of chemicals and will remain infective in the soil for at least 1 year.

Oocysts ingested by transport hosts (earthworms, snails, arthropods, birds) are spread throughout the environment. If ingested by humans or other mammals (including herbivores), the oocysts release the sporozoites in the intestine. They rapidly penetrate the intestinal wall, are phagocytized by macrophages, and are distributed throughout the body. Inside the macrophages, the parasites (tachyzoites) reproduce at the expense of the

Toxoplasma gondii

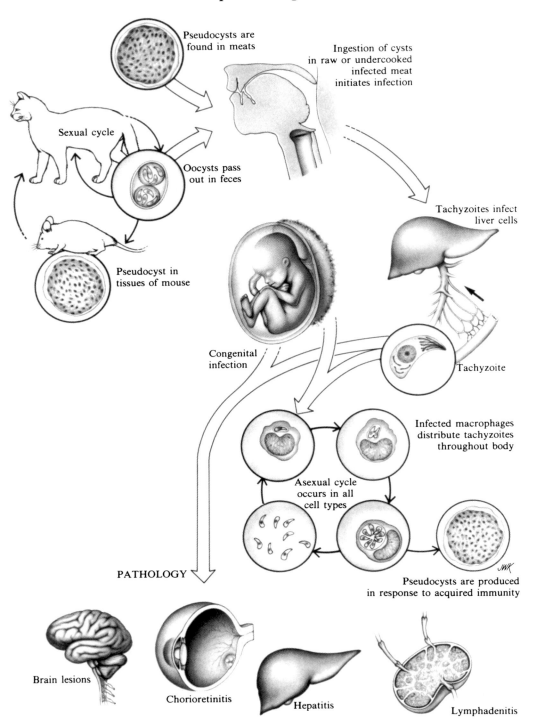

Pseudocysts are found in meats

Ingestion of cysts in raw or undercooked infected meat initiates infection

Sexual cycle

Oocysts pass out in feces

Tachyzoites infect liver cells

Pseudocyst in tissues of mouse

Tachyzoite

Congenital infection

Infected macrophages distribute tachyzoites throughout body

Asexual cycle occurs in all cell types

PATHOLOGY

Pseudocysts are produced in response to acquired immunity

Brain lesions

Chorioretinitis

Hepatitis

Lymphadenitis

Figure 24–4 ■ Life cycle of *Toxoplasma gondii*. (From Katz, M., Despommier, D. D., and Gwadz, R. W.: Parasitic Diseases. Springer-Verlag, New York, 1982, with permission. Illustration by John W. Karapelou.)

host cell. The parasites are not destroyed by the macrophage microbicidal mechanisms, in part because the parasite is able to prevent the fusion of lysosomes with the vacuole containing them. As the parasite numbers increase, the cell lyses, releasing tachyzoites, which are able to penetrate any cell in the body (including red blood cells). During this acute phase, any tissue or organ in the body can be infected with *Toxoplasma* parasites. With the appearance of antibody, the parasites remain in infected cells, forming pseudocysts. Each pseudocyst contains hundreds of infectious units (bradyzoites) that can be liberated when immunity wanes (e.g., during immunosuppression) or when ingested by a naive host. Humans can acquire *Toxoplasma* infection by ingesting pseudocysts in the flesh of improperly cooked meat. This route of transmission is very common among carnivores. The life cycle in humans is the same as described earlier when oocysts are ingested. A third form of transmission is congenital. If pregnant women in their second or third trimester acquire a primary infection in which there is a parasitemia, parasites can cross the placenta and multiply in the tissues of the fetus, causing serious damage. Infection acquired before pregnancy induces immunity and prevents congenital transmission.

PATHOGENESIS AND SYMPTOMATOLOGY

The large numbers of humans with serum antibodies to *Toxoplasma* suggest that most infections are asymptomatic. The most seriously affected are newborns who acquire the infection transplacentally, usually from an asymptomatic mother. Approximately 40 percent of infants born of females acquiring *Toxoplasma* infection during pregnancy show signs of disease. At birth or shortly thereafter, these infants commonly have evidence of retinochoroiditis, cerebral calcification, and occasionally hydrocephalus or microcephaly. Psychomotor disturbances are also common. Severe damage in the central nervous system, stillbirth, and abortion can occur.

Acquired infections are manifested by lymphadenitis, fever, headache, myalgia, and splenomegaly. The symptoms are often confused with those of infectious mononucleosis. However, since during acute infection the parasites can infect any cell in the body, inflammation can occur in any organ, in the form of myocarditis, pneumonitis, or encephalitis. Retinochoroiditis may result in some cases. Recrudescence in toxoplasmosis occurs when a patient with pseudocysts is immunosuppressed or immunocompromised. Clinically, this form of toxoplasmosis is identical to the acquired acute infection. *Toxoplasma* infection is a major cause of death in AIDS patients.

DIAGNOSIS AND TREATMENT

Specific diagnosis is made by serologic tests or demonstration of the organisms in tissues. Clinical symptoms alone are not sufficient to make the diagnosis. Serologic tests include the Sabin-Feldman dye test, the indirect fluorescent antibody (IFA) test, the ELISA test, the indirect hemagglutination test, and the complement fixation (CF) test. Serum titers for the Sabrin-Feldman dye test, IFA, and ELISA tests appear early in infection, reach a higher level, and drop much later than those obtained with the CF test. Occasionally diagnosis can be made from smears of biopsy material. However, in certain laboratories body fluids or ground tissue are inoculated into mice free of *Toxoplasma*, and 7 to 10 days later their tissues examined for the proliferating parasite.

Patients with acute toxoplasmosis who appear normal may not require treatment. When treatment is required clindomycin plus sulfadiazine and pyrimethamine are recommended drugs; the last drug causes side effects.

In pregnant women diagnosed as having acute toxoplasmosis, the possibility of congenital infection must be considered; in some cases chemotherapy that is teratogenic or therapeutic abortion may be recommended.

EPIDEMIOLOGY AND CONTROL

The high prevalence of *Toxoplasma* in the human population (approximately half of the population in the United States) can be explained by the continuous exposure to the risk of infection by ingesting improperly cooked meat and ingestion of oocysts introduced in the environment by cats. As expected, prevalence of infection increases with age.

Congenital transmission accounts for relatively little of the high prevalence observed in humans. However, toxoplasmosis acquired by the mother during pregnancy (two to six cases per 1000 pregnancies in the United States) may result in severe or fatal damage to the fetus.

Immunocompromised individuals such as transplant patients and those with debilitating disease such as AIDS also account for those with serious disease.

Control measures are to cook meat (from sheep, cattle, and swine) properly. Freezing is not as dependable as adequate heating to destroy infectivity. The principal mode of transmission is by ingestion of oocysts shed into the environment in the feces of cats. These stages remain viable for 1 year and are a source of infection for mice, birds, and other prey that return the infections to cats. Protection of sandboxes where children play is advisable. A vaccine for cats, which has recently become available, has shown some success.

Pneumocystis carinii

Pneumocystis carinii is a ubiquitous parasite found in many species of mammals including humans. The organism maintains itself in an immune population, and clinical disease presents itself in those few who are immunosuppressed or immunologically compromised. *Pneumocystis* causes an interstitial plasma cell pneumonia. At one time pneumocystis pneumonia was associated with newborns or individuals who were immunosuppressed by underlying disease or chemotherapy. Today, it is a well-known disease because of its association with acquired immune deficiency syndrome (AIDS).

MORPHOLOGY AND LIFE CYCLE

P. carinii inhabits the lungs, where it is found in either the alveoli or the alveolar walls. The organism exists in two forms: as trophozoites and as cysts. The trophozoites, which are ameboid, range from 1 to 5 μm in size. They consist of a small nucleus surrounded by a mass of protoplasm, enclosed in a double-layered pellicle. Fine filopodia project from the trophozoite, apparently functioning like pili to facilitate attachment to one another and to the alveolar walls of the lungs. The cysts are 3.5 to 5 μm in diameter, with a thick wall. Within the cyst are typically found eight trophozoites, each 1 to 2 μm in size. The life cycle is unknown.

It is thought that the cyst is the infective form and that transmission is more likely from human to human than from animal to human.

PATHOGENESIS AND SYMPTOMATOLOGY

The lungs, which appear grayish to tan, are firm and airless. Microscopically the alveoli are filled with a foamy, honeycomb material. Within this exudate are found various stages of parasite, histiocytes, lymphocytes, plasma cells, and cellular debris. In advanced cases, most of the alveoli are filled and the alveolar septa are thickened. The material in the alveoli persists with little phagocytosis or other inflammation, and expectoration is deficient. At autopsy the thickened alveolar septa are infiltrated with plasma cells; hence the name "interstitial plasma cell pneumonia." The infiltrate also consists of lymphocytes and histiocytes. Parasites may not be numerous in the thickened septa, even though many are in the alveoli.

Dyspnea is the most common symptom observed, followed by fever and a nonproductive cough. *Pneumocystis* infection may be suspected in any patient with a diffuse or nodular bilateral pulmonary infiltrate that is disproportionate with the minimal physical findings consisting of malaise, anorexia, slight fever, dyspnea, or nonproductive cough, with lungs clear to percussion and auscultation except for scattered rales. Patients with *P. carinii* pneumonia but no immunodeficiency disease show normal serum immunoglobulin levels.

The incubation period is 6 to 8 weeks. Death, almost always occurring in untreated cases, is usually by asphyxia.

DIAGNOSIS AND TREATMENT

Clinical signs and symptoms have been used to make a diagnosis, especially when immunosuppressed or immunocompromised individuals develop a pneumonitis that cannot otherwise be explained. However, the demonstration of the parasite in affected lung tissue or secretions is necessary to confirm the diagnosis. Transbronchial lung biopsy via fiberoptic bronchoscopy is safer than open lung biopsy and more effective than brush-biopsy by bronchoscopy. Staining tissue imprints or tissue sections with methenamine-silver is useful for screening purposes. To differentiate the thick-walled cysts from yeast cells, a follow-up stain with Gram's, Giemsa's, or trichrome is necessary. Serologic tests are not satisfactory and still need development.

Drug treatment is available. The drug of choice for adults and children is the fixed combination of trimethoprim-sulfamethoxazole. Supportive measures such as administering antibiotics and oxygen are also important. Recurrent infection in immunosuppressed individuals is a problem.

EPIDEMIOLOGY AND CONTROL

Pneumocystis is a very common parasite of humans and numerous species of mammals. Overt disease is rare except in immunocompromised individuals. Clinical infections occur usually in infants who are premature or malnourished; in older children and adults, the disease is associated with hypogammaglobulinemia, debilitating diseases such as malignancies (e.g., leukemia), or the administration of immunosuppressive drugs such as corticosteroids. AIDS patients are particularly prone to this opportunistic infection.

At present no preventative measures are available. Infection should be anticipated in immunocompromised individuals (e.g., AIDS patients) so that treatment can be given early.

Cryptosporidium

Cryptosporidium is a cosmopolitan parasite that inhabits the human intestinal tract. In the gastrointestinal tract of immunocompromised individuals, *Cryptosporidium* causes a severe diarrheal disease known as cryptosporidiosis.

MORPHOLOGY AND LIFE CYCLE

Cryptosporidium is a coccidian parasite, with a life cycle similar to that of *Toxoplasma*, except that the sexual and asexual developmental stages occur in the same host. There appears to be no obligate intermediate host. All known stages of this parasite are found in the brush border of the mucosal epithelium of the stomach and intestine. The oocysts (4 to 5 μm in diameter), which are passed in the feces, represent the infective stage for humans. The freshly passed oocyst contains four sporozoites. Infection begins

when sporozoites released from ingested oocysts enter the brush border of the mucosal epithelium. The sporozoite grows into a trophozoite and then undergoes asexual division (schizogony) to produce a schizont (2 to 5 μm in diameter) that contains eight crescent-shaped merizoites that are released to repeat the schizogonic cycle. Some may form macro- and microgametocytes that mature and by fertilization produce a zygote. The zygote will eventually develop into the oocyte, the transmission stage. The wall of the oocyte protects the parasite from environmental stresses.

PATHOGENESIS AND SYMPTOMATOLOGY

In immunocompetent individuals, *Cryptosporidium* causes a short-term flu-like, gastrointestinal illness with minimal histologic changes. Illness results in self-limiting (1 to 2 weeks) episodes of watery diarrhea. Parasite multiplication is interrupted by T-cell–dependent immune mechanisms.

In immunocompromised individuals (e.g., AIDS patients) the unchecked cycle of multiplication of the parasite results in heavy parasite burdens producing a chronic infection with profuse debilitating diarrhea, malabsorption syndrome, anorexia, weight loss, and signs of cachexia.

The incubation period ranges from one to several weeks. Onset of illness may be accompanied by fever, malaise, nausea, and vomiting; this is followed by abdominal cramps and diarrhea.

DIAGNOSIS AND TREATMENT

Diagnosis is made by demonstrating the oocysts in the feces. They are usually present in sufficient numbers for a direct fecal smear. However, standard concentration methods are employed as well. Biopsy specimens of intestinal mucosa have also been used to detect *Cryptosporidium*.

No good treatment has been identified for immunocompromised individuals. In immunocompetent individuals the disease is self-limiting and therefore only supportive treatment is necessary.

EPIDEMIOLOGY AND CONTROL

Cryptosporidium is a cosmopolitan parasite found in many mammals including humans.

Infection is acquired through the ingestion of oocysts from human or animal feces. Oocysts are infective when passed and are resistant to ordinary disinfectants. Control measures include those for all fecal-orally transmitted diseases. Immunocompromised patients are at risk. As of April 1986, 19,182 persons with AIDS had been reported to the CDC. Of these 697 (3.6 percent) had confirmed cases of cryptosporidiosis. The reported case fatality rate for this group of patients was 61 percent. The case fatality rate for AIDS patients without reported cryptosporidiosis was slightly but significantly lower than that for patients with this disease. The high incidence of *Cryptosporidium* in homosexual males compared with other groups (e.g., heterosexuals) is consistent with the hypothesis that oral-anal contact contributes to the transmission of *Cryptosporidium*.

REFERENCES

Beaver, P. C., and Jung, R. C.: Animal Agents and Vectors of Human Disease. Lea and Febiger, Philadelphia, 1985.

Beck, J. W., and Davies, J. E.: Medical Parasitology. C. V. Mosby, St. Louis, 1981.

Brown, H. W., and Neva, F. A.: Basic Clinical Parasitology. Appleton-Century-Crofts, Norwalk, CT, 1983.

Erlandsen, S. L., and Meyer, E. A.: *Giardia* and Giardiasis. Plenum Press, New York, 1984.

Katz, M., Despommier, D. D., and Gwardz, R.: Parasitic Diseases. Springer-Verlag, New York, 1982.

Martinez-Paloma, A.: Human Parasitic Diseases. Vol. 2, Amebiasis. Elsevier, New York, 1986.

section IV

Oral health and disease

IV

chapter 25

Ecology of the oral flora

W. J. Loesche, D.M.D., Ph.D.

The mucous membranes of animals are normally colonized by a large and diverse microbial flora. These bacteria are constantly interacting with the host and with each other in competition for survival. In this chapter some of the parameters of these interactions will be discussed.

Bacterial Populations on the Surfaces of Animals

Bacteria colonize all surfaces of an animal, but are particularly dense in the oral cavity and lower gastrointestinal tract, where they achieve densities of 100 million bacteria per milligram plaque wet weight or fecal wet weight. Numbers of this magnitude put a severe constraint upon bacteriologic isolation and taxonomic procedures. An additional problem is that these bacterial populations can fluctuate with the changing conditions of their environment. Thus, a considerable amount of investigation is necessary before even simple statements can be made about the flora of the surfaces of the various body cavities.

Researchers have sought to establish some order by defining the flora in terms of numerical dominance of various organisms in certain sites, under certain well-recognized conditions. The best examples of this approach are found in the study of the rumen flora, present in various grazing animals, exposed to a standard dietary regimen. Information and concepts obtained from these studies have been transposed to the human situation, particularly to the oral flora. It should be remembered, however, that this information has never been unequivocally established for the oral flora, as it has not been possible to study the oral flora under standard conditions of diet and frequency of eating. Thus, when we speak in the following paragraphs of indigenous, transient, and supplemental flora, we are doing so in the hope of imposing a modicum of order upon a system about which we have only fragmentary knowledge.

The Oral Flora

Bowden and his colleagues have listed, as of 1979, about 21 genera of bacteria comprising about 60 species, which have been isolated from the oral cavity. This is an underestimation, as many new species have been described in the succeeding years and it is now estimated that there may be over 200 different species that can be isolated from dental plaque alone. Of these, some such as *Actinomyces, Bacterionema, Rothia,* and *Leptotrichia* (all gram-positive rods or filaments) appear to be autochthonous genera, as they have not been isolated from any other habitat. Others, like *Actinobacillus actinomycetemcomitans* and *Streptococcus mutans,* are species that were described 60 to 70 years ago but only recently have been reisolated and associated with dental pathology.

In order to deal with this degree of taxonomic diversity, many bacteriologists recognize a normal and a transient bacterial species simply on the basis of prevalence. A normal species is almost always present, whereas a transient species is only occasionally present. A normal species can be present in numerically dominant numbers, in which case it is defined as an indigenous species, or it can be present in low numbers and is then called a supplemental species. The distinction between an indigenous and a supplemental species can change with the environment, as will be illustrated with *S. mutans* and the *Lactobacillus* species.

THE INDIGENOUS FLORA

The indigenous flora comprise those indigenous species that are almost always present in high numbers, that is, greater than 1 percent, in a particular site, such as the supragingival plaque or the surface of the tongue. Their numerical dominance implies that they are compatible with the host and have entered into a stable relationship with the host. They do not compromise the host's survival.

The environments found in the oral cavity of various animals must share some similarities, as the indigenous oral flora of these animals bear some resemblances to each other. Thus, the oral flora is dominated by anaerobic and facultative bacteria, which exhibit optimal growth at about body temperature (37°C). Also many of these organisms have complex nutritional requirements that can only be met in a rich organic milieu such as exists in or on animal surfaces. Beyond these similarities, however, there are apparently pressures that select for a characteristic oral flora. Thus, certain genera, such as the *Streptococcus, Actinomyces,* and *Neisseria,* appear to be found in the oral cavity of all animals tested (Table 25–1), whereas other genera, such as the *Bacteroides* and the *Enterobacteriaceae,* are characteristically intestinal organisms. This is not to say that genera such as the *Bacteroides* are not found in the oral cavity, for indeed, *Bacteroides* species can be isolated regularly from the subgingival plaques of humans and lower primates (Table 25–1). The distinction, rather, is that they have not been isolated from the oral cavities of all animals.

SUPPLEMENTAL FLORA

The supplemental flora are those bacterial species that are nearly always present, but in low numbers, that is, less than 1 percent of the total viable count. These organisms may become indigenous if the environment changes. For example, *Lactobacillus* species are normally found in low levels in plaque (i.e., 0.00001 to 0.001 percent of the viable flora). If a carious lesion develops under this plaque, the plaque pH will become acidic. In

Table 25–1 ■ Genera that appear to be indigenous to the tooth surfaces

Animal	Genera			
	Streptococcus	*Actinomyces*	*Neisseria*	*Bacteroides*
Humans	+ +*	+ +	+	+
Primates	+ +	+ +	+	+
Herbivores	+ +	+ +	+	0
Carnivores	+ +	+ +	±	0
Others†	+	+	±	0

*+ + = present in all animals examined; + = usually isolated; ± = occasionally isolated; 0 = not isolated.
†Others include Indian fruit bat, spinny tenrec, bushbaby, and red mantled tamarin.
(Adapted from Bowden et al., 1979.)

this new environment the lactobacilli, because they are acid tolerant, will be selected for and can become numerically dominant in the carious lesion. In this case one may consider the lactobacilli as being indigenous to the carious lesion, a finding that has pathologic significance.

A single bacterial species can be an indigenous species in one mouth and a supplemental species in another. This is often the case with *S. mutans*. For example, in an epidemiologic investigation of an entire school system, involving 500 first-grade students, *S. mutans* was found in the occlusal fissure plaque of all children. In this sense it was a normal organism in these children. In most subjects, *S. mutans* was a member of the supplemental flora. Statistical analysis revealed that *S. mutans* was a member of the indigenous plaque flora when decay was present.

Thus, as with the lactobacilli, the transition of *S. mutans* from the supplemental flora into the indigenous flora was associated with dental pathology. This pattern is repeated in periodontal disease, in which increases in the levels of spirochetes, *B. gingivalis*, and *A. actinomycetemcomitans* in the subgingival plaque are associated with inflammation and bone loss. From this we may deduce that the supplemental flora contains most of the potential dental pathogens found in the plaque. When we speak of dental decay and periodontal disease as endogenous infections, we concede that some new factor(s) have imposed themselves into the microbial ecosystem on the dentogingival surfaces, which allow the emergence of the odontopathogens.

TRANSIENT FLORA

Transient flora comprise organisms "just passing through" a host. At any given time a particular species may or may not be represented in the flora. Bacteria present in food or drink may be temporarily established in the mouth. However, as these transients normally do not have mechanisms for persisting in the crowded oral environment, they quickly disappear. Overt pathogens of the type that are medically important are exceptions to this general concept, in that they appear to quickly pass, under certain circumstances, from a transient stage to a predominant stage on the mucous membrane. These medically important pathogens do not dominate in plaque, but often can be isolated in high numbers from many periapical, pericoronal, and periodontal abscesses.

Host-Bacteria Inter-Relationships

The preceding discussion described the quantitative nature of the mucous membrane flora. However, this flora cannot be adequately understood independent of its host environment. The relationship of a host to its flora can be described in one of three ways.

SYMBIOSIS

When both the host and the bacteria benefit from their inter-relationship, it is termed "symbiotic." A classic example of symbiosis is found in the digestive tract of ruminants and termites. These two hosts subsist on diets containing a large proportion of cellulose, yet lack the enzyme to degrade the cellulose. This enzyme is supplied by the gut bacteria, which secrete an extracellular cellulase that breaks down the cellulose to residues that can be absorbed by the host. In return, the bacteria receive a supportive environment with optimal temperature, nutrients, water, and the absence of inhibiting agents. This relationship is extremely stable, as the survival of both members is dependent upon it. In fact, from an evolutionary standpoint this has been a very stable solution, as evidenced by the universal success of grazing animals.

ANTIBIOSIS

An antibiotic relationship is the opposite of a symbiotic relationship. Instead of helping each other, the bacteria and the host are antagonistic to each other. When bacteria cause an infection that is combatted by the defense systems of the host, the relationship is said to be antibiotic.

This antibiotic relationship is very unstable for both the host and the pathogenic bacteria. If the host is killed by the pathogen, the pathogen also dies unless it is able to make its way to another host. If the pathogen can be passed from host to host, killing as it goes, it will eventually eliminate its host populations, which again results in death for the pathogen. On the other hand, if the pathogen is not virulent enough to withstand the host's defense systems, such as antibodies and phagocytic cells, it will be eliminated. Thus, an antibiotic relationship will not be a permanent one.

In some instances a balance is struck between the virulence of a pathogen and the ability of the host population to contend with the organisms. An example of such a balance is the measles virus, which causes a mild illness in the inhabitants of most industrialized nations. Hosts in which this balance has not been achieved are readily susceptible to the viral pathogen. When the American Indians were first exposed to the measles virus by European colonists, they had no defense systems prepared. As a result, the same pathogen that caused a relatively minor illness in the colonists decimated the Indian populations. This problem is seen today, as humans living in isolated communities succumb readily to what are mild infectious diseases in westernized humans.

AMPHIBIOSIS

The new relationship described between the measles virus and the host appears to be a general rule in biology. An unstable relationship, such as the antibiotic one, will clearly be discriminated against by the evolutionary selection process. Recent medical history has shown a decreased virulence for all the classic pathogens, such as the *tubercle bacillus*, *Treponema pallidum*, and others. This means that these organisms have entered into a new, more stable relationship with the host. Rosebury introduced the term ''amphibiotic'' to describe an intermediate state in which the host and its flora exist in a form of stable balance with each other. Most of the oral flora are thought to exist in an amphibiotic relationship with their host, as there has been no demonstration, yet, of their being harmful or beneficial.

This balance can change, as when *S. mutans* or *B. gingivalis* increases proportionally in the plaque, causing evidence of dental pathology. This overgrowth does not compromise the survival of the host, so that from an evolutionary perspective this type of low-grade infection is inconsequential.

In many instances members of the indigenous flora are related to overt pathogens. For example, the indigenous oral spirochetes resemble morphologically and serologically the virulent spirochete, *T. pallidum*, the causative agent of syphilis. The bacteria now recognized as indigenous varieties probably evolved from more virulent species. Organisms would be selected on the basis of reduced virulence. Eventually the species that came to dominate on a mucous membrane would be those with minimal, if any, virulence for the host. With further time, some of these bacteria might become beneficial to the host.

Such symbiotic interactions undoubtedly have occurred but, with the exception of the example of cellulase-producing bacteria in the rumen, little is known of them, because in nature the host and its flora cannot be separated. However, in recent years a unique research animal, the germ-free animal, has become available to aid in this type of research. At present, it is possible to raise a large number of mammalian species in the absence of detectable bacteria. These animals permit the study of a host in the presence of one or more known organisms.

Germ-Free Animals

The fetus grows and matures in a bacteria-free uterus. Contamination of the fetus occurs during passage through the birth canal, handling by hospital personnel and family, and exposure to atmospheric and surface bacteria. If these sources of contamination can be avoided, the neonate should remain bacteria- or germ-free. A germ-free animal is obtained by a cesarean section in which the neonate is delivered and placed aseptically into a sterile chamber. Once obtained, a newborn can be kept sterile by preventing any contact with environmental contaminants.

The air, food, water, and other objects are sterilized before being placed in the chamber and given to the animal. All research animals can be raised for at least one generation in such a sterile environment. The rat and mouse are the only germ-free species that can be bred, for reasons to be discussed shortly. The germ-free animal requires the introduction of new definitions. The normal animal, harboring an unknown flora, is referred to as a conventional animal. Animals that have a known flora are called gnotobiotic animals. Gnotobiotic animals may be germ-free or colonized with one or more known bacterial species.

DEFENSE SYSTEMS

One of the most obvious differences between germ-free and conventional animals is the lack of development of lymphoid tissue in the former, particularly along the gastrointestinal tract. The antibody levels in germ-free animals, compared with those of conventional animals, are significantly depressed. A few antibodies are produced in reaction to the remnants of bacteria remaining in the sterilized food, but the level is much below that of conventional animals.

The rate of synthesis of antibody, as determined chemically as serum gamma globulin levels, was about 1/200 of the rate of synthesis observed in conventional animals living under crowded conditions. The reduction of lymphoid tissue and antibody levels was predictable, as the normal flora and environment provide the host with a considerable amount of antigenic stimulation. Germ-free animals are somewhat sluggish in their response to antigens but, if suitably challenged, they make antibody in a normal manner. They clearly are not immunologically incompetent.

The second major distinction between germ-free and conventional animals is found in the lining of the digestive system. The lower portion of the small intestine in the germ-free animal is atrophied, with a significant reduction in the total mucosal surface area. But, the most obvious change in the morphology of the digestive tract is the greatly enlarged cecum in the germ-free animals. The cecum lies at the junction of the large and small intestines and is about 1 percent of the body weight in a conventional animal.

The cecum of the germ-free animal, however, may exceed 18 percent of the animal's body weight. This greatly enlarged cecum prevents normal gestation in all germ-free animals except the rat and mouse, which explains why these two are the only animals capable of breeding in a sterile environment.

The enlargement of the germ-free cecum is a direct result of the disruption of normal digestive mechanisms by the lack of appropriate flora. In conventional animals the large quantities of proteins and glycoproteins present in the secretions and surface cell sloughings from the duodenum and jejunum are degraded by the gut flora into a form that can be absorbed in the ileum and reused by the animal. Without this degradation, the animal loses the protein equivalent of a diet that contains 15 percent protein. This endogenous protein accumulates in the cecum of the germ-free animal, where it is further degraded by endogenous proteolytic enzymes, such as trypsin and chymotrypsin, to osmotically active, low molecular weight compounds that retain water. The failure to reabsorb this endogenous protein forces the germ-free animal to eat more dietary protein in order to remain in nitrogen balance.

The enlarged cecum came as a surprise to the early investigators of germ-free animals, as they did not realize that the indigenous flora played a role in the digestion of host-derived proteins. This demonstrated a symbiotic relationship between the host and the intestinal flora that was not identified until the flora was eliminated.

DENTAL DISEASE

Germ-free animals do not develop dental decay, despite the ingestion of high sucrose diets. This observation confirmed the essential role of bacteria in the decay process. Germ-free animals also have reduced inflammation in the periodontal tissues. However, germ-free animals will form calculus and may exhibit what appear to be genetically related patterns of bone loss. The germ-free rat and mouse have been successfully utilized to test the virulence of odontopathic organisms such as *S. mutans, A. viscosus, A. naeslundii, A. actinomycetemcomitans,* and *Capnocytophaga* strains. Potentially periodontopathic organisms such as *B. gingivalis* and various spirochetes cannot be evaluated in these animals because of their inability to grow on the mucous membranes of these animals. This surprising observation brought attention to the fact that a sterile mucous membrane is essentially an aerobic surface and is not capable of supporting anaerobic bacteria.

The demonstration of dental pathology in a germ-free animal, infected with a single species, should be interpreted with some caution given the peculiarities of the germ-free animal. First, the germ-free animal's immune system would be hypofunctional at the time of the initial colonization. Second, all the available sites on the dentogingival surfaces are unoccupied, so that the introduced species would have exclusive access to those niches which, in the conventional animal, would already be occupied by an established bacterial community. Third, the introduced species would not have to contend with the competition and antagonisms related to survival, which exist in any densely and diversely populated microbial community. Fourth, the altered metabolism and eating patterns of the host that are secondary to cecal enlargement could introduce various factors that would not be operable in conventional animals. Even after these peculiarities are accounted for, the germ-free animal has proved to be an invaluable animal model for the demonstration of the virulence of *S. mutans*.

Selection Forces Operating on the Oral Flora

The oral flora had, until the mid-1960s, been regarded as a homogeneous bacterial community that was accurately represented by the bacteria found in the saliva. In this chapter we will find that salivary cultures reflect the flora found on the oral soft tissues and, only minimally, the flora found on the teeth. First, however, we shall discuss the main environmental selection forces, which serve to shape the normal oral flora into distinct ecosystems—namely, the anaerobic nature of the oral mucous membranes and the available nutrient sources.

Anaerobiosis

The transit of air through the mouth would seem to preclude any possibility that the oral cavity contained niches where anaerobes could thrive. Although evidence to the contrary was apparent by the presence of "fusospirochetal" organisms in subgingival plaques taken from sites of periodontal inflammation, this was ignored, probably because salivary and plaque samples that were cultured aerobically always yielded ample growth. However, when quantitative culturing procedures were first employed, about 10 percent of the organisms observed microscopically could be cultured aerobically, whereas about 20 percent could be cultured when anaerobic jars were used. These recoveries increased to about 50 to 70 percent when investigators used procedures such as the roll tube or anaerobic chamber in which oxygen was eliminated from the gas atmosphere. The conclusion was obvious. If anaerobes dominated in the flora, the oral mucous membranes must constitute an anaerobic environment.

OXYGEN TENSIONS IN THE MOUTH

Little attention had been given to the oxygen tension of the oral cavity as an ecologic determinant. The oxygen tension, which is a measure of the amount of oxygen in a gas, is about 21 percent (160 mm Hg) for air. When an oxygen electrode was placed in the mouth and then the lips were closed so as to provide a seal, the gas space over the tongue had an oxygen tension of 12 to 14 percent. When the electrode was placed in the buccal cavity lateral to the buccal surfaces of the molar teeth, the oxygen tension was about 1 percent. When a miniaturized electrode was placed into a periodontal pocket, the oxygen tension was about 1 to 2 percent oxygen.

These data indicate that the gaseous atmosphere over the dentogingival surfaces is mainly anaerobic, particularly in the sites where subgingival plaques would form. The oxygen tensions in the atmosphere over supragingival plaques, especially those on the labial, lingual, and occlusal surfaces, could range from 1 to about 20 percent. Thus, it should come as no surprise that anaerobic species are found primarily in subgingival plaques, while facultative and microaerophilic species dominate in supragingival plaques.

OXIDATION-REDUCTION POTENTIAL (Eh)

Another measure of anaerobiosis is the level of the electrical potential of a site relative to a standard hydrogen electrode. This potential, called the Eh, is the tendency for a medium or compound to oxidize or reduce an introduced molecule by the removal or addition of electrons. Tissues or microbes that need a positive Eh for viability are termed "aerobes," and those that need a negative Eh are "anaerobes."

Experience has shown that media that are "prereduced" with sulfhydryl compounds (i.e., cysteine, dithiothreitol, and glutathione), so as to have a negative Eh, permit the reliable growth of anaerobes, and yield the highest recoveries of viable bacteria from plaque samples. If a low Eh is beneficial for the in vitro growth of these organisms, then it is likely that similar low Ehs exist in their "in vivo" habitat. Such Ehs would be expected in any crowded microbial community that performs a fermentative metabolism, as fermentation results in the formation of reduced end products. Thus, one could conclude that the Eh in oral sites where microbes accumulate would eventually become negative. This was verified by the in vivo measurement of Eh in plaque in which subjects wore artificial teeth (pontics) containing Eh electrodes (a platinum wire) for several days. The patients came in on different days, and the electrodes were connected to a pH meter, which measured the Eh potential of the plaque that had accumulated on the pontic. On the first day, the potential was much the same as saliva, $+200$ millivolts (mv). As the plaque got older, the Eh dropped to -112 mv and eventually, in some, reached an Eh of -141 mv.

The study indicated that portions of plaque are indeed changing over time from an aerobic to an anaerobic environment, with a corresponding drop in Eh. This change in Eh in undisturbed plaque coincides with a shift in the flora from entirely facultative microaerophilic bacteria to one in which anaerobes such as spirochetes can be detected. Indeed, in subgingival plaques associated with periodontitis, these anaerobic spirochetes can account for half of the flora (see Chapter 19).

SUPEROXIDE RADICAL

Before leaving this section of anaerobiosis, some mention should be made about how oxygen kills a cell and how aerobic cells avoid this fate. First, oxygen can react with the double bonds in lipids, forming peroxides that irreversibly alter the lipids. Since lipids are found in membranes, their oxidation would destroy the integrity of the cell. Second, oxygen can react with sulfhydryl groups of enzymes, forming a disulfide bond. The oxidation of an enzyme in this way may inactivate the enzyme, shutting down the related metabolic pathways, resulting in death for the cell. These effects have not been proved in cells but have been observed using pure enzymes and lipid membranes.

Recent evidence indicates that molecular oxygen reacts with reduced flavoprotein to form a superoxide radical (Fig. 25–1). This superoxide radical rapidly destroys the lipids and enzymes of living cells. Oxygen by itself, as well as hydrogen peroxide, reacts with lipids and enzymes, but at such low rates that the superoxide radical appears to be the actual lethal form of oxygen in biologic systems.

SUPEROXIDE DISMUTASE

How do bacteria and other organisms, including tissue cells exposed to oxygen, protect themselves against this superoxide radical? Humans have a copper-containing blood protein called hemocuprine, which acts to remove the superoxide radical. Hemocuprine (or, as called by its enzymatic function, superoxide dismutase) converts the superoxide radical to hydrogen peroxide, which in turn is reduced by the cell to water by a reaction

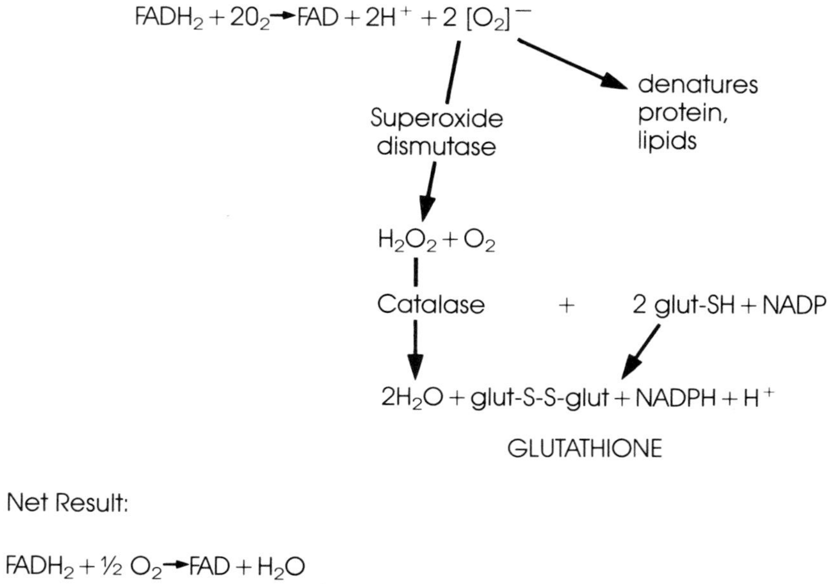

$$FADH_2 + 2O_2 \rightarrow FAD + 2H^+ + 2\,[O_2]^-$$

Superoxide dismutase

denatures protein, lipids

$$H_2O_2 + O_2$$

Catalase $+$ 2 glut-SH + NADP

$$2H_2O + glut\text{-}S\text{-}S\text{-}glut + NADPH + H^+$$

GLUTATHIONE

Net Result:

$$FADH_2 + \tfrac{1}{2}\,O_2 \rightarrow FAD + H_2O$$

Figure 25–1 ▪ Inactivation of O_2 by superoxide dismutase.

involving glutathione (see Fig. 25–1). The oxidized glutathione is subsequently reduced by a reaction involving NADPH.

Bacteria that are normally exposed to oxygen (facultative aerobes) also have a superoxide dismutase that destroys the superoxide radical. Anaerobes generally do not have a superoxide dismutase and are killed by oxygen via the superoxide radical. In fact, the absence of this enzyme may be the functional definition of an anaerobe. Several investigators have surveyed various fermentative bacteria for the presence of superoxide dismutase and found a significant positive relationship between the absence of this enzyme and the inability to grow in the presence of oxygen.

BIOLOGIC SIGNIFICANCE OF AN ANAEROBIC FLORA

Anaerobes dominate in the mucous membrane flora of all animals from insects to humans. The universality of this occurrence states that there is some unequivocal advantage to both the host and the flora in this arrangement. The advantage to the host is so obvious that it is amazing that it has gone so long unrecognized. Anaerobes cannot survive in aerobic tissues because they lack enzymes such as superoxide dismutase. If anaerobes penetrate the physical barrier of the mucous membrane epithelium, as has been shown for the periodontium, they are quickly killed by the molecular oxygen present in the aerobic host tissue, before they can propagate. This would imply that an anaerobic mucous membrane flora should be nonpathogenic and thus selected for by the host during evolutionary time. The universal success of anaerobes on the mucous membranes indicates that this relationship is so stable that it should be considered a symbiotic relationship.

But why symbiotic? The defense mechanisms of the host include the physical barrier of the lining epithelial cells, the phagocytic actions of the white blood cells, and the finely tuned response of the immune system (Fig. 25–2). The last two mechanisms respond to those organisms capable of both invading and propagating in the host tissue. This response is not needed when anaerobes invade the host because they cannot survive in the tissues. When an anaerobe moves from a mucous membrane locale where the Eh is about -100 mv to an oxidized host cell environment where the Eh is about $+100$ mv, its enzymes are quickly inactivated and its lipid membranes are disrupted. Thus, when the host is colonized by an anaerobic flora, an electrical potential of about 200 mv difference is created between the mucous membranes and the underlying, highly vascularized host tissues. Electrical barriers of this magnitude ensure that the anaerobic bacteria and the aerobic host cells remain physically separated. In this manner the host benefits from its anaerobic flora and provides, in exchange, the nutrient base essential to the survival of the normal flora.

The importance of Eh in regard to the growth of anaerobes is demonstrated by the inability of anaerobes to establish on the mucous membranes of germ-free animals. This is because the Eh of the sterile secretions is positive, resembling that of the host tissues. Anaerobes cannot grow at these Ehs and, therefore, do not colonize the mucous membranes. A similar situation occurs each time a newborn confronts life. In this case,

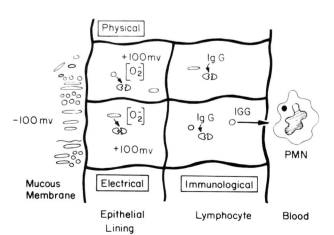

Figure 25–2 ■ Barrier systems in the host against bacterial invasion include the physical barrier composed of the surface epithelium, the electrical barrier that reflects the Eh difference between the host cell and the microbial layer, the immunologic barrier composed of the antibody-forming cells, and the reticuloendothelial system. (From Loesche, W. J. L.: Dental Caries: A Treatable Infection. University of Michigan, 1986, with permission.)

the sterile mucous membranes are first colonized by facultative organisms. The metabolism of these organisms quickly lowers the Eh to negative values that permit the establishment and eventual domination of the anaerobic flora.

Thus, nature exploits the incompatibility of anaerobic and aerobic forms of life to establish a stable symbiotic relationship between the host and its flora.

Nutrient Sources in the Oral Cavity

The host's contribution to this symbiotic relationship is, of course, to provide a ready supply of usable nutrients, which permits the normal flora to survive on the mucous membranes. In this regard the oral flora has access to a wider range of nutrients than perhaps the normal flora in any other mucous membrane niche. Nutrients are derived from at least five sources. The food eaten by a person is quantitatively probably the most important nutrient source for the oral flora. Nutrients also are present in saliva and the gingival crevice fluid. Epithelial cells are shed from the oral surfaces and some of these cells lyse in the hypotonic saliva, thereby releasing nutrients into the saliva. In some cases, the bacteria themselves add nutrients to their surrounding environment, which in turn are used by other organisms (Table 25–2).

MAGNITUDE OF MICROBIAL NUTRIENT NEEDS

The nutrients available to the oral flora must provide an energy source, such as fermentable carbohydrates or amino acids, or both, as well as biosynthetic compounds necessary for the growth and maintenance of the various organisms. The quantitative nutrient needs per day for the entire oral flora can be estimated, if we make the assumption that the total number of bacteria that reside in the oral cavity remains constant. Then we need only to know the total number of bacteria that exit from the oral cavity and calculate from this number the amount of nutrient matter needed to replace them. The number of organisms swallowed per milliliter of saliva is approximately 100 million, which corresponds to 1 mg wet weight of bacteria. If about 1 liter of saliva is swallowed per day, then 100 billion bacteria, corresponding to 1

Table 25–2 ■ Nutrient sources available to the oral microbial ecosystems

Nutrient Source	Microbial Ecosystems On or In
Diet	Tongue
	Soft tissue
	Supragingival plaque
Saliva	Tongue
	Soft tissue
	Supragingival plaque
Gingival crevicular fluid	Subgingival plaque
	Supragingival plaque
Microbial products	Subpragingival plaque
	Subgingival plaque
	Tongue
	Soft tissue
	Tongue
Host products	Subgingival plaque
	Supragingival plaque
	Soft tissue
	Tongue

g wet weight, exit from the oral cavity per day. In order to keep the oral bacteria mass constant, enough nutrients must be consumed to replace this 1 g wet weight bacteria. Studies with *E. coli* show that 80 percent of a nutrient source is expended in energy metabolism and 20 percent is converted to bacterial mass. If this 4:1 ratio holds for the way the oral flora metabolizes its substrates, then 1 g wet weight of cell mass would require 5 g wet weight of nutrients. This is a small amount, which can easily be met in the oral environment.

GROWTH RATE(S) OF THE ORAL FLORA

The 100 billion bacteria that are shed into the saliva daily come from all the oral surfaces. The teeth constitute a relatively small surface area for washoff and, accordingly, their flora are poorly represented in the saliva. Studies in which volunteers rinsed with a mouth rinse containing radioactive carbon-14–labeled chlorhexidine before and after extraction of diseased teeth indicated that the tooth surfaces composed about 5 percent of the surface area of the mouth. From this we can estimate that the total plaque flora, if shed rates from hard and soft surfaces are similar, constitutes about 5 percent of the salivary flora. This value allows the calculation of the approximate growth rate of the oral flora, if we consider this flora a single entity, and if we know the weight of the plaque present at any given time on the teeth.

If the plaque on all the teeth at any given time weighs 10 mg wet weight, which is about what one would find on teeth subjected to reasonable levels of oral hygiene, then the biomass of the oral flora would be about 200 mg wet weight (10 mg plaque = 5 percent of the salivary flora; therefore, 100 percent of the salivary flora = 200 mg). If this biomass remains constant, then in order for 1 g wet weight of bacteria to be shed daily into the saliva, the oral bacteria must divide about five times per day, i.e., 5×200 mg = 1 g that is shed.

According to this calculation the generation, or doubling time, of the oral flora in vivo is just under 5 hours. This is considerably slower than the 30- to 50-minute generation times that pure cultures of oral bacteria, such as the streptococci, exhibit in vitro. From this it is apparent that the oral flora is growing at a relatively slow rate in vivo. The rate limiting step(s) could be either a nutrient deficiency or an inhibitory environment. Whenever a new site becomes available for colonization, such as a clean tooth surface or a new epithelial cell surface, it seems to be populated rapidly by the oral flora. This suggests that the overall growth rate of the oral flora is regulated by physiochemical considerations, such as pH, Eh, or accumulations of toxic products, rather than by nutrient needs.

An analogous situation is seen in the colonization of a gnotobiotic animal by a facultative organism. The bacterium grows rapidly after its introduction into the animal, often obtaining growth rates observed in vitro, until its population density approaches the maximum normally observed on the mucous membranes. Thereafter, the organism grows at a much slower rate but one that is adequate to maintain a constant density. Thus, population size is maintained within a finite range in which cell loss, because of death or shedding, is balanced by new cell divisions. These slow-growing bacterial cells, however, are metabolically quite active. Resting cell suspensions of supragingival plaques were on a per CFU (colony-forming units) basis, 8- to 62-fold more active in fermenting sucrose than any of six pure cultures of species isolated from the plaque.

These considerations suggest that although the oral flora is not growing rapidly in vivo, it does have the potential to do so (at least some of its members have this potential) and that it is able to utilize nutrients rapidly once they are sequestered. This latter capability may be of great survival value, as it enables the oral flora to remove the maximal amount of nutrients from a flowing stream, such as the saliva or the gingival crevicular fluid.

DIET AS A NUTRIENT SOURCE

Three factors influence the effectiveness of the diet as a microbial nutrient source. These are the chemical composition of the diet, the physical consistency of its components, and the frequency of its presentation. The macromolecular nutrients such as starches, proteins, and lipids are normally not available to the oral flora, as their transit time through the oral cavity is too short for them to be degraded to usable nutrients. However, if the physical consistency of the foods that contain them permits retention, such as fibrous foods between the teeth or sticky foods in fissures, pits, and contact points, then some utilization of the starches and proteins could occur. Low molecular weight, soluble carbohydrates such as sucrose (sugar) and lactose (milk sugar) are readily metabolized by the oral flora. It is this bioavailability of these simple sugars that make them cariogenic.

In dental decay the consistency of the diet and the frequency of ingestion may be more important than diet composition. Both consistency and frequency influence the length of time that food remains in contact with plaque and thus is available for bacterial use. The longer bacteria have food available, the more they can grow, the more acid they will produce, and the greater the plaque mass that will accumulate. When snacks are interspersed between meals, they augment the time of nutrient availability, allowing further growth of the plaque organisms. If the plaque is only partially debrided by toothbrushing prior to retiring, the plaque mass remaining on the teeth of the snackers may metabolize stored polysaccharides and produce an appreciable pH drop on the tooth surfaces during sleep. In experimental animals and in clinical studies, frequent eating of a high sucrose diet is associated with high caries activity.

The consistency of food also influences the plaque flora. Liquid foods, such as fruit juices and tonics, are usually swallowed quickly, and are therefore not readily available to the oral flora. Sticky and fibrous foods, however, are retained in those areas that trap food (e.g., fissures, missing contacts, pockets, and cavities) and can be used by the flora in these areas for extended periods of time. It is no mere coincidence that these sites usually are associated with dental pathology. Hard candy, in this context, would be an exceptionally cariogenic foodstuff. The sucrose that is slowly released would bathe the supragingival plaque and lead to the selection of organisms, such as *S. mutans*, which can efficiently utilize sucrose.

The importance of between-meal eating of sucrose and the consistency of sucrose-containing foods in dental disease was unequivocally demonstrated by a clinical study conducted in adult residents of a mental hospital in Vipeholm, Sweden. The 5-year caries attack rate in these subjects on the institutionalized diet—that is, the control group—was about 0.2 DMF (decayed-missing-filled) teeth per year. The addition of about one-half pound of sucrose per day in the form of toffees, caramels, chocolates, or bread at meal times caused less than one decayed tooth per year. However, the ingestion of the same forms of sucrose between meals led to an explosive increase in DMF teeth, in that five to seven newly decayed teeth were observed per year. The frequent ingestion of sucrose was shown to cause an elevation in the levels of salivary sugars and in the length of time that sugars could be detected in the saliva.

Thus, for those subjects who ate between meals, sugar could be detected in their salivas during most of the day. This meant that some microbial fermentation was ongoing in the plaque for most of the day and accordingly, the pH at the plaque-enamel interface probably was below pH 5.5, the critical pH for enamel demineralization. This long exposure of the tooth surface to an acidic pH could easily account for the increased decay rate observed in these adults.

Diet is the single most important nutrient source for the plaque found on the coronal surfaces of teeth. Dietary restriction of carbohydrates, especially sucrose, should profoundly influence the composition of the supragingival microbial flora. Detailed bacteriologic studies on individuals maintaining such a restricted diet have yet to be performed. The salivary lactobacilli levels and the plaque levels of intracellular polysaccharide-forming bacteria decrease appreciably on low-carbohydrate diets. These low-carbohydrate diets are difficult for patients to maintain and are therefore essentially impractical for caries control.

However, dietary reduction of caries by replacement of sucrose with noncariogenic sugar substitutes, such as xylitol, mannitol, or sorbitol, may be possible. Xylitol, in particular, has been shown in human studies to reduce caries either when a total substitution for sucrose was made or when chewing gum sweetened with xylitol was taken between meals. The xylitol either is not fermented by the plaque flora or, if fermented, does not lower the pH. The use of such a sucrose substitute should change the microbial composition of plaque, and indeed the proportions of efficient sucrose-fermenting organisms such as *S. mutans* decline in the plaque when xylitol is substituted for sucrose.

SALIVA AS A NUTRIENT SOURCE

Saliva is quite properly considered a homeostatic fluid that buffers the plaque. However, saliva can provide nutrients to the flora that resides on the surface it bathes. Saliva contains about 1 percent solids, which include glycoproteins, inorganic salts, and most importantly for the plaque flora, milligram amounts of amino acids and glucose, and microgram amounts of certain vitamins. These quantities are sufficient to sustain some bacterial growth during periods when a person does not eat, such as between meals and overnight during sleep. Some investigators suggest that the glycoproteins present in saliva could also serve as nutrient sources, if they are trapped in plaque. Some plaque bacteria possess neuraminidases, which break down the terminal sugar residues on certain glycoproteins, but no evidence exists that shows that the neuraminic acid (sialic acid), which is released, can be used by the plaque flora. Those bacteria that can utilize and have access to the salivary nutrients always have a good source available. This advantage is meaningless, however, for those bacteria that do not grow on surfaces exposed to saliva. The bacteria that reside in the gingival crevices and periodontal pockets have limited access to salivary nutrients and do not appear to be influenced by them.

GINGIVAL CREVICE FLUID

The gingival crevice is bathed by microliter amounts of a serum transudate that contains tissue and serum proteins, as well as free amino acids, vitamins, glucose, and so forth.

Under healthy gingival conditions, this gingival crevice fluid is protective, flushing out nonadherent plaque from the sulcus and bringing phagocytic cells and antibodies into the area. The presence of certain serum components may act as a strong selection factor for some of the gingival crevice microbes such as the spirochetes and black-pigmented bacteroides (see section on Nutrient Needs later in this chapter).

SHED CELLS

The epithelial surfaces of the oral cavity undergo a turnover, shedding their surface cells; also, phagocytic cells enter the oral cavity from the gingival crevice area. These mammalian cells can be lysed by the hypotonicity of saliva and their contents are then available for microbial nutrition. The magnitude of this food source for microbial metabolism is not known.

BACTERIA

The bacteria themselves can provide nutrients for each other. In a dense microbial population, such as plaque, one would expect considerable microbial interactions. One well-documented interaction is the relationship between lactic-acid–producing bacteria, such as the streptococci and a lactate-utilizing species, such as *Veillonella alkalescens*. *V. alkalescens* has lost the enzyme, hexose kinase, which means that it cannot phosphorylate glucose. Under most conditions this would be a lethal mutation and the mutant never observed. However, if this mutation occurred in nature in the presence of lactic acid, the mutant could survive because this acid is absorbed by *V. alkalescens* and fermented so as to yield ATP.

Many organisms in plaque, including the streptococci, form lactic acid. This would suggest that the *Veillonella* parasitize the lactate producers. However, the relationship between the *Veillonella* and organisms such as streptococci may be symbiotic, as the lactic acid is converted to propionate, acetate, and carbon dioxide, with a resultant elevation in pH. This shift away from low pHs would be beneficial for acid-sensitive streptococci such as *S. sanguis*. Other examples of plaque-microbial interactions exist. *Treponema denticola* is dependent upon cohabitant plaque species for isobutyrate and spermine. *Bacter-oides melaninogenicus'* requirement for vitamin K can be provided by a variety of other oral bacteria, such as *C. sputorum* and *B. oralis*.

These microbial interactions indicate that some of the oral flora are microbe dependent—that is, they will not grow in the absence of the provident microbes. This is indeed the case, as none of the cited organisms will easily establish in pure cultures in germ-free animals. *Veillonella* can be grown in germ-free animals after prior establishment of a streptococcus. No one has yet established the spirochetal species in gnotobiotic animals under any circumstances, indicating that parameters other than nutrient availability, such as Eh, may be preventing colonization.

Ecologic Niches

Thus far we have discussed the oral flora as if it were a single entity. Now it is known that microorganisms that live on the tongue are not necessarily the same organisms that are found in the plaque. Moreover, organisms like the spirochetes and gram-negative anaerobic rods inhabit the subgingival plaque but are rarely found in supragingival plaque or in high numbers in the saliva. Clearly, there is some heterogeneity within the "oral" flora.

Prior to 1963 most bacteriologists had considered the "oral" flora to be uniformly distributed throughout the mouth, and they concentrated their efforts on the culturing of saliva on the assumption that the saliva reliably reflected the "oral" flora. This approach ignored the unique contributions to the saliva of the bacteria shed from the different anatomic sites within the mouth and, accordingly, delayed the understanding of the role of specific microbes in both dental caries and in periodontal disease. For example, if an organism such as *S. mutans* composed less than 1 percent of the salivary flora, it is difficult to conceive how it could be a cariogenic organism. However, if *S. mutans* constituted 25 percent of the flora in an occlusal fissure, then its role as a cariogenic organism is plausible.

PLAQUE

In the late 1950s and early 1960s quantitative culturing procedures were introduced in which plaques and saliva were dispersed, serially diluted, and cultured under an anaerobic atmosphere. Gibbons, Socransky, and their colleagues collected plaque from either the coronal or subgingival surfaces of all the teeth in a mouth and pooled them so as to give a single sample for each subject. The pooled plaques from the coronal surfaces contained mainly gram-positive saccharolytic organisms (carbohydrate fermenters), whereas the pooled plaques from the subgingival surfaces contained, in addition, gram-negative saccharolytic and asaccharolytic (proteolytic) organisms. Neither plaque contained *S. salivarius,* although this organism had until this time been considered to be the numerically dominant streptococcus in the oral cavity because of its prominence in the saliva.

When Krasse, in the early 1950s, reported that *S. salivarius* was not present in the plaque, he said that a discrepancy must exist between salivary sampling techniques and the technique of sampling material from the tooth surface. This discrepancy is now known to be the incorrect assumption that plaque and saliva are bacteriologically identical. The washoff of bacteria from all the surfaces in the oral cavity are found in the saliva. Since the tongue and cheeks constitute most of the mouth's surface areas, the flora shed from their surfaces is highly prominent in the salivary flora. As *S. salivarius* is the predominant streptococcus on these surfaces, it becomes also the predominant streptococcus in the saliva.

These quantitative culturing studies were extended to look at other sites in the mouth and to look for specific bacterial types, so that eventually the geographic localization of many oral species was determined (Table 25–3). The flora on the tongue, on the buccal mucosa, and in the saliva are similar, whereas the plaque flora differs by having almost undetectable levels of *S. salivarius* and appreciable levels of *Actinomyces* and gram-negative species. The gram-negative species are mainly confined to the subgingival plaque so that it is not even valid to think of plaque as a homogeneous entity.

Not only do microbial populations differ from location to location in the mouth, but the plaque flora in the same location also may show definitive changes over time. For example, following cleaning of the teeth, the plaque that initially forms at the dentogingival margin after 1 day is made up primarily of cocci. If the plaque remains undisturbed for a few weeks, some gram-negative, motile species are observed (see section on Plaque Formation in Chapter 26).

These studies with pooled plaques demonstrated the differences between subgingival and supragingival flora and their respective differences from salivary flora. However, they did not demonstrate appreciable differences between patients with and without dental diseases. This is because the pooled plaques contained mostly plaque from non-diseased sites, which would dilute out the plaque obtained from single sites that were

---

Table 25–3 ■ Intraoral site distribution of various indigenous and supplemental members of the oral flora

Species	Saliva	Tongue	Plaque Supragingival	Plaque Subgingival
S. salivarius	+ + +	+ + +		
S. sanguis	+ +	+ +	+ + +	+
S. mitior	+ +	+ +	+ +	+ +
S. milleri	±	±	+ to + + +	0
S. mutans	± to +	±	+ to + + +	0
Lactobacillus sp.	± to +	+	+	±
Actinomyces sp.	+	+	+ +	± to + +
Fusobacterium sp.	0	0	±	± to + +
Capnocytophaga	0	0	±	± to +
Treponema sp.	0	0	±	± to + + +
B. melaninogenicus	0	0	±	± to +
B. gingivalis	0	0	0	0 to + +
A. actinomycetemcomitans	0	0	±	0 to +
Veillonella	+	+	+ +	+ +

0 = not usually detected; ± = rarely present; + = usually present in low proportions; + + = usually present in moderate proportions; + + + = usually present in high proportions.

Adapted from following sources: Gibbons, R. J., and van Houte, J.: J. Periodontol. 44:347, 1973; Loesche, W. J.: J. Periodontol. 6:245, 1968; Mejare, B., and Edwardsson, S.: Arch. Oral Biol. 20:757, 1975; Slots, et al.: Infect. Immun. 29:1013, 1980; Loesche, W. J., and Syed, S. A., unpublished data.

diseased. It is only in the last few years that plaques from single diseased pockets or single carious fissures have been cultured and compared with plaques from nondiseased sulci or fissures.

ECOLOGIC DETERMINANTS

What phenomena can explain the microbial diversity that exists in different anatomic sites in the mouth? What ecologic differences exist between the teeth and the soft tissue that results in the establishment of distinct flora in these sites? Why does plaque in the supragingival area contain fewer gram-negative species than does the subgingival plaque? Bacteria establish themselves in sites where they can fulfill their nutrient requirements and do not encounter inhibitory or adverse conditions for their growth. Could these factors be the determinants responsible for the different microbial ecosystems?

NUTRIENT NEEDS

The nutrient sources in the mouth are diverse and should provide a wide variety of organic compounds capable of supporting the growth of the most fastidious organisms, yet it is possible that some unique growth factor needed by *S. salivarius*, for instance, is not present in the plaque microenvironment. Carlsson explored this possibility by developing chemically defined media for *S. salivarius*, *S. sanguis*, and *S. mutans*. The three species had similar nutrient requirements except for differences in single amino acids. Thus, nutrient needs could not account for the absence of *S. salivarius* in the plaque.

Nutrient availability, however, could explain the localization of certain gram-negative species to the subgingival plaque. *B. melaninogenicus*, *B. gingivalis*, and *Capnocytophaga* either have a requirement for or were stimulated by hemin. Many isolates of the black-pigmented bacteroides were also stimulated by vitamin K, estradiol, and progesterone. *Treponema denticola* has a requirement for spermine.

All of these compounds would be present in serum but not in saliva, foods, or shed cells. The only site in the mouth where microbes would have access to these nutrients would be in the flow bed of the gingival crevicular fluid. Thus, the aforementioned species could thrive only in the subgingival

plaque. If gingival pathology occurs and the transudate increases in volume, a proliferation of these organisms might occur. In fact, when gingivitis has progressed to the point when bleeding occurs, these organisms can be found among the indigenous flora of the site. This can be documented in pregnancy gingivitis, where a specific increase in *B. intermedius* was found after bleeding occurred. The specificity of this increase could be correlated with the ability of this organism to utilize estradiol and progesterone, both of which would increase in the gingival crevice fluid during pregnancy. Thus, in the case of the spirochetes and the black-pigmented bacteroides, nutrient supply appears to be of paramount importance in their localization and actual levels in the plaque.

INHIBITORY FACTORS

A variety of inhibitory factors of either host or microbial origin could be responsible for the distinct ecosystems observed in the plaque and soft tissues. The host factors would include specific antibodies, lysozymes, lactoperoxidase, lactoferrin, and high molecular weight adhesins—all of which are present in the saliva. These host antibacterial mechanisms do not appear to be responsible for the establishment or maintenance of the various oral ecosystems.

Bacteria produce factors such as organic acids, which lower the pH; reduced end products, which lower the Eh; hydrogen peroxide, which oxidizes certain enzymes and membranes; and fatty acids and bacteriocins, which prevent the growth of certain species. All of these could shape the microbial composition in a niche. The role of these factors in regulating microbial populations in vivo has not been adequately investigated.

Acidic pHs ■ Members of the oral flora grow best in vitro at about pH 7.0. This is the level found in saliva and maintained by the carbonate buffer in the saliva. However, the plaque pH can drop to below 5.0 during eating. This low pH could select for aciduric organisms, which could account for the absence of species such as *S. salivarius* in the plaque. This possibility was investigated by observing the relative abilities of several oral species, including *S. salivarius*, to initiate growth in media with acid pHs.

All tested species grew luxuriantly when the initial pH was 7.0 but exhibited diminished growth when the initial pH was 5.5

(Table 25–4). When the pH was dropped to 5.0, only *S. mutans* and *L. casei* were capable of growth. There was no difference in acid tolerance between *S. salivarius* and such prominent plaque organisms as *S. sanguis*, *S. mitis*, and *A. viscosus*. Thus, the absence of *S. salivarius* from the plaque could not be related to its being more sensitive to low pH than *S. sanguis* or *S. mitis*. Tolerance of low pH can explain the selection of *S. mutans* and *L. casei* in the cariogenic plaques and lesions, and this trait, known as aciduricity, may be the single most important determinant in the cariogenicity of these organisms.

Reduced products and pO$_2$ ▪ Bacterial metabolism results in the formation of reduced end products that lower the Eh. In the dentogingival area and in the pockets, the Eh may be as low as -100 mv and the oxygen tension as low as 1 percent. Only anaerobes and certain facultative organisms could survive in this environment. The oxygen tension over the dorsum of the tongue and perhaps on certain coronal tooth surfaces would be considerably higher and supportive of more oxygen tolerant organisms, such as the streptococcal species. Organisms such as the spirochetes, *B. gingivalis*, *B. melaninogenicus*, *B. oralis*, and *F. nucleatum* cannot survive in well-aerated areas such as the tongue and many supragingival sites but are well adapted to the anaerobic crevicular environment. All streptococcal species tested could grow in air. Thus, oxygen sensitivity cannot explain the absence of *S. salivarius* from the dental plaque.

The absence of *S. salivarius* from the plaque is best explained by its inability to attach to the tooth and plaque-covered surface. The importance of adherence to attachment in oral microbial ecology is covered elsewhere in this volume.

Summary

The host supports a large and diverse bacterial population on its surfaces. Powerful selection pressures such as anaerobiosis, temperature, and nutrient availability shape this flora into distinct microbial communities on the various anatomic surfaces and orifices of the body. Each community contains, as its characteristic members, those species that have no, or low, virulence for the host. This so-called normal flora separates out into those species that are numerically dominant, or the indigenous flora, and those that persist in low numbers and are known as the supplemental flora. The indigenous flora probably interacts with the host in a symbiotic fashion, whereas some members of the supplemental flora interact in an amphibiotic or unstable fashion. In the oral cavity overgrowth of certain members of the supplemental flora can be associated with either dental caries or periodontal disease. These common dental afflictions appear then to be specific, albeit chronic, endogenous infections.

Nutritional and inhibitory factors, to the extent that they could be identified, can explain the localization of anaerobic and certain fastidious organisms to the subgingival plaque. They explain why saccharolytic-microaerophilic organisms dominate in the supragingival and soft-tissue sites. They do not explain why certain organisms such as *S. salivarius* dominate in the soft tissue but are absent from the plaque. Clearly, other ecologic determinants are operative. One of these, the ability of an organism to adhere to a surface, will be described in Chapter 26.

Table 25–4 ▪ Effect of initial pH of broth media on growth of various plaque bacteria

Bacteria	Initial pH of Media		
	7.0	5.5	5.0
S. salivarius	0.9	0.20	NG†
S. sanguis	0.9	0.40	NG
S. mitis	0.7	0.04	NG
A. viscosus	1.3	0.20	NG
S. mutans	1.1	0.50	0.2
L. casei	0.8	0.70	0.6

*Terminal optical density after 53 hours of anaerobic incubation.

†NG = no growth.

Adapted from Harper, D. S., and Loesche, W. J.: Arch. Oral Biol. 29:843, 1984.

REFERENCES

Alexander, M.: Microbial Ecology. John Wiley and Sons, New York, 1971.

Bonesvoll, P., and Olson, I.: Influence of teeth, plaque and dentures on the retention of chlorhexidine in the human oral cavity. J. Clin. Periodontol. 1:214, 1974.

Bowden, G. H. W., Ellwood, D. C., and Hamilton, I. E.: Microbial ecology of the oral cavity. In Alexander, M. (ed.): Advances in Microbial Ecology. Plenum Publishing, New York, 1979, pp. 135–217.

Burnett, M., and White, D. O.: Natural History of Infectious Disease, ed 4. Cambridge University Press, Cambridge, 1972.

Carlsson, J.: Nutritional requirements of *Streptococcus sanguis*. Arch. Oral Biol. 17:1327, 1972.

Gibbons, R. J., and van Houte, J.: On the formation of dental plaque. J. Periodont. 44:347, 1973.

Gustafsson, B. E., Quensel, C. E., Lanke, L. S., Lundquist, C., Grahnen, H., Bonow, B. E., and Krasse, B.: The Vipeholm dental caries study. The effect of different levels of carbohydrate intake on caries activity in 436 individuals observed for five years. Acta Odontol. Scand. 11:232, 1954.

Harper, D. S., and Loesche, W. J.: Growth and acid tolerance of dental plaque bacteria. Arch. Oral Biol. 29:843, 1984.

Hungate, R. E.: The Rumen and its Microbes. Academic Press, New York, 1966.

Kenney, E. B., and Ash, M. M.: Oxidation reduction potential of developing plaque, periodontal pockets and gingival sulci. J. Periodont. 40:630, 1969.

Kornman, K. S., and Loesche, W. J.: Effects of estradiol and progesterone on *Bacteroides melaninogenicus* and *Bacteroides gingivalis*. Infect. Immun. 35:256, 1982.

Krasse, B.: The proportional distribution of *Streptococcus salivarius* and other streptococci in various parts of the mouth. Odont. Rev. 5:203, 1954.

Loesche, W. J.: The rationale for caries prevention through the use of sugar substitutes. Int. Dent. J. 35:1, 1985.

Loesche, W. J., Eklund, S., Earnest, R., and Burt, B.: Longitudinal investigation of human fissure decay: Epidemiological studies in molars shortly after eruption. Infect. Immun. 46:765, 1984.

Luckey, T. D.: Germfree Life and Gnotobiology. Academic Press, New York, 1963.

Minah, G. E., and Loesche, W. J.: Sucrose metabolism in resting-cell suspensions of caries-associated and non-caries-associated dental plaque. Infect. Immun. 17:43, 1977.

Morris, J. G.: Oxygen and growth of the oral bacteria. In Kleinberg, I., Ellison, S. A., and Mandel, I. D. (eds.): Proceedings of Saliva and Dental Caries. Sp. Supp. Microbiol. Abstr. pp. 293–306, 1979.

Rogosa, M., Krichevsky, M. I., and Bishop, F. S.: Truncated glycolytic system in *Veillonella*. J. Bacteriol. 90:164, 1965.

Rosebury, T.: Microorganisms Indigenous to Man. McGraw-Hill, New York, 1962.

Tally, F. P., Stewart, P. R., Sutter, V. L., and Rosenblatt, J. E.: Oxygen tolerance of fresh clinical anaerobic bacteria. J. Clin. Microbiol. 1:161, 1975.

chapter 26

Dental plaque and calculus

Mariano Sanz, M.D., D.D.S. □ *Michael G. Newman, D.D.S.*

CHAPTER OUTLINE

- **DENTAL PLAQUE**
- **DENTAL CALCULUS**

Dental Plaque

The importance of bacteria in dental plaque and its key role in the development of both dental caries and gingival and periodontal disease has evolved in the last 20 years. In 1963, Socransky and colleagues demonstrated that human dental plaque contains 1.7×10^{11} organisms per wet weight per gram, showing that plaque consists predominantly of bacteria rather than food remnants as had been previously thought. At the same time, several clinical longitudinal studies showed conclusively that plaque control can arrest and prevent dental caries and periodontal disease, and evidence has shown that in compromised patients, poor plaque control and dental pathology may have even more serious local and systemic consequences.

Therefore, a thorough understanding of the structure and composition of dental plaque is required to fully understand the major dental diseases, dental caries and periodontal disease.

DEFINITION

The term *plaque* is used universally to describe the association of bacteria to the tooth surface. Dental plaque may be defined as bacterial aggregations on the teeth or other solid oral structures. *Materia alba* is another term used to describe bacterial aggregations, leukocytes, and desquamated oral epithelial cells accumulating at the surface of plaque and teeth, but lacking the regular internal structure observed in dental plaque. The differentiation between both deposits is determined by the strength of the adherence of the deposit. If it is removed by the mechanical action of a strong water spray, the deposit is then termed "materia alba," but if it withstands the water spray, it is called "dental plaque."

Based on its relationship to the gingival margin, plaque is differentiated into two categories: *supragingival* and *subgingival* plaque. Supragingival plaque is sometimes further differentiated into *coronal plaque,* or plaque in contact only with the the tooth surface, and *marginal plaque,* in association with both tooth surface and gingival margin.

PHYSICAL AND CLINICAL DESCRIPTION

Supragingival plaque can be clinically detectable once it has reached a certain thickness. Small amounts of plaque are not clinically visible unless they are disclosed by

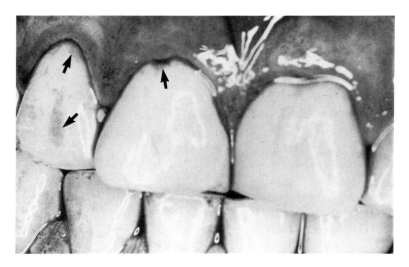

Figure 26–1 ■ Small amounts of dental plaque can only be seen if stained with a disclosing solution *(arrows).*

pigments, from within the oral cavity or stained by disclosing solutions (Fig. 26–1). As plaque develops and accumulates, it becomes a visible globular mass with a nodular surface and a whitish to yellowish color (Fig. 26–2).

Dental plaque can also grow on other hard surfaces in the mouth, mainly if the site is protected from the normal mechanical cleansing action of the tongue, cheeks, and lips. Therefore, plaque deposits regularly occur in pits and fissures of occlusal surfaces, on restorations and artificial crowns, orthodontic bands, dental implants, removable orthodontic appliances, and dentures.

Measurable amounts of supragingival plaque may form within 1 hour after the teeth have been cleaned, with maximum ac-cumulation in about 30 days. The rate of formation and location vary among individuals and is influenced by diet, age, salivary factors, oral hygiene, tooth alignment, systemic disease, and host factors.

Subgingival plaque cannot be detected by direct observation, since it occurs below the gingival margin. Its presence can be proved only by running the end of a probe around the gingival margin or by means of a disclosing solution.

CLINICAL IMPORTANCE

The relationships among improper oral hygiene, formation of dental deposits, and development of dental diseases have been rec-

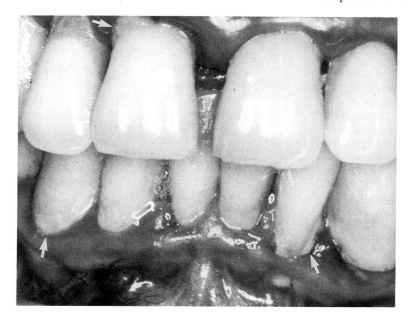

Figure 26–2 ■ Gross accumulations of plaque can be seen forming globular masses of white-yellow color *(arrows).*

ognized for centuries. There is substantial scientific evidence implicating dental plaque as the most important factor in the development of periodontal diseases (Table 26–1).

In the middle of this century, well-designed epidemiologic studies were performed to relate different epidemiologic variables with periodontal disease. From these studies, oral hygiene and age were the only variables with a significant relationship to the prevalence and severity of periodontal disease. An almost linear relationship exists between severity of periodontal disease and lack of oral hygiene and accumulation of dental deposits.

In experimental studies using germ-free animals, periodontal tissue loss was accelerated after infection with microorganisms.

Final evidence was gathered when gingivitis was experimentally developed in humans when oral hygiene measures were purposely abolished. When oral hygiene was reinstituted, gingivitis resolved within a week, restoring gingival health.

The transition from gingivitis to periodontitis has not been demonstrated experimentally in humans. However, in dogs gingivitis develops as the result of plaque accumulation and, if allowed to continue, causes loss of attachment and destruction of the supporting tissues of the teeth, similar to typical human periodontal disease (periodontitis).

Additional evidence for the role of dental deposits in the development of periodontal disease in humans has been derived from longitudinal clinical studies in which the progression of periodontal disease has been retarded by the introduction of oral hygiene practices and with the use of antimicrobials such as chlorhexidine. These measures inhibit plaque formation and therefore prevent the development of experimental gingivitis.

Table 26–1 ■ Etiologic importance of dental plaque: scientific evidence

1. Epidemiologic studies—poor oral hygiene increases prevalence and severity of periodontal disease
2. Experimental studies in germ-free animals— monoinfection with suspected pathogen: signs of periodontal disease
3. Experimental gingivitis in humans (Löe 1965); experimental periodontitis in dogs (Lindhe 1976)
4. Longitudinal clinical studies—oral hygiene + mechanical or chemical plaque control therapy arrest and/or prevent the progression of periodontal disease

---

COMPOSITION OF DENTAL PLAQUE—MICROBIOLOGY

Dental plaque consists primarily of proliferating microorganisms along with a scattering of epithelial cells, leukocytes, and macrophages, in an adherent intercellular matrix. Bacteria make up approximately 70 to 80 percent of this material. One cubic millimeter of dental plaque weighing about 1 mg contains more than 10^8 bacteria. These bacteria exist in an extremely complex arrangement. There may be as many as 200 to 400 different species of microorganisms in one particular site; some species have not been currently identified. Dental plaque may contain microorganisms other than bacteria; *Mycoplasma*, fungi, protozoa, and viruses have been demonstrated in different proportions.

Improved bacteriologic sampling techniques, anaerobic culturing, and complex species identification matrices have identified several patterns of dental plaque composition.

SUPRAGINGIVAL PLAQUE

Formation and Biochemistry

Supragingival plaque has been examined in multiple studies with different microscopic techniques. Plaque formed on artificial or natural surfaces does not significantly differ in structure or microbiology. However, the first layer of organic material that forms on artificial surfaces differs significantly from the one that forms on natural tooth. This first layer is called the *pellicle.*

Pellicle is the initial distinct organic structure on surfaces of teeth and/or artificial splints, formed prior to colonization by bacteria. After bacterial colonization, the pellicle is regarded as part of the dental plaque, which then consists of pellicle, bacteria, and intercellular matrix. The composition of pellicle is dependent on the nature of the solid on which it is formed. Therefore, in vitro models of pellicle formation on glass or plastic surfaces are of questionable value compared with hydroxyapatite matrices.

The first stage in pellicle formation involves adsorption of salivary proteins to apatite surfaces. This involves electrostatic ionic interaction between calcium ions and phosphate groups in the enamel surface and opposite-charged groups in the salivary macromolecules. The structure of the pellicle is heterogeneous. Initially the pellicle develops by adsorption of small globules or aggregations of amorphous material to the apatite surface. In later stages, it can adopt a globular, fibrillar, or granular morphology. The mean pellicle thickness ranges from about 100 nm at 2 hours to 500 to 1000 nm at 24 to 48 hours.

This structural heterogeneity reflects a complex composition, consisting mainly of high molecular weight blood group reactive glycoproteins, immunoglobulins, virus hemagglutination inhibition factors, and different carbohydrates. However, recent studies suggest the main proteins are low molecular weight phosphoproteins and sulphoglycopeptides. These phosphate and sulphate groups may attach to the apatite surface by ion displacement through direct ionic and hydrophobic interaction. In a second stage, the remaining salivary glycoproteins are adsorbed through different intermolecular interactions including ionic, hydrogen-bonding, hydrophobic, and van der Waal's.

The transition between pellicle and dental plaque is extremely rapid. The first constituents include mainly cocci with small numbers of epithelial cells and polymorphonuclear leukocytes. The individual bacteria initially adhere to small irregularities, fissures, or areas with imperfections (roughness, cracks) that are relatively sheltered from oral cleansing forces.

Generally, the first organisms form a monolayer of cells, either singly or in small groups. Bacterial growth extends beyond surface defects and increases in volume. At the periphery the growth continues, eventually coalescing with neighboring patches of plaque. During the first few hours, the attached bacteria proliferate and form small colonies of cocci. With time, other types of microorganisms proliferate, giving rise to different microcolonies. Eventually, dental plaque becomes characteristically complex (Fig. 26–3).

The material among bacteria in dental plaque is termed *intermicrobial matrix* and accounts for approximately 25 percent of plaque volume. Its composition includes microbial substances, salivary material, and gingival exudate. The organic matrix is mainly a polysaccharide protein complex produced by plaque microorganisms. Several oral streptococci synthesize levans and glucans from dietary sucrose (see Chapter 6). The levans (fructans) provide mainly energy, while the glucans, mainly dextran, act not only as a source of energy but also as the organic skeleton of plaque, playing a role in bacterial adhesion and interbacterial coaggregation reactions. Other matrix carbohydrates are galactose and methylpentose in the form of rhamnose. The small amount of lipids present in the plaque matrix is mainly composed of small extracellular trilaminar vesicles from gram-negative microorganisms, representing lipopolysaccharide endotoxins. The matrix protein component is provided by salivary glycoproteins, which promote bacterial adherence if adsorbed to the tooth surface or to agglutinate other bacteria. Other proteins are also provided by lysed bacteria.

Inorganic components of supragingival plaque matrix include primarily calcium and

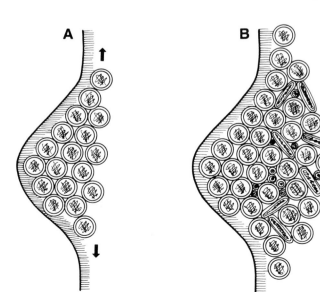

Figure 26–3 ■ Initial colonization of bacteria in dental plaque. *A,* Gram-positive cocci are able to adhere to irregularities in pellicle covered enamel sheltered from oral cleansing mechanisms. *B,* Once adherent, subsequent bacterial colonization (rods) is facilitated in the direction of the arrows and becomes part of the plaque mass. (Adapted from Lie, T.: J. Perio. Res. 12, 73, 1977.)

phosphorus, with small amounts of magnesium, potassium, and sodium. The inorganic content of early plaque is very low but greatly increases as plaque is transformed into calculus.

The formation of dental plaque involves two major processes: initial adherence of salivary organisms to the acquired pellicle and proliferation of attached bacteria and further aggregation of bacteria to already attached cells. In both processes, the two primary ecologic determinants are bacterial adherence and growth.

Bacterial Adherence

Oral bacteria vary markedly in their ability to attach to different surfaces. There is a preference of various oral bacteria for colonizing different oral surfaces, which is not due to differences in growth rate. *S. mutans*, *S. sanguis*, *Lactobacillus* sp., and *A. viscosus* have been preferentially found colonizing tooth surfaces; *S. salivarius* and *A. naeslundii* the dorsum of the tongue; and *Bacteroides* and spirochetes the gingival crevice or periodontal pocket.

In dental plaque development, two adhesive processes are required. First, bacteria must adhere to the pellicle surface and become sufficiently attached to withstand oral cleansing forces. Second, they must grow and adhere to each other to allow plaque accumulation.

During initial adherence, interactions occur mainly between specific bacteria and the pellicle. In subsequent phases of plaque formation, bacteria, bacterial products, interbacterial matrix, host, and dietary factors are involved.

Electrostatic forces ■ All oral bacteria bear an overall net negative charge, which is probably due to the outward orientation of some cell wall components, such as anionic residues on surface glycoproteins (see Chapter 3). Bacterial attachment to the enamel pellicle may occur via electrostatic attractions in which negatively charged components of the bacterial cell surface and negatively charged tooth surface constituents become linked via cations such as calcium. In order to overcome the electrostatic repulsive forces, bacterial appendages such as fimbriae and flagella extend a distance from the bacterial cell wall (approximately 10 to 20 nm), permitting cation bridging or other adhesive mechanisms to take place (Fig. 26–4).

Bacterial adhesion is a very complex proc-

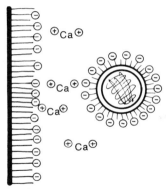

Figure 26–4 ■ Bacterial attachment via electrostatic interactions. Negatively charged components of the bacterial surface and pellicle become linked by cations, such as calcium.

ess. Conditions such as pH and ionic strength have a variable effect on bacterial adhesion. Studies of zeta potentials of different oral bacteria show that species such as *S. sanguis* and *S. salivarius*, differing only slightly in zeta potential, are able to elicit a completely different pattern of bacterial adhesion.

Hydrophobic interactions ■ The hydrophobic association is based on a close structural fit between molecules. The nature of bacterial cell wall constituents contributing to the hydrophobicity of the cell is not clearly known, although several oral bacteria have hydrophobic properties at their surface. A contributing factor might also be LTA, with its hydrophilic linear polymer of glycerophosphate and a nonpolar tail of fatty acids that provide a long hydrophobic area. Such a molecule could contribute to the hydrophobic properties of the cell wall in addition to its anionic properties if the lipid moiety is properly oriented (Fig. 26–5).

Organic components ■ The organic components in saliva and other tissue fluids have a profound influence on adhesion and colonization. Depending on the bacterial species, salivary proteins may either inhibit or promote adhesion. As a general rule, proteins of saliva are inhibitors of bacterial adhesion, through interaction with the bacterial and tooth surface or through alterations in the ionic or hydrophobic/hydrophilic balance of both surfaces. However, in specific bacteria, saliva promotes bacterial adherence by a specific reaction between the bacterial surface and the organic pellicle on the tooth. This specificity has been suggested as a mechanism to explain the selective nature of the attachment of bacteria to oral surfaces. In studies of competitive binding among strep-

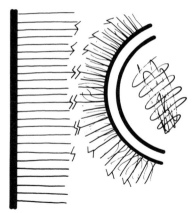

Figure 26–5 ■ Bacterial attachment via hydrophobic interactions. These interactions are based on the close structural fit between molecules on the pellicle (⤙) and bacterial surfaces (⤚).

tococci to saliva-coated hydroxyapatite, no competition for binding sites was evident among strains of *S. mutans, S. sanguis, S. mitis,* and *S. salivarius,* which may indicate that these organisms interact with different receptor sites on the pellicle. The interactions between different bacteria involved in coaggregation are also highly specific; the aggregation of *S. sanguis* with *A. naeslundii* is strain specific. The receptors responsible for these highly specific interactions are associated with the fibrillar coating or fimbriae on the bacterial cell surface.

In view of the specificity characteristic for bacterial adhesion to different oral tissues, it has been postulated that biochemical differences in cell surface coatings must exist among different bacteria. Recently, different binding sites or biochemical bonds have been identified, allowing interaction of molecules on the bacterial cell surface with specific receptors on the pellicle-covered tooth surface. These molecules are termed *adhesins.* These biochemical bonds have been demonstrated in vitro and have shown to be inhibited by certain sugars, which has suggested the presence of *lectin-like* substances in oral bacteria. These lectins (proteins) would recognize specific carbohydrate structures in the pellicle (carbohydrate groups of glycoproteins). Lectin-like interactions have been demonstrated by selective inhibition of adherence with the addition of sugars. The adherence of *S. mutans* to saliva coated hydroxyapatite is strongly inhibited by galactose but not by lactose, galactosamine, and mannosamine. *S. mutans* cells bind to α-galactoside residues of salivary glycoprotein in the pellicle, whereas *S. sanguis* cells require

sialic acid residues. Lectin-like interactions also appear to play a role in bacterial coaggregations. Strains of *A. viscosus* and of *S. sanguis* coaggregate through a β-galactose–specific lectin, as well as *S. salivarius* and *Veillonella* (Fig. 26–6).

In 1984, Rolla and associates proposed another specific interaction for adherence of *S. mutans.* The adhesion of this bacteria involves the production of glycosyltransferase (GTF) by the bacteria. GTF is adhesive and adsorbs to tooth surfaces, where it produces glucans when exposed to sucrose. The interaction between the rigid α-1-3 glucans and adsorbed GTF on the surface may thus cause a strong, specific sucrose dependent colonization of *S. mutans.*

Multiple binding sites ■ Evidence suggests that oral bacteria each possess different cell surface-binding sites responsible for their attachment and accumulation on oral surfaces. *S. mutans* cells interact with high molecular weight salivary glycoproteins, which adsorb selectively to hydroxyapatite and which may be responsible for its direct attachment to the pellicle. This process is very inefficient, probably owing to a low number of binding sites in the pellicle for this organism. *S. mutans* cells also possess other binding sites such as GTF and nonenzyme glucan-binding proteins, which are responsible for their attachment to glucans bound to the tooth surface.

Multiple binding sites involved in interactions with salivary glycoproteins, extracellular polysaccharides, and direct cell-to-cell adhesion are probably necessary for the survival of these organisms in such a complex environment.

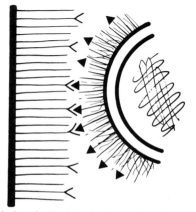

Figure 26–6 ■ Bacterial attachment via specific lectin-like interactions. Lectins (proteins) (▶) in the bacterial surface recognize specific carbohydrate structures in the pellicle (❮) and become linked.

Growth and Accumulation of Supragingival Plaque

Once bacteria originating from saliva or contiguous surfaces adhere to the pellicle surface, saturation of bacterial binding sites takes place. As a result, subsequent growth leads to bacterial accumulation and increased plaque mass. Although adhesion processes dominate in the initial phase of plaque formation, the total plaque mass that develops is mainly determined by multiplication of the attached bacteria. The relative importance of adhesion versus multiplication has been demonstrated experimentally with the use of antibacterial treatments with no or negligible effects on adhesion. Plaque accumulation, however, is almost negligible in the absence of cell division (Fig. 26–7).

Accumulations of dental plaque also require cohesion of bacterial cells. This is accomplished by the formation of the plaque matrix, which is dependent on bacterial metabolic activities and salivary and host-derived components. Therefore, factors influencing the ultimate composition and pathogenicity of dental plaque depend on (1) bacterial factors and (2) host and environmental factors (Table 26–2).

Bacterial factors ■ Apart from bacterial adhesive mechanisms, already discussed, other bacterial mechanisms play an important role in plaque growth and accumulation.

Role of extracellular products ■ Variety of oral microorganisms such as *S. mutans, S. sanguis, S. mitis, S. salivarius,* and *Lactobacillus* species have the capability to form extracellular polymers from sucrose. The role of these extracellular polysaccharides has been most intensively studied with *S. mutans,* because of its demonstrated importance as an etiologic agent of dental caries (see Chapter 27). This is mainly due to the synthesis by this microorganism of large amounts of ex-

Table 26–2 ■ Factors influencing the composition and maturation of dental plaque

I. *Factors of Bacterial Origin*
  A. Extracellular Products: Glucans (skeleton of plaque)
    Fructans (energy resources)
  B. Bacterial Interactions: Coaggregation reactions
  C. Plaque Ecology:
    Dietary changes: Sucrose intake—aciduric bacteria
    Oxygen environment—anaerobic bacteria
    Nutritional interactions—bacterial succession
    Bacteriocin production
II. *Host-Derived Factors*
  A. Mechanical Oral Cleansing Mechanisms
  B. Saliva:
    pH, lactoperoxidase, lactoferrin, lysozyme
    Salivary glycoproteins: adhesion mechanisms
  C. Host-Immune Responses:
    Oral secretions—IgA
    Crevicular fluid: leukocytes, IgG, IgM, complement, etc.

tracellular glucans (dextran or mutan) from sucrose and by extracellular enzyme complexes, glucosyltransferases (GTF).

These extracellular glucans are insoluble and result in increased bacterial adhesion. Generally, glucan-induced aggregation does not occur with other streptococcal species, even though they may synthesize glucans. However, *S. mutans* has the capacity to bind glucan molecules, resulting in aggregation and accumulation of these organisms. Furthermore, synthesis of sticky insoluble glucans by *S. mutans* may mediate nonspecific entrapment of other microorganisms from oral fluids, promoting the accumulation of bacteria other than *S. mutans. Actinomyces* species can also form copious amounts of plaque in the presence of a variety of carbohydrates. *A. viscosus* synthesizes an extracellular heteropolysaccharide composed of *N*-acetylglucosamine, glucose, and galactose.

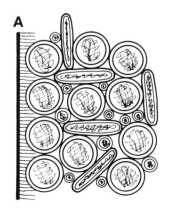 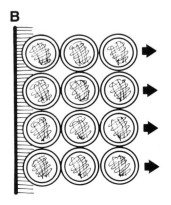

Figure 26–7 ■ Dental plaque growth depends on *(A)*, growth via adhesion of new bacteria, and *(B)*, growth via multiplication of attached bacteria.

Role of bacterial interactions ■ Electron microscopic studies have shown direct interactions between bacteria, with the attachment of one species to the surface of others. This may have special importance for organisms incapable of attaching *directly* to the tooth surface. *Veillonella*, for example, is unable to attach to glass surfaces in vitro, but adheres and accumulates on preformed plaque of *A. viscosus*. Certain *Actinomyces* species aggregate specifically with *S. sanguis* through β-galactosil residues. The presence of dental plaque containing *Actinomyces* or other gram-positive bacteria may be beneficial for the attachment and colonization of some black-pigmented *Bacteroides* species (Table 26–3).

Plaque ecology ■ Changes in dietary carbohydrate alter the microbial composition of dental plaque. Carbohydrate fermentation produces a low pH and an aciduric environment. Among the oral bacteria that grow in this aciduric environment are lactobacilli and certain streptococcal species, mainly *S. mutans*.

Certain bacteria also store intracellular glycogen-like materials known as IPS. These bacteria exhibit prolonged acid production when exogenous carbohydrates are depleted, giving them a better chance of survival. Other exogenous factors, such as the production of ammonia from urea provoked by bacterial ureases and the presence of lactic acid–fermenting organisms such as *Veillonella* and *Neisseria* also modify the final plaque pH and consequently its pathogenicity.

Oxygen and oxygen products are very important ecologic determinants because they influence the ability of plaque bacteria to grow and multiply. Streptococci and lactobacilli can grow under facultative conditions, consuming large quantities of oxygen and producing highly reactive and potentially destructive products. Superoxide anions (O_2), hydroxen peroxide (H_2O_2), and hydroxyl radicals (OH^-) that are formed may damage cell membranes and enzyme systems. In order to survive, bacteria must have enzymatic systems that inactivate these oxygen products. The presence of these oxygen products is bactericidal for several oral bacteria and may affect the ultimate bacterial composition of plaque. When there is a heavy accumulation of bacteria, as in mature plaque, the oxygen level and the redox potential are especially low, allowing the growth of obligate anaerobes, unable to survive in an aerobic environment.

Table 26–3 ■ Coaggregation reactions between oral bacteria	
Gram-Positive	Gram-Positive
Streptococcus sp.	*Actinomyces viscosus*
	Actinomyces naeslundii
or	*Actinomyces odontolyticus*
Actinomyces sp.	*Bacterionema matruchottii*
	Propionibacterium acnes
	Gram-Negative
	Bacteroides sp.
	Capnocytophaga sp.
	Fusobacterium nucleatum
	Eikenella corrodens
	Veillonella sp.
Gram-Negative	
Bacteroides melaninogenicus	*Fusobacterium nucleatum*
	Capnocytophaga

(Adapted from Cisar, 1982.)

In order to grow, bacteria must be supplied with sources of nutrients and energy. In the formation of supragingival plaque, most nutrients are provided by saliva. The initial colonizers must have a high capacity to utilize nutrients available at low concentrations. Once established, specific members of the supragingival ecosystem produce compounds that are essential nutrients and growth factors for other microorganisms. Lactate, formate, and hydrogen excreted from carbohydrate fermentation by streptococci and *Actinomyces* species are used by *Veillonella* as an energy source. In the catabolism of lactate by *Veillonella*, hydrogen gas is formed, which is used by a number of organisms such as *Campylobacter*, *Wolinella*, and *Bacteroides gracilis*. Some oral spirochetes require spermine, spermidine, or putrescine, which can be provided by gram-positive rods and fusobacteria. *Veillonella* and other gram-positive rods are able to produce vitamin K, which, together with hemin, is an essential requirement for the growth of some black-pigmented *Bacteroides* species.

The nutritional interactions among bacteria are essential for the microbial succession that takes place in the maturation of supragingival plaque (Fig. 26–8).

The last bacterial factor is bacteriocin production. Animal experiments have shown that strains of *S. mutans* capable of producing bacteriocins can prevent the establishment of *A. viscosus*, but the corresponding nonbacteriocin mutant does not. Therefore, bacteriocin production may influence the microbial ecol-

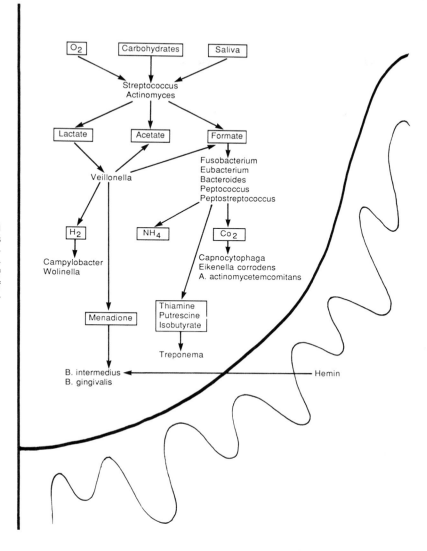

Figure 26–8 ■ Interbacterial and host nutritional interactions influence the maturation of dental plaque. (Adapted from Carlsson, J.: The Microbiology of plaque. In J. Lindhe (ed.): Text of Clinical Periodontology. Munksgaard, 1984.

ogy by promoting implantation by the producing bacteria replacing the indigenous flora or preventing accumulation of other bacteria.

Role of host factors ■ Oral cleansing mechanisms such as salivary flow, mastication, and movements of the tongue and cheek are very important in controlling the rate of supragingival plaque formation. Furthermore, the saliva exerts a major effect on the metabolism and microbial composition of this dental plaque.

Saliva influences the plaque pH through several mechanisms, including clearance of carbohydrates, neutralization of plaque acids by salivary buffers, and supply of essential nutrients for specific bacteria such as salivary oxygen, carbon dioxide, and carbohydrates.

Several salivary bacterial inhibitory substances have been identified. Saliva contains the enzyme lactoperoxidase (LPO), which, in combination with a salivary cofactor (salivary thiocyanate -SCN⁻) and H_2O_2, generates hypothiocyanate (OSCN), which is much less toxic to the cells than hydrogen peroxide and is a potent inhibitor of bacterial glycolytic enzymes, mainly streptococcal.

Iron is another essential nutrient for bacterial growth. Lactoferrin is an iron-binding protein present in saliva and in other exocrine secretions. The high iron-binding ability of this compound may deprive plaque organisms of iron affecting their growth.

Lysozyme, like lactoferrin, is found in saliva. This enzyme splits the bond between *N*-acetylglucosamine and *N*-acetyl muramic acid in the bacterial cell wall. At salivary concentrations most of the plaque organisms are not sensitive to lysis.

As mentioned earlier, salivary components including high molecular weight glycoproteins and immunoglobulins can bind to bacterial surfaces and induce their aggregation. This would limit their initial attachment to tooth surfaces or to previously attached bacteria. But the same salivary components are also involved in initial attachment and aggregation of bacteria to saliva-coated oral surfaces. Salivary effect on bacterial adsorption and desorption appears to occur continuously during plaque formation. Glycoproteins adsorbed to oral surfaces or to firmly attached bacteria in the periphery of plaque may protrude and promote the specific attachment of selected species and prevent adherence of others. On the other hand, salivary polymers adsorbed to bacteria may also promote or inhibit attachment to preexisting plaque. The composition of saliva

plays an important role in attachment of bacteria and subsequent accumulation (Fig. 26–9).

Finally, the host immune responses affect the composition of dental plaque. There are two main sources of immune components in the oral cavity: those present in oral secretions and those derived from mainly gingival crevice fluid. The first category involves antibodies, predominantly IgA secreted by the salivary glands, which act mainly in supragingival plaque by coating bacterial surfaces, promoting their aggregation and thus preventing their attachment, and by interacting with specific receptors on oral surfaces and on bacteria and thus competing with their adherence. In addition, antibodies that have reacted with bacteria already present on tooth surfces may influence their metabolism and therefore prevent their growth and accumulation. Antibodies in the crevicular fluid, in combination with leukocytes and other immune components, such as complement, function predominantly in subgingival areas as a response to the large antigenic challenge in this microenvironment (see Chapter 2).

Clinical Significance

The ecologic mechanisms discussed earlier permit the colonization of oral bacteria in a predictable succession, with organisms altering the environment, thus allowing new organisms to become established or certain existing bacteria to achieve dominance. If this microbial community on tooth surfaces is prevented from maturing, it may be compatible with gingival health. However, if it is allowed to grow and mature it usually produces inflammatory changes characteristic of gingivitis.

Clear evidence that supragingival plaque growth and maturation are the direct cause of gingivitis was derived from the experimental gingivitis model (Fig. 26–10). When specific bacteria were studied during the development of gingivitis, young plaque revealed almost entirely gram-positive cocci and rods. At 3 days of plaque accumulation, gram-negative cocci and rods, as well as filaments and fusobacteria, began to appear. By day 9, there was a further increase in gram-negative forms, and spiral forms and spirochetes were also detected. Subsequent cultural studies have confirmed these early reports.

At clinically healthy sites, streptococci and facultative species of *Actinomyces*, especially *A. viscosus* and *A. naeslundii*, account for up

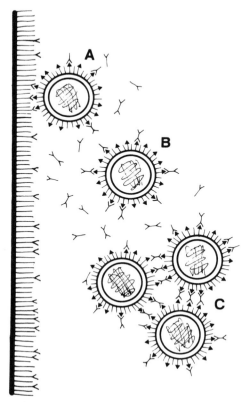

Figure 26–9 ■ Role of saliva in the development and maturation of dental plaque. *A*, Promoting adherence between bacteria and the tooth surface; *B*, inhibiting bacterial adherence by coating their surface receptors; *C*, inhibiting adherence by promoting bacterial agglutination.

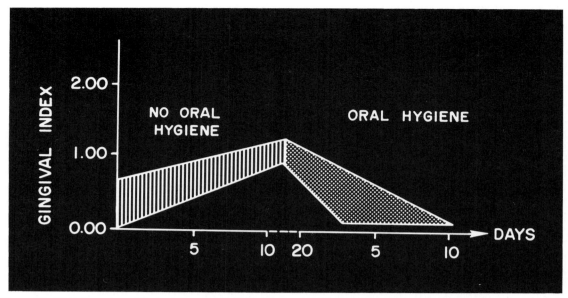

Figure 26–10 ■ Experimental gingivitis model. Note direct correlation between plaque accumulation and gingival inflammation. (Adapted from Löe, H. et al.: Experimental gingivitis in man. J. Periodontol. 36:177, 1965.)

to 85 percent of the total cultivable flora. During 3 weeks of plaque accumulation, there is an increase of gram-positive rods, especially *A. israelii,* and also of *Fusobacterium, Veillonella,* and *Treponema* species. At this stage, bacterial species directly associated with periodontitis lesions can be identified in sites with gingivitis. *Eikenella corrodens, Fusobacterium,* and *Capnocytophaga gingivalis* also are elevated in sites with gingivitis. These cultural studies indicate that the development of gingivitis is not just a mere increase in the amount of plaque, but also requires a sequential colonization of additional specific species. Thus, the bacterial succession that takes place in the development of supragingival plaque is ultimately responsible for the inflammatory changes associated with gingivitis.

SUBGINGIVAL PLAQUE

Structure and Development

Supragingival plaque directly and indirectly influences the establishment and relative proportions of subgingival microorganisms.

In association with supragingival plaque maturation and accumulation, there are inflammatory changes that modify the anatomic relationships of the gingival margin and the tooth surface (see Chapter 28). When inflammatory changes occur in the gingiva, edema causes gingival enlargement, which increases the capacity of the subgingival area for bacterial colonization. This space may protect bacteria from normal oral cleansing mechanisms. At the same time, there is a concomitant increase in the crevicular fluid flow and in pocket epithelial cell turnover. The end result is a new ecologic environment, protected from the supragingival oral environment, bathed with gingival crevicular fluid, desquamated epithelial cells, and bacterial end products, which influence the establishment and relative proportions of subgingival microorganisms. Many of these microorganisms lack the ability to be first colonizers and have evolved mechanisms that can utilize supragingival bacteria as a means of colonization of the subgingival area.

Once these microorganisms have colonized the subgingival area, they have access to nutrients (mainly proteins) present in the gingival fluid. This environment has a low oxidation-reduction potential, which allows the most fastidious anaerobic bacteria to become established. Under these conditions, local environmental changes and local host defense reactions allow specific subgingival microorganisms to increase or decrease to a point where they can elicit pathology.

Light and electron microscopic studies of extracted teeth and adjacent tissues from humans have provided information about the internal structure of subgingival plaque. These studies have differentiated tooth-associated plaque, epithelium-associated plaque, and connective tissue–associated plaque.

Tooth-Associated Subgingival Plaque

The structure of this portion of the subgingival plaque is very similar to the supragingival plaque. Bacteria are densely packed, adjacent to the cuticular material covering the tooth surface. In the inner layers, close to the tooth surface, the flora is dominated by gram-positive filamentous bacteria. Gram-positive cocci and rods are also present, and some gram-negative cocci and rods can always be found (Fig. 26–11).

This flora is associated with calculus formation, root caries, and root resorption areas in animal models. The apical border of tooth-associated plaque is always found some distance away from the junctional epithelium, and leukocytes are regularly interposed between the plaque and the epithelial surface. In this apical portion, the filamentous organisms are fewer and the bacterial deposit is dominated by gram-negative rods, without a particular orientation.

Epithelium-Associated Subgingival Plaque

This loosely adherent component of subgingival plaque is in direct association with the gingival epithelium, extending from the gingival margin to junctional epithelium. It contains one layer in contact with the epithelial cells and another loose in the sulcular or pocket lumen.

This plaque contains predominantly gram-negative rods and cocci, as well as a large number of flagellated bacteria and spirochetes. The organisms are not oriented in any specific manner, and they are very loosely adherent to the surface owing to the absence of a definite intermicrobial matrix (Fig. 26–12).

The relative proportions of the subgingival plaque components appear to be related to the nature and activity of the periodontal condition (see Chapter 28). In rapidly advancing lesions, such as localized juvenile periodontitis, the tooth associated component of the subgingival plaque appears to be minimal. These periodontal pockets contain almost exclusively gram-negative, motile organisms (Fig. 26–13). A similar pattern of

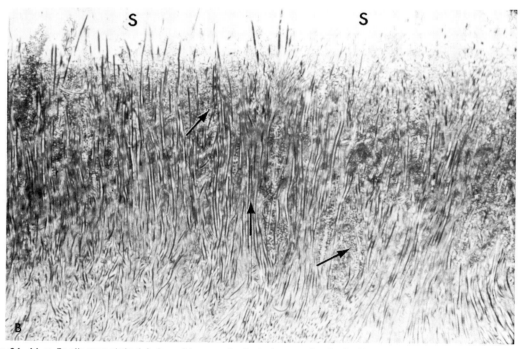

Figure 26–11 ■ Tooth-associated 1-day-old supragingival plaque, dominated by gram-positive cocci microcolonies *(arrows)* and gram-positive filamentous bacteria extending perpendicularly away from the tooth surface. (S = surface bathed with saliva.) (Courtesy of Dr. Max Listgarten. From Carranza, F. A. Jr.: Glickman's Clinical Periodontology, ed. 6. W. B. Saunders, Philadelphia, 1984, with permission.)

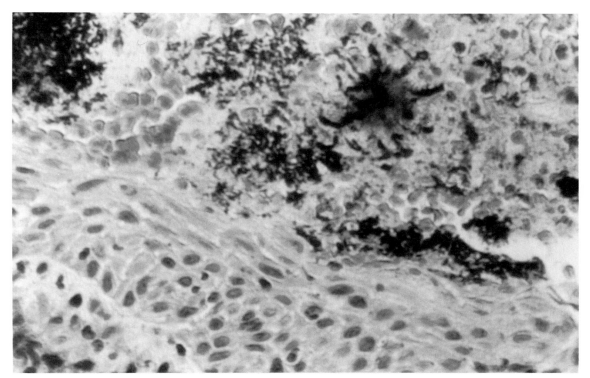

Figure 26–12 ■ Epithelium-associated plaque, showing no specific orientation and organization, being loosely adherent to the epithelial cells.

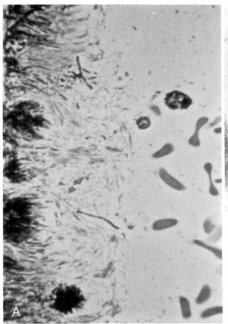

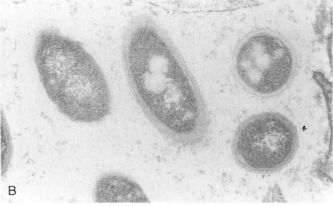

Figure 26–13 ■ Subgingival plaque in juvenile periodontitis. *A,* The tooth-associated component is scarce. It is dominated by loosely adherent plaque. (Courtesy of Dr. Max Listgarten.) *B,* Detail of this subgingival microbiota showing gram-negative rods and cocci as the dominant bacteria.

subgingival bacterial colonization occurs in rapidly progressing periodontitis. It has been suggested that plaque adjacent to the *junctional epithelium* may be the *"advancing front"* of the periodontal lesion. Recent morphologic data from advanced periodontitis cases suggests a direct relationship of the bacteria in this "advancing front" and connective tissue–associated bacteria present inside the gingival tissue (Fig. 26–14).

Electron microscopic studies of the soft tissue wall of periodontal pockets have shown the presence of distinct areas of heavy bacterial accumulation. Other areas along the epithelium exhibit signs of a strong host response consisting of emergence of leukocytes and leukocyte bacterial interactions. Areas of tissue destruction as evidenced by hemorrhage and ulceration can also be seen. The presence of these distinct areas suggests that the pocket wall is constantly changing as a result of the interaction between the epithelium, the epithelium-associated bacteria, and host factors. These different microen-

vironments may be important in allowing colonization and growth of specific bacteria and, most likely, allowing bacterial penetration into the tissues by some of the subgingival bacteria (Fig. 26–15).

Connective Tissue-Associated Subgingival Plaque

Microscopic studies have shown the presence of subgingival bacteria inside gingival connective tissue in different periodontal conditions (see Chapter 28). This bacterial presence, has been demonstrated in acute ulcerative gingivitis, advanced periodontitis, and localized juvenile periodontitis (Fig. 26–16). The clinical significance is unclear (see Chapter 28).

Dental Calculus

Since ancient times calculus has been etiologically linked with periodontal diseases.

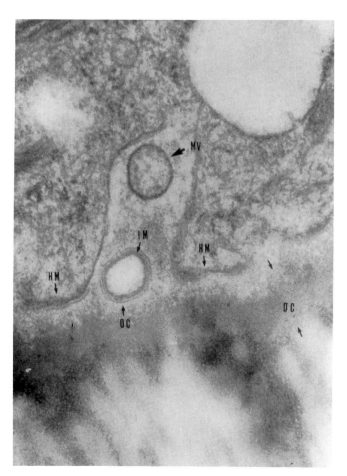

Figure 26–14 ■ Apical progression of subgingival bacteria in advanced periodontitis. In this micrograph a typical gram-negative bacterium is seen penetrating between junctional epithelial cells and the tooth surface. MV = microvilli; OC = outer coat; IM = inner membrane; HM = hemidesmosome; DC = dental cuticle.

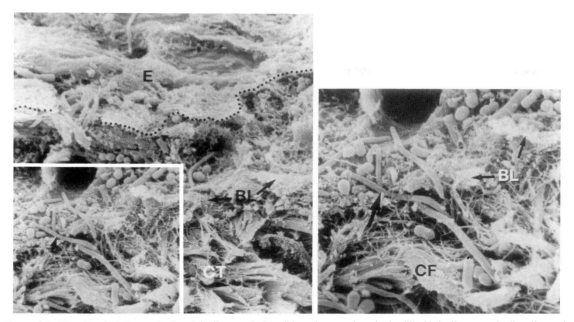

Figure 26–15 ■ Bacterial penetration into the pocket wall in advanced periodontitis. Note the penetration through the pocket epithelium and basement lamina into the connective tissue *(arrows)*. E = epithelium; BL = basement lamina; CT = connective tissue; CF = collagen fibers. (Courtesy of Dr. R. Saglie.)

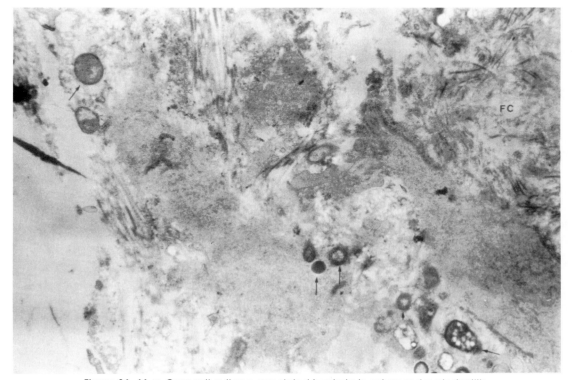

Figure 26–16 ■ Connective tissue associated bacteria in advanced periodontitis.

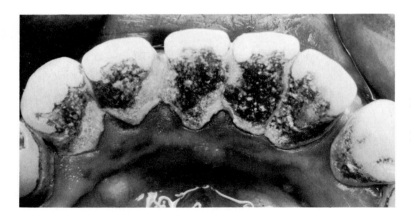

Figure 26–17 ■ Calculus forming a bridge-like structure on the lingual surface of the mandibular anterior teeth. (From Carranza, F. A. Jr.: Glickman's Clinical Periodontology, ed. 6. W. B. Saunders, Philadelphia, 1984, with permission.)

In the last 25 years it has been clearly demonstrated that calculus per se does not have *direct* etiologic significance in periodontal disease and acts to favor plaque accumulation. However, it may play a major role in *maintaining* and *accentuating* periodontal disease by keeping plaque in close contact with the gingival tissue and creating areas where plaque removal is impossible. Subgingival plaque may also facilitate ulceration of the periodontal pocket wall in periodontitis.

This concept has become clear mainly through two lines of research:

1. Experimental and electron microscopic studies of developing plaque and calculus that demonstrated that supragingival and subgingival calculus consisted of mineralized plaque covered by an unmineralized bacterial layer.

2. Epidemiologic studies that displayed a strong correlation between calculus and periodontal disease.

DEFINITION AND CLASSIFICATION

Dental calculus may be defined as adherent calcified or calcifying deposits on teeth and other solid structures in the oral cavity. Ordinarily it consists of mineralized bacterial plaque.

Calculus is classified according to its relation to the gingival margin. *Supragingival calculus* refers to calculus coronal to the gingival margin and visible in the oral cavity. It is usually white or whitish yellow, although the color may change to brown as a result of secondary staining. It may localize on a single tooth or a group of teeth or be generalized throughout the mouth forming bridge-like structures along adjacent teeth (Fig. 26–17). Supragingival calculus occurs more fre-

quently and in greatest quantity on the buccal surfaces of the maxillary molars, opposite Stensen's duct, and on the lingual surfaces of the mandibular anterior teeth opposite Warton's duct of the submandibular and Bartholin's duct of the sublingual salivary glands (Fig. 26–18).

Subgingival calculus refers to calculus that forms below the crest of the marginal gingiva, usually in periodontal pockets, so that it is not visible upon oral examination. It is usually dense and hard, dark-brown or greenish-black, flint-like in consistency, and firmly attached to the tooth surface. Subgingival calculus is more evenly distributed on the various teeth than supragingival calculus, but on the individual tooth subgingival cal-

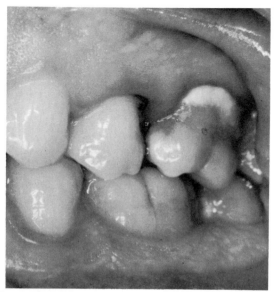

Figure 26–18 ■ Calculus on a molar opposite to the Stensen's duct. (From Carranza, F. A. Jr.: Glickman's Clinical Periodontology. W. B. Saunders, Philadelphia, 1984, with permission.)

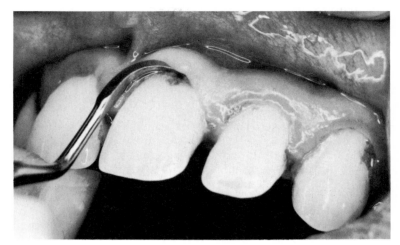

Figure 26–19 ■ Subgingival calculus seen by detachment of the gingival margin. (From Carranza, F. A. Jr.: Glickman's Clinical Periodontology, ed. 6. W. B. Saunders, Philadelphia, 1984, with permission.)

culus is more prevalent on the approximal and lingual tooth surfaces than on the buccal surfaces. It is often difficult to detect by visual inspection. It may be seen by detachment of the gingival margin from the tooth by air blast or with an instrument (Fig. 26–19). It can also be detected by tactile detection with a periodontal probe or a fine explorer, although this method has proved inefficient.

Gross deposits of calculus on the approximal surfaces of teeth can also be visible on radiographs, although its appearance is dependent on its density and radiographic technique (Fig. 26–20).

Supragingival and subgingival calculus generally occur together, but one may be present without the other. Microscopic studies have demonstrated that the calcified deposits usually extend near but do not reach the base of periodontal pockets in chronic periodontal lesions.

COMPOSITION

Supragingival calculus consists of 70 to 90 percent inorganic salts, with calcium and phosphorus the major constituents, mainly in the form of calcium phosphate ($Ca_3(PO_4)_2$); although calcium carbonate ($CaCO_3$) and magnesium phosphate ($Mg_3(PO_4)_2$) also occur. At least two thirds of the inorganic component is crystalline in structure, with four main crystal forms: hydroxyapatite [$Ca_{10}(PO_4)_6 (OH)_2$] approximately in 58 percent; magnesium whitlockite [$Ca_9 (PO_4)_6 \times PO_7$] and octacalcium phosphate [$Ca_4H (PO_4)_3 \times 2H_2O$] approximately 21 percent each; and brushite [$CaOHP_4 \cdot 2H_2O$] approximately 9 percent.

Generally two or more crystal forms occur in calculus, and their incidence varies according to the age and location of calculus. Brushite is more common in supragingival calculus

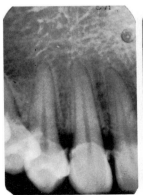
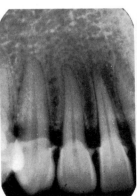
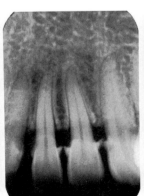
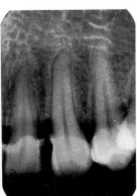

Figure 26–20 ■ Gross deposits of calculus can be seen interproximally on radiographs. Buccally and lingually, their image is superimposed on teeth. (From Carranza, F. A. Jr.: Glickman's Clinical Periodontology, ed. 6. W. B. Saunders, Philadelphia, 1984, with permission.)

and in the mandibular anterior region, while magnesium whitlockite is present particularly in the subgingival variety and in the posterior areas.

The organic component of calculus consists of a mixture of protein-polysaccharide complexes, desquamated epithelial cells, leukocytes, and various types of microorganisms and is comparable to that of dental plaque.

The composition of subgingival and supragingival calculus is different. It has similar hydroxyapatite content, but it has more magnesium whitlockite and less brushite and octacalcium phosphate, as well as a higher ratio of calcium to phosphate.

STRUCTURE

A clearer understanding of the structure of calculus is provided by electron microscopy. Calculus is a layered structure in which the degree of calcification varies among the different layers (Fig. 26–21). Its structure is dominated by small, needle-shaped, inorganic crystals, which by electron diffraction show a pattern of apatite. These crystals are randomly oriented and contain outlines of calcified microorganisms.

Both scanning and transmission electron microscopic studies have shown consistently that its surface is very rough and is covered by a layer of unmineralized bacterial plaque (Fig. 26–22). This bacterial covering is different between supragingival and subgingival calculus. On supragingival calculus, filamentous organisms oriented at right angles to the surface usually dominate. Subgingival calculus is usually covered by cocci, rods, and filamentous organisms, with no distinct pattern of orientation.

The porous nature of calculus deposits is also observed with tubular holes or orifices usually representing areas of uncalcified bacteria surrounded by calcified matrix.

Different experimental studies have also proved its porous nature. In 1970, Baumhammers showed that calculus can be completely permeated by dyes within 24 hours. Therefore, it has been hypothesized that dental calculus acts as a reservoir for irritating substances from microbial plaque and tissue lysis. Patters and coworkers recently showed a higher bone resorption activity and higher *Bacteroides gingivalis* antigen in samples from calculus than from cementum. These studies have suggested an intrinsic pathogenic potential of dental calculus.

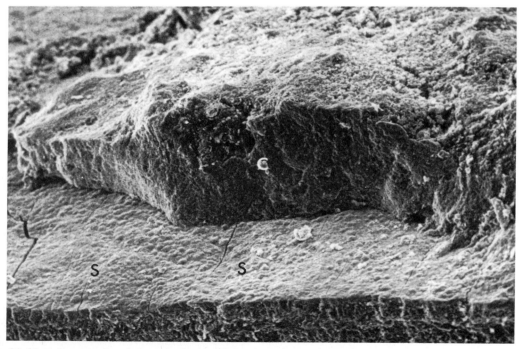

Figure 26–21 ■ Cross-sectional view of calculus (C) showing a layered structure attached to the cementum surface (S). (Courtesy of Dr. Sottosanti.) (From Carranza, F. A. Jr.: Glickman's Clinical Periodontology, ed. 6. W. B. Saunders, Philadelphia, 1984, with permission.)

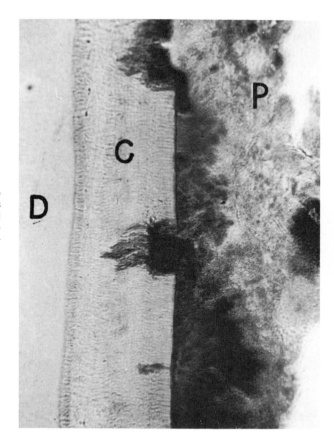

Figure 26-22 ■ Subgingival calculus attached to the cementum surface. Note that its surface is covered by a layer of nonmineralized bacterial plaque. (From Carranza, F. A. Jr.: Glickman's Clinical Periodontology, ed. 6. W. B. Saunders, Philadelphia, 1984, with permission.)

CALCULUS FORMATION

As stated before, calculus is dental plaque that has undergone mineralization. The plaque accumulation serves as an organic matrix for the subsequent mineralization. The precipitation of mineral salts usually begins in 1 to 14 days after plaque formation.

All plaque does not necessarily undergo calcification, and microorganisms are not always essential in calculus formation, as its formation has been demonstrated in germ-free rats. The mineral source for calculus is saliva for supragingival calculus and gingival fluid or exudates for subgingival calculus. Biochemical studies show that plaque from heavy calculus formers contains three times more phosphorus and less potassium than that of nonformers.

Calcification begins by binding of calcium ions to the carbohydrate-protein complexes of the organic matrix and follows with the precipitation of crystalline calcium phosphate salts. Crystals form initially in the intercellular matrix and on bacterial surfaces and finally within the bacteria (i.e., *Bacterionema*). Calcification begins as foci along the inner surface of the supragingival plaque and in the attached component of the subgingival plaque adjacent to the tooth. It increases in size by coalescence to form solid masses of calculus.

Calculus is formed in layers, often separated by a thin cuticle that becomes embedded in it as calcification progresses.

The time required for the formation of supragingival calculus in some persons is less than 2 weeks. However, the development of a hard deposit with a crystal composition characteristic of old calculus may require months.

ETIOLOGIC SIGNIFICANCE OF CALCULUS

Although the presence of calculus is invariably associated with periodontal disease, it is difficult to separate the effects of calculus and plaque upon the gingiva, because calculus is always covered with an unmineralized layer of plaque.

From epidemiologic data, there is a positive correlation between calculus and the prevalence of gingivitis, although the correlation between plaque and gingivitis is much stronger. Therefore, it is assumed that the unmineralized plaque on the calculus surface is the primary irritant, although the underlying calcifying portion may be a contributing factor because its rough surface will provide a fixed nidus for the continuous accumulation of plaque and a means to hold this plaque against the gingiva. However, it has been clearly demonstrated that roughness per se does not cause gingivitis, and calculus without bacteria may permit an epithelial attachment to form. Calculus may also become encapsulated in connective tissue without causing a marked inflammatory reaction.

REFERENCES

Ainamo, J.: Concomitant periodontal disease and dental caries in young adult males. Soumen Hammaslaakariseuran Tomituksia 66:301, 1970.

Allen, D. L., and Kerr, D. A.: Tissue response in the guinea pig to sterile and non-sterile calculus. J. Periodontol. 36:121, 1965.

Axelsson, P. and Lindhe, J.: The effect of a preventive programme on dental plaque, gingivitis, caries in schoolchildren. Results after one and two years. J. Clin. Peridontol. 1:126, 1974.

Baumhammers, A., and Rohrbaugh, E. A.: Permeability of human and rat dental calculus. J. Periodontol. 41:39, 1970.

Bladen, H., Hageage, G., Pollock, F., and Harr, R.: Plaque formation in vitro on wires by Gram negative oral microorganisms (Veillonella). Arch. Oral Biol. 15:127, 1970.

Bowden, G. H., Mulnes, A. R., and Boyar, R.: Streptococcus mutans and caries. In Guggehein, B. (ed.): Cariology Today. Karger, Basel, 1984, pp. 173–181.

Brecx, M., Ronstrom, A., Theilade, J., and Attstrom, R.: Early plaque formation of dental plaque on plastic films. J. Periodont. Res. 16:213, 1981.

Carranza, F. A., Saglie, F. R., Newman, M. G., and Valentin, P.: Scanning and transmission electron microscopic study of tissue invading microorganisms in localized juvenile periodontitis. J. Periodontol. 54:598, 1983.

Cisar, J. O.: Coaggregation reactions between oral bacteria. In Genco, R. J., and Mergenhagen, S. E. (eds.): Host-Parasite Interactions in Periodontal Diseases. ASM, Washington, D.C., 1982, pp. 121–131.

Egelberg, J.: Local effect of diet on plaque formation and development of gingivitis in dogs. Odontologysk Revy 16:31, 1965.

Eide, B., Lie, T., and Selvig, K. A.: Surface coatings on dental cementum incident to periodontal disease. I. A scanning electron microscopic study. J. Clin. Periodontol. 10:157, 1983.

Ellen, R. P., and Balcerzak-Raczkowski, I. B.: Interbacterial aggregation of Actinomyces naeslundii and dental plaque streptococci. J. Periodont. Res. 12:11, 1973.

Embery, G., Hogg, S. D., Heaney, T. G., Stanbury, J. B., and Green, D. R. J.: Some considerations on dental pellicle formation and early bacterial colonization. In Ten Cate, J. M., Arens, J., and Leach, S. A. (eds.): Bacterial Adhesion and Preventive Dentistry. IRL, Oxford, 1984, pp. 73–84.

Frank, R. M., and Houver, G.: An ultrastructural study of human supragingival dental plaque formation. In McHugh, W. D. (ed.): Dental Plaque. Churchill-Livingstone, Edinburgh, 1970, pp. 85–108.

Frank, R. M.: Bacterial penetration in the apical pocket wall of advanced human periodontitis, J. Periodont. Res. 15:563, 1980.

Friskopp, J., and Hammarstrom, L.: A comparative, scanning electron microscopic study of supragingival and subgingival calculus. J. Periodontol. 51:553, 1980.

Gibbons, R. J., and Engle, L. P.: Vitamin K compounds in bacteria that are obligate anaerobes. Science 146:1307, 1964.

Gibbons, R. J., and Qureshi, J. V.: Inhibition of adsorption of Streptococcus mutans strains to saliva treated hydroxyapatite by galactose and certain amines. Infect. Immun. 26:1214, 1979.

Gillet, R., and Johnson, N. W.: Bacterial invasion of the periodontium in a case of juvenile periodontitis. J. Clin. Periodontol. 9:93, 1982.

Gonzalez, F., and Sognnaes, R. F.: Electron-microscopy of dental calculus. Science 131:156, 1960.

Gustafsson, B. E., and Krasse, B.: Dental calculus in germ free rats. Acta Odontol. Scand. 20:135, 1962.

Huis in't Veld, J. H. J.: Ecological aspects of dental plaque development. In Leach, S. A. (ed.): Dental Plaque and Surface Interactions in the Oral Cavity. IRL, London, 1980, pp. 123–143.

Jordan, H. V., and Keyes, P. H.: Aerobic gram positive filamentous bacteria as etiologic agent of experimental periodontal disease in hamsters. Arch. Oral Biol. 9:401, 1964.

Kleingerg, I., Kanapka, J. A., and Craw, D.: Effect of saliva and salivary factors on the metabolism of the mixed oral flora. In Stiles, Loesche, and O'Brien (eds.): Microbial Aspects of Dental Caries. Microbiology Abstr. (Suppl.) Vol. 11, 1976, pp. 433–464.

Leach, S. A., and Agalamany, E. A.: Hydrophobic interactions that may be involved in the formation of dental plaque. In Ten Cate, J. M., Leach, S. M., and Arens, J. (eds.): Bacterial Adhesion and Preventive Dentistry. IRL, Oxford, 1984, pp. 43–49.

Lie, T.: Early dental plaque morphogenesis. J. Periodont. Res. 12:73, 1977.

Lie, T.: Ultrastructural study of early dental plaque formation. J. Periodont. Res. 13:391, 1978.

Liljemark, W. F., and Schauer, S. V.: Competitive binding among oral streptococci to hydroxyapatite. J. Dent. Res. 56:157, 1977.

Lindhe, J., Hamp, S.-E., and Loe, H.: Experimental periodontitis in the Beagle dog. J. Periodont. Res. 8:1, 1973.

Lindhe, J., Haffajjee, A. D., and Socransky, S. S.: Progression of periodontal disease in adult subjects in the absence of periodontal therapy. J. Clin. Periodontol. 10:433, 1983.

Lindhe, J., and Nyman, S.: Long-term maintenance of patients treated for advanced periodontal disease. J. Clin. Periodontol. 11:504, 1984.

Listgarten, M. A.: Electron microscopic observations on the bacterial flora of acute necrotizing ulcerative gingivitis. J. Periodontol. 36:328, 1965.

Listgarten, M. A.: Structure of the microbial flora associated with periodontal health and disease in man. A light and electron microscope study. J. Periodontol. 47:1, 1976.

Listgarten, M. A., and Ellegard, B.: Electron microscopic evidence of a cellular attachment between junctional epithelium and dental calculus. J. Periodont. Res. 8:143, 1973.

Listgarten, M. A., Mayo, H., and Amsterdam, M.: Ultrastructure of the attachment device between coccal and filamentous microorganisms in corn cob formations in dental plaque. Arch. Oral Biol. 8:651, 1973.

Listgarten, M. A., Mayo, H., and Tremblay, R.: Development of dental plaque on epoxy resin crowns in man. A light and electron microscope study. J. Periodontol. 46:10, 1975.

Little, M. F., and Hazen, S. P.: Dental calculus composition. II. Subgingival calculus: ash, calcium, phosphorus and sodium. J. Dent. Res. 43:645, 1964.

Loe, H.: Epidemiology of periodontal disease, and evaluation of the relative significance of the etiologic factors in light of recent epidemiological research. Odontologisk Tidskrift 71:479, 1963.

Loe, H. E., Theilade, E., and Jensen, S. B.: Experimental gingivitis in man. J. Periodontol. 36:177, 1965.

Loesche, W. J., and Syed, S. A.: The bacteriology of human experimental gingivitis. Infect. Immun. 21:830, 1978.

Lovdal, A., Arno, A., and Waehaug, J.: Incidence of clinical manifestations of periodontal disease in light of oral hygiene and calculus formation. J. Amer. Dent. Assoc. 56:21, 1958.

Mandel, I. D.: Histochemical and biochemical aspects of calculus formation. Periodontics 1:43, 1963.

Moore, W. E., Holdeman, L. V., Smibert, R. M., Good, I. J., Burmeister, J. A., Palcanis, K., and Ranney, R. R.: Bacteriology of experimental gingivitis in young adult humans. Infect. Immun. 38:651, 1982.

Newman, H. N.: Ultrastructure of the apical border of dental plaque. In Lehner, T. (ed.): The Borderland Between Caries and Periodontal Disease. Academic Press, London, 1977, pp. 78–103.

Olsson, J., Glantz, P.-O., and Krasse, B.: Surface potential and adherence of oral streptococci to solid surfaces. Scand. J. Dent. Res. 84:240, 1976.

Oste, R., Ronstrom, A., Birkhed, D., Edwardsson, S., and Stemberg, M.: Gas-liquid chromatographic analysis of aminoacids in pellicle formed on tooth surface and plastic film in vitro. Arch. Oral Biol. 26:635, 1981.

Østravik, D.: Initial bacterial adhesion to surfaces: ecological implications in dental plaque formation. In Ten Cate, J. M., Leach, S. A., and Arens, J. (eds.): Bacterial Adhesion and Preventive Dentistry. IRL, Oxford, 1984, pp. 153–166.

Patters, M. R., Landersberg, R. L., Johansson, L. A., Trummel, C. L., and Robertson, P. B.: Bacteroides gingivalis antigens and bone resorption activity in root surface fractions of periodontally involved teeth. J. Periodont. Res. 17:122, 1982.

Pollock, J. J., Iacono, V. J., Goodman Bicker, H., McKay, B., Katona, L. I., Taichman, L. B., and Thomas, E.: The binding, aggregation and lytic properties of lysozyme. In Stiles, Loesche, and O'Brien (eds.): Microbial Aspects of Dental Caries. Microbiol. Abstr. 11(Suppl.):325, 1976.

Ramfjord, S. P.: The periodontal status of boys 11–17 years old in Bombay, India. J. Periodontol. 32:237, 1961.

Ramfjord, S. P., Knowles, J. W., Nissle, R. R., Schick, R. A., and Burgett, F. G.: Longitudinal study of periodontal therapy. J. Periodontol. 46:66, 1973.

Rogers, A. H., van der Hoeven, J. S., and Mikx, F.: Effect of bacteriocin production by Streptococcus mutans on the plaque of gnotobiotic rats. Infect. Immun. 23:571, 1979.

Rolla, G.: Formation of dental integuments—some basic chemical considerations. Swed. Dent. J. 1:241, 1977.

Rolla, G., Bonesvoll, P., and Opermann, T.: Interaction between oral streptococci and salivary proteins. In Kleinberg, Ellison, and Mandel (eds.): Proceedings of Saliva and Dental Caries (sp. supp.) Microbiology Abstr. 1979, pp. 227–241.

Rolla, G., Ciardi, J. E., Deas, M., Lau, A., and Bowen, W. H.: Adherence of active glycosyltansferase from Streptococcus mutans to ionic, hydrophobic and dextran surfaces. In Ten Cate, J. M., Leach, S. A., and Arens, J. (eds.): Bacterial Adhesion and Preventive Dentistry. IRL, Oxford, 1984, pp. 133–142.

Rowles, S. L.: The inorganic composition of dental calculus. In Blackwood, H. J. J. (ed.): Bone and Tooth. Pergamon Press, Oxford, 1964, pp. 175–183.

Saglie, R., Newman, M. G., Carranza, F. A., and Pattison, G. L.: Bacterial invasion of gingiva in advanced periodontitis in humans. J. Periodontol. 53:217, 1982.

Sanz, M., Herrera, I., Bascones, A., Newman, M. G., and Saglie, R.: Association of bacterial invasion with the advancing front of the periodontitis lesion. J. Dent. Res. 65, Spec Iss. AADR A#116, 1986.

Schroeder, H. E.: Inorganic content and histology of early calculus content in man. Helv. Odontol. Acta 7:17, 1963.

Schroeder, H. E., and Baumbauer, H. U.: Stages of calcium phosphate crystallization during calculus formation. Arch. Oral Biol. 11:1, 1966.

Silverman, G., and Kleinberg, I.: Fractionation of human dental plaque and the characterization of its cellular and acellular components. Arch. Oral Biol. 12:1387, 1967.

Slots, J., and Gibbons, R. J.: Attachment of Bacteroides melaninogenicus subsp. asaccharolyticus to oral surfaces and its possible role in colonization of the mouth and of periodontal pockets. Infect. Immun. 19:254, 1978.

Socransky, S. S., Gibbons, R. J., Dale, A. C., Bortnick, L., Rosenthal, E., and McDonald, J. B.: The microbiota of the gingival crevice in man. Arch. Oral Biol. 8:275, 1963.

Sonju, T., and Glantz, P.-O.: Chemical composition of salivary integuments formed in vivo on solids with some established surface characteristics. Arch. Oral Biol. 20:687, 1975.

Tanner, A. C. R., Haffer, C., Brathall, G. T., Visconti, R. A., and Socransky, S. S.: Wolinella gen. nov., Wolinella succinogenes comb. nov. and description of Bacteroides gracilis sp. nov., Wolinella recta sp. nov., and Eikenella corrodens from humans with periodontal disease. Int. J. Syst. Bacteriol. 31:432, 1981.

Theilade, E., Wright, W. H., Jensen, S. B., and Loe, H.: Experimental gingivitis in man. II. A longitudinal clinical and bacteriological investigation. J. Periodont. Res. 1:1, 1966.

Theilade, J.: The microscopic structure of dental calculus. Thesis. University of Rochester, Rochester, NY, 1960.

Theilade, J.: Development of bacterial plaque in the oral cavity. J. Clin. Periodontol. 4 (extra issue No. 5):1, 1977.

Turesky, S., Renstrup, G., and Glickman, I.: Histologic and histochemical observations regarding early calculus formation in children and adults. J. Periodontol. 32:7, 1961.

van Houte, J.: Bacterial Adhesion in the mouth. In Leach, S. A. (ed.): Dental Plaque and Surface Interactions in the Oral Cavity. IRL, London, 1980, pp. 69–99.

van Houte, J.: Colonization mechanisms involved in the development of the Oral Flora. In Genco, R. J., and Mergenhagen, S. E. (eds.): Host-Parasite Interactions in Periodontal Diseases. ASM, Washington, DC, 1982, pp. 86–97.

Waerhaug, J.: Healing of dento-epithelial junction following subgingival plaque control. II. As observed on extracted teeth. J. Periodontol. 49:119, 1978.

Waerhaug, J.: The infrabony pocket and its relationship to trauma from occlusion and subgingival plaque. J. Periodontol. 50:355, 1979.

Warl, W.: Role of oral hygiene practices in oral health and general health. In Loe, H., and Kleinman, D. (eds.): Dental plaque—control measures and oral hygiene practices. IRL, Oxford, 1986.

Weerkamp, A. H., van der Mei, H. C., Engelen, D. P. E., and de Windt, C. A. E.: Adhesion receptors (adhesins) of oral streptococci. In Ten Cate, J. M., Leach, S. A., and Arens, J. (eds.): Bacterial Adhesion and Preventive Dentistry. IRL, London, 1984.

Westergaard, J., Frandsen, A., and Slots, J.: Ultrastructure of the subgingival flora in juvenile periodontitis. Scand. J. Dent. Res. 86:421, 1978.

World Health Organization (WHO): Periodontal Disease. Geneva WHO Technical Report Series No. 207, 1961.

chapter 27

Caries and cariology

L. E. Wolinsky, Ph.D., D.M.D.

CHAPTER OUTLINE

- CARIES MICROBIOLOGY
- CARIES PHYSIOLOGY
- CARIES THEORIES
- CARIES HISTOPATHOLOGY
- PLAQUE FORMATION

- PLAQUE BIOCHEMISTRY
- HOST FACTORS AND CARIES
- CARIES CONTROL AND PREVENTION
- ROOT CARIES

Dental caries in simplest terms is a slow decomposition of teeth resulting from the loss of hydroxyapatite crystals. This dissolution of the mineralized matrix leads to reduced structural integrity of the teeth. The bacterial nature of this process may result in a chronic infection of the tooth. The eventual loss of teeth and supporting alveolar bone may result from progressive caries lesions. Current understanding supports the "plaque-host-substrate" theory, whereby caries has a bacterial etiology interdependent on (1) the host defense systems, (2) dietary factors, and (3) time. Caries occurs when all the aforementioned factors are operating together (Fig. 27–1). This chapter will consider the microbiology, physiology, and immunology of dental caries. In addition, an examination of recent developments in the treatment of caries will be presented.

Caries Microbiology

There is a large body of in vitro and in vivo data to support the belief that caries can only occur in the presence of microorgan-

isms. First, germ-free animals develop caries only in the presence of bacteria. Second, oral bacteria can cause demineralization of enamel in vivo. Third, histologic studies have shown bacteria within the enamel and dentin of carious lesions. However, there are differing opinions as to which bacteria are the primary etiologic agents in various types of dental caries.

In order to look more closely at this question, one must realize there are three types of caries: enamel, dentin, and root surface caries. Enamel surface caries can be further divided into smooth surface, and pit and fissure caries. The smooth-surface lesion has a well-characterized microbiology (Table 27–1). The most consistently found organisms in this lesion are the gram-positive facultative cocci, specifically *Streptococcus mutans* and *S. salivarius*. *S. mutans* is the primary etiologic organism in the formation of this carious lesion based upon several observations. This microorganism effectively ferments sugars to lactic acid, a fermentation product thought responsible for dissolution of the enamel matrix. *S. mutans* is also a prolific producer of insoluble extracellular dextrans, which allow

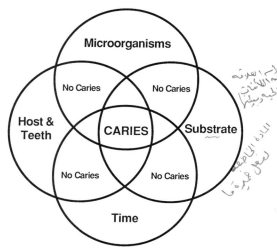

Figure 27–1 ■ Diagrammatic representation of the parameters involved in the development of human caries. All individual factors must be present before caries can occur.

bacteria to stick to the tooth surface. Furthermore, this organism shows a high selectivity for the pellicle-coated enamel surface. While *S. mutans* is a minor smooth-surface plaque component consisting of no more than 2 to 7 percent of the total, it is particularly virulent with respect to caries-producing potential and is therefore considered the primary etiologic organism. *S. salivarius* is also present in smooth surface caries and has been shown to produce caries in animal models. How-

ever, its role in the overall production of the carious lesion is not yet fully known. Although the facultative streptococci are the most predominant organisms, the microbial ecology of the smooth-surface plaque is quite complex. The microbial population of plaque changes dramatically with time. During the early stages of plaque development, the gram-positive cocci predominate, owing to their preferential affinity for pellicle-bound salivary components on the tooth. During this early period the environment is fairly rich in oxygen. However, as the plaque matures a phenomenon of bacterial succession is seen (see Chapter 26). The relative percentage of cocci decreases and after approximately 7 days filaments and rods constitute about 50 percent of the total bacterial counts. The coccal organisms have thus changed the local environment to allow the growth of other organisms. The rapid growth of the streptococci changes factors such as pH, nutrients, and oxidation-reduction potentials in the deepest portions of the plaque matrix favoring the growth of these other organisms.

Pit and fissure caries comprise the greatest proportion of human lesions. However, much less is known about its microbiology compared to smooth surface caries. In addition, a good model for this lesion is not available. One would expect to find a wide variety of bacterial types because of the var-

Table 27–1 ■ Bacteria associated with caries type

Caries Type	Organisms Isolated	Possible Significance in Caries
Pit and fissure	*Streptococcus mutans*	Highly significant
	Streptococcus sanguis	Slight significance
	Streptococcus mitis	No significance
	Lactobacillus sp.	Highly significant
	Actinomyces sp.	May be significant
Smooth-surface	*Streptococcus mutans*	Highly significant
	Streptococcus salivarius	Little significance
Dentinal caries	*Lactobacillus* sp.	Highly significant
	Actinomyces viscosus	Significant
	Actinomyces naeslundii	Highly significant
	Streptococcus mutans	May be significant
	Filamentous rods	Significant
Root caries	*Actinomyces viscosus*	Highly significant
	Actinomyces naeslundii	Highly significant
	Streptococcus mutans	Some significance
	Streptococcus sanguis	Significance unclear
	Streptococcus salivarius	No clear significance
	Filamentous rods	Highly significant

(From Newbrun, Cariology, 2nd ed., 1983, p. 52, with permission.)

ied environment present. However, the microbiology of this area has remained elusive, owing to the difficulties in accurately sampling these areas. Attempts have been made to mimic this area of the tooth by folding mylar strips to imitate fissures. These "artificial fissures" were inserted in the mouth and bacterial sampling performed. It was found that coccoid forms constituted 75 to 95 percent of the organisms, with S. sanguis being the predominant bacteria. As the age of the plaque increased, the relative numbers of S. mutans and lactobacilli increased. The validity of the mylar strip model for pit and fissure plaque formation is questionable since the mylar surface characteristics are very different from those of enamel. Of the several species of bacteria isolated from these lesions S. mutans and lactobacilli are suspected as etiologic organisms.

Dentinal caries exhibit a somewhat different microbial ecology related to the location of this lesion. The organisms found here must grow in a more anaerobic environment with most of their food source being derived from the tooth itself. The most commonly found pathogens in this region are lactobacilli. However, other gram-positive anaerobic rods and filaments such as Bifidobacterium, Eubacterium, and Propionibacterium have been identified. In addition Actinomyces and Bacillus species have been noted at the invasive front of the deep dentinal lesion.

The root surface lesion is also associated with a particular microbial ecology. This lesion is initiated on pellicle-coated cementum with a different flora than in the smooth surface lesions. Bacterial sampling of the plaque from cemental caries reveals high numbers of Actinomyces sp. including A. viscosus, A. naeslundii, and A. odontolyticus. Other organisms including Nocardia and S. mutans have also been identified (Table 27–1).

STREPTOCOCCUS MUTANS SEROTYPES

Studies performed in the 1960s indicate that Streptococcus mutans is a heterogeneous family of bacteria. In order to classify this organism two identification methods have been applied. The first method involves serotyping the bacteria to specific cell wall carbohydrate antigens (the Lancefield method). Applying this method, seven different serotypes of S. mutans have been identified and given the designation of a lowercase letter, a

through g. A second method based upon DNA homology reveals five distinct groups of S. mutans. Among the seven serotype strains, serotype c (homology group I) is the most frequent isolate from human dental plaque samples obtained in the United States. The other serotypes have been isolated from some human plaque samples but at a much lower frequency. Each of the serotypes is capable of producing caries in an animal model and is therefore thought to be cariogenic. However, in the human it may well be that only serotype c is a key pathogen in caries initiation.

Caries Physiology

Dental caries has been a prevalent disease since the first recorded history of mankind. Observations of "demons" and "tooth worms" can be found in ancient writings at about the time of Christ. Although the existence of this malady was well documented, the basic understanding of the disease process was not understood until the end of the 18th century. Dr. W. D. Miller (1890) first described dental caries as the action of organic acids upon the calcium phosphate of the teeth. He showed that when teeth were incubated with saliva and carbohydrates, acids formed that dissolved the mineralized portion of the teeth. He concluded that acid formed by bacteria in the saliva resulted in the breakdown of the teeth. From this work he formulated the "chemo-parasitic" theory of dental caries. Since then, data support a lowering of pH by bacterial acid production causing dissolution of the enamel. Dr. Miller's work has formed the basis for the modern "plaque-host-substrate" theory of caries formation.

To understand why the acidity of the area adjacent to the enamel is so important to the carious process, the structure of enamel must be considered. Enamel, which is 95 percent calcified, is the most highly mineralized structure in the human body. The majority of the mineral is hydroxyapatite, a large family of calcium phosphate salts. The commonly represented formula for hydroxyapatite is $Ca_{10}(PO_4)_6OH_2$. Pure hydroxyapatite has a unique structure (Fig. 27–2). There is a sixfold axis of symmetry surrounding a threefold axis of symmetry. The crystals are arranged in a hexagonal configuration with calcium and phosphorus atoms placed on the outer crystal. In the center of the crystal, hydroxyl

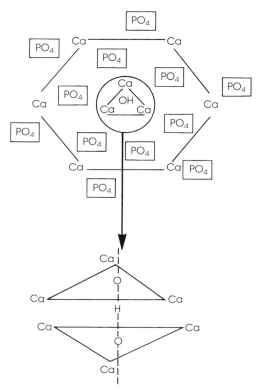

Figure 27–2 ■ Crystal structure diagram of pure hydroxyapatite found in enamel.

groups are surrounded by three calcium atoms. The relationship of each hydroxyl group in the crystal plays an important role in the crystal stability. In fact, replacement of some of these hydroxyl groups with other atoms such as fluoride results in increased crystal stability. The hexagonal crystals are grouped together into rods. The enamel is made up of many rods packed together, as illustrated in Figure 27–3. These rods extend from the surface of the enamel to the dental junction. Density measurements on the enamel show that the outer surface has a slightly greater density than the remaining structure. Explanations for this may be the lower carbonate concentration or the higher fluoride concentration noted in the surface enamel. Interspaced between each enamel rod is an organic matrix. Although the enamel appears extremely hard and well mineralized, its surface is porous to small ions including sodium, potassium, magnesium, and fluoride. The presence of these interprismatic spaces has been used to explain the observed permeability of the enamel.

Hydroxyapatite has a finite solubility constant dependent upon the temperature, pH, and ionic strength of the solvent surrounding the crystal. Alterations in these parameters can result in a solubilization of the crystals. For example, a tooth placed in a container of distilled water would eventually undergo a finite dissolution of the hydroxyapatite until the ionic strength of the solution reached a favorable equilibrium. In the oral cavity the saliva is supersaturated with respect to calcium and phosphate which favors the crystalline state of enamel, and as a result the teeth do not eventually dissolve over a lifetime. Because of the nature of the equilibrium reaction in the oral cavity, enamel is under a constant state of mineralization and demineralization at physiologic conditions (saturated Ca^{+2}, PO_4, pH 6.8). At this pH, the solubility is extremely small and, for practical purposes, insignificant; however, if the pH

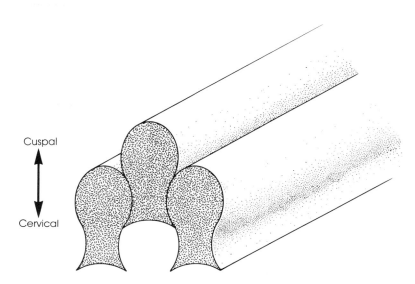

Cuspal

Cervical

Figure 27–3 ■ Diagrammatic representation of a microscopic cross section of enamel showing some enamel rods.

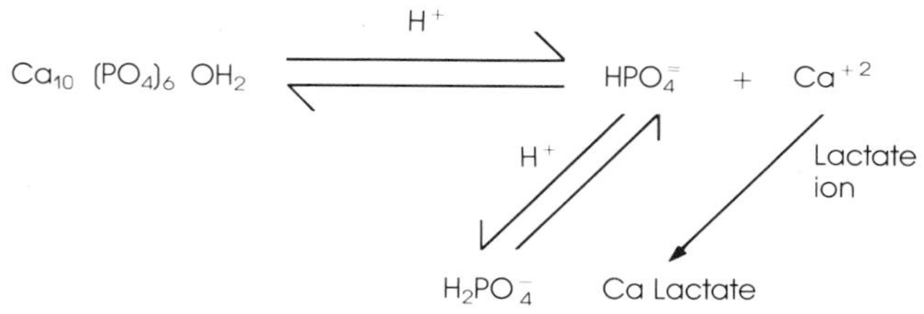

$$Ca_{10}(PO_4)_6\,OH_2 \underset{\longleftarrow}{\overset{H^+}{\longrightarrow}} HPO_4^= + Ca^{+2}$$

Figure 27–4 ■ The chemical equation for the acid catalyzed demineralization of hydroxyapatite.

H^+ — Lactate ion

$H_2PO_4^-$ — Ca Lactate

is lowered approximately 1.3 log units to 5.5, the solubility is then increased to the point where dissolution occurs. It is thought that at this pH (the "critical" pH) the hydroxyapatite is destabilized by the reaction of the acid with the hydroxyl groups in the center of the crystal resulting in the formation of water (Fig. 27–4). The dissociated form of calcium phosphate then becomes favored and the crystal dissolves. Like all acid-base reactions, the dissolution of the hydroxyapatite is an equilibrium process, so that the deformation of the crystal can occur with the resultant precipitation of hydroxyapatite. For example, if the local calcium concentration is increased and/or the pH increases the hydroxyapatite could be reformed.

Caries Theories

Since Dr. Miller's observations considerable experimental evidence has appeared which supports the acid theory: that acids produced by plaque bacteria result in the demineralization of enamel. Some of the experimental evidence for this is as follows:

1. Plaque pH measurements can drop below 5.5 for extended periods following the production of bacterial organic acids.

2. pH measurements made in carious lesions are lower than in surrounding tissues.

3. There is a correlation between caries incidence and the presence of S. mutans and and Lactobacillus, bacteria capable of producing organic acids upon consumption of fermentable sugars.

4. In germ-free rats, caries can be induced by oral bacteria capable of producing acid without proteolytic capacity.

There have been other hypotheses proposed for enamel breakdown by plaque bacteria.

The proteolysis-chelation theory ■ This theory is based upon the concept that demineralization of enamel can occur without acid if complexing agents such as lactate remove enough calcium ions surrounding the enamel

crystal to shift the equilibrium toward dissolution. If this is true, demineralization could occur at neutral or even alkaline pH. Although there is some experimental support for this theory, the overwhelming evidence supports the acid hypothesis.

The proteolytic theory ■ This theory assumes that caries are initiated by proteolytic enzymes produced by the plaque bacteria which destroy the inter-rod organic material and destabilize the enamel crystals. There is not much support for this theory.

The phosphoprotein theory ■ This theory is based upon experimentation in rats, which showed that plaque bacteria produce enzymes capable of removing phosphate from enamel phosphoproteins. The removal of these proteins is thought to destabilize the enamel matrix leading to enamel breakdown. However, phosphoprotein concentrations in human enamel are not high enough to play a role in caries formation.

Caries Histopathology

Let us now examine the histopathology of the carious lesion in enamel and dentin. Macroscopic examination of initial enamel caries usually reveals a white-chalky area that appears to have an intact surface. In general, bacterial plaque will be present over this lesion. Microscopic examination of ground sections reveals a relatively intact enamel surface with an area of subsurface demineralization. The lesion can be described as having four characteristic microscopic zones (Fig. 27–5): the innermost translucent zone representing approximately 1.2 percent mineral loss; a dark zone with 6 percent mineral loss; the body of the lesion, with about 24 percent mineral loss; and the surface layer which appears intact. In actuality there has been some demineralization of the surface, which appears as pitting. Upon radiographic examination, the smooth-surface lesion appears as a cone with its tip pointing toward the dentin. Photodensity tracings of micro-

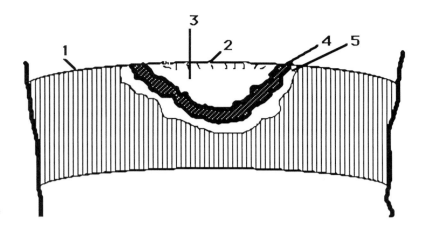

Figure 27–5 ■ Diagrammatic representation of a microscopic thin ground section showing enamel caries. Major zones are (1) sound enamel, (2) surface enamel slightly demineralized, (3) body of the lesion, (4) dark zone, and (5) translucent zone.

radiographic sections of sound and carious enamel supports the observation of the relatively intact surface and demineralized subsurface (Fig. 27–6).

It is thought that non-ionized acid diffuses through the porous enamel surface through the interprismatic junctions. The acid then dissociates and interacts with the subsurface hydroxyapatite crystals at the rod surface. In time, small gaps develop between the enamel rods. As the number of dissolved hydroxyapatite crystals increases, the lesion becomes progressively more porous. These porous spaces become filled with fluid, which results in the clinically observed change in the enamel translucency. With the more advanced destruction of the subsurface hydroxyapatite, the surface enamel becomes weakened and breakdown occurs leading to the ingression of bacteria. Therefore, early enamel caries is an aseptic lesion resulting from the chemical reaction of acids with hydroxyapatite. As such, it has a high potential for remineralization. Once the bacteria have entered the lesion, treatment by mechanical means becomes a necessity. Following the spread of

caries into the dentin, the lesion spreads laterally along the dentin-enamel junction. Radiographically this appears as a less well-defined hemispherical lucency. The apparent rapid spread of the lesion in dentin is related to several factors. First, the dentin is less mineralized than the enamel, so acids will destroy more of the mineralized matrix. Second, the dentin is cellular, which allows for easy movement of the bacteria into the deeper portions of the lesion. Microscopic examination of the dentin lesion reveals several distinct zones described by Newbrun (1983) (Fig. 27–7). The innermost zone (first) contains retreating odontoblasts. The second zone is an area of what appears as fatty degeneration. The next zone (third) consists of dentinal sclerosis where peritubular dentin is being laid down to block the bacterial insult. The fourth zone is the area of demineralization, which is similar to the "body of the lesion" zone in the enamel caries. The most superficial zone (fifth) is the area of bacterial invasion and this is followed by the zone of bacterial necrosis (sixth).

The next logical step in understanding the

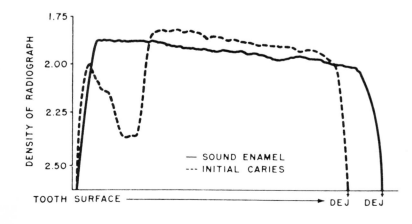

Figure 27–6 ■ Photodensity tracing of microradiographs of sound enamel (—) and initial enamel caries (----). (Courtesy of E. Newbrun. From Newbrun's Cariology, ed. 2, p. 240, Williams and Wilkins, Baltimore, 1983, with permission.)

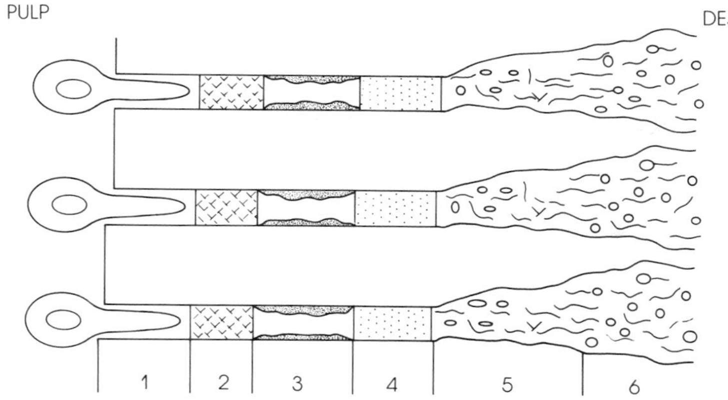

PULP   DEJ

Figure 27–7 ■ Diagrammatic illustration of Newbrun's six zones seen in microscopic sections of dentinal caries. Zone 1, retreating odontoblastic process; zone 2, fatty degeneration; zone 3, dentinal sclerosis; zone 4, dentinal demineralization; zone 5, bacterial invasion; and zone 6, necrotic dentin.

physiology of dental caries is to examine bacterial plaque formation, since without the bacterial plaque the typical carious lesion can not exist.

Plaque Formation

The production of acids from plaque bacteria and subsequent formation of dental caries is the culmination of a highly selective process of bacterial adherence and colonization of the tooth surface. In order for oral bacteria to survive in the mouth they must be able to firmly attach and colonize a host surface.

Research has shown that a high degree of selectivity occurs with plaque formation (see Chapter 26). Despite the relatively wide variety of oral flora normally found in the mouth, only select organisms are present on a particular oral surface (Table 27–2). The high degree of bacterial selectivity seems related to the nature of the salivary pellicle adsorbed onto the surface of the enamel. The enamel pellicle is an acellular material derived from specific salivary components. The interaction of the saliva with the teeth results in a rapid selective adsorption of highly charged proteins and glycoproteins. This occurs through electrostatic interactions between the highly charged surface of the enamel and the charged proteins (Fig. 27–8). The formation of the pellicle occurs within minutes of enamel exposure to the oral cavity. The interaction of these molecules with the hydroxyapatite is quite strong. It is believed that the salivary pellicle is directly responsible for the subsequent adherence of oral bacteria. There are two major theories for how this occurs. The first, supported by Rølla (1979), proposes that the interaction of bacteria with the pellicle-coated tooth occurs through electrostatic charges (Fig. 27–9). The highly negative surface of most oral bacteria can interact with calcium ions complexed to the surface of the pellicle. There is some experimental support for such a theory. Most streptococci possess outer cell walls that are highly anionic. The surface of the enamel pellicle also carries a negative charge density from the selective adsorption of anionic salivary glycoproteins. Interaction of the oral streptococci with the pellicle happens in

	Location				
Table 27–2 ■ Percentage distribution of bacteria in different sites in the oral cavity					
Bacterium	Tongue	Gingival Crevice	Saliva	Cheek	Supragingival Plaque
S. mutans	0.3	—	0.2	0.5	3.9
S. sanguis*	9.0	—	47.0	29.0	75.0
S. salivarius*	55.0	0.5	47.4	10.7	0.7
B. melaninogenicus†	0.4	4.5	0.4	0.3	0.3
Treponema sp‡	—	1.5	—	—	>0.1
Lactobacillus sp.	—	—	0.01	—	>0.01

(Data taken from Socransky and Manganiello: J. Periodontol., 42:486, 1971, with permission.)
*% of facultative streptococci.
†% of total cultivable flora.
‡% of microscopic counts.

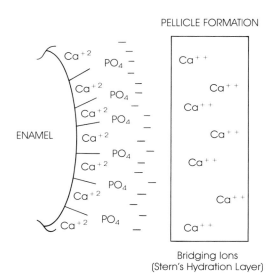

PELLICLE FORMATION

CHARGED SALIVARY GLYCOPROTEINS

Bridging Ions
(Stern's Hydration Layer)

Figure 27–8 ■ The interaction of host-derived salivary glycoproteins with the charged surface of enamel. This electrostatic interaction is believed to occur through bridging calcium ions found in the "Stern hydration layer."

much the same fashion as the binding of salivary components to the enamel; that is, bridging cations such as calcium support the interaction and allow initial adherence to occur. This theory has several drawbacks. First, it does not explain the selectivity among several strains of streptococci which possess similar anionic surface charges. Second, it is known that some strains of oral bacteria which do not possess negatively charged cell wall components still bind to the enamel surface. An alternative hypothesis proposed by Gibbons (1977) is that bacterial attachment occurs through a "lectin-like" interaction of specific bacterial surface receptors with pellicle-bound glycoproteins (Fig. 27–9). This theory is also supported by experimental evidence. The adsorption of oral bacteria to saliva-treated hydroxyapatite is inhibited by specific sugars suggesting sugar-protein interactions. In vitro studies have shown that the number of binding sites for bacterial strains on saliva-treated hydroxyapatite differs markedly. In addition, more than one bacterial strain can bind to the surface of the hydroxyapatite without competing for the same binding sites. In general, recent opinion favors the Gibbons hypothesis.

Once initial bacterial attachment and colonization have occurred, secondary adherence processes begin. This involves production of extracellular bacterial products which act as intracellular glue to protect the bacteria and supply them with a food source during times of need. These polymeric sugars are commonly known as glucans and levans.

Dental plaque has three phases of development as described by Newbrun: (1) initial colonization, (2) rapid bacterial growth, and (3) remodeling. The formation of the enamel pellicle occurs within minutes after exposure to the saliva and is followed by the initial stages of bacterial adherence within a few hours. The streptococci, which are the first bacterial colonizers, have a short doubling time of approximately 2 hours. Therefore, within 12 to 24 hours after initial adherence, a well-defined bacterial colonization has formed a thin plaque mass covering the exposed enamel surface. During this time the bacteria, with appropriate substrate, are producing copious amounts of extracellular glucans, which add to the overall plaque matrix. If allowed to continue, the plaque forms up to the height of contour of the tooth and fills the interproximal areas. Growth above these areas is somewhat limited by mastication. The consumption of fibrous foods can have an effect upon the overall distribution of plaque, but the chewing of these foods seems to have little if any effect upon the plaque growth in the cervical and interproximal areas of the teeth. Unfortunately, these are the areas of high caries prevalence. After 2 to 3 days, if left undisturbed, the plaque begins to change. The innermost environment of the plaque becomes more anaerobic and other bacterial forms begin to appear. The overall plaque mass has now increased by 10 to 200 percent. It now appears as a thick jelly-like mass on the enamel (Fig. 27–10). If allowed to remain on the tooth surface, calcium phosphate deposition can occur, leading to the transformation of the plaque into calculus.

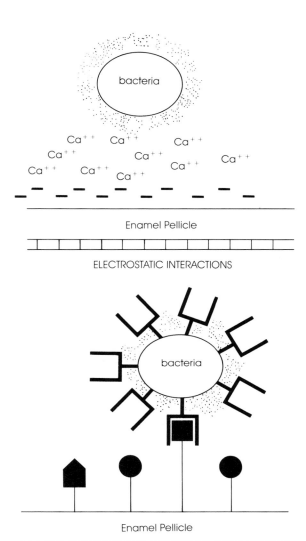

ELECTROSTATIC INTERACTIONS

LECTIN-LIKE INTERACTIONS

Figure 27–9 ■ The diagrammatic representation of the proposed interaction of oral bacteria with pellicle-coated enamel surfaces. The upper figure illustrates the electrostatic hypothesis, while the lower shows the "lectin-like" interactions.

Plaque Biochemistry

The single most important feature of dental plaque is its unique ability to selectively utilize fermentable sugars in the diet and rapidly convert them to destructive organic acids and sticky insoluble dextrans. There is a unique way in which oral bacteria handle these substrates. Focusing on this concept, let us now examine some of the chemical aspects of the process.

Like all living organisms bacteria must be able to produce energy by various biochem-

ical processes. Humans and other higher organisms use a complex biochemical pathway which first requires the breakdown of molecules into pyruvate anion. Pyruvate is then converted enzymatically to acetate, which serves as the primary substrate for the pathway known as the tricarboxylic acid cycle. This biochemical pathway results in the production of high energy molecules used to power the individual cells. Bacteria also have energy-producing pathways, the most common of which is glycolysis (see Chapter 3). In this process, glucose is enzymatically broken down into two molecules of lactate. Therefore, glucose is a very important substrate for the maintenance and growth of common oral bacteria. To accommodate their need for this substrate, bacteria possess enzymes capable of breaking down and transporting sugars into the cell cytoplasm. Obviously, the production of small organic acids from the fermentation of glucose plays a key role in the development of dental caries. However, the ability of oral bacteria to produce extracellular polysaccharides is probably the single most important feature in plaque development and the caries process.

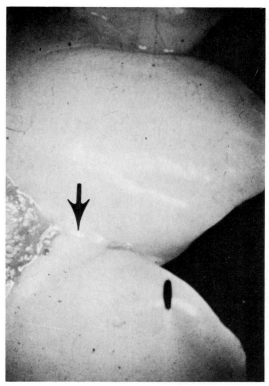

Figure 27–10 ■ Clinical photograph of supragingival plaque formed on the cervical area of the teeth. Note the white "gelatinous" appearance.

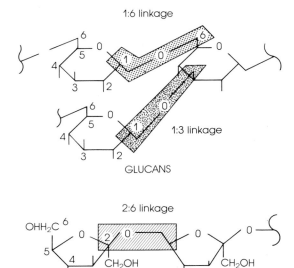

1:6 linkage

1:3 linkage

GLUCANS

2:6 linkage

LEVANS

Figure 27–11 ■ Molecular diagrams of bacterial dextrans and levans, two common types of polysaccharides produced by oral plaque-producing streptococci.

Oral bacteria, specifically the streptococci, possess a unique set of enzymes called transferases which are capable of rapidly converting disaccharides, particularly sucrose, into long-chain polysaccharides. They produce glucans, composed of glucose units, and levans, composed of fructose moieties (Fig. 27–11). The glucans, specifically the water-insoluble fraction, serve as a structural component of the plaque matrix. More simply, they are the "biologic glue" holding the plaque mass together and allowing the adherence of the plaque to the tooth surface. The soluble levans and glucans also serve as a carbohydrate food reserve, which is readily available in times of carbohydrate deprivation. These enzyme systems are primarily cell-membrane bound and show a high specificity for sucrose. They function by binding sucrose and cleaving the high-energy dihemiacetal linkage resulting in the formation of one glucose

and one fructose molecule. The glucose molecule is then transferred to a previously bound glucose moiety to yield a dextran primer. Sequential addition of glucose residues will then occur to yield the long-chain glucans. Other glucosyl-bearing disaccharides such as maltose and lactose are not utilized by these enzymes and therefore will not produce dextrans. This can be explained on examination of the high-energy bond found in the sucrose molecule. The glucose and fructose moieties are linked together by a dihemiacetal bond, which has a very high free energy of hydrolysis (Fig. 27–12). When this bond is broken, a significant amount of energy is released to the environment (Table 27–3). This energy may be conserved by the oral bacteria through enzymatic coupling reactions and used to power the transferase enzyme systems.

Host Factors and Caries

Another important factor in caries formation is the host. Caries, which is selective for humans, occurs relatively slowly, requiring 1 to 2 years for progression through the enamel. There appear to be host mechanisms that inhibit the development of caries.

The first host factors that favor caries are the **dental anatomic contours** and **arch form** in the human. In humans, the height of contour of the teeth is found above the gingival margin, which lends itself to bacterial growth as a result of stagnation. The molar teeth frequently contain deep pits and fissures favoring plaque development. The evolutionary development of the human arch form has led to the proximal contact of the teeth and the appearance of tooth crowding. Each of these features again favors the development of plaque as a result of stasis. The second and most obvious host factor that affects caries incidence is the **saliva**. This unique secretion contains a wide variety of

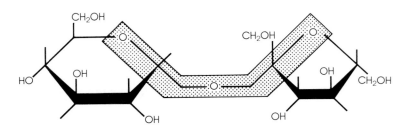

Figure 27–12 ■ Molecular structure of sucrose. Shaded area indicates the high-energy di-hemiacetal bond thought to be important to the production of extracellular glucans.

Table 27–3 ■ Free energy of hydrolysis of glucosyl donors and some polysaccharide

Compound	Standard Free Energy of Hydrolysis (ΔG_H, cal/mole)
Glucose 1-phosphate	−5000
UDP-glucose*	−7600
Sucrose	−6600
Maltose	−3000
Lactose	−3000
Glycogen	−4300
Dextran	−2000
Levan	−4600

*UDP = uridine diphosphate.
(From Newbrun, Cariology, 2nd ed., 1983, p. 105, with permission.)

substances that are thought to act in unison to serve as the host's primary defense for the development of dental caries. Most dental practitioners are well aware of rampant caries occurring when saliva production ceases. The important role of saliva in the host defense mechanisms has led to the isolation and identification of many unique chemical components. For discussion purposes these defense components will be divided into two types: (1) active defense molecules and (2) passive defense agents (Table 27–4). Active agents, similar to antibiotics, are bacteriocidal or bacteriostatic toward oral flora. The passive defense agents disrupt or prevent plaque formation by modifying the microbial environment to reduce the bacteria's chances for survival rather than actually destroying the bacteria.

Table 27–4 ■ Proposed salivary bacterial defense components

Component	Mode of Action
Active	
Lysozyme	Bacterial cell wall lysis
Lactoperoxidase	Catalyzes OSCN⁻ formation, which disrupts bacterial proteins
Lactoferrin	Binds up Fe leading to cell growth inhibition
Passive	
Secretory IgA	Interferes with bacterial attachment
Salivary glycoproteins	Can act as specific bacterial agglutinins
Salivary bicarbonate	Can buffer organic acids produced during sugar fermentation

ACTIVE SALIVARY COMPONENTS

Characterization of whole saliva has led to the isolation of several enzymes thought to be antibacterial. **Lysozyme**, first identified by Flemming in nasal fluids, has been isolated from parotid saliva. This molecule is quite effective in killing several types of gram-positive bacteria. As its name implies, it causes bacterial death by promoting cell wall disruption and subsequent cell lysis. It was first believed that this enzyme played a key role in the destruction of oral bacteria. However, recent microbiologic studies on pure strains of plaque-producing bacteria have shown that lysozyme is not that effective and is probably of lesser importance. Two other enzymes have been identified and characterized from saliva—lactoperoxidase and lactoferrin. **Lactoperoxidase** is found in other animal products such as milk. In the presence of hydrogen peroxide and thiocyanate ion, this enzyme catalyzes the formation of hypothiocyanate ion ($OSCN^-$). This compound reacts rapidly with sulfhydryl groups within proteins, leading to disruption of the bacterial metabolic systems. **Lactoferrin**, a sulfur-containing enzyme, binds iron that is essential for bacterial growth. Therefore, the presence of this compound reduces iron availability and results in the inhibition of bacterial growth.

PASSIVE SALIVARY COMPONENTS

Salivary Buffers

One of the essential functions of saliva is as a buffer. This is also an important component for the passive defense of the host against caries. The major buffer system found in saliva is bicarbonate-carbonate. This buffer can rapidly neutralize strong acids in the pH range of 6.1 and lower. Therefore, it can efficiently handle the production of lactic and acetic acids by plaque bacteria and can reduce enamel demineralization. Although phosphate is also present in the saliva and can act as a buffer, bicarbonate appears to be of greater importance. There are several explanations for this:

1. Bicarbonate buffers can react rapidly by losing CO_2.

2. It has a dissociation constant (pK) effective in the range at which plaque acids are produced.

3. As salivary flow increases, the bicarbon-

ate concentration also increases. This is in contrast to phosphate, which falls slightly.

Pellicle Components

The salivary pellicle proteins may also serve a protective function for the host. Surface enamel is more resistant to bacterial acids than the subsurface mineral. It is thought that the surface salivary pellicle stabilizes the surface hydroxyapatite, increasing its acid resistance. This hypothesis is supported by the observation that acid demineralization of hydroxyapatite in vitro does not give the same sort of carious lesion as seen in vivo unless bacterial plaque and salivary pellicle are both present on the tooth surface.

Immunoglobulins

Like most other glandular excretions, saliva contains immunoglobulins. The major immunoglobulin found in saliva is secretory IgA (see Chapter 2). This molecule differs from serum IgA in both structure and stability. Serum IgA is found as a monomer, whereas secretory IgA is a dimer consisting of two IgA monomers connected by a protein "J" chain. The secretory IgA also contains a secretory associated protein. Apparently, dimeric IgA is synthesized by plasma cells that reside in the connective tissues surrounding the salivary glands. Glandular cells found in the intercalated ducts are thought to synthesize the glycoprotein secretory unit. The immunoglobulins are assembled in the tight junctions below the glandular epithelium and then are secreted into the lumen of the gland duct. The secretory unit is thought to facilitate the transport of the immunoglobulin into the saliva. In addition, this protein makes the immunoglobulin resistant to the oral proteolytic enzymes. It has been suggested that salivary IgA may protect the host from oral pathogens by acting as a specific agglutinin. As mentioned earlier, the ability of bacteria and other pathogens to survive in the oral cavity is dependent upon their ability to adhere to an oral surface. Secretory IgA binds and agglutinates specific oral bacteria, rendering them unable to bind to host tissues. This results in a removal of oral flora from the mouth.

The host has a wide variety of defense mechanisms in the oral cavity. However, protection from localized oral infections is dependent upon the functioning of all these systems acting in unison to achieve a balance. No single mechanism can effectively protect the host at the expense of another.

DIET, NUTRITION, AND DENTAL CARIES

The role of diet is also important when considering the etiology of dental caries. Diet, which relates to the consumption of foods, has a local effect upon the oral structures rather than a systemic one, as in the case of nutrition. Nutrition is defined as that process by which foods are assimilated and metabolized in the body. The effects of nutrition on the teeth are greatest during the developmental stages. The best example of this is the systemic incorporation of fluoride during tooth formation, which results in a more caries-resistant tooth. Other nutritional factors such as calcium and phosphorus would be expected to play an important role in tooth development. However, the present experimental evidence is inconclusive about the effects of these and other nutritional factors on the caries susceptibility of the dentition.

Dietary factors, on the other hand, have dramatic effects upon the caries incidence. The role of dietary sugars, particularly sucrose, in the prevalence of dental caries has been examined in human and animal studies. One of the earliest experiments with sugars was performed by Stephan (1940). Using antimony electrodes Stephan measured the effects of glucose rinses upon the pH of dental plaque. Within 2 to 3 minutes following a sugar rinse, the plaque pH rapidly fell from about 6.8 to 5.0. This fall lasted 20 minutes and took about 40 minutes to return to the original, "resting pH" (Fig. 27–13). Similar experiments with repeated sucrose rinses show that multiple exposures to sugar have an additive effect upon the acid production of plaque (Fig. 27–14). Animal studies in rodents to assess the relative cariogenicity of human foods and drinks have shown a direct relationship between sucrose concentration and caries scores. Several human studies have also examined the relationship of diet to caries incidence. In one of the first controlled studies, Sognnaes (1948) examined the caries incidence among European schoolchildren during World War II. During the rationing of sugar the caries score significantly decreased. When rationing ceased the caries scores increased to prewar levels. Although this work is well quoted, there are

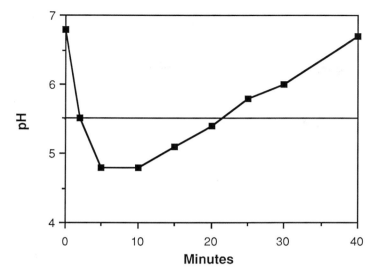

Figure 27–13 ■ The pH of plaque after rinsing the mouth with 10 percent glucose solution. The line at pH 5.5 is the value at which decalcification of enamel will occur. This is termed the "critical pH." The curve is commonly called a "Stephan curve."

some questions concerning the validity of the conclusions drawn from the experimental design. The Sognnaes study was based upon routine examinations rather than research surveys and were relatively crude. It is believed that the reduced caries rate noted by Sognnaes would not have occurred until several years after rationing had been present. Therefore, one would expect the lowered caries score to be delayed until sometime after rationing had begun. Some scientists have suggested that the observed lowered caries rate was due instead to an increased consumption of unrefined carbohydrates and fibrous foods.

The Vipeholm study (Gustafsson et al., 1954) examined institutionalized patients in Sweden. The investigators studied the effects of frequency and form of carbohydrate consumed upon the caries experience. The researchers found that caries increased significantly when the frequency of sucrose-containing food was increased. Therefore, extended consumption of carbohydrates increased the chances for acid demineralization and caries. They also found that sticky or adhesive forms of carbohydrates resulted in a delayed clearance time from the mouth and an increased caries risk.

Another human study examined a group of children in an Australian orphanage. The children were on restricted diets that did not contain processed sugar. Their caries experience was significantly lower (about 10 percent) than that of other children in the state school system. However, after the children left the orphanage and were no longer under strict dietary control, the amount of their DMFT (decayed, missing, and filled permanent teeth) approximated that of the general population. This implied that the potential for caries is always present and that teeth do

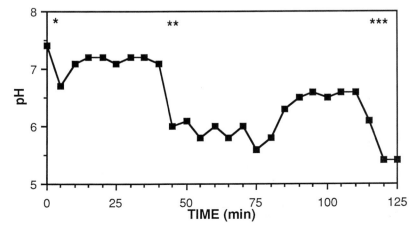

Figure 27–14 ■ The effect of plaque pH following the application of repeated ingestion of 0.5 percent glucose solutions at 2 minute intervals. Note the additive effects of repetative glucose applications which results in an overall drop in the plaque pH to well below the "critical pH" of 5.5. *One addition 0.06 ml of 0.5 percent glucose; **0.06 of 0.5 percent glucose per 2 minute intervals; ***5 percent glucose added similarly.

not acquire any permanent resistance to caries. Another study examined a group of individuals with hereditary fructose intolerance, in which there is a reduced enzymatic activity of fructose 1-phosphate aldolase, resulting in an inability to metabolize fructose. These individuals become very sick upon ingestion of foods containing fructose or sucrose, forcing them to restrict their sugar intake carefully. An examination of the DMFS caries score of 17 individuals with hereditary fructose intolerance showed a greater than 90 percent reduction in caries incidence when compared with a control group.

Several other epidemiologic studies have examined isolated human populations such as Eskimos, Aborigines, and the Bantu tribes in Africa. When the diets of these populations were modified to contain more refined carbohydrate, their DMFS scores increased proportionately. Thus, the type and amount of carbohydrate exposure has a direct effect upon the caries experience of humans.

Other dietary components have also been thought to play a role in caries incidence. The phosphates are thought to have some anticaries activity because animals on diets supplemented with inorganic phosphates have reduced caries. Organic phosphates have also been suggested as having some cariostatic properties. While the mechanism of this anticaries activity is unknown, the effects are local rather than systemic. Several mechanisms for this activity have been proposed:

1. Increased phosphate ions in the saliva may shift the equilibrium dissociation of hydroxyapatite to favor the mineralized salt in the presence of acids.

2. Phosphate could act as a buffer reacting with organic acids produced by oral bacteria.

3. Phosphate ions are able to desorb pellicle proteins, which may alter the ability of oral bacterial adherence.

Although the results in the animal models are encouraging, similar studies in humans have not been conclusive. Further studies are indicated to investigate fully the anticaries potential of phosphates.

Another dietary component with anticariogenic activity is lipid. Addition of lipids to a cariogenic diet reduces dental caries in animals. Medium-chain fatty acids and their salts also have some antibacterial properties in vitro and in animal models. Whether these materials might work in humans has not yet been established. Studies by Gibbons and Dankers (1981), Wolinsky and Sote (1984), and Staat and associates (1978) have reported on plant extracts that act as specific bacterial agglutinins. The results of these studies suggest that "lectin-like" components in specific foods may affect plaque formation in the mouth and could alter the caries susceptibility of an individual. Wolinsky and Sote have found that natural plant polyphenolic compounds known as **tannins** are quite effective bacterial agglutinins.

The last area of consideration in dietary factors that may affect dental caries are the trace elements. A number of trace elements including barium, vanadium, strontium, selenium, and molybdenum have been thought to have some influence upon dental caries. Enamel is permeable to small ions, which can change the surface composition. The adsorption of these ions may alter the surface characteristics of the enamel and cause changes in the pellicle. This in turn may alter plaque formation.

Caries Control and Prevention

Despite our knowledge of dental caries and its prevention, a large portion of the general population still suffers from dental caries. There have been great strides made in the prevention of the disease, the most notable one being water fluoridation. More recently, attention has focused upon the possibility of a caries vaccine. In this section we will examine several approaches to the control of dental caries, including chemotherapeutic agents that are effective in controlling dental plaque and caries.

IMMUNOLOGIC CONTROL OF CARIES

The development of immunologic vaccines has resulted in the control of many viral and bacterial diseases. These past successes have generated much interest in the concept of a caries vaccine. As mentioned earlier, the saliva is known to contain immunoglobulins. The concentration of immunoglobulins in saliva is approximately 1 to 3 percent. The major source of these immunoglobulins is the salivary secretions which produce secretory IgA. However, saliva also contains the humoral immunoglobulins IgG and IgM from the gingival sulcular fluid. In addition, cellular components of the immune system such as lymphocytes, macrophages, and neutrophils are present in the gingival sulcus (Fig. 27–15). The immunoglobulin host defense system is not totally understood. However, it is believed that the control of cariogenic bacteria by these molecules does play an important role in the overall maintenance of oral health. There are two possible ways antibodies might control bacterial growth:

1. The salivary immunoglobulins may act as specific agglutinins interacting with bacterial surface receptors and inhibiting colonization and subsequent caries formation. They might also inactivate surface glucosyltransferases, which would then reduce the synthesis of extracellular glucans resulting in reduced plaque formation.

2. The antibodies might also opsonize bacteria leading to phagocytosis by lymphocytes and PMNs.

The stimulation of salivary immunoglobulins generally occurs through the small intestine. The Peyer's patches populating the lamina propria contain B cells, which can be stimulated by the commonplace swallowing of oral bacteria. Plasma cells sensitized to the oral bacteria are then produced and migrate to the excretory glands. The plasma cells in the salivary glands produce S-IgA to specific bacteria. The current basis for a caries vaccine suggests stimulation of secretory IgA via the gut. The question arises, how can IgA stimulation be maintained when there are low levels of a particular bacteria? Animal and human studies have examined the use of salivary immunoglobulins for control of caries incidence.

Animal Studies

In gnotobiotic rats ingestion of whole *Streptococcus mutans* selectively produces S-IgA. The appearance of S-IgA correlated with reduced caries incidence. In another study, hamsters fed bacterial surface proteins from *S. mutans* developed antibodies and had a lowered incidence of caries when fed high-sucrose diets. Animal studies were indicated to determine if stimulation of serum antibodies to cariogenic bacteria could also reduce the caries incidence. Animals injected with high doses of streptococci had elevated serum IgG, however, the incidence of caries was not consistently reduced. This may be due to serum antibodies not reaching sufficient levels in the saliva to have significant effects. In addition, serum antibodies excreted into the oral cavity through the gingival sulcus do not have a secretory associated protein. Therefore, their activity is rapidly destroyed by oral proteolytic enzymes. Lehner and coworkers do not agree with this view and feel that serum IgG probably accounts for most of the caries reduction noted in immunized animals. This is based upon the fact that IgG levels are quite high in plaque—about three times IgA levels.

Human Studies

Currently, clinical trials are underway to test the use of a "pill" of *S. mutans* for control of caries. There have been some conflicting results thus far in human studies. Some workers have actually reported a negative correlation between S-IgA and caries preva-

Figure 27–15 ■ Illustration of the sources of immunoglobulins in the oral cavity. (Courtesy of E. Newbrun. From Newbrun's Cariology, ed. 2, p. 31, Williams and Wilkins, Baltimore, 1983, with permission.

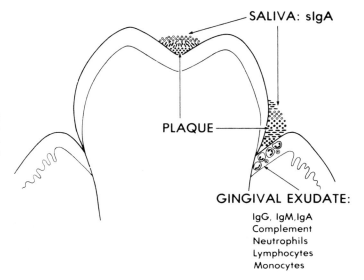

SALIVA: sIgA

PLAQUE

GINGIVAL EXUDATE:

IgG, IgM, IgA
Complement
Neutrophils
Lymphocytes
Monocytes

lence. However, this result could be the result of the experimental design. It has been shown that ingestion of capsules containing *S. mutans* stimulates the production of S-IgA. In a study of individuals who could not produce any salivary immunoglobulins, the caries rates were much higher than in the normal control group. Stimulation of serum immunoglobulins in humans has also produced mixed results and no correlation could be made between caries experience and serum immunoglobulin stimulation.

The idea of a caries vaccine is a good one. However, several problems must be resolved to ensure the desired results. First, bacteria have the ability to rapidly change antigenic properties, which could render the immunity ineffective. In addition, the removal of a particular strain of oral flora will not ensure against the repopulation with another more virulent organism. One must be certain that the antigens injected will not result in cross-reactivity of the humoral antibodies with other body tissues. For example, it is thought that *S. mutans* possess antigenic components shared with heart muscle. Induction of these antibodies could be disastrous, leading to heart damage. Last, if a vaccine is developed, would it be necessary to remove most of the oral flora and then allow for a repopulation to occur following antibody stimulation? How long would the immunity last? These are questions still to be answered.

FLUORIDES

The routine use of fluorides in the maintenance of oral hygiene remains the most effective chemotherapeutic method currently used in the United States. Extensive data show significant reduction in enamel caries when fluoride is used topically or systemically. As a result of the widespread use of fluorides in the drinking water and home dentifrices, there has been a 50 to 60 percent reduction of the DMFS in children and teenagers. Several mechanisms have been proposed to explain the anticaries effects of the fluoride ion. The proposed hypotheses are summarized in Table 27–5. The first and most widely accepted concept is that the incorporation of fluoride ions into the developing enamel increases its acid resistance. Experiments have shown that systemic incorporation of fluoride in developing hydroxyapatite crystals occurs readily leading to the formation of a mixed fluorhydroxyapatite. The

Table 27–5 ■ Proposed hypotheses for the anticaries effects of fluoride

1. Substitution of fluoride for hydroxyl ion in apatite makes the crystal less soluble at low pH, therefore, making the enamel more resistant to bacterial demineralization. Fluoride occupies some of the voids created by improper stacking of the hydroxyl groups resulting in stabilization of the lattice.
2. Fluoride in the developing hydroxyapatite influences the solubility of the enamel matrix proteins. This results in a slower crystal formation and an increased stability of the hydroxyapatite.
3. Fluoride may compete for carbonate ion which makes the apatite crystals smaller and may provide "seed" sites for dissolution.
4. Fluoride can act as an effective antibacterial agent. Concentrations of 30 ppm and greater have been shown to inhibit glycolytic enzymes in plaque bacteria.
5. Systemic fluoride during tooth formation can result in altered tooth formation. The teeth can be smaller and the pit and fissures of the posterior teeth may be more coalesced. This may increase their resistance to caries.

fluoride ion is thought to replace hydroxyl groups or fill voids found in the center of the crystal structure (see Fig. 27–2). This results in a more stable crystal structure which results in a less soluble crystal. An alternative explanation has been proposed by Simmons (1972). He believes that the incorporation of fluoride into the hydroxyapatite crystal changes the surface pH of the crystal. This in turn reduces the rate of growth of the crystal into the enamel matrix proteins. The slower the rate of crystal formation, the more stable the fluorhydroxyapatite crystal. Elemental analysis of enamel has shown that the outermost surface of the enamel contains higher levels of fluoride than the remaining crystal. It has been proposed that this changes the charge characteristics of the surface influencing the nature of the salivary pellicle. This in turn may alter the plaque.

Another property of fluoride is its antibacterial activity. Fluoride ion is a potent inhibitor of many bacterial enzymes including enolase, which is required for bacterial metabolism of sugars. Concentrations of 10 ppm or greater in the plaque reduces plaque acid. These levels of fluoride can easily be attained in plaque because the ion accumulates following repeated exposures. Therefore, very high levels of fluoride in the plaque can result from the daily application of a topical gel, rinse or use of a fluoridated dentifrice.

One other important anticaries property of fluoride may be its ability to cause remineralization of incipient enamel caries. Fluoride ion is rapidly converted to calcium fluoride in the oral cavity. This salt is not very soluble and will precipitate out onto the tooth surface. If demineralization of the enamel occurs, the calcium fluoride can act as a reservoir and release fluoride ion which can react with the hydroxyapatite. This will result in a remineralization of the enamel. Some researchers believe that acid demineralization microscopically occurs frequently at the tooth-plaque interface but the teeth remineralize keeping the development of caries to a reasonably slow rate. Therefore topical fluorides are extremely important to an overall caries prevention program and should be emphasized to all patients for routine home care. The recommended fluoride supplementation dosage is given in Table 27–6.

OTHER CHEMOTHERAPEUTIC ANTICARIES AGENTS

Other chemical agents have recently appeared that have the potential to be effective anticaries agents. These agents are antibacterial and are effective at reducing the overall plaque formation in the oral cavity. The most widely known agents in present use in Europe are chlorhexidine and its chemical analogue alexidine (Fig. 27–16). These bisguinide aromatic compounds are excellent antimicrobial agents for gram-positive streptococci. These cationic compounds are believed to bind to the negatively charged surfaces of gram-positive bacteria, resulting in a disruption of the cell membrane leading to cytoplasmic leakage and cell death. The bisguinides also have the interesting property of being substantive; that is, they are bound to the tooth pellicle where they act as a reservoir for the chemical and are released slowly over a long time, extending their plaque-inhibiting

Figure 27–16 ■ Chemical structural illustrations of chlorhexidine and its chemical analogue alexidine. The microbiologic activity of these molecules is related to the presence of the vicinal guanidine moieties giving this molecule a highly cationic nature.

properties. The disadvantage of these agents is that they stain the teeth over time. They are also bitter tasting. Last, they have been known to modify the taste perception in certain individuals. Chlorhexidine (Peridex) is now available in the United States as a prescription mouthwash at 0.12 percent concentration; this concentration minimizes the staining effects.

There are many other agents that have produced some antiplaque activity. As yet, none of the agents replace the need for judicious oral hygiene with mechanical devices. However, the daily use of antimicrobial agents in conjunction with mechanical debridement and fluoride may prove to be the most effective means of controlling this dental disease.

CARIES ACTIVITY TESTS

Knowledge of caries etiology has led to the development of tests which attempt to measure a patients' individual susceptibility to dental caries. Although a multitude of tests are described in the literature none is at present thought to be an ideal indicator of disease activity. This is due to the multifactorial nature of the disease. All the current assay methods focus on one feature of the caries process and attempt to draw strong positive correlations to actual caries experi-

Table 27–6 ■ Recommended fluoride supplementation dosage schedule*			
	Concentration of Fluoride in water (ppm)		
Age (yr)	0.0.3	0.3–0.7	0.7–1.0
0 to 2	0.25	0.0	0.0
2 to 3	0.50	0.25	0.0
3 to adult	1.00	0.50	0.0

*Adjusted allowance in mg of fluoride/day; 2.2 mg sodium fluoride contains 1 mg F⁻.
From Newbrun, Cariology, 2nd ed., 1983, p. 312, with permission.

ence. This approach precludes many other variables which may affect the overall caries experience of an individual. Perhaps it may be necessary to use several tests simultaneously to provide the high degree of correlation ($r = 0.9$) necessary to give a valid indication of caries prediction. However, these assays can act as a valuable aid for patient motivation in a well-designed plaque control program.

An ideal caries test should have the following characteristics: validity, reliability, and feasibility. **Validity** simply means that the test accurately measures what it says it does. In order to measure test validity properly a prediction of caries experience must be made in a group of test patients. The patients must then be followed for some period of time—perhaps 1 or 2 years—and the caries occurrence must be recorded. If a high percentage of positive test responders develops caries, the test is then said to exhibit validity.

Reliability is a second characteristic necessary for a good predictive test. Reliability means that the test will yield the same results under varied conditions and among several independent observers.

Finally, **feasibility** of the assay must also be considered. The ease and costs of performing the test are important to the overall acceptance of the method to clinical situations. Ideally, a test that is noninvasive, inexpensive, and easily run is desired.

Among the large number of caries tests that have been developed in research laboratories several have gained some acceptance among dental practitioners. The first group of tests are based upon the microbiologic vector of the disease. These tests attempt to correlate oral bacteria and/or their metabolic products to caries incidence. The older test of this type is the lactobacillus colony count, in which salivary samples are obtained and incubated in selective media for lactobacilli. The numbers of lactobacillus colonies per milliliter of saliva are quantitated and related to caries activity. Although this test has been used as a standard assay for many years it has some drawbacks, including a relatively high cost per test. This method also requires several days to run and requires tedious counting of bacterial colonies. A newer, more convenient method for estimating oral lactobacilli is now available.* This test measures lactobacilli present by comparison to a standard optical density chart that has been cor-

related to the number of organisms per milliliter. This method is relatively simple to use and can be adapted to most dental offices. However, once again this method requires several days to complete.

The Snyder test is another relatively inexpensive caries prediction test. It measures the salivary acid production over a 3-day period. The test uses pH color indicators, which make it quite easy to determine bacterial acid production. Snyder and others who have used this assay report a strong correlation between clinical caries activity and a positive test result. Table 27–7 indicates how the results of the Snyder test may be interpreted. Although this test is relatively inexpensive to run, it also requires 3 days to obtain the results and is therefore somewhat time-inefficient for the clinical dental setting.

The reductase test, a colorimetric assay that measures the activity of the salivary enzyme reductase, has also been used as a caries predictive test with some success. It has the advantage of giving results in the relatively short time of 15 minutes. However, there has been some question as to the validity of this test, since results have not been confirmed among several independent investigators.

The buffering capacity of whole saliva has also been used as a means of predicting caries experience. This method measures the ability of a salivary sample to neutralize a standard acid solution. It is based upon the hypothesis that increased acid production by plaque bacteria leads to increased enamel demineralization and caries. Therefore, an inverse relationship between buffering capacity of the saliva and caries activity should exist. Although there is some validity to this test, the results obtained cannot be adequately correlated to caries activity. Table 27–8 conveniently lists these and other proposed caries predictive tests that are based upon chemical or bacteriologic assays.

---

*Orion Diagnostica (Helsinki, Finland).

Table 27–7 ■ Interpretation of Snyder caries test results

	Time (hr)		
	24	*48*	*72*
Color	Yellow	Yellow	Yellow
Caries activity	High	Definite	Limited
Color	Green	Green	Green
Caries activity	Continue test	Continue test	Inactive

(From Newbrun, Cariology, 2nd ed., 1983, p. 259, with permission.)

Table 27–8 ■ Caries activity tests: basis, method, and clinical correlation

Test	Basis	Method	Clinical Correlation
Lactobacillus count	Aciduric bacteria (saliva)	Quantitative counts/ml	Group correlation only
Synder	Aciduric bacteria (saliva)	Qualitative colorimetric	Group correlation only
Swab	Aciduric bacteria (plaque)	Qualitative colorimetric	Unsatisfactory
Fosdick	Total bacteria (saliva)	Quantitative Ca demin. of enamel	None established
Dewar	Total bacteria (saliva)	Quantitative modified Fosdick	Unsatisfactory
Rickles	Total bacteria (saliva)	Quantitative buffering capacity	Unsatisfactory
Reductase	Total bacteria (saliva)	Qualitative color indicator	Group correlation only
Amylase	Starch hydrolysis (saliva)	Qual./Quant. color indicator	Unsatisfactory
Buffer capacity	Buffer capacity (saliva)	Quantitative titration	Some extreme deviations
Streptococcus mutans screening	S. mutans (plaque)	Semiquantitative	Best correlation for high caries group

(From Newbrun, Cariology, 2nd ed., 1983, p. 266, with permission.)

Another approach to predicting caries activity is to examine an individual's previous caries experience and try to formulate future trends. This type of method has been successfully applied to groups of children and was shown to be a predictable means of identifying children with high and low caries activity.

The role of dietary carbohydrate in the carious process has been clearly established. Furthermore, sucrose is implicated as the key substrate for caries-producing bacteria and the relationship of the percent of sucrose in foods and their caries-producing activity is shown in Table 27–9. Therefore, the correlation of sucrose ingestion to caries experience may be another method for predicting caries potential. The variability of caries among individuals raises the question of what differences, if any, exist between caries-prone and caries-resistant individuals. Early studies focused upon the saliva, since its protective role in caries development was somewhat understood. Researchers looked at calcium-to-phosphate ratios in caries-resistant humans. Although some caries-resistant individuals did show higher calcium-to-phos-

phate ratios, no definite conclusions could be made. Investigators also looked at the resting salivary pH and found the pH to be significantly higher in people who were caries free. Other studies examining specific salivary components such as salivary IgA, lysozyme,

Table 27–9 ■ Correlation of sucrose content of selected foods to caries score in rats*

Food*	Sucrose Conc. (%)	Caries Score
Sucrose	99.5	62
Milk chocolate	42	34
Dates	47	33
10% sucrose/water	10	32
Raisins	14	31
Candy mints	78	25
Bananas	9	21
Apples	3	19
Figs	0.1	10
Milk	0	0
Soda crackers	0	0

(Data adapted from Table 4–3 in Newbrun, Cariology, 2nd ed., 1983, Williams & Wilkins, p. 99, with permission.)
*Rats fed a noncariogenic diet for 1 hour twice a day. Test food was continuously available.

amylase, and lactoperoxidase have shown some differences among caries-free and caries-prone humans. Still other studies have focused upon plaque in these two groups, supporting the concept that caries occurs at the enamel-plaque interface and that examination of the saliva may not be as useful for comparison. Examination of plaque samples from caries-resistant and -susceptible groups was shown generally to produce equivalent amounts of lactic acid after sucrose ingestion. Therefore, the basic nature of the plaque is the same. However, plaque from caries-free individuals was shown to contain lower numbers of *S. mutans* and *L. acidophilus*. The variability in the results of these and other studies supports the concept that no single factor is common to all caries-free humans. It seems likely that in some caries-free individuals, salivary antibodies may be inhibiting cariogenic bacteria; however, this single effect is not enough to totally eliminate caries, and other salivary and host factors must work in unison to afford the individual overall caries protection. Furthermore, clinical observations suggest that different combinations of factors operate in each person resulting in a specific caries risk.

Root Caries

Root caries comprise the group of carious lesions that affect the cementum and dentin of the root surface. It is a lesion generally found in the adult. The prevalence of root caries increases significantly after the age of 35 and has been noted in more than 50 percent of the population between the ages of 40 and 50. The nature of root caries is somewhat different from that of enamel caries. Many lesions are associated with gingival recession. This recession can be the result either of periodontal therapy or of natural aging. It is a soft progressive lesion of the root surface, which is associated with microbial plaque. It should be distinguished from abrasion, erosion, and idiopathic resorption. Caries on the root surface usually appears as a shallow, ill-defined area, often discolored, and quite soft. Lesions are thought to start at the cemental-enamel junction. The progression of this lesion usually extends laterally rather than in depth. However, lesions can spread rather rapidly and pulpal involvement can occur in a few months' time. Diagnosis of root caries is based upon the clinical features of location, color, surface roughness, softness of the root, and/or obvious cavitation. As yet no clear diagnostic tests are available for root caries detection.

The etiology of root caries is primarily microbial. Plaque-sampling studies have identified gram-positive filamentous *Actinomyces* species as a predominant bacteria. Animal studies in rodents have supported this finding and bacteria such as *A. viscosus* were shown to be essential for the development of cemental caries in these animals. Other microorganisms such as *A. naeslundii*, *S. mutans*, *S. salivarius*, *S. sanguis*, and *B. cereus* have all been shown to produce root caries in animal models. Although *A. viscosus* remains a favored etiologic bacteria in this lesion, no specific microorganism or particular group of oral flora has been clearly associated with the initiation or progression of root caries.

As with other caries, the role of the host is important in the overall development and progression of root caries. Specifically, decreased salivary function (xerostomia) can result in a dramatic increase in the incidence of root surface caries. Xerostomia can be associated with individuals undergoing head and neck radiation therapy, patients taking a variety of medications, and those suffering from Sjögren's syndrome. Therefore, persons with reduced salivary function must be carefully watched and maintained in order to prevent the rapid occurrence of root caries. Probably the most effective means of reducing the incidence of root carries is by dietary control, strict oral hygiene, and the daily use of topical fluorides. The consumption of fermentable carbohydrates should be closely monitored. These patients should be given repeated home care instruction to ensure excellent plaque control. Fluoride therapy will usually consist of a daily application of a fluoride gel using a custom-fitted stent. The most common formulations are a 0.4 percent stannous fluoride gel, which provides about 1000 ppm of fluoride ion, or a 1.1 percent neutral sodium fluoride gel which yields about 5000 ppm of fluoride ion.

REFERENCES

Gibbons, R. J.: Adherence of bacteria to host tissue. *In* Schlessinger, D. (ed.): Microbiology. A series of monographs. ASM, Washington, D.C., 1977, p. 395.
Gibbons, R. J., and Dankers, I.: Patterns of lectin-like reactivity of selected oral bacteria. J. Dent. Res. (spec. iss. A), 547, 1981.
Gustafsson, B. E., Quensel, C. E., Lanke, L. S., Lund-

qvist, C., Grahnen, H., Bonow, B. E., and Krasse, B.: The Vipeholm dental caries study. The effect of different levels of carbohydrate intake on caries activity in 436 individuals observed for five years. Acta. Odontol. Scand. 11:232, 1954.

Miller, W. D.: The microorganisms of the human mouth, edited by K. Konig. S. Karger, Basel, p. 205, 1890 (reprinted 1973).

Newbrun, E.: Cariology, ed 2. Williams and Wilkins, Baltimore, p. 246, 1983.

Rolla, S., Bonesvoll, P., and Opermann, R.: Interactions between oral streptococci and salivary proteins. In Kleinberg, Ellison, and Mandel (eds.): Saliva and Dental Caries. (sp. suppl.) Microbiology Abstr. 1979, p. 227.

Simmons, N. S.: Extraction of enamel rods and apatite ribbons from embryo teeth. J. Dent. Res. 51(sp. iss.):252, 1972.

Sognnaes, R. F.: Analysis of war-time caries reduction in European children, with special regard to observations in Norway. Am. J. Dis. Child. 75:795, 1948.

Staat, R. H., Doyle, R. J., Langley, S. D., and Studdick, R. P.: Modification of in vitro adherence of Streptococcus mutans by plant lectins. Adv. Exp. Med. Biol. 107:639, 1978.

Stephan, R. M.: Changes in the hydrogen ion concentration on tooth surfaces and in carious lesions. J. Am. Dent. Assoc. 27:718, 1940.

Wolinsky, L. E., and Sote, E. O.: Isolation of natural plaque-inhibiting substances from "Nigerian Chewing Sticks." Caries Res. 18:216, 1984.

chapter 28

Periodontal disease

Russell J. Nisengard, D.D.S., Ph.D □ *Michael G. Newman, D.D.S.*
Joseph J. Zambon, D.D.S., Ph.D.

CHAPTER OUTLINE

- ■ MICROBIOLOGY OF PERIODONTAL DISEASE— GENERAL ASPECTS
- ■ IMMUNOLOGY OF PERIODONTAL DISEASE— GENERAL ASPECTS
- ■ GINGIVAL HEALTH
- ■ SPECIFIC DISEASES
- ■ DIAGNOSTIC TESTS FOR PERIODONTAL DISEASE

The term *periodontal disease* describes a number of distinct clinical entities that affect the periodontium including the gingiva, gingival attachment, periodontal ligament, cementum, and supporting alveolar bone.

The most common periodontal diseases, gingivitis and periodontitis, as well as many other less common periodontal diseases, are chronic bacterial infections. Like other infections, the bacterial-host interactions determine the nature of the resulting disease. The pathologic microorganisms may produce disease indirectly (e.g., through the effects of toxins), or by direct invasion of the tissues. The host response to microorganisms may be protective or destructive or both, which accounts for the wide variety of patterns of tissue changes observed in patients. Periodontal diseases may be generalized or site-specific (affecting isolated areas) and may contribute to the development and course of certain systemic disease.

Gingivitis, or inflammation of the gingiva, is characterized clinically by gingival changes in color, form, position (see pocket formation further on), and surface appearance. Bleeding and exudate from the gingival crevice are also sometimes apparent.

Periodontitis occurs by the extension of inflammation into the deeper structures of the periodontium. Pocket formation, bone loss, and mobility are usual clinical features. Periodontitis may be generalized or localized. It is classified into adult forms and juvenile forms depending on the specific clinical, microbiologic, and host factors that are present at the time of diagnosis (Table 28–1).

A periodontal pocket is pathologically deepened gingival sulcus and it is one of the key clinical features of periodontitis (Fig. 28–1). Pocket formation may occur by the apical migration of the junctional epithelium along the root. Destruction of the periodontal ligament and alveolar bone occurs as a result of bacterial and host factors described later in this chapter.

CLASSIFICATION

Periodontics emphasizes the maintenance of gingival health through identification and

Table 28–1 ■ Classification of periodontal diseases

I. Gingival Disease
  A. Gingivitis
    1. Nonspecific gingivitis
    2. Acute necrotizing ulcerative gingivitis (ANUG)
  B. Manifestations of systemic diseases and hormonal disturbances—e.g., desquamative gingivitis, primary herpetic gingivostomatitis, "pregnancy gingivitis" and other hormonally mediated changes, diabetes and other metabolic diseases
  C. Drug-associated gingival inflammation—e.g., dilantin hyperplasia
II. Mucogingival conditions—e.g., gingival recession and aberrant frena and/or muscle attachment
III. Periodontitis
  A. Adult Periodontitis
    1. Slight
    2. Moderate
    3. Advanced
    4. Refractory and rapidly progressive
  B. Juvenile Periodontitis (JP)
    1. Prepubertal
    2. Generalized juvenile periodontitis (GJP)
    3. Localized juvenile periodontitis (LJP)
  C. Periodontal abscess
IV. Pathology Associated With Occlusion
V. Other Conditions—Miscellaneous (e.g., infection, trauma)

Adapted from *Current Procedural Terminology for Periodontics*, ed. 5. Am. Acad. Periodontol. 1986.

elimination of the etiologic factors. An understanding of the classification of periodontal diseases is important in any consideration of the effects of the host-bacterial interactions. The classification is based on the clinical, bacterial, host, and environmental factors. The contribution of each factor determines the course and treatment of the particular disease process. With the discovery of new bacterial etiologic agents, more specific diagnosis will permit refinement of the present classification and treatments (Table 28–1). In the future, some of the descriptive clinical names for periodontal diseases may be supplanted by bacterial names in recognition of their role in the etiology of the diseases.

Among the periodontal diseases, several are considered "aggressive" forms (Table 28–2). These forms of periodontitis frequently demonstrate rapid bone loss, sometimes measured in millimeters per year. This contrasts with adult periodontitis in which bone loss is usually in tenths of a millimeter per year.

PREVALENCE OF PERIODONTAL DISEASE

The most common inflammatory periodontal diseases, nonspecific gingivitis and periodontitis, occur in the United States and throughout the world. Gingivitis involving at least one site per patient affects more than 80 percent of the population and in some instances nearly 100 percent. It is seen in all age groups. Similarly, periodontitis affects approximately 75 percent of the adult American population. Alveolar bone loss due to periodontitis may start as early as the teen years, although it usually begins in adulthood, and progresses with age. Sex, socioeconomic factors, race, and the sensitivity of the methods used for detecting periodontitis all contribute to the reported prevalence. The

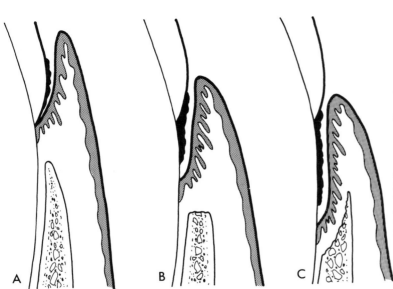

Figure 28–1 ■ Types of periodontal pockets. *A,* Normal gingival sulcus, where there is only soft tissue inflammation associated with plaque. *B,* Suprabony pocket. The base of the pocket is coronal to the alveolar bone. The alveolar bone loss is horizontal in nature. *C,* Infrabony pocket. The base of the pocket is apical to the level of the alveolar bone. The alveolar bone loss is vertical in nature. (From Carranza, F. A., Jr.: Glickman's Clinical Periodontology, 6th ed. Philadelphia, W. B. Saunders Co., 1984.)

Table 28–2 ■ "Aggressive" periodontal disease
Localized juvenile periodontitis
Generalized juvenile periodontitis
Rapidly progressive periodontitis
Refractory periodontitis

other forms of periodontal disease, including periodontal abscesses, acute necrotizing ulcerative gingivitis, prepubertal periodontitis, herpetic gingivostomatitis, juvenile periodontitis, rapidly progressive adult periodontitis, and drug or systemic-induced gingival conditions, are not as well studied but are considerably less common and account for less than 10 percent of all periodontal disease. These other diseases often require special diagnostic and treatment procedures.

CONCEPT AS AN INFECTION

The primary cause of the most common forms of gingivitis and periodontitis are bacteria. Bacteria attach to the tooth surface above and below the gingival margin as an organized mass referred to as bacterial plaque (see Chapter 26). Plaque is necessary to initiate these diseases. The pathogenic potential of the particular bacteria within the plaque varies from individual to individual and from one gingival site to another within the same mouth. A small but varying amount of plaque can be controlled or tolerated without causing periodontal disease probably as a result of host defense mechanisms. When specific bacteria within the plaque increase to significant numbers or produce virulence factors or both, the "controlled environment" or balance shifts toward the development of disease. Disease also occurs by a reduction in the host defensive capacity. These host factors can be local or systemic (see further on).

Early theories regarding the role of dental plaque in periodontal disease suggested that it consisted of a complex, homogeneous bacterial mass, which caused disease wherever it was allowed to grow. It was thought to be purely a quantitative change resulting from increased numbers rather than an alteration in the types of bacteria. It was later discovered that bacterial plaque associated with gingival health differed from that seen in periodontal disease and most periodontal diseases had their own characteristic flora (Table 28–3). In general, gram-negative, an-

Table 28–3 ■ Principal bacteria associated with periodontal disease	
Adult periodontitis	*Bacteroides gingivalis, B. intermedius*
Refractory periodontitis	*Bacteroides forsythus, B. gingivalis, Wolinella recta, B. intermedius*
Localized juvenile periodontitis (LJP)	*Actinobacillus actinomycetemcomitans, Capnocytophaga*
Periodontitis in juvenile diabetics	*Capnocytophaga, A. actinomycetemcomitans*
Pregnancy gingivitis	*B. intermedius*
ANUG	*B. intermedius,* intermediate-sized-spirochetes

aerobic microorganisms are the principal bacteria associated with most periodontal diseases with a bacterial etiology. *Bacteroides gingivalis, B. intermedius,* and *Actinobacillus actinomycetemcomitans* are the three most common bacteria identified to date. These are thought to be important because of their pathogenic capabilities and the increased numbers associated with disease states. Other bacteria found in lower numbers may also be important but have not been studied to the same extent as the principal bacteria.

At present, the etiologic relationship of bacteria to different periodontal diseases is based on several factors, as summarized in Table 28–4:

1. An organism thought to be important in the disease process should be commonly found in high numbers and absent or infrequently found in health.

2. Elimination or suppression of the organism by treatment should have a positive influence.

3. While host responses are influenced by the immunogenicity of the organism, there should usually be an elevated immune re-

Table 28–4 ■ Identification of the bacterial etiology in periodontal disease
1. Large numbers of the bacteria are *associated* with the disease state and absence or reduced numbers associated with health
2. *Elimination* or suppression of the organism reverses or reduces the disease
3. Elevated *host responses* are associated with the disease
4. *Animal pathogenicity* similar to periodontal disease occurs upon implantation of the organism(s) into germ-free animals
5. The bacteria possess potentially *pathogenic mediators* that could contribute to the disease process

sponse to the organism. This may be an elevated antibody response or cellular response.

4. Experimental implantation of the organism into the gingival crevice of an animal should lead to development of at least some of the characteristics of the naturally occurring disease (e.g., inflammation, connective tissue disruption, and bone loss).

5. The purported pathogen should possess pathogenic or virulent factors.

TREATMENT OF PERIODONTAL DISEASE

The rationale for treatment depends upon the identification of as many environmental and host factors as possible, as well as knowledge of the currently available therapies and their limitations.

Control of environmental or local factors is the major emphasis of current periodontal treatment modalities. Bacterial plaque is the primary etiologic agent while calculus and other factors are secondary local factors. These components elicit and perpetuate the vast majority of pathologic changes in the periodontium. Therapy is aimed at first identifying, removing, and controlling the etiologic factors and then correcting the defects these pathogens have created. Therapy for many periodontal diseases caused by bacterial plaque includes oral hygiene education and instruction, instrumentation for removal of calculus (scaling) and toxic root substances (root planing), chemotherapy (see Chapter 29), periodontal surgery (if pockets remain), and maintenance therapy.

Other environmental and local factors such as occlusion and iatrogenic factors can modify the progression of the local disease state. Diagnosis, detection, and treatment of each of these factors includes occlusal analysis and therapy, control of temporomandibular joint (TMJ) factors, orthodontics, repair or replacement of lost periodontal tissues, repair or replacement of existing restorations or prosthesis, and replacement of implanted materials.

HOST FACTORS

Alterations in the periodontium and other oral tissues are caused or influenced by a variety of systemically associated conditions. Factors such as age, occurrence of systemic disease, immune status, and stress greatly influence the nature of periodontal pathology. Assessment of these contributing factors significantly influences the therapeutic regimen. Physiologic and psychologic factors, chemotherapy, and hormones influence both the observed periodontal pathology and the associated therapy. Often, control of systemic etiologic factors greatly improves periodontal health. Similarly, periodontal pathology, especially acute gingivitis and periodontitis, affects the patient's general health. In some systemically compromised patients, periodontal disease can be a source of systemic infections. The control of metabolic diseases, such as diabetes, may also be adversely affected by periodontal disease.

Hereditary, genetic, and developmental factors influence every aspect of the periodontal tissues. Recognition and detection of contributing factors are essential to successful maintenance of periodontal health and prevention of disease.

Microbiology of Periodontal Disease— General Aspects

Bacterial infectious diseases are a result of one or more mechanisms (Table 28–5). The direct effects include invasion, exotoxins, cell constituents, and enzymes, which will be considered in the section on the microbiology of periodontal disease. The indirect response to the bacteria including immunologic and other host responses are considered subsequently in the section on the immunologic aspects of periodontal disease.

Periodontal microbiology has been examined by several approaches: cultural, taxonomy, microscopy, and immunodiagnosis. All these methods have led to an improved understanding of the etiology and pathogenesis of periodontal disease as well as further clarification of periods of disease activity. These studies have also extended periodontal therapy to include changing the subgingival flora to that associated with disease inactivity.

Table 28–5 ■ Potential bacterial mechanisms in periodontal disease

1. Invasion
2. Exotoxins
3. Cell constituents (such as endotoxins)
4. Enzymes
5. Immunologic—host responses

Table 28–6 ■ Bacterial factors important in direct tissue damage

Enzymes
   Collagenase
   Hyaluronidase
   Phospholipase
   Phosphatases
Endotoxin
Cell inhibitors
Ammonia

One of the important advances in the field of periodontal microbiology is the concept of specificity. Periodontal disease is now considered to be a group of diseases or infections. Each disease has its own associated group of microorganisms. Disease specificity was first identified with the advent of anaerobic microbiology techniques and their application in identifying "unusual" gram-negative rods associated with localized juvenile periodontitis. Since then, characteristic microfloras have been associated with the different periodontal diseases and stages of disease.

The mechanisms by which subgingival bacteria may contribute to the pathogenesis of periodontal disease is varied. The periodontopathogens possess numerous factors that permit them to directly damage the periodontium (Table 28–6) or indirectly compromise the host response (Table 28–7).

BACTERIAL INVASION

Studies of acute necrotizing ulcerative gingivitis have clearly demonstrated the invasive nature of spirochetes in this disease. It is thought that this invasion contributes to the disease in a similar fashion to spirochetal invasion in syphilis.

Our concepts of periodontitis are changing. In early studies of periodontitis, bacteria were identified microscopically in gingival tissue. However, later studies could not confirm this, leading to the conclusion that the bacteria were artifacts introduced into the tissues as a result of sectioning or local trauma. As a result, the consensus was that bacteria did not actively invade the periodontium. Instead, they were thought to infiltrate passively following routine, mild gingival trauma such as toothbrushing, chewing hard substances, and subgingival scaling.

Recently, more sophisticated techniques including immunofluorescence, anaerobic culture, and electron microscopy have led to a reconsideration of the idea that bacteria can routinely be identified in gingival tissues in periodontal disease.

Bacteria were first identified by transmission electron microscopy within the gingival tissues and close to resorbing bone surfaces in over half of the cases of advanced human periodontitis. Bacteria-leukocyte interactions on the surface of pocket epithelium, bacteria between junctional epithelial cells and the epithelium lining the lateral wall of pockets, as well as within the connective tissue are also observed (Fig. 28–2). Some of the bacteria observed within the gingival tissues in periodontitis have been identified. Along with the bacterial invasion, alteration in the epithelial basement membrane of the pocket epithelium can be observed with a discontinuous absence of basement membrane antigen. This suggests basement membrane disruption associated with bacterial invasion.

In localized juvenile periodontitis, bacteria, particularly *Actinobacillus actinomycetemcomitans*, have been identified within the gingival connective tissue. The presence of this organism within the tissues appears to make the disease more resistant to treatment and necessitates antibiotic therapy.

EXOTOXINS

Many bacteria produce exotoxins such as *Corynebacterium diphtheriae* and *C. botulinum* which contribute to the pathogenesis of their respective diseases. Production of exotoxins by subgingival bacteria is rare. Those bacteria that produce exotoxins are only transiently found subgingivally at the time of a systemic infection. Exotoxins are therefore not normally considered important in the pathogenesis of periodontal disease. However, one type of exotoxin directed toward human

Table 28–7 ■ Bacterial factors important in evasion of host defenses

Inhibition of PMN
   Leukotoxin
   Chemotaxis inhibitors
   Decreased phagocytosis and
   intracellular killing
   Resistance to C-mediated killing
Lymphocyte alterations
Endotoxicity
IgA, IgG proteases
Fibrinolysin
Superoxide dismutase
Catalase

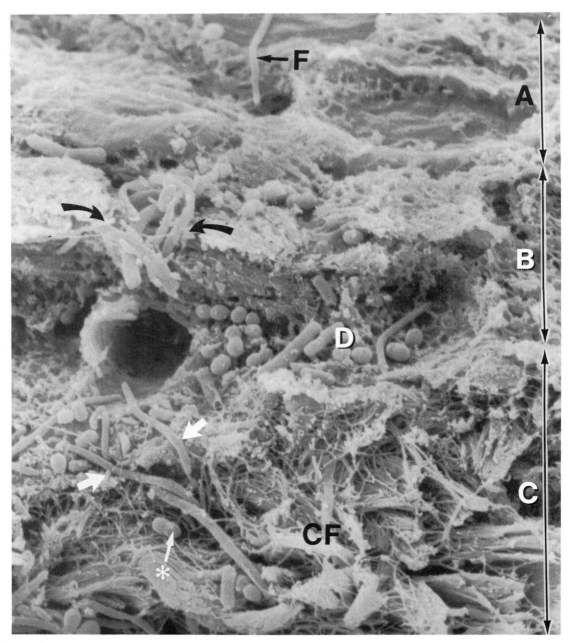

Figure 28–2 ■ Cross-sectional electron micrograph of pocket wall from a patient with advanced periodontitis. View of surface of pocket wall *(A)*, sectioned epithelium *(B)*, and sectioned connective tissue *(C)*. *Curved arrows* point to areas of bacterial penetration into the epithelium. *Thick white arrows* point to bacterial penetration into the connective tissue through a break in the continuity of the basal lamina. F, filamentous organism on surface of epithelium; D, accumulation of bacteria (rods, cocci, filaments) on basal lamina; CF, connective tissue fibers. Asterisk points to coccobacillus in connective tissue. (From Carranza, F. A., Jr.: Glickman's Clinical Periodontology, 6th ed. Philadelphia, W. B. Saunders Co., 1984.)

polymorphonuclear leukocytes is produced by *Actinobacillus actinomycetemcomitans.* This leukotoxin may enable *A. actinomycetemcomitans* to destroy leukocytes in the gingival crevice, which assists the microorganism in its ability to colonize and invade the gingival tissues.

CELL CONSTITUENTS

Cellular constituents of both gram-positive and gram-negative bacteria may also play a role in periodontal disease. These include endotoxins, bacterial surface components, and capsular components.

The predominance of gram-negative bacteria within pockets in periodontal disease leads to high concentrations of endotoxin, a constituent of cell walls of gram-negative bacteria. Endotoxin is a lipopolysaccharide complex commonly shared by all gram-negative bacteria which is released upon cell disintegration. Endotoxins are highly potent, toxic substances affecting tissues directly and through activation of host responses. Important in considering their role in periodontal disease is their ability to (1) produce leukopenia; (2) activate factor XII or Hageman factor, which affects the clotting system, thus leading to intravascular coagulation; (3) activate the complement system by the alternate pathway which begins with C3 activation and bypasses C1, 4, and 2; (4) lead to a localized Shwartzman phenomenon with tissue necrosis following two or more exposures to endotoxin; (5) produce cytotoxic effects on cells such as fibroblasts; and (6) induce bone resorption in organ culture. Endotoxins have been shown to penetrate gingival epithelium. Entrance into the underlying tissue would allow their full pathogenic potential to be manifested.

Both gram-positive and -negative subgingival bacteria produce a variety of toxic end products that are also capable of tissue destruction. These include fatty and organic acids such as butyric and propionic acids, amines, volatile sulfur compounds, indole, ammonia, and glycans.

Peptidoglycan, a cell wall component, affects the host in a variety of ways including complement activation, immunosuppressive activity, stimulation of the reticuloendothelial system, and immunopotentiating properties. Peptidoglycans also appear capable of stimulating bone resorption and stimulating macrophages to produce prostaglandin and collagenases.

Capsular material and slime constituents also are capable of tissue destruction.

ENZYMES

Some of the enzymes produced by oral bacteria such as hyaluronidase are capable of influencing gingival permeability and allowing apical proliferation of the junctional epithelium along the root surfaces.

Hyaluronidase occurs in higher concentrations in periodontal pockets than in normal sulci. In addition, a greater number of isolates from pockets produce hyaluronidase. Experimental studies have demonstrated that topical application of hyaluronidase to gingival epithelium leads to widening of the intercellular spaces and increased permeability. Injection of hyaluronidase into the gingiva causes disruption of gingival connective tissue and apical migration of the gingival epithelium along the cementum, the initial phases of pocket formation.

Disruption of collagen seen in periodontal disease, while mainly a result of release of tissue collagenase, can also result from bacterial collagenase. Black-pigmented *Bacteroides* and some strains of *A. actinomycetemcomitans* produce collagenase.

Other bacterial enzymes produced by suspected periodontal pathogens that potentially cause periodontal destruction include gelatinase, aminopeptidases, phospholipase A, alkaline phosphatase, acid phosphatase, DNase, and RNase. Phospholipase A may initiate alveolar bone resorption as a precursor for prostaglandin. Alkaline and acid phosphatases may also cause alveolar bone loss.

Bacterial factors also help in evasion of host defenses, as previously discussed (Table 28–7). These factors influence both the cellular and humoral responses. Polymorphonuclear leukocytes, for example, are influenced by leukotoxins, chemotactic factors, and inhibitors. Immunoglobulins are inactivated or destroyed by proteases. The combination of direct effects of the bacteria on the periodontal tissues and indirect effects achieved by influencing host responses both influence the response of the periodontium to the periodontal pathogens.

Immunology of Periodontal Disease—General Aspects

Host responses play an important role in the pathogenesis of many types of periodontal diseases (Table 28–8). In the bacterial- or plaque-associated diseases they may contribute to the disease process or modulate the effects of the bacteria. In desquamative gingivitis, they are either the cause or the result of the disease.

In the bacterial-associated periodontal diseases, immune responses may be both beneficial (protective) and detrimental (destructive). Several components of the immune system are active in periodontal disease (Table 28–9). The neutrophils, lymphocytes, plasma cells, and macrophages vary in number depending on the disease status of the tissues. Localized and systemic antibodies to the oral bacteria and complement also are of significance. These functions are thought to influence (1) bacterial colonization, (2) bacterial invasion, (3) tissue destruction, and (4) healing and fibrosis (Table 28–10).

BACTERIAL COLONIZATION

Antibodies to bacteria confer protection in many systemic bacterial diseases. This results from bacterial destruction by lysis or phagocytosis or both. Antibody interactions with bacteria also prevent the initial bacterial attachment or colonization. In periodontal disease, the subgingival area is the major environment of concern. In contrast to supragingival sites where secretory IgA (S-IgA) from saliva can reduce or inhibit specific bacteria within plaque, there is little if any subgingival S-IgA. Subgingivally, the major source for immunoglobulins and complement is gingival or crevicular fluid, which contains systemically and locally produced antibodies. These could potentially modulate the types and numbers of microorganisms through inhibition of colonization or lysis or both. However, in bacterial-associated periodontal disease, there is an "explosion" in the numbers of subgingival bacteria compared with the situation in gingival health. This heavy antigen load in an "external" environment may overwhelm the immune system, distorting or obviating any apparent positive effects.

BACTERIAL INVASION

As indicated earlier, invasion of the tissue occurs by whole bacterial cells and products in bacterial-associated periodontal diseases. In comparison to the large numbers of bacteria within the gingival crevice or pocket, relatively few reach beneath the basal lamina of the epithelium. This reduction probably is a combination of the physical barrier pro-

Table 28–8 ■ Significant immune findings in periodontal diseases

Disease	Finding
ANUG	PMN chemotactic defect
	Elevated antibody titers to *B. intermedius* and intermediate-sized spirochetes
Pregnancy gingivitis	No significant findings reported
Adult periodontitis	Elevated antibody titers to *B. gingivalis* and other periodontopathogens
	Occurrence of immune complexes in tissues
	Immediate hypersensitivity to gingival bacteria
	Cell-mediated immunity to gingival bacteria
Juvenile periodontitis	
LJP	PMN chemotactic defect and depressed phagocytosis
	Elevated antibody levels to *A. actinomycetemcomitans*
GJP	PMN chemotactic defect and depressed phagocytosis
	Elevated antibody levels to *B. gingivalis*
Prepubertal	PMN and monocyte chemotactic defects
Rapid periodontitis	Suppressed or enhanced PMN or monocyte chemotaxis
	Elevated antibody levels to several gram-negative bacteria
Refractory periodontitis	Reduced PMN chemotaxis
Desquamative gingivitis	Diagnostic or characteristic immunopathology in two thirds of cases
	Autoimmune etiology in cases resulting from pemphigus and pemphigoid

Table 28–9 ■ Components of immune system affecting periodontal disease

System	Function
Secretory immune system	Decreases bacterial colonization on surfaces exposed to saliva
Neutrophil, Antibody, Complement	Bacteriocidal
Lymphocyte, Macrophage, Lymphokine	Tissue destruction
Immunoregulatory	Controls immune responses to bacteria

Adapted from Genco and Slots: J. Dent. Res. 63:441, 1984.

vided by the junctional epithelium and the host protective responses. The gingival tissues are bathed with antibodies to the oral bacteria and complement, which could lead to bacterial lysis. In addition, chemotactic factors could lead to polymorphonuclear leukocyte and monocyte infiltration with phagocytosis and lysis.

Recently, the importance of polymorphonuclear leukocytes and macrophages as phagocytes in defense against periodontopathic microorganisms has become evident. Even in clinically normal gingiva, small numbers of neutrophils are seen in the gingival crevice. Increasing numbers of neutrophils infiltrate within and directly below the dentogingival epithelium. Phagocytes are usually chemotactically attracted to invading bacteria where they attach to the bacteria via C3b and other receptors. After phagocytosis, the bacteria are usually lysed. Functional neutrophil or macrophage defects in chemotaxis predispose to periodontal disease. Patients with systemic diseases where there are chemotactic defects frequently have severe periodontitis (Table 28–11). Similarly, several periodontal diseases have characteristic chemotactic defects (Table 28–12).

TISSUE DESTRUCTION

Several bacterial mechanisms could contribute to the pathogenesis of periodontal disease. These include anaphylactic or reagin-dependent reactions, cytotoxic reactions, immune complex or Arthus reactions, and cell-mediated or delayed hypersensitivity reactions. In anaphylactic reactions, IgE produced by plasma cells fixes to or sensitizes mast cells and basophilic leukocytes. Subsequent antigenic exposure leads to antigen-antibody complexes on the cell surface with the degranulation of mast cells and basophils with release of mediators including histamine. Cytotoxic reactions occur when IgG and IgM antibodies react with cell or tissue antigens. Consequent complement activation further contributes to the pathogenesis. In immune complex reactions, microprecipitates of antigen with IgG and IgM antibodies occur in tissues in and around blood vessels. Microcomplexes that form in moderate antigen excess activate the complement system leading to hormonal, vascular, and cytotoxic effects. Associated with the reaction is a leukocytic infiltrate which releases lysozymes causing further tissue damage. Cell-mediated reactions occur when sensitized T lymphocytes react with the sensitizing antigen leading to the lymphocytic release of lymphokines such as osteoclast activating factor (OAF). While host mechanisms leading to tissue destruction could be activated in any of the bacterial-associated periodontal diseases, most research has focused on gingivitis and periodontitis. Details will therefore be considered later in the section on gingivitis and periodontitis.

HEALING AND FIBROSIS

Macrophages influence fibroblast activity. They play a role in healing through their

Table 28–10 ■ Influence of host responses on periodontal disease

Aspect of Disease	Host Factors
Bacterial Colonization	Subgingivally, antibody-C' in crevicular fluid inhibits adherence and coaggregation of bacteria and potentially reduces their numbers by lysis
Bacterial Invasion	Antibody-C' mediated lysis reduces bacterial counts; neutrophils as a consequence of chemotaxis, phagocytosis, and lysis reduces bacterial counts
Tissue Destruction	Antibody-mediated hypersensitivity; cell-mediated immune responses; activation of tissue factors such as collagenase
Healing and Fibrosis	Lymphocytes and macrophage-produced chemotactic factors for fibroblasts; fibroblast-activating factors

Table 28–11 ■ Neutrophil disorders associated with periodontal disease

Diabetes mellitus
Papillon-LeFevre syndrome
Down's syndrome
Chédiak-Higashi syndrome
Drug-induced agranulocytosis
Cyclic neutropenia

release of fibronectin, which is chemotactic for fibroblasts and other factors that influence fibroblast function and lead to fibroblast activation. Lymphocytes also release lymphokines capable of activating and recruiting fibroblasts.

Immunoregulation appears to play a role in periodontal disease. One important immune mediator is interleukin-1 (IL-1), a monokine produced by macrophages, B cells, and squamous epithelial cells. IL-1 release is stimulated from these cells by lipopolysaccharides of periodontal pathogens such as *B. gingivalis*. It influences thymocytes, T cells, B cells, and fibroblasts, as well as other cells. IL-1 induces the proliferation of thymocytes, T cells, B cells, and fibroblasts. It also enhances the production of lymphokines including T-cell growth factor (IL-2) and osteoclast activating factor. Furthermore, IL-1 enhances antibody production by B cells and production of collagenase and prostaglandin by fibroblasts. IL-1 is found in gingival fluid in greater amounts in inflamed sites, suggesting it may play a role in periodontal disease by influencing the host immunologic and inflammatory responses to bacterial antigens and mitogens. Lymphocytes from chronically inflamed gingival tissues have also been shown to be capable of producing IL-2. However, no relationship has been shown between IL-2 and severity of periodontal disease.

The role of bacteria in modulating the immune response and connective tissue function has also been demonstrated. Leukocyte activity can be affected by the subgingival bacteria. Some periodontopathogens chemotactically attract leukocytes, reduce chemo-

Table 28–12 ■ Periodontal diseases with neutrophil disorders

Acute necrotizing ulcerative gingivitis
Localized juvenile periodontitis
Prepubertal periodontitis
Rapid periodontitis
Refractory periodontitis

tactic ability, elaborate leukotoxins, resist phagocytosis, inhibit their own phagocytic killing, and interfere with fibroblast proliferation. For example, lipopolysaccharide from *Bacteroides* species and other gram-negative bacteria activate the complement system by the classical and alternate pathways inducing PMN chemotaxis. However, soluble products of *Bacteroides* can also block receptors on leukocytes, reducing the chemotactic response. A distinguishing difference between pathogenic and less-pathogenic strains on *Bacteroides* is that the pathogenic strains are more resistant to phagocytosis. Resistance to PMN killing appears to derive from capsular material, an unknown mechanism dependent on serum and ability to split PMN-derived hydrogen peroxide and superoxide dismutase.

The humoral response to subgingival bacteria can be nonspecifically altered by the bacterial production of IgG, IgA, IgM, C3, and C5 proteases. Enzymes to some or all of the humoral components are elaborated by black-pigmented *Bacteroides* and *Capnocytophaga*. The *Bacteroides* species completely degrade the immunoglobulins, while *Capnocytophaga* splits the immunoglobulin into Fab and Fc fragments, which may still have some biologic activity. This protease activity may inhibit the local host response, allowing penetration and spread within the tissues.

Subgingival bacteria also affect the humoral immune response by polyclonal B-cell activation. Bacteria nonspecifically induce multiple clones of B lymphocytes to produce immunoglobulins so that B cells stimulated by one microorganism produce antibodies to other microorganisms. The immunoglobulin production by B cells is under the regulatory control of T cells. Extracts of *B. gingivalis*, *B. intermedius*, *B. melaninogenicus*, *F. nucleatum*, *A. actinomycetemcomitans*, *A. viscosus*, *A. naeslundii*, and *C. ochracea* stimulate polyclonal antibody responses and osteoclast-activating factors in cultures of normal human peripheral blood lymphocytes. These bacterial activators may play a role in the pathogenesis of periodontal disease.

Bacterial factors affect lymphocytes and other cellular constituents via suppression, activation, and mitogenicity. A factor from *A. actinomycetemcomitans* selectively activates human T suppressor cells. Sonic extracts of *F. nucleatum* lead to immunosuppression either by altering T-helper cell activity or by direct effects on the effector or responding cell population. *F. nucleatum* also suppresses mitogen activation of peripheral leukocytes. Extracellular polysaccharide from *Capnocytophaga ochracea* exerts immunosuppressive activity through macrophages, possibly with the participation of T-suppressor cells.

Gingival Health

Gingival health is defined clinically and histologically. Clinically, the gingival tissues are usually pale pink, firm, and scalloped with knife-edge margins and stippling on the surface. Histologically, health is characterized by an absence of an inflammatory infiltrate. It is common to observe clinical health when there is histologically a minimal inflammatory infiltrate. Histologic health is usually achieved in "supernormals" in whom there is repeated scaling and root planing as well as heavy emphasis on patient home-care plaque control.

Gingival health usually is maintained when there is a balance between the subgingival microflora and host resistance factors active in the gingival crevice and tissues.

MICROBIOLOGY

The gingival crevice is not sterile but harbors a microbial flora both in health and in disease. During health, the flora is relatively simple and sparse (Tables 28–13 and 28–14). It tends to reflect the bacterial types found in the early stages of plaque formation (see Chapter 26).

In healthy sulci from young adults, gram-positive cocci are the major morphotype and compose almost two thirds of the total flora.

Table 28–13 ■ Predominant subgingival bacteria associated with gingival health

Streptococcus mitis
Streptococcus sanguis
Staphylococcus epidermidis
Rothia dentocariosa
Actinomyces viscosus
Actinomyces naeslundii
Small spirochetes

Filamentous forms, small spirochetes, fusiforms, and motile rods are also identified. In general, gram-negative species and motile forms are considerably less frequent and in smaller numbers. Similar bacterial findings occur in aged subjects with healthy gingival sulci. However, gram-negative bacteria may be slightly more common.

IMMUNOLOGY

Except in "supernormal" individuals where the gingival tissues exhibit maximum health as a result of comprehensive, ideal plaque control and frequent professional cleaning, the gingival tissues are usually infiltrated by chronic inflammatory cells, primarily lymphocytes. Leukocytes are also common within the junctional epithelium and in the gingival crevice. This cellular infiltrate, part of the host defense, is thought to be a direct response to the plaque. In "supernormals," in whom there is essentially no plaque, the cellular infiltrate is absent.

Serum antibodies to the microbial flora also occur. The titers to many oral bacteria are usually low in health, reflecting the minimal antigenic stimulation of plaque via the gin-

Table 28–14 ■ Bacterial types in health, gingivitis, and periodontitis

	Health		Gingivitis		Periodontitis	
	Freq*	Prop*	Freq	Prop	Freq	Prop
Small spirochetes	25%	2%	82%	13%	100%	32%
Medium spirochetes	0	0	41	3	100	8
Large spirochetes	0	0	24	1	38	2
Small motile rods	13	1	12	1	75	7
Large motile rods	6	1	47	2	50	3
Curved motile rods	19	1	71	5	94	16
Filaments	31	4	53	4	63	2
Fusiforms	44	7	94	17	81	9
Small nonmotile rods	69	18	100	38	94	13
Cocci	94	66	92	15	50	4
Other nonmotile rods	5	2	3	2	4	7

*Freq = frequency (percent) of detection in sites by dark-field microscopy; Prop = proportion (mean percent) of dark-field groups per site.

Adapted from Savitt, E. D., and Socransky, S. S.: J. Periodontol. Res. 19:111, 1984.

gival tissues. When antibody titers are higher to some organisms, it is thought to reflect extragingival sites of antigenic stimulation in addition to the gingival tissues.

Specific Diseases

GINGIVITIS AND PERIODONTITIS

Gingivitis, or inflammation of the gingiva, affects virtually the entire population to some degree. It is primarily a response to the bacteria in plaque. The earliest clinical signs of gingivitis are usually color and texture changes accompanied by slight enlargement of the tissues with some loss of firmness and adaptation to the teeth. The tissues often appear red, glossy, and edematous. The disease may remain in this state or, with continued presence of pathogenic plaque bacteria, progress to a loss of attachment of the gingiva to the tooth and the formation of periodontal pockets. This is termed periodontitis. However, it is important to stress that not all gingivitis conditions proceed to periodontitis.

Periodontitis, the major cause of tooth loss in adults, is the usual sequela to untreated gingivitis. It is an extension of the inflammatory process into the periodontal ligament, cementum, and the alveolar bone surrounding the teeth, leading to progressive destruction of these tissues and loss of teeth. The critical "last step" that permits this transition is currently unknown but appears to involve bacteria and host interactions.

When microorganisms accumulate and grow adjacent to the gingiva, they elicit gingival inflammation. Clinically this low-level response may not be apparent, but histologically there is a vascular response consisting of capillary dilation and increased blood flow. Pocket formation starts as an inflammatory change in the connective tissue wall of the gingival sulcus caused by bacteria of the epithelial-associated subgingival plaque (Chapter 26) and may be exacerbated by the presence of subgingival calculus. The resulting cellular and fluid exudate causes further breakdown of the adjacent connective tissue, epithelium, and the gingival fibers. In the early stages of gingivitis, the inflammatory infiltrate is mostly lymphocytic with T cells predominating. In advanced gingivitis and periodontitis, the plasma cells are the most common inflammatory cells. Lymphocytes found in periodontitis are predominantly B

cells. T cells constitute less than 6 percent of the lymphoid population. The helper-to-suppressor T-cell ratio in naturally occurring gingivitis in children and in experimental gingivitis is approximately 2:1. In contrast, the ratio in periodontitis is lower, approximately 1:1. This suggests a local alteration in the immunoregulatory mechanisms. The organisms present in the pocket are capable of synthesizing an array of products that can cause *direct* tissue damage. In some periodontitis lesions, bacteria can be found within the lateral wall of the periodontal pocket, the junctional epithelium, and periodontal ligament (see Fig. 28–2). As a result of the host-bacterial interactions, the periodontal pocket is formed. Once formed, this deepened area provides a specialized "protected" environment for further disease and diminishes the ability of the patient to cleanse the area.

The perpetuation of the periodontal lesion is controlled by both local and systemic factors. The significant feature associated with progressive periodontitis is the continued loss of periodontal ligament and bone support referred to as periodontal attachment loss. Attachment loss, an indication of disease "activity," may occur rapidly and last for days, weeks, or months. Active disease is associated with increased proportions of pathogenic bacteria, changes in the host response and possibly bacterial invasion within the tissues. The exact triggering mechanisms are not known. Periodontal disease is no longer thought to be a continuously progressive disease. Instead, there appears to be bursts of active periodontal destruction followed by periods of slower activity or quiescence. Ultimately, the periods of activity, which are additive, result in irreversible periodontal destruction—periodontitis. This ultimately causes loss of teeth.

Microbiologic Findings

The role of bacteria in the etiology of gingivitis and periodontitis has been well established on the basis of multiple factors.

Epidemiologic studies ■ Numerous epidemiologic studies throughout the world have established that plaque is the primary etiologic factor in both gingivitis and periodontitis. In cross-sectional studies, with increasing plaque scores, there is increasing severity of periodontal disease. In longitudinal studies of several years' duration, poor plaque control leads to increased severity of periodontal disease. In contrast, good plaque control prevents such periodontal breakdown.

Antimicrobial studies ■ Antimicrobial agents including antibiotics, disinfectants, and antiseptics directly affect microorganisms, with minimal effects if any on host tissue. Penicillin, tetracyclines, and other antibiotics, while not usually clinically recommended as the sole means of treatment, significantly reduce gingival inflammation. Antimicrobials such as chlorhexidine in mouthwash are also very effective and are used clinically for control of gingival inflammation.

Oral hygiene studies ■ The classic experimental gingivitis model demonstrates the direct relationship between gingivitis and plaque accumulations. When all forms of plaque control are stopped, plaque rapidly forms and reaches a plateau. Within 7 to 9 days, early gingivitis occurs. When oral hygiene is again instituted and the plaque is removed, the gingivitis disappears within 3 days. Thus, by simply controlling plaque, gingivitis can be induced or eliminated. When plaque is allowed to accumulate for years in dogs rather than for less than a month in humans, periodontitis can also be induced. Along with the development of human experimental gingivitis, three phases are observed in plaque composition (Table 28–15). The initial phase, from 0 to 2 days after ending plaque control, is characterized by a flora of gram-positive cocci. The second phase from 2 to 4 days is one with increased filaments and fusiform bacilli. The third phase from 4 to 9 days when gingivitis is seen is characterized by increased vibrios and spirochetes.

Pathogenicity studies ■ Numerous subgingival bacteria can induce one or more aspects of periodontal disease when orally implanted into germ-free and conventional animals or injected subcutaneously. The pathology observed includes inflammation, destruction of connective tissue, vasculitis, osteoclastic bone resorption, and apical migration of the junctional epithelium. These responses can often be induced by a culture of a single organism such as *A. actinomycetemcomitans*, which leads to rapid bone loss in a germ-free animal within a few months. Selected "mixed cultures" can also induce rapid tissue destruction and periodontitis. However, models of experimental periodontal disease in germ-free animals and soft tissue abscesses must be carefully interpreted and only considered as pathogenic potential. Bacterial interactions in the complex subgingival flora and environmental and host factors in the pocket can either inhibit or stimulate bacterial growth.

The viability of the bacteria appears necessary for such responses. When freshly collected plaque is injected subcutaneously, transmissible, sometimes fulminating, abscesses occur. If the plaque is first autoclaved to prevent bacterial growth, subcutaneous injection only induces a mild inflammatory response.

Scaling and root planing experience ■ Clinical experience and studies have demonstrated the efficacy of scaling and root planing in periodontal therapy. Thorough removal of the bacterial deposits quickly and effectively reduces gingival inflammation. This coupled with plaque control at home can completely reverse gingivitis to the healthy state. A similar approach in patients partially reverses the pathology.

With the accumulation of plaque and development of gingivitis, there is both a quantitative and a qualitative change in plaque. There is a shift in the flora from gram-positive cocci seen in health to a condition characterized by increased numbers of filamentous bacteria, gram-negative rods, and spirochetes (see Table 28–13). In the earlier stages of gingivitis, *Actinomyces* species are common. In longstanding gingivitis, gram-negative bacteria including *Veillonella* and *Fusobacteria* increase until they constitute approximately 25 percent of the flora.

In periodontitis, there is a continued change in the flora to one increasingly characterized by gram-negative, anaerobic rods (see Table 28–13). The flora is much more varied and complex than seen in health or gingivitis.

Recent studies have demonstrated qualitative differences in the subgingival flora in "active" sites, defined on the basis of recent

Table 28–15 ■ Phases associated with experimental gingivits

Phase	Time Period	Characteristic Bacterial Flora
1	0–2 days	Predominantly gram-positive cocci
2	2–4 days	Increased filaments and fusiform bacilli
3	4–9 days	Increased vibrios and spirochetes

loss of alveolar bone or attachment, compared with "inactive" sites, with no recent bone or attachment loss. Active sites usually have elevated numbers of *B. gingivalis*, *B. intermedius*, *A. actinomycetemcomitans*, "fusiform" *Bacteroides*, *Wolinella recta*, and small spirochetes. Conversely, successfully treated sites have small numbers of *B. gingivalis*, *B. intermedius*, and *A. actinomycetemcomitans*.

Immunologic Findings

The continued exposure to bacterial antigens in the gingival crevice and within the gingival tissues induces systemic and local host responses. In gingivitis and adult-onset periodontitis, these immune responses have both protective and destructive functions (Fig. 28–3). The mechanisms summarized in this figure are potentially active in periodontitis. Their relative importance may vary from patient to patient and from site to site.

Protection ■ There is little evidence to demonstrate a significant protective immune function, since plaque accumulation inevitably leads to gingivitis. However, crevicular fluid contains immunoglobulins and complement, which constantly bathe the subgingival bacteria. Antibodies in the crevicular fluid are reactive with some of the bacteria and also bind to the subgingival bacteria in vivo along with complement. This reactivity may modulate or alter the composition of the subgingival microflora. The bacterial masses could be reduced via antibody-antigen reactions with complement activation leading to bacterial cytolysis and phagocytosis. The important role of the neutrophil in control of the periodontopathogens is evident in systemic diseases with reduced neutrophil function where there usually is severe periodontal disease.

Humoral responses ■ The importance of B-cell responses in the pathogenesis of peri-

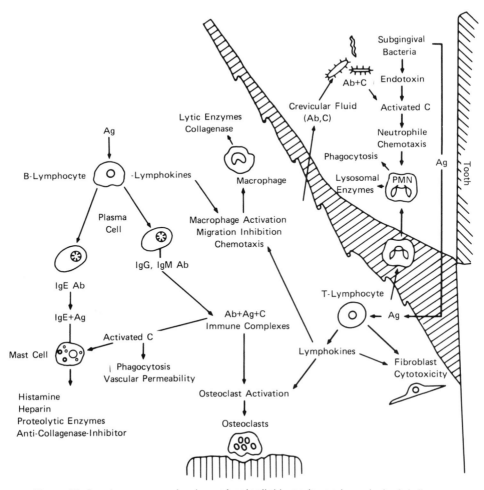

Figure 28–3 ■ Immune mechanisms of potential importance in periodontal disease.

odontal disease has been demonstrated experimentally in athymic rats devoid of T cells. Athymic rats with predominantly B cells in their gingival tissues show increased bone loss. In contrast, when T cells predominate in athymic rats reconstituted by injection of T cells, or in normal animals, there is less bone loss. Progressive periodontal disease, therefore, appears to be associated with B-cell lesions.

The immunopathology of gingivitis and periodontitis indicates that the gingival tissues contain the necessary elements for humoral responses. IgG-, IgA-, IgM-, and IgE-containing plasma cells are found in the inflammatory infiltrate where IgG and IgM predominate.

It is clear that local and systemic antibody responses to the crevicular microflora commonly occur. Early animal experiments demonstrated that when antigenic stimulation is minimal, there is only a local plasma cell infiltration and antibody response at the site of injection. Higher antigen levels induce both a local and a systemic response.

As a measure of local antibody response, crevicular fluid and supernates from gingival explants have been assayed for antibody levels and compared with serum antibody levels. Frequently, higher levels of antibodies to periodontopathogens occurred locally, suggesting local antibody production in response to local challenge. Local production of antibodies to *A. actinomycetemcomitans, B. gingivalis, F. nucleatum,* and *Wolinella recta* has been demonstrated. Indirect evidence for a local antibody response is further provided by the finding that many subgingival bacteria are "coated" in vivo with immunoglobulins and complement.

Because of the ease of assay, systemic serum responses to oral bacteria have been extensively studied. Levels of serum antibodies to some organisms are uniformly high, while to other organisms they are uniformly low, regardless of periodontal status. Antibody levels to most periodontopathogens are usually high, often correlating with the severity or type of periodontal disease, and are relative to the bacterial numbers. For example, patients with adult periodontitis usually have high numbers of *B. gingivalis* and significantly elevated antibody levels to this organism compared with subjects with healthy gingiva. Similarly, higher antibody levels also occur in periodontitis patients to *Capnocytophaga ochracea,* other gram-negative anaerobic bacteria, *A. naeslundii, Fusobacter-*

ium, and *Leptotrichia buccalis,* which often occur in high numbers.

Dental treatment such as scaling and root planing commonly elicits a humoral response to some but not all the subgingival bacteria. The serum antibody response generally peaks 2 to 4 months after scaling and root planing and gradually decreases to the pre-scaling level within 8 to 12 months. After scaling and root planing, elevated antibody levels occur to black-pigmented *Bacteroides* including *B. gingivalis* and *B. intermedius,* as well as *Eikenella corrodens, Campylobacter concisus,* and *A. actinomycetemcomitans.* It has been suggested that this elevated humoral response may play a role in the success of therapy.

Many responses to antigen-antibody interactions are complement dependent. Complement activation is important in bacterial lysis, phagocytosis, bone resorption, chemotaxis, and other biologically significant events. Thoroughly washed gingival tissues from patients with periodontitis reveal significantly reduced complement within the tissues, compared with unwashed samples, suggesting that most of the complement represents extravasated serum rather than immune precipitates. The small amount of C3 and C4 remaining after washing is frequently located in foci, suggesting that while most complement is soluble, small amounts may be tissue bound in immune complexes. Quantitative studies of gingival fluid from periodontitis patients demonstrate significantly reduced C3 levels and marked depression of C4 in comparison to serum. This may indicate complement activation by the classical pathway; however, the role of the complement system is not well established.

The immunopathology of periodontal disease may result from anaphylactic reactions, cytotoxic reaction, immune complex reactions, and cell-mediated reactions playing a role in the pathogenesis.

Anaphylactic reactions ■ Anaphylactic or immediate hypersensitivity reactions occur when IgE fixed to mast cells or basophils reacts with antigens and leads to the release of histamine and other mediators. The necessary components for such reactions are all associated with periodontitis.

IgE-containing plasma cells occur in the gingival tissues, though in fewer numbers than IgG-, IgA-, and IgM-containing cells. Mast cell numbers increase from gingival health to moderate periodontitis and then decrease in advanced periodontitis. It has been suggested that the decrease is a result of anaphylactic reactions leading to the degranulation of mast cells. Histamine levels in chronically inflamed gingivae are significantly higher than in normal tissues, and in vitro challenge of inflamed gingival tissues with anti-IgE leads to histamine release, suggesting IgE is already fixed to gingival mast cells.

The traditional method of identifying immediate hypersensitivity with skin tests has been applied to studies of periodontal disease. Intradermal skin tests with extracts of *Actinomyces* have revealed immediate and, less commonly, delayed reactions in humans. There is a significant correlation between the incidence of immediate hypersensitivity to this organism and severity of periodontal disease. The greatest incidence occurs in periodontitis. Similar immediate skin test responses have been demonstrated to *Bacterionema matruchotii*, *Bacteroides melaninogenicus*, and *Fusobacterium nucleatum*.

Repetitive challenge of the gingival tissues to induce immediate hypersensitivity reactions in monkeys experimentally evokes an inflammatory response. It is characterized by a chronic inflammatory infiltrate of plasma cells and lymphocytes along with connective tissue breakdown. Osteoclastic bone loss is not apparent.

The role of anaphylactic reactions in the pathogenesis of gingivitis and periodontitis has not been definitively shown. While the potential for this mechanism exists, it is not thought to be a major factor, because of the small numbers of IgE-containing cells in the gingival tissues.

Cytotoxic reactions ■ Cytotoxic reactions occur when antibodies react with cell or tissue antigens, activating complement. The antigens can be either host cell constituents or bacterial antigens attached to host cells via receptor sites. An example of cytotoxic reactions is humoral autoimmune disease. There is no evidence, however, for considering cytotoxic reactions in the pathogenesis of gingivitis and periodontitis.

Immune complex reactions ■ Immune complex or Arthus reactions occur when antigen forms microprecipitates with IgG or IgM antibodies, or both, in or around blood vessels in tissues. Microcomplexes in moderate antigen excess activate the complement system, leading to hormonal, vascular, and cytotoxic reactions depending on where the complexes lodge.

The elements for immune complex disease are present in the gingival tissues: bacterial antigen, antibodies to the bacteria, and complement activation. The constant shower of bacterial antigens within inflamed gingival tissues, as seen by bacteremias resulting from gingival manipulation and by bacterial invasion, serves to both sensitize and subsequently challenge the host. These bacterial antigens encounter tissue fluids containing bacterial antibodies, permitting immune complex formation. Recent studies with the Raji cell assay have shown immune complexes commonly occur in soluble extracts of human gingival tissue from patients with periodontitis.

Experimental Arthus reactions in monkey gingivae are similar to those found in human periodontitis. Repetitive reactions lead to chronic inflammatory infiltrates of macrophages, lymphocytes, and plasma cells. Accompanying this is collagen breakdown and osteoclastic bone loss.

Cell-mediated reactions ■ Cell-mediated reactions or delayed hypersensitivity are dependent on T lymphocytes and the release of lymphokines. Numerous studies have demonstrated that peripheral leukocytes from patients with periodontitis blast or proliferate in response to some oral bacteria.

There are three basic types of responses. One pattern is characterized by a low blastogenic response in normal, healthy persons and a uniformly strong blastogenic response in gingivitis and periodontitis, which does not discriminate between the severity of disease. An example is the response to *Actinomyces* antigens. The second pattern is characterized by infrequent blastogenic response upon stimulation, which does not relate to disease severity. This pattern occurs with *Streptococcus sanguis* and *Eikinella corrodens*. The third pattern is one in which blastogenic responses are significantly greater in patients with destructive periodontitis than in individuals with healthy gums or gingivitis. Such responses occur in association with *B. gingivalis* and *Treponema denticola*. This last pattern suggests that patients with periodontitis are specifically immune to these organisms as a result of the periodontal infection.

The lymphoproliferative response in the gingival tissues is thought to release potent lymphokines including osteoclast-activating factor (OAF). Gingival lymphocytes isolated from nondiseased gingiva produce low levels of the lymphokines including chemotactic factor, leukocyte migration inhibition factor, and mitogenic factor in response to plaque and specific plaque bacteria. In contrast, lymphocytes from gingivitis and periodontitis tissues produce more lymphokines upon challenge with plaque and specific plaque bacteria suggesting the lymphocytes are sensitized to the bacterial antigens.

Experimental induction of cell-mediated immunity in the periodontium of monkeys is characterized by massive tissue destruction including marked bone loss, reduced fibroblasts, and collagen breakdown. It has been suggested that the bone loss in cell-mediated immune responses results directly from T-cell effects or enhanced B-cell activation.

Experimental depression of cell-mediated immunity with antithymocyte globulin, however, does not influence development of gingivitis or alter existing gingivitis. In addition, patients receiving immunosuppressive therapy, such as transplant patients, have been evaluated for periodontal status. Most longitudinal studies indicate there is no difference in the rate of periodontitis between immunosuppressed patients and normal controls.

The contribution of cell-mediated immunity to the immunopathology of gingivitis and periodontitis is unknown; however, with the relatively low numbers of T cells in the tissue, it is not thought to be a major contributor.

PREGNANCY GINGIVITIS AND HORMONALLY RELATED GINGIVITIS

An increased incidence of gingivitis sometimes occurs during pregnancy, puberty, menstruation, postmenopause, and oral contraceptive use.

Clinical Findings

In pregnancy gingivitis, there is erythema, edema, and increased gingival bleeding when a patient brushes and flosses or a dentist probes. The inflammation is a heightened or exacerbated response to plaque during periods of progesterone and estrogen imbalance. The degree of inflammation peaks in the second trimester and decreases following parturition. When there is no plaque-associated gingivitis prior to pregnancy and plaque control is maintained, the gingivitis does not develop. As a consequence, preventive measures are directed toward meticulous plaque control.

During puberty, menstruation, and oral contraceptive use, gingival inflammation is a hyper-response to plaque, just as occurs during pregnancy. Postmenopausal women sometimes exhibit shiny, red gingivae that can be irritated by spicy food.

Microbiologic Findings

Bacteriologically, during pregnancy, the changes in hormone levels influence the composition of the plaque. There is a shift toward a greater percentage of anaerobic bacteria, particularly *Bacteroides intermedius*. It appears that *B. intermedius* can substitute progesterone or estradiol for vitamin K as a growth factor. Steroid hormones occur in crevicular fluid and may parallel serum concentrations which dramatically change during pregnancy, puberty, and menstruation, and after menopause.

Immunologic Findings

Changes in the immune responses to the oral flora during pregnancy have not been evaluated.

PERIODONTITIS IN JUVENILE DIABETICS

Clinical Findings

Patients with insulin-dependent diabetes mellitus (IDDM), or juvenile diabetes, frequently have more severe periodontal disease than the general population. This is related to the degree of metabolic control and plaque factors. Periodontitis begins near puberty with a prevalence of 9.8 percent in 13- to 18-year-old diabetics and increases to 39 percent in IDDM patients 19 years of age or older. IDDM patients may have more severe bone loss. Also, patients with uncontrolled or undiagnosed diabetes who have periodontitis often have multiple periodontal abscesses.

Microbiologic Findings

In IDDM associated gingivitis, the predominant cultivable organisms include *Actinomyces* (33 percent), streptococci (36 percent), *Veillonella parvula* (12 percent), and *Fusobacterium* (10 percent).

The predominant cultivable flora in IDDM-associated periodontitis includes *Capnocytophaga* and anaerobic vibrios averaging 24 percent and 13 percent of the cultivable flora respectively. This pattern differs from adult periodontitis, in which *B. gingivalis* frequently predominates and localized juvenile periodontitis (LJP), in which *A. actinomycetemcomitans* usually predominates.

Immunologic Findings

As in other aggressive forms of periodontal disease, IDDM diabetics frequently have a leukocyte chemotactic defect (Table 28–10). This deficiency is thought to contribute directly to the pathogenesis of the disease.

PERIODONTAL ABSCESSES

Clinical Findings

Periodontal abscesses occur in patients with pre-existing periodontitis. This acute infection occurs in the walls of periodontal pockets as a result of the invasion of bacteria into the periodontal tissues. While abscesses usually spontaneously occur in patients with untreated periodontitis, it is more common in periodontitis patients with a systemic disease such as diabetes, in which there is a reduced ability to combat infections. In some cases an abscess can even occur within a few days after a dental cleaning as a result of mechanical disruption of junctional epithelium, allowing the bacteria to gain entrance into the tissues.

Microbiologic Findings

Early animal studies demonstrated that fulminating, transferrable abscesses could be induced by subcutaneous injections of plaque. A limited number of bacteria were necessary for this and the abscesses were termed "mixed anaerobic infections." *Bacteroides* species, probably *B. gingivalis*, were necessary constituents.

Cultural examination of human abscesses reveal a similar microbiota with gram-negative anaerobic rods predominating. *B. gingivalis*, *Fusobacterium* species, *Capnocytophaga*, and *Vibrio* species were the most common gram-negative isolates, making up over 30 percent of the total cultivable microbiota.

LOCALIZED JUVENILE PERIODONTITIS (LJP)

Clinical Findings

LJP occurs in patients approximately 12 to 20 years of age. Clinically, there is usually little gingival inflammation and minimal supragingival plaque. The hallmark of the disease is marked, localized, alveolar bone loss involving the permanent first molars and often the incisors. The bone loss is so discrete that the distal aspect of a second bicuspid may have no bone loss while the adjacent mesial aspect of a first molar can have several millimeters of loss (Fig. 28–4). LJP has a genetic component in that there is a familial inheritance and it is more common in females. The incidence of this disease has been estimated to be approximately 0.1 percent of the United States population, although in certain groups it has been found in up to 10 percent of the population. Prior to recognition of the bacterial factors, the affected teeth were usually extracted. Now the prognosis is greatly improved by scaling, root planing, surgery, and antibiotic therapy.

Microbiologic Findings

Early anaerobic cultural studies of first molar sites exhibiting localized bone loss in LJP patients characterized a unique bacterial flora consisting of gram-negative anaerobic rods. These organisms were less frequently isolated and in significantly lower numbers in healthy subgingival sites in LJP patients and their non-LJP siblings or other adolescents. These organisms have been identified as *Actinobacillus (Haemophilus) actinomycetemcomitans* (Table 28–3, see also Chapter 17).

A. actinomycetemcomitans has been implicated in the etiology of LJP as a result of several factors:

1. The prevalence and the humoral immune response to this organism are elevated in patients with LJP. *A. actinomycetemcomitans* has been isolated in up to 97 percent of LJP patients, compared with 21 percent of adult periodontitis patients and 17 percent of healthy individuals. Not only is the prevalence of this organism six times greater in LJP than in health, but their proportion of the cultivable subgingival flora is also elevated. Among the three serotypes, serotype B is the most common, followed by serotype A.

2. The incidence of *A. actinomycetemcomitans* is greater in younger LJP patients than in older LJP patients. If the age is considered representative of the duration of the disease, the younger patients had destructive disease within a short period. This suggests that this organism correlates with disease activity.

3. Large numbers of *A. actinomycetemcomi-*

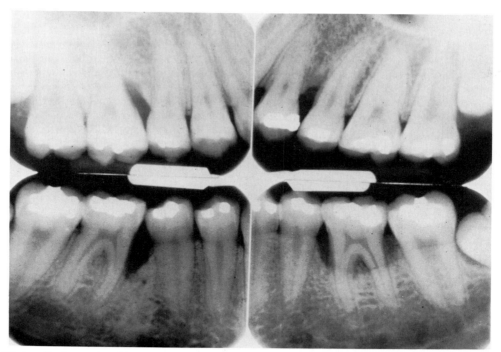

Figure 28–4 ■ Radiographs of teenage female patient with localized juvenile periodontitis. Alveolar bone loss is typically localized to the first molars or incisors or both.

tans occur in lesions in LJP patients but are absent or found in small numbers in healthy sites.

4. *A. actinomycetemcomitans* can be identified by electron microscopy and immunofluorescence, and can be cultured from the gingival connective tissues of LJP lesions.

5. The organism is quite virulent, producing a leukotoxin, collagenase, phosphatases, and bone-resorbing factors, as well as other factors important in evasion of host defenses and destruction of periodontal tissues.

6. There is a positive correlation between the elimination of this organism from the subgingival flora and the successful clinical treatment of LJP.

The source of *A. actinomycetemcomitans* in LJP has not been well studied. It is known that early bacterial colonizers are derived maternally and from other family members. An intrafamily transmission of *A. actinomycetemcomitans* is also suggested by observations that the same biotype and serotype of *A. actinomycetemcomitans* can be isolated in family members of LJP patients, though in smaller numbers. This may explain the apparent familial tendency for this disease. It appears that the transmissibility of this organism is difficult and probably requires ex-

tended exposure. Periodontal probes contaminated with *A. actinomycetemcomitans* from LJP lesions during routine examinations can transfer the organism from infected to healthy, noninfected sulci. However, the organism does not permanently colonize the healthy sites and is eliminated within a matter of weeks.

It has been suggested that development of LJP is dependent on both bacterial and host factors. An explanation for primary involvement of first molars and incisors is not clear. The time of eruption of these teeth, coupled with hormonal factors, host immune factors, and colonization by this organism, are all believed to play a role.

Prior to recognizing the role of *A. actinomycetemcomitans* in LJP, there was usually a poor response to periodontal therapy. Home care procedures for plaque control, scaling and root planing followed by surgery for pocket elimination which usually were successful in treating adult periodontitis rarely achieved beneficial results in LJP. It is now understood that this organism cannot be eradicated by mechanical methods alone, as it occurs not only in the pocket but also within the gingival tissues. This intragingival location allows rapid repopulation of the pocket. Thus, clinical studies suggest that the best therapeutic approach is a combination of surgery to eliminate the pocket and antibiotic therapy to suppress the organism. The antibiotic of choice is tetracycline (250 mg qid for 3 weeks). Tetracycline can suppress *A. actinomycetemcomitans* for periods of 6 to 18 months.

Immunologic Findings

Studies of LJP were the first to demonstrate the importance of neutrophils in periodontal disease. Approximately 75 percent of patients with LJP exhibit a polymorphonuclear neutrophil chemotactic defect and depressed phagocytosis in peripheral blood. The chemotactic defect is a cellular abnormality that is not associated with serum factors or neutrophil ability for random migration, deformation, or adherence. The demonstration of reduced receptor sites for chemotactic peptides and C5a in patients with LJP further points to a genetic factor in this disease. In addition to altered systemic neutrophil function, neutrophil migration into the gingival crevice is slower in response to in vivo casein challenge than in healthy individuals. The gingival crevicular neutrophils also appear to have grossly altered morphology and diminished phagocytosis. It is not clear if this altered phagocytosis is inherent or reflects blockage of C3 receptors by surface C3 or they already contain a high amount of previously phagocytosed material.

The role of the neutrophil chemotactic defect in LJP has been clarified by studying families of patients with LJP. In many cases, brothers and sisters of patients with LJP may also exhibit a chemotactic defect without clinical signs of LJP. This has led to the conclusion that the chemotactic defect is a predisposing factor in LJP. The failure in neutrophil chemotactic responsiveness diminishes the host's ability to ward off the effects of periodontopathogens associated with LJP. Coupled with the chemotactic defect, the leukotoxin produced by *A. actinomycetemcomitans* which destroys the reduced numbers of neutrophils that are chemotactically attracted into the gingiva further complicates the situation.

Associated with the high numbers of *A. actinomycetemcomitans* in LJP, the serum, crevicular fluid, and saliva from LJP patients have elevated antibody levels to this organism. Nearly 60 to 90 percent of patients have serum IgG antibodies and to a lesser extent

IgM, IgA, and IgE antibodies. While the antibody levels in serum and crevicular fluid are usually similar, crevicular fluid antibody levels may exceed serum levels during periods of ongoing attachment loss. This suggests local antibody production within the gingival tissues. As expected, scaling patients with *A. actinomycetemcomitans* introduces bacterial antigens into tissues, leading to a hyperimmune response. Within 2 to 3 months after scaling, IgG serum and salivary antibodies increase.

Capnocytophaga species are also common inhabitants of the subgingival flora in LJP. In contrast to the immune response to *A. actinomycetemcomitans*, the level of antibodies to this organism is low, possibly because of suppressor cell activation or tolerance to the *Capnocytophaga* antigens.

GENERALIZED JUVENILE PERIODONTITIS (GJP)

Clinical Findings

Patients with GJP have clinical findings similar to those of patients with LJP, except that in GJP the bone loss is generalized rather than localized.

Microbiologic Findings

The predominant cultivable microorganisms in GJP differ from those in LJP. *B. gingivalis* is the most common isolate, constituting 13 to 20 percent of the total cell counts. Other common isolates include *Eikenella corrodens*, *B. intermedius*, *Capnocytophaga*, and *Neisseria*. In contrast to LJP, *A. actinomycetemcomitans* is present only in low numbers.

Immunologic Findings

Similar to LJP patients, GJP patients frequently have a neutrophil chemotactic defect and reduced phagocytosis. The chemotactic defect is cellular in nature but the neutrophils have normal random migration and oxidative metabolic activity. While the incidence of chemotactic defects is similar but somewhat less in GJP than in LJP, GJP patients are less likely to exhibit decreased phagocytosis. Twenty-nine percent of GJP patients and 62 percent of LJP patients have decreased phagocytosis, compared with healthy control subjects.

Reflecting the high incidence and numbers of *B. gingivalis* in GJP, patients exhibit high IgG antibody titers to this organism. Approximately two thirds of GJP patients have elevated antibody levels. Antibodies to *A. actinomycetemcomitans* are less frequent in GJP than in LJP, with low titers to serotypes A and B and unexpectedly high titers to serotype C, approximating levels in LJP patients.

RAPID PERIODONTITIS

Clinical Findings

Rapid periodontitis, sometimes termed rapidly progressive periodontitis or early-onset periodontitis, is a rare form of periodontitis. Frequently, patients have a history of LJP. This disease is clinically similar to adult-onset periodontitis but occurs in a younger age group, usually from postpubertal to 35 years of age. During the active phase, patients exhibit severe alveolar bone loss, and gingival bleeding with acutely inflamed, proliferative gingival tissue (Fig. 28–5). The disease may become inactive with no signs of clinical inflammation in spite of severe bone loss as a result of spontaneous regression or therapy. Treatment usually consists of thorough scaling and root planing, surgery, and antibiotic therapy.

Microbiologic Findings

Limited microbiologic examination has been performed on the subgingival flora in pockets from patients with rapid periodontitis. *Bacteroides gingivalis*, *B. intermedius*, and spirochetes—particularly small spirochetes—are major subgingival components in this disease.

Immunologic Findings

The majority of patients with rapid periodontitis have functional defects in either neutrophils or monocytes. This manifests as either a suppression or an enhancement of chemotaxis. Neutrophils and, to a lesser extent, monocytes may play a role in the adverse response to the associated microflora.

While the exact significance of antibodies to oral bacteria is not known, elevated antibody titers occur to *B. gingivalis*, *A. actinomycetemcomitans*, *C. sputigena*, *W. recta*, *Eubac-*

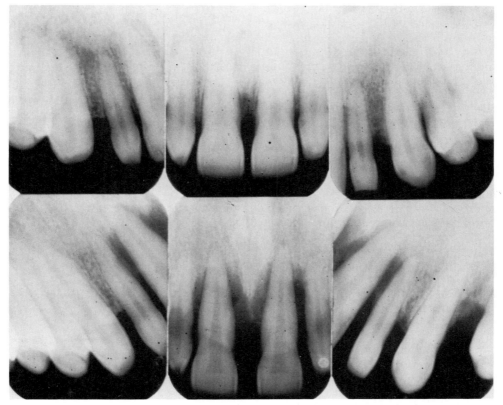

Figure 28–5 ■ Radiographs from a male patient 40 years of age with rapid periodontitis. The lower set of three radiographs taken 15 months after the upper set demonstrate rapid progressive bone loss.

terium brachy, Fusobacterium nucleatum, and *Peptostreptococcus micros.*

PREPUBERTY PERIODONTITIS

Clinical Findings

Prepuberty periodontitis, a rare form of periodontal disease, occurs during or immediately after the eruption of the primary teeth. In addition to bacterial and immunologic factors, there appears to be a genetic component, since family members may have the disease and females are more commonly involved than males. There are generalized and localized forms of the disease.

In the generalized form, the gingiva is intensely red, often with proliferation and cleft formation. Accompanying this is very rapid destruction of alveolar bone and, in some cases, root resorption. While all the deciduous teeth are usually involved, the permanent teeth may not be affected. These children frequently have skin and upper respiratory infections as well as otitis media (middle ear infections). Because only a few cases have been well characterized, treatment is not adequately documented. It appears that the generalized form of the disease is resistant to antibiotic treatment.

In the localized form, a limited number of teeth are involved with minimal gingival inflammation. Frequent systemic infections are not common, as they are in patients with the generalized form. Although reports on treatment are scanty, curettage with antibiotic therapy appears beneficial.

Microbiologic Findings

The microflora seen in prepubertal periodontitis differs from that seen in juvenile periodontitis and rapid periodontitis. Species of *Fusobacterium, Selenomonas, Wolinella, Bacteroides,* and *Capnocytophaga* are frequently found in prepubertal periodontitis, while *A. actinomycetemcomitans, Haemophilus aphrophilus,* and *Bacteroides gingivalis* are infrequent subgingival inhabitants.

Immunologic Findings

Generalized form ■ Although the peripheral white cell counts are elevated, these patients suffer from pronounced depression in neutrophil and monocyte chemotaxis and ability to adhere to surfaces. Whereas gingi-

val biopsies from adult periodontitis usually reveal inflammation including extravascular leukocytes, leukocytes are rare in patients with generalized prepubertal periodontitis. It is thought that these functional defects play a role in the pathogenesis of this disease.

Localized form ■ In comparison to the generalized form, defects in neutrophil and monocyte function in the localized form are less frequent, less severe, and do not occur simultaneously.

REFRACTORY PERIODONTITIS

Clinical Findings

For many years it has been obvious that periodontitis could not always be successfully treated. A small number of patients suffer continued periodontal breakdown. This is called refractory periodontitis, as the disease does not respond to current conventional therapy. It is assumed that this breakdown is a response to poorly understood bacterial factors or host factors, or both. Some clinicians have observed that patients receiving long-term antibiotic therapy (such as tetracycline for months to years) do not experience continued breakdown.

Bacterial Findings

Several microorganisms commonly are isolated from refractory periodontitis pockets. In active sites, these include *B. forsythus, B. gingivalis, W. recta,* and *B. intermedius.* Inactive sites are characterized by increased numbers of aerobic bacteria, including *S. sanguis* and *Actinomyces.* The numbers of *S. sanguis* also increase in treated pockets.

Immunologic Findings

Refractory periodontitis appears to have a reduced neutrophil chemotaxis. This has not been well studied.

ACUTE NECROTIZING ULCERATIVE GINGIVITIS (ANUG)

Clinical Findings

ANUG is a disease with rapid onset characterized by painful, necrotic, ulcerative gingival lesions. In most cases, particularly during the early stages, the lesions are limited to the tips of the gingival papillae. Occasionally in longstanding disease, the necrotic ulcerative lesions may extend into the attached gingiva and alveolar mucosa. Patients with ANUG frequently have associated physiologic stress or psychologic stress, or both. Two stereotypical candidates for ANUG are military personnel under battle conditions (leading to an early name for the disease of "trench mouth") and college students studying for examination. Patients with ANUG often have a history of lack of sleep, poor eating patterns, and failure in plaque control. The stress in ANUG patients leads to elevated serum cortisol levels.

Treatment is focused on reinstitution of proper plaque control procedures and debridement, usually with ultrasonic instrumentation, to remove the necrotic tissue and reduce the bacterial counts. If there is systemic involvement, such as fever, antibiotics may be prescribed. Several follow-up appointments are necessary for thorough scaling and root planing and to assess whether there are residual soft tissue craters that would necessitate periodontal surgery.

Bacterial Findings

There is ample evidence to demonstrate that bacteria play an important role in the pathogenesis of ANUG. While rarely recommended for treatment, antibiotics such as penicillin lead to almost complete healing within a matter of days.

Early observations of smears from ANUG patients suggested that ANUG was caused by an intermediate-sized spirochete called *Borrelia vincentii* and fusiform bacilli. Ultrastructural classification of spirochetes by Listgarten (1965) indicated that this spirochete was found only superficially rather than within the lesion.

The principal bacteria now found to be associated with ANUG are *Bacteroides intermedius* and an unnamed intermediate-sized spirochete. *B. intermedius* constitutes a significant part of the microflora in ANUG, making up 8 to 15 percent of the total cell counts.

Ultrastructurally, the disease is characterized by four major zones extending from the surface to the depths of the lesions:

1. *Bacterial Zone*—This is the most superficial zone and contains small, intermediate-sized, and large spirochetes, as well as other bacteria.

2. *Neutrophil-Rich Zone*—This zone contains numerous spirochetes and rod-shaped bacteria interspersed between neutrophils.

3. *Necrotic Zone*—In addition to necrotic tissue, there are numerous spirochetes and rod-shaped bacteria in this zone.

4. *Zone of Spirochetal Infiltration*—In this deepest area, intermediate-sized and large spirochetes are located between areas of normal collagen fibrils. The intermediate-sized spirochetes in this zone, however, are not *Borrelia vincentii.*

Although the roles of the microorganisms in the pathogenesis are not fully understood, both direct bacterial effects and indirect host responses may be important. Along with the direct invasion of the gingival tissues, the bacterial counts and associated endotoxin concentrations may be important. The host responses are considered subsequently.

Immunologic Findings

In ANUG, both the cellular and humoral responses are affected. Sera collected from patients within a few days after onset of ANUG (acute phase) have elevated IgG and IgM antibody titers to intermediate-sized oral spirochetes and elevated IgG titers to *B. intermedius.* These elevated titers suggest that these organisms proliferated weeks to months before the development of the lesions and indicate that they are pathogenically significant agents. The significance of the elevated bacterial antibody titers in the pathogenesis of ANUG is unknown. The histopathology, the large numbers of bacteria within the tissues, and the elevated levels of antibodies suggest the possibility of an immune complex type of disease. However, further studies are necessary.

Cellularly, patients with ANUG have reduced PMN chemotaxis and phagocytosis. Although not proven, such dysfunction could play a role in the pathogenesis of ANUG. Whether the leukocyte dysfunction results from the bacterial infection in ANUG or develops first, thus allowing the "explosion" in the bacterial flora to occur, is unknown.

DESQUAMATIVE GINGIVITIS

Desquamative gingivitis is a chronic gingival disease characterized by erythematous, erosive, vesiculobullous, and/or desquamative lesions of the free and attached gingivae. Instead of a single etiology, it is a clinical manifestation of several disease processes, as summarized in Table 28–16. Because of the

Table 28-16 ■ Diseases associated with desquamative gingivitis

I. Dermatoses (75.4%)
  Cicatricial pemphigoid
  Lichen planus
  Pemphigus
  Psoriasis
  Bullous pemphigoid
  Epidermolysis bullosa acquisita
  Contact stomatitis
II. Endocrine imbalance
  Estrogen deficiencies following oophorectomy and in postmenopausal women
  Testosterone imbalance
  Hypothyroidism
III. Aging
IV. Abnormal response to bacterial plaque
V. Idiopathic
VI. Chronic infections
  Tuberculosis
  Chronic candidiasis
  Histoplasmosis

multiple etiologies, desquamative gingivitis may be better called desquamative gingival lesions. The majority of cases or approximately 75 percent are dermatologic diseases. Among the total cases, approximately 49 percent are cicatricial pemphigoid, 24 percent are lichen planus, 2 percent are pemphigus, and 1 percent are psoriasis. Among the dermatologic diseases, pemphigus and pemphigoid are autoimmune diseases, psoriasis has characteristics of an autoimmune disease, and lichen planus with an unknown etiology has characteristic immunopathology (Table 28-17).

Clinically, most desquamative gingival lesions occur in middle-aged females. Half the time, lesions are localized solely to the gingivae and in the others, lesions concurrently involved other intraoral and extraoral sites including the buccal mucosa, palate, tongue, lips, skin, and the conjunctiva of the eye.

Table 28-17 ■ Immunopathology in dermatoses associated with desquamative gingivitis

Disease	Immunopathology
Cicatricial Pemphigoid	Basement membrane deposits of IgG and C3*
Lichen planus	Globular deposits or cytoid bodies and/or fibrin deposits along the basement membrane zone†
Pemphigus, all forms	Intercellular IgG in gingival epithelium*
Psoriasis	Stratum corneum deposits†

*Findings are diagnostic.
†Findings are suggestive but not diagnostic.

The diagnosis and treatment of desquamative gingivitis is dependent on identifying the underlying etiology through (1) clinical observation, (2) histologic examination, and (3) immunologic examination (direct immunofluorescence tests on biopsies and sometimes indirect immunofluorescence tests on sera) (see Chapter 34). The newest of the three criteria, immunofluorescence, has led to a more precise identification of the underlying etiology and has permitted a dermatologic diagnosis to be made in a greater percentage of desquamative gingival lesions. The rapid identification of patients with cicatricial pemphigoid and pemphigus is of the utmost importance, since cicatricial pemphigoid can cause blindness and pemphigus is a life-threatening disease.

The examination of sera from patients with desquamative gingivitis by indirect immunofluorescence usually yields negative results, except in pemphigus and in less than one third of the cases of cicatricial pemphigoid. Because of this, serum tests are not usually recommended.

The association of desquamative gingival lesions with different diseases as determined by direct immunofluorescence is summarized in Table 28-17. On the basis of direct immunofluorescence, approximately one half of the desquamative lesions are cicatricial pemphigoid, one quarter are lichen planus, and one quarter have no significant immunopathology, suggesting an unknown or nondermatologic etiology. In addition, a small number are pemphigus and psoriasis.

Desquamative Gingivitis Associated With Cicatricial Pemphigoid

Approximately 50 percent of the cases of desquamative gingivitis are associated with cicatricial pemphigoid.

Histologically, the presence of a subepithelial blister is indicative of the pemphigoid group of diseases.

Immunologically, immunofluorescence yields diagnostic findings in both gingival biopsy specimens and sera. In biopsy specimens, basement membrane zone deposits of IgG and C3 are most common. In approximately 10 percent of the cases, IgG antibodies to the basement membrane occur in the sera.

Desquamative Gingivitis Associated With Pemphigus

Approximately 2 percent of the cases of desquamative gingivitis are associated with pemphigus. While most pemphigus vulgaris cases first develop intraorally, the gingiva does not appear to be a major intraoral site.

Histologically, acantholysis of epithelial cells with the resultant intraepithelial blisters occur.

Immunologically, desquamative gingivitis associated with pemphigus is identical to pemphigus involving any part of the body. Biopsies have intercellular deposits of IgG in the gingival epithelium and sera contains IgG antibodies reactive with the intercellular substance of squamous epithelium in most if not all specimens.

Desquamative Gingivitis Associated With Lichen Planus

Approximately 25 percent of the cases of desquamative gingivitis are associated with lichen planus.

Histologically, there is a band-like infiltrate below the epithelium, degeneration of the basal cells, and a "saw-tooth" interdigitation of the epithelium and lamina propria.

Immunologically, desquamative gingivitis associated with lichen planus reveals characteristic but not diagnostic findings including cytoid bodies in the epidermis and dermis and fibrin (fibrinogen) deposits along the basement membrane.

Desquamative Gingivitis Associated With Psoriasis

A few rare cases of desquamative gingivitis are associated with psoriasis.

Histologically, there is epithelial hyperplasia with a thickened stratum corneum, parakeratosis, hyperplasia of the stratum malpighi, and epidermal microabscesses.

Immunologically, desquamative gingival biopsy specimens reveal antibodies and complement bound in vivo to the stratum corneum antigen.

Diagnostic Tests for Periodontal Disease

Numerous assays have been used in studies of periodontal disease (Table 28–18). Details on test methodology are provided in Chapter 34. Several of these assays may also have applications as clinical tests. With periodontal diseases now mainly considered as bacterial infections with characteristic subgingival flora, it is reasonable to identify perio-

Table 28–18 ■ Assays for studying periodontal disease

I. *Plaque Assays*
  1. Phase and dark field microscopy
  2. Culture and isolation
  3. Identification of bacterial enzymes and products in subgingival specimens
  4. Immunofluorescence
  5. Latex agglutination
  6. Immunoperoxidase
  7. ELISA
  8. Immunoblotting
II. *Indirect Assays on Sera*
  1. Immunofluorescence
  2. ELISA

dontopathogens as aids for determining disease activity and effectiveness of clinical therapy. Based on current knowledge, assays on plaque appear to have more clinical relevance than immunologic tests on sera (with the exception of desquamative gingivitis). Commercial laboratories are already offering cultural and immunofluorescence tests. Second generation tests that can be performed in the clinical office with minimal training, such as latex agglutination tests, are under consideration. These and other tests will emerge to help dental personnel in the future.

REFERENCES

Altman, L. C., Page, R. C., Vandesteen, G. E., Dixon, L. I., and Bradford, C.: Abnormalities of leukocyte chemotaxis in patients with various forms of periodontitis. J. Periodont. Res. 20:553, 1985.

Asikainen, S.: Occurrence of *Actinobacillus actinomycetemcomitans* and spirochetes in relation to age in localized juvenile periodontitis. J. Periodontol. 57:537, 1986.

Bick, P. H., Carpenter, A. B., Holdeman, L. V., Miller, G. A., Ranney, R. R., Palcanis, K. G., and Tew, J. G.: Polyclonal B-cell activation induced by extracts of Gram-negative bacteria isolated from periodontally diseased sites. Infect. Immun. 34:43, 1981.

Bolton, R. W., Kluever, E. A., and Dyer, J. K.: In vitro immunosuppression mediated by an extracellular polysaccharide from *Capnocytophaga ochracea*. J. Periodont. Res. 20:251, 1985.

Chung, C. P., Nisengard, R. J., Slots, J., and Genco, R. J.: Bacterial IgG and IgM antibody titers in acute necrotizing ulcerative gingivitis. J. Periodontol. 54:557, 1983.

Cogen, R. B., Stevens, A. W. Jr., Cohen-Cole, S., Kirks, K., and Freeman, A.: Leukocyte function in the etiology of acute necrotizing ulcerative gingivitis. J. Periodontol. 54:402, 1983.

Christersson, L. A., Slots, J., Zambon, J. J., and Genco, R. J.: Transmission and colonization of *Actinobacillus actinomycetemcomitans* in localized juvenile periodontitis patients. J. Periodontol. 56:127, 1985.

Dzink, J. L., Tanner, A. C. R., Haffajee, A. D., and

Socransky, S. S.: Gram negative species associated with active destructive periodontal lesions. J. Clin. Periodontol. 12:648, 1985.

Ebersole, J. L., Taubman, M. A., Smith, D. J., and Haffajee. A. D.: Effect of subgingival scaling on systemic antibody responses to oral microorganisms. Infect. Immun. 48:534, 1985.

Frank, R. M., and Voegel, J. C.: Bacterial bone resorption in advanced cases of human periodontitis. J. Periodont. Res. 13:251, 1978.

Genco, R. J., and Slots, J.: Host responses in periodontal disease. J. Dent. Res. 63:441, 1984.

Holt, S. C.: Bacterial surface structures and their role in periodontal disease. In Genco, R. J., and Mergenhagen, S. E. (eds.): Host-Parasite Interactions in Periodontal Diseases. Washington, DC, American Society of Microbiology, 1982, p. 139.

Kilian, M.: Degradation of immunoglobulins A1, A2, and G by suspected principal periodontal pathogens. Infect. Immun. 34:757, 1981.

Kornman, K. S., and Loesche, W. J.: The subgingival microbial flora during pregnancy. J. Periodont. Res. 15:111, 1980.

Kornman, K. S.: Age, supragingival plaque, and steroid hormones as ecological determinants of the subgingival flora. In Genco, R. J., and Mergenhagen, S. E. (eds.): Host-Parasite Interactions in Periodontal Diseases. Washington, DC, American Society of Microbiology, 1982, p. 132.

Listgarten, M. A.: Electron microscopic observations on the bacterial flora of acute necrotizing ulcerative gingivitis. J. Periodontol. 36:328, 1965.

Loesche, W. J., Syed, S. A., Laughon, B. E., and Stoll, J.: The bacteriology of acute necrotizing ulcerative gingivitis. J. Periodontol. 53:223, 1982.

Loesche, W. J., Syed, S. A., Schmidt, E., and Morrison, E. C.: Bacterial profiles of subgingival plaques in periodontitis. J. Periodontol. 56:447, 1985.

Mashimo, P. A., Yamamoto, Y., Slots, J., Park, B. H., and Genco, R. J.: The periodontal microflora of juvenile diabetics: Culture, immunofluorescence, and serum antibody studies. J. Periodontol. 54:420, 1983.

Mergenhagen, S. E.: Thymocyte activating factor(s) in human gingival fluids. J. Dent. Res. 63:461, 1984.

Newman, H. N., and Addison, I. E.: Gingival crevice neutrophil function in periodontosis. J. Periodontol. 53:578, 1982.

Newman, M. G., Socransky, S. S., Savitt, E. D., Propas, D. A., and Crawford, A.: Studies of the microbiology of periodontosis. J. Periodontol. 47:373, 1976.

Newman, M. G., Grinenco, V., Weiner, M., Angel, I., Karge, H., and Nisengard, R.: Predominant microbiota associated with periodontal health in the aged. J. Periodontol. 49:553, 1978.

Newman, M. G., and Sims, T. N.: The predominant cultivable microbiota of the periodontal abscess. J. Periodontol. 50:350, 1979.

Newman, M. G.: Current concepts of the pathogenesis of periodontal disease. J. Periodontol. 56:734, 1985.

Nisengard, R. J.: The role of immunology in periodontal disease. J. Periodontol. 48:505, 1977.

Nisengard, R. J., and Neiders, M.: Desquamative lesions of the gingiva. J. Periodontol. 52:500, 1981.

Nisengard, R. J., and Blann, D. B.: Detection of immune complexes in gingiva from periodontitis patients. J. Dent. Res. 64:361, 1985.

O'Neil, P. A., and Woodson, D. L.: Lymphokine production by human gingival lymphocytes. J. Periodont. Res. 21:338, 1986.

Oshrain, H. I., Telsey, B., and Mandel, I. D.: A longitudinal study of periodontal disease in patients with reduced immunocapacity. J. Periodontol. 54:151, 1983.

Page, R. C., Altman, L. C., Ebersole, J. L., Vandesteen, G. E., Dahlberg, W. H., Williams, B. L., and Osterberg, S. K.: Rapidly progressive periodontitis: A distinct clinical condition. J. Periodontol. 54:197, 1983.

Page, R. C., Bowen, T., Altman, L., Vendesteen, E., Ochs, H., Mackenzie, P., Osterberg, L., Engel, D., and Williams, B. L.: Prepubertal periodontitis. I. Definition of a clinical disease entity. J. Periodontol. 54:257, 1983.

Preus, H. R.: Possible exogenous source of Aa in rapid destructive periodontitis in man (abstr). J. Dent. Res. 66:709, 1987.

Saglie, R., Newman, M. G., Carranza, F. A., Jr., and Pattison, G. L.: Bacterial invasion of gingiva in advanced periodontitis in humans. J. Periodontol. 53:217, 1982.

Savitt, E. D., and Socransky, S. S.: Distribution of certain subgingival microbial species in selected periodontal conditions. J. Periodont. Res. 19:111, 1984.

Seymour, G. J.: Possible mechanisms involved in the immunoregulation of chronic inflammatory periodontal disease. J. Dent. Res. 66:2, 1987.

Seymour, G. J., Cole, K. L., Powell, R. N., Lewins, E., Cripps, A. W., and Clancy, R. L.: Interleukin-2 production and bone-resorption activity in vitro by unstimulated lymphocytes extracted from chronically-inflamed human periodontal tissues. Arch. Oral Biol. 30:481, 1985.

Schenkein, H. A.: The complement system in periodontal disease. In Genco, R. J., and Mergenhagen, S. E. (eds.): Host-Parasite Interactions in Periodontal Diseases. Washington, DC, American Society of Microbiology, 1982, p. 299.

Shenker, B. J., and DiRienzo, J. M.: Suppression of human peripheral blood lymphocytes by Fusobacterium nucleatum. J. Immunology 132:2357, 1984.

Slots, J.: Importance of black-pigmented Bacteroides in human periodontal disease. In Genco, R. J., and Mergenhagen, S. E. (eds.): Host-Parasite Interactions in Periodontal Diseases. Washington, DC, American Society of Microbiology, 1982, p. 27.

Slots, J., and Rosling, B. G.: Suppression of the periodontopathic microflora in localized juvenile periodontitis by systemic tetracycline. J. Clin. Periodontology 10:465, 1983.

Slots, J., and Genco, R. J.: Black-pigmented Bacteroides species, Capnocytophaga species, and Actinobacillus actinomycetemcomitans in human periodontal disease: Virulence factors in colonization, survival, and tissue destruction. J. Dent. Res. 63:412, 1984.

Slots, J., Bragd, L., Wikstrom, M., and Dahlen, G.: The occurrence of Actinobacillus actinomycetemcomitans, Bacteroides gingivalis and Bacteroides intermedius in destructive periodontal disease in adults. J. Clin. Periodontol. 13:570, 1986.

Sundqvist, G., Carlsson, J., Herrmann, B., and Tarnvik, A.: Degradation of human immunoglobulins G and M and complement factors C3 and C5 by black-pigmented Bacteroides. J. Med. Microbiol. 19:85, 1985.

Suzuki, J. B., Collison, B. C., Falker, W. A., Jr., and Nauman, R. K.: Immunologic profile of juvenile periodontitis. II. Neutrophil chemotaxis, phagocytosis and spore germination. J. Periodontol. 55:461, 1984.

Taubman, M. A., Ebersole, J. L., Smith, D. J.: Association between systemic and local antibody and periodontal disease. In Genco, R. J., and Mergenhagen, S. E. (eds.): Host-Parasite Interactions in Periodontal Diseases. Washington, DC, American Society of Microbiology, 1982, p. 283.

Taubman, M. A., Yoshie, H., Ebersole, J. L., Smith, D. J., and Olson, C. L.: Host response in experimental periodontal disease. J. Dent. Res. 63:455, 1984.

Tew, J. G., Marshall, D. R., Moore, W. E. C., Best, A. M., Palcanis, K. G., and Ranney, R. R.: Serum antibody reactive with predominant organisms in the subgingival flora of young adults with generalized severe periodontitis. Infect. Immun. 48:303, 1985.

Van Dyke, T. E., Horoszewicz, H. U., Cianciola, L. J., and Genco, R. J.: Neutrophil chemotaxis dysfunction in human periodontitis. Infect. Immun. 27:124, 1980.

Van Dyke, T. E., Schweinebraten, M., Cianciola, L. J., Offenbacher, S., and Genco, R. J.: Neutrophil chemotaxis in families with localized juvenile periodontitis. J. Periodont. Res. 20:503, 1985.

Vandesteen, G. E., Williams, B. L., Ebersole, J. L., Altman, L. C., and Page, R. C.: Clinical, microbiological and immunological studies of a family with a high prevalence of early-onset periodontitis. J. Periodontol. 55:159, 1984.

Whal, S. M.: Mononuclear cell-mediated alterations in connective tissue. In Genco, R. J., and Mergenhagen, S. E. (eds.): Host-Parasite Interaction in Periodontal Disease. Washington, DC, American Society of Microbiology, 1982, p. 132.

Wilson, M. E., Zambon, J. J., Suzuki, J. B., and Genco, R. J.: Generalized juvenile periodontitis, defective neutrophil chemotaxis and Bacteroides gingivalis in a 13-year old female. J. Periodontol. 56:457, 1985.

Zambon, J. J., Christersson, L. A., and Slots, J.: Actinobacillus actinomycetemcomitans in human periodontal disease—Prevalence in patient groups and distribution of biotypes and serotypes within families. J. Periodontol. 54:707, 1983.

chapter *29*

Control and prevention of periodontal disease

Sebastian G. Ciancio □ *Russell J. Nisengard, D.D.S., Ph.D.*

With the significant reduction in dental caries during the past decade, attention has turned to new methods of control, prevention, and treatment of periodontal disease. This is being extensively investigated through research supported by the National Institute of Dental Research and commercial companies. This chapter will focus on chemotherapeutic and immunologic approaches to periodontal therapy. (See Chapter 28 for further details.)

Plaque Control

The role of plaque in the etiology of gingivitis and periodontitis has been known for several decades. While the exact organisms causing periodontal diseases and their mechanisms of action have not been conclusively identified, plaque control definitely aids in the prevention and treatment of these diseases. This has been the backbone of preventive dentistry whereby plaque is removed by mechanical means—brushing and flossing by patients, scaling and root planing by dentists.

Because of the relatively high incidence of periodontal disease indicating a failure in prevention by traditional (demonstrably successful but difficult to motivate) mechanical means, other methods of plaque control are being explored. The major thrust so far has been toward finding a chemical agent that would control plaque. This could be incorporated in a mouthwash, toothpaste, pill, or other delivery system. The chemotherapeutic agents could be (1) nonspecific, affecting all plaque bacteria uniformly and leading to a quantitative reduction in plaque, or (2) specific, acting as a "silver bullet" to qualitatively reduce only the periodontopathic plaque bacteria. The simpler approach of reducing all plaque is closer to reality. Chemical agents could reduce plaque by (1) affecting initial colonization, (2) inhibiting plaque development and metabolism, or (3) reducing existing plaque.

The Council on Dental Therapeutics of the American Dental Association (ADA) has established guidelines for accepting an agent for control of plaque and gingivitis. To receive the seal of approval of the ADA, an

Table 29–1 ■ Ideal chemotherapeutic agent
Clinically effective in plaque control
Clinically effective in control of inflammation
Maximum effect on pathogens
Highly substantive to minimize dosage
Minimal adverse effects
No bacterial resistance
Stable for prolonged time periods

agent must not only reduce plaque, particularly supragingival plaque, it must also reduce gingival inflammation when used in conjunction with routine home care procedures such as brushing and flossing. To this end, most companies with products capable of reducing plaque are performing clinical studies in an attempt to extend claims for their products that they also reduce gingival inflammation. It is quite possible that some agents that reduce plaque quantitatively would not significantly reduce the periodontopathic bacteria and therefore have little, if any, effect on gingival inflammation. In considering different agents, they should be evaluated not only in terms of efficacy but also on the basis of specificity, substantivity (adherence to teeth or gingival tissue), safety, and stability. Two mouth rinses are currently approved by the ADA for control of plaque and gingivitis: Peridex and Listerine, chlorhexidene and phenol solutions, respectively. The characteristics of an ideal agent are listed in Table 29–1.

DELIVERY SYSTEMS

Topical, local delivery of chemotherapeutic agents for control of periodontal disease is considered most desirable, since the incidence of side effects is far less by this method than by the systemic route. Solutions used as mouthwashes offer advantages in ease of use. However, they mainly affect supragingival plaque with little subgingival activity. This may limit their efficacy in treating gingivitis and cause them to be of minimal value in treating periodontitis. A number of studies have evaluated delivery directly into the gingival crevice using various types of devices. Additionally, antibiotics have been placed into hollow fibers that are positioned subgingivally, leading to some improvement in periodontal health; antimicrobials have also been placed on acrylic strips inserted subgingivally; and the subgingival area has been irrigated with chemotherapeutic agents.

These systems offer promise for future therapy.

Korman divided chemotherapeutic agents into first-generation and second-generation agents, based on their efficiency in plaque control and substantivity. Agents included in these two groups either are nonspecific, affecting all plaque similarly, or have minimal specificity, such as antibiotics. A third-generation agent may eventually be developed that has high specificity for the periodontopathogens. Some topical agents currently of interest are listed in Table 29–2.

FIRST-GENERATION AGENTS

These agents demonstrate limited substantivity and are therefore not retained intraorally for any significant amount of time after use. As a consequence, they must be taken frequently and have a limited efficacy of 20 to 50 percent in reducing plaque and gingivitis. This group includes topical antibiotics, quaternary ammonium compounds, phenolic compounds, and sanguinarine.

SECOND-GENERATION AGENTS

These agents demonstrate significant substantivity, so they are retained and released in a prolonged fashion beyond the time of use. They can therefore be used less frequently than first-generation agents—once or twice a day—and achieve a greater reduction in plaque and gingivitis of 40 to 70 percent. Chlorhexidine and its analogues, and possibly stannous fluoride, are included in this group. Tetracycline, an antibiotic with recently demonstrated substantivity, may also be in this group.

Table 29–2 ■ Chemotherapeutic agents for control of plaque*
First-Generation
Antibiotics
Cetylpyridinium chloride
Essential oils
Fluorides
Salicylanilides
Sanguinarine
Zinc compounds
Second-Generation
Alexidine
Chlorhexidine
Antibiotics (tetracyclines)

*Agents are listed in alphabetical order. (See text for efficacy.)

THIRD-GENERATION AGENTS

These agents have yet to be developed. Instead of no bacterial specificity as occurs with antiseptics or limited specificity as with antibiotics, agents may be identified that are effective against only one or a few periodontopathogens. For such an agent to be of value, three major criteria would have to be fulfilled: (1) only a limited number of organisms could be responsible for disease; (2) elimination of the small group of periodontopathogens would not lead to increased growth of a usually nonpathogenic organism that is converted to a pathogen by its increased numbers (superinfection); and (3) bacterial resistance does not develop. Considerable research into the pathogenesis of periodontal diseases and nature of antibacterial agents would be necessary before third-generation agents could be given serious consideration.

ANTIBIOTICS

Some antibiotics, when taken systemically or topically, have the ability to inhibit plaque and plaque-induced disease for short time periods. In limited situations, their use has been advocated for treatment of some types of periodontal diseases (see Chapter 28). However, the potential for hypersensitivity reactions and microbial antibiotic resistance limits the use of antibiotics for long-term plaque control. Even more important, since antibiotics are often essential for control of serious infections, their use may best be reserved for treatment of systemic infection rather than for control of plaque.

A number of systemically administered antibiotics have been evaluated as aids to periodontal therapy, such as tetracyclines, clindamycin, and metronidazole (see Chapter 33). These drugs offer some promise as adjuncts to periodontal therapy but, as with any antibiotic, it is necessary to monitor various body functions for adverse effects. For instance, tetracyclines have reportedly caused kidney and liver disorders; clindamycin can cause serious gastrointestinal disorders including colitis; and metronidazole initiates tumors in rats and causes bacterial mutagenicity. The risk-benefit ratios of these and other antibiotics must be evaluated before use in periodontal therapy.

As more antibiotics are employed, the development of resistance is an increased prob-ability. With the tetracyclines, the development of multi-drug–resistant bacteria (termed plasmid factor resistance) has been documented with *Escherichia coli*. In view of this, microbiologic monitoring of bacterial resistance may be part of future therapy.

CHLORHEXIDINE

Chlorhexidine, a bisbiquanide, in a concentration of 0.2 percent is currently the most extensively tested and most effective antiplaque and antigingivitis agent. It has been available in Europe for over 20 years in toothpastes and mouthwashes. Its efficacy has been clearly demonstrated in short-term trials with and without any mechanical means of plaque control. In a long-term study, plaque and gingivitis scores were reduced by approximately 50 percent for 2 years. It may be of value as an agent for selected populations requiring short-term plaque control. Tooth staining, mucosal irritation (especially in children), and a bitter taste are common side effects. The brownish stain is removed by a routine dental prophylaxis.

Chlorhexidine is now available as a mouthwash (Peridex) at a concentration of 0.12 percent in the United States. This lower concentration minimizes the side effects without altering its effectiveness on plaque and gingivitis. Peridex is marketed by Proctor and Gamble as a prescription drug. It is the first chemotherapeutic agent to receive Food and Drug Administration (FDA) and ADA approval for treatment of gingivitis. Six-month studies have shown clinically significant reductions in plaque and gingivitis with the use of this agent. In addition, chlorhexidine is also effective in treatment of oral candidiasis.

Alexidine, another drug with a similar chemical structure, has shown promise in short-term studies but has not been adequately investigated. As with chlorhexidine, tooth staining and taste alteration can occur.

DENTIFRICES

Most dentifrices claim to be of value in plaque reduction. These claims are based not on chemotherapeutic agents but on the observation, from clinical studies, that brushing with a dentifrice is more effective in plaque removal than brushing without a dentifrice.

The incorporation of effective chemotherapeutic agents into dentifrices must overcome the problems of bioavailability of the agent and compatibility with other dentifrice ingredients.

ENZYMES

At present, enzymes directed against pellicle, plaque, or its components have not been effective.

FLUORIDE

The efficacy of fluorides in control of caries is without question. Fluoride preparations have also been recently investigated in short-term studies for efficacy as antiplaque and antigingivitis agents. Stannous fluoride has some substantivity. Stannous fluoride in a 0.4 to 1.64 percent concentration may be of value for control of plaque. While the relative effectiveness of stannous fluoride versus sodium fluoride is not clear, short-term data suggest a distinct advantage of stannous fluoride. Tooth staining and an unpleasant taste have been reported as frequent side effects of some fluoride preparations. Long-term studies have not shown efficacy.

PHENOLS

Listerine, a mouthwash that contains a mixture of phenolic compounds and methylsalicylate, has moderate antiplaque activity with no reported side effects other than a temporary burning sensation. Two long-term 6-month trials in conjunction with routine oral hygiene have shown plaque reduction. In another study of 9 months' duration, lower gingivitis scores were seen after 9 months but not after 6 months. The average plaque reduction has been 25 percent and gingivitis reduction has been 30 percent. The effect of phenols on gingival inflammation must be further evaluated. This product has also been shown to control candidiasis in the oral cavity.

QUATERNARY AMMONIUM COMPOUNDS

Quaternary ammonium compounds such as cetylpyridinium chloride mouthwashes exhibit moderate antiplaque activity, reducing plaque by an average of about 25 percent. They rapidly absorb to the tooth surface in high concentrations but have limited substantivity and are therefore quickly released. Some side effects include burning tongue, mucosal irritations, and minor reversible tooth staining. Cepacol (Merrill-Dow), Scope (Proctor and Gamble), and some Amway products contain these agents.

OXYGENATING AGENTS

Oxygenating agents that raise the oxygen tension of the gingival sulcus were proposed as agents that would reduce the anaerobic periodontopathogens. Short-term studies on the value of such agents have been contradictory, and long-term studies have not been performed. Serious questions of safety have also been raised in view of the fact that there have been reports of burns and tissue irritation with chronic use and co-carcinogenic effects in animals.

SANGUINARINE

Sanguinarine, a benzophenanthradine alkaloid, has been evaluated in several short-term studies, generally of 6 weeks or less. The agent appears to reduce plaque and gingival inflammation from 20 to 60 percent in short-term studies, but its long-term effectiveness on plaque and disease reduction is unclear. In a recent study evaluating sanguinarine's effects on the development of experimental gingivitis, no differences from the placebo were observed. Additional long-term studies on the prevention of plaque and gingivitis, as well as the agent's side effects, are warranted. Viadent mouthwash, commercially available from Vipont Laboratories, contains 0.03 percent of sanguinarine extract (0.01 percent pure sanguinarine). It is also manufactured as a dentifrice.

Sodium Benzoate

This chemical, found in Plax, has surface-active properties and may aid plaque removal by mechanical methods. However, studies have been too limited to draw any conclusions.

Comparisons among antiplaque agents are sometimes difficult to make, as their actions are usually compared with placebos rather than with other antiplaque agents. Some

Table 29–3 ■ Comparison of chemotherapeutic agents in studies 6 months or longer				
	Frequency Use	Number of Subjects	Plaque Reduction	Gingivitis Reduction
Cetylpyridinium chloride				
Chlorhexidine 0.2%	Twice daily	99	14%	24%
0.12%	Twice daily	150	50%	50%
0.1%	Twice daily	430	61%	45%
	Once daily	158	60%	67%
Phenol	Twice daily	145	20%	28%
	Twice daily	109	34%	34%
	Twice daily	85	20%	24%
	Twice daily	104	25%	28%
Sanguinarine	Twice daily	100	0%	0%*
	Twice daily	115	0%	0%
Stannous fluoride	Twice daily	268	0%	0%

*In this dentifrice study, the gingival index scores increased by 71% in the placebo group and 49% in the sanguinarine group.

comparisons have been made and more will certainly follow. Table 29–3 compares the effectiveness of several agents on plaque formation and development of gingivitis, in studies of 6 months' duration or longer. Without a doubt, chlorhexidine was significantly more effective than phenolic compounds, quaternary ammonium compounds, and sanguinarine, earning its reputation as a second-generation agent. Another concern with mouthwashes is their alcoholic content. Table 29–4 summarizes the alcoholic concentrations, which range approximately 11 to 27 percent and their pH's.

Since chemotherapeutic agents have resulted in significant plaque reduction, they definitely have a role in periodontal therapy. At this time they can be recommended as adjuncts to oral hygiene in patients experiencing difficulty in mechanical plaque control, those with extensive splinting of teeth, and those with refractory cases or who are considered unsuitable for periodontal surgery.

IMMUNOLOGIC CONTROL OF PLAQUE

Numerous animal studies have demonstrated the effectiveness of immunization as

Table 29–4 ■ Alcohol and pH of mouthwashes		
	Alcohol	pH
Cepacol	14.0%	6.0
Listerine	26.9%	5.0
Peridex	11.6%	5.6
Scope	18.5%	5.5
Viadent	11.5%	3.0

a means of controlling S. mutans caries (see Chapter 27). Secretory IgA is stimulated by local sensitization in the salivary glands or intestinal tract with S. mutans antigens. Currently, several groups are undergoing human clinical trials of this novel approach to prevention. Secretory IgA occurs only in saliva and not in crevicular fluid. Thus, if immunization were considered for blocking the colonization of periodontopathogens in plaque, two routes of immunization may be required: salivary stimulation for supragingival plaque and systemic stimulation for subgingival plaque. There has been little research in this area.

Chemotherapeutic Agents for Treatment of Periodontal Disease

ANTIBIOTICS

Antibiotics have demonstrable efficacy for the treatment of some forms of periodontal disease. For example, tetracyclines are now part of the routine therapy for patients with localized juvenile periodontitis (see Chapter 33) presumably because of their effects on A. actinomycetemcomitans.

Recently, Golub and coworkers have demonstrated another potentially important role for tetracycline in addition to its antibacterial activity. Tetracyclines appear to inhibit tissue collagenase and therefore retard the breakdown of collagen that normally occurs in periodontal disease. They have suggested that reduction in collagen breakdown may reduce the chemotactic effect associated with collagen fragments; this results in a reduction of polymorphonuclear leukocytes in gingival crevicular fluid, with the end point being a reduction in inflammation. It is possible that agents such as these may become a part of therapy in the "defense of collagen."

ANTI-INFLAMMATORY AGENTS

Research in animals has demonstrated that flurbiprofen, a nonsteroidal anti-inflammatory drug, may aid in bone regeneration. Since this substance is a prostaglandin inhibitor, further studies may prove it to be useful in therapy. In contrast, nonsteroidal anti-inflammatory drugs appear to have no significant effect on gingival inflammation. One possible conclusion is that these agents may be effective in diseases of oral hard tissues but not oral soft tissues.

REATTACHMENT AGENTS

Coronal reattachment of connective tissue and epithelium in patients with periodontitis would be quite beneficial. Citric acid, fibronectin, and tetracycline have been evaluated as topical agents to be applied to root surfaces during periodontal surgery as aids in soft tissue reattachment. Tetracyclines have the added benefit of being substantive and maintaining their bacteriocidal activity for some time after topical application.

Results of studies of various root surface modifiers to date have been mixed, with some demonstrating reattachment and others showing no differences from untreated controls. Some studies have even reported irreversible resorption and ankylosis of the root. Longer time periods are needed to answer the question of their therapeutic value.

Agents for Control of Calculus

The incidence of calculus formation ranges from 45 to 66 percent, depending to some degree on sex and age. Some patients are "calculus formers" and appear to form heavy calculus in spite of reasonable plaque control. Recently, dentifrices and mouth rinses have been introduced that reduce calculus *formation* to a limited extent (approximately 30 to 40 percent). They are not effective against calculus already present nor do they affect gingival inflammation, as do antiplaque agents.

Crest Tartar Control, Colgate Tartar Control, and Prevent toothpastes are advertised as reducing the formation of dental calculus. The active ingredients in Crest are 3.4 percent tetrasodium pyrophosphate and 1.37 percent disodium, dihydrogen pyrophosphate. Colgate's active agent is 5 percent tetrasodium pyrophosphate. Similar ingredients are found in Crest and Colgate Tartar Control mouth rinses. Prevent contains 2 percent zinc chloride as its tartar-reducing ingredient. These chemicals block receptor sites on enamel for calcium phosphate (found in food and saliva), and inhibit crystal growth of calculus. All of these dentifrices contain sodium fluoride and are formulated so that the fluoride is available.

The practitioner must decide if calculus formation is an esthetic problem for the patient, or if it interferes with good oral hygiene, or both. For selected patients, especially those with intracoronal splints or extensive fixed bridgework, a reduction of calculus by 30 to 40 percent might be of value.

REFERENCES

Accepted Dental Therapeutics, ed. 39. American Dental Association, 1982.

Addy, M., Rawle, L., Handley, R., Newman, H. N., and Coventry, J. F.: Development and in vitro evaluation of acrylic strips and dialysis tubing for local drug delivery. J. Periodontol. 53:693, 1985.

Braatz, L., Garrett, S., Claffey, N., and Egelberg, J.: Antimicrobial irrigation of deep pockets to supplement non-surgical periodontal therapy. II. Daily irrigation. J. Clin. Periodontol. 12:630, 1985.

Caffesse, R., Holden, M., Kon, S., and Nasjleti, C.: Citric acid/fibronectin in treating periodontitis in beagle dogs. IADR Progr. Abstr. J. Dent. Res. 63:221, 1984.

Ciancio, S. G., Mather, M. L., and Bunnell, H. L.: Clinical evaluation of a quaternary ammonium-containing mouthrinse. J. Periodontol. 46:397, 1975.

Ciancio, S. G., Slots, J., Reynolds, H. S., et al.: The effect of short-term administration of minocycline HCl on gingival inflammation and subgingival microflora. J. Periodontol. 53:557, 1982.

Ciancio, S. C.: Chemotherapeutic agents and periodontal therapy—their impact on clinical practice. J. Periodontol. 57:108, 1986.

Crigger, M., Renvert, S., and Bogle, G.: The effect of topical citric acid application on surgically exposed periodontal attachment. J. Periodontal Res. 18:303, 1983.

Dunn, R. K., Perkins, B. H., and Goodson, J. M.: Controlled release of tetracycline from biodegradable fibers. IADR Progr. Abstr J. Dent. Res. 62:289, 1983.

Flota, L., Gjermo, G., Rolla, G., and Waerhaug, J.: Side

effects of chlorhexidine mouth washes. Scand. J. Dent. Res. 79:119, 1971.

Golub, L. M., Ramamurthy, N., McNamara, T., et al.: Tetracyclines inhibit tissue collagenase activity: A new mechanism in the treatment of periodontal disease. J. Periodontal Res. 19:651, 1984.

Gordon, J., Walker, C., Lamster, I., et al.: Evaluation of clindamycin in refractory periodontitis. IADR Progr. Abstr. J. Dent. Res. 63:268, 1984.

Gordon, J. M., Lamster, I. B., and Seiger, M. C.: Efficiency of Listerine antiseptic in inhibiting the development of plaque and gingivitis. J. Clin. Periodontol. 12:697, 1985.

Kornman, K. S.: The role of supragingival plaque in the prevention and treatment of periodontal diseases: A review of current concepts. J. Periodontal Res. 21 (Suppl.):5, 1986.

Lang, N. P., and Brecx, M. C.: Chlorhexidine digluconate—an agent for chemical plaque control and prevention of gingival inflammation. J. Periodontal Res. (Suppl.):74, 1986.

Linde, J., Heijl, L., Goodson, J. M., and Socransky, S. S.: Local tetracycline delivery using hollow fiber devices in periodontal therapy. J. Clin. Periodontol. 6:141, 1979.

Linde, J.: Clinical assessment of antiplaque agents. Comp. Cont. Educ. Dent. (Suppl.)5:s78, 1984. Lobene, R. R., Kashket, S., Soparkar, P. M., et al.: The effect of cetylpyridinium chloride on human plaque bacteria and gingivitis. Pharmacol. Thera. Dent. 4:33, 1979.

Mazza, J. E., Newman, M. G., Perry, D. A., and Carranza, Jr., F. A.: The effect of daily self-applied SnF_2 on clinical parameters of periodontitis. IADR Progr. Abstr. J. Dent. Res. 63:268, 1984.

Menaker, L., Weatherford, T. W., III, Pitts, G., et al.: The effects of Listerine antiseptic on dental plaque. Ala. J. Med. Sci. 16:71, 1979.

Nygaard, P., and Persson, I.: Evaluation of sanguinarine chloride in control of plaque in the dental practice. Comp. Cont. Educ. Dent. (Suppl.)5:s90, 1984.

Pallasch, T. J.: Drugs and periodontal therapy. Dent. Clin. North. Am. 20:23, 1976.

Valtonen, M. Y., Valtonen, Y. Y., Salo, O. P., et al.: The effect of long-term tetracycline treatment for acne vulgaris on the occurrence of R factors in the intestinal flora of man. J. Dermatol. 95:311, 1976.

Vogel, R. I., Cooper, S. A., Schneiders, L. G., and Goteiner, D.: The effects of topical steroidal and systemic nonsteroidal anti-inflammatory drugs on experimental gingivitis in man. J. Periodontol. 55:247, 1984.

Wikesio, U. M. E., Baker, P. J., Christersson, L. A., et al.: A biochemical approach to periodontal regeneration: Tetracycline treatment conditions dentin surfaces. J. Periodontal Res. 21:322, 1986.

Zacheryl, W. A., Pfeiffer, H. J., and Swancar, J. R.: The effects of soluble pyrophosphates on dental calculus in adults. J.A.D.A. 110:737, 1985.

/

chapter 30

Periapical infections

Anthony D. Goodman, D.D.S., M.Sc.D.* □ *Russell J. Nisengard, D.D.S., Ph.D.*
Benjamin Schein, D.D.S., M.Sc.D.

CHAPTER OUTLINE

- **DIAGNOSIS**
- **MICROBIOLOGY**
- **IMMUNOLOGY**

- **TREATMENT**
- **SUMMARY**

The dental pulp is a loose connective tissue with collagen fibers, amorphous ground substance, intercellular fluid, arterioles, venules, lymphatics, and a nerve supply. During tooth development, the pulp is active in the calcification process. Once the tooth is fully developed, it communicates with the periapical tissues permitting maintenance of normal physiologic health. This physiologic functioning is particularly dependent on the pulpal blood supply and a normal tissue osmotic and hydrostatic pressure.

The dental pulp is surrounded by the unyielding, calcified dentinal walls which physically restricts the tissue. Even minimal inflammation with edema and cellular infiltrates causes pressure which cannot be easily alleviated. In some cases, pain and pulpal necrosis may ensue.

Periapical infections of endodontic origin are subdivided into acute and chronic disease. A common acute form is acute apical periodontitis or acute alveolar abscess. Examples of the chronic form are periapical granulomas and periapical cysts. These are not distinct entities but actually a continuum of pathologic processes.

Periapical infections result from pulpal trauma by bacteria, temperature extremes, and physical forces. *The most common cause is bacterial contamination of the pulp from carious lesions extending through the enamel and dentin.* Bacteria and their products may also gain entrance to the pulp via accessory foramina, which communicate with periodontal pockets. Restorative dentistry can also traumatize the dental pulp. Temperature generated during tooth preparation and impression-taking, as well as from chemicals in some restorative materials, may also irritate the dental pulp. Physical trauma to the dentition such as a sudden blow to the face can compromise the pulpal blood supply leading to pulpal death and subsequent bacterial colonization of the root canal. This phenomenon is termed *anachoresis*. Anachoresis is the attraction of bacteria via the bloodstream into inflamed areas or necrotic tissue, or both.

The host response begins when bacteria invade the dentin. The response becomes more acute and intense after cariogenic bacteria invade the pulp. Because the pulp is enclosed by unyielding dentin, continued presence of bacteria and their antigens causes the pulp rapidly to become necrotic.

It is obvious that the inflammatory response, while often protective, may also cause unwanted deleterious effects. Accompanying the inflammatory infiltrate is complement and immunoglobulins. These lesions are also surrounded by type II collagen, as the body attempts to wall off the area. The specific means by which the bacteria cause pulpal inflammation, degeneration, and destruction is not completely understood but involves an interaction of the host with the bacteria. Once degeneration occurs, large numbers of viable and nonviable bacteria accumulate in the root canal system leading to high concentrations of toxins and enzymes. Periapical disease is an infectious process with direct and indirect microbial damage to tissue cells and blood vessels, leading to release of inflammatory substances.

If the bacterial irritant is removed early (e.g., excavation of caries and restoration with a filling), pulpal tissues can return to normal. However, if caries remains for an extended time, the inflammatory response may reach a critical, irreversible, self-sustaining stage with necrosis continuing in an apical direction.

Diagnosis

Periapical infections are diagnosed on the basis of clinical symptoms, radiographic findings, and pulp testing. Conventional radiographs of chronic cases usually show apical or lateral bone loss, while those of acute cases often show little or no abnormality.

Pulp testing performed by applying an electrical stimulus, heat, or cold to the crown of a tooth is a clinical method for determining pulp vitality. In teeth with vital pulp tissue, pulp testing elicits a sensation. In nonvital pulp there is no response. Single-rooted teeth with chronic periapical infections almost invariably fail to respond to pulp testing stimuli or have a delayed response. Multirooted teeth with chronic infections sometimes yield mixed responses—for instance, the teeth may respond to pulp testing yet be sensitive to percussion, indicating periapical inflammation. This occurs when there are both vital and necrotic canals. Teeth with acute, painful symptoms commonly respond to lower levels of stimuli or are hyper-responsive to pulp testing.

Restorative procedures on asymptomatic teeth with either chronic periapical lesions or necrotic pulps can cause pain during or immediately following treatment. This results from acute pulpal inflammation and edema within the confined root canal system. In many cases, this can be avoided by pulp testing prior to treatment to identify problematic teeth and performing appropriate endodontic treatment first. In some cases, restorative procedures on vital teeth can also evoke pulpal inflammation with acute, painful symptoms. In such situations, the pulp either heals or becomes necrotic within a period of a few months, leading to cessation of symptoms. Pulp testing and radiographs are necessary to determine which outcome has occurred.

Frequently, periodontal therapy may be compromised by asymptomatic *undetected necrotic* teeth. Teeth with large carious lesions, large restorations, or bone loss in the furcations should be endodontically evaluated and treated when indicated prior to periodontal therapy.

MICROBIOLOGY

It is well established that bacteria and their products are the main causative factors in pulp disease. Kakehashi and coworkers (1965) in a classic study conclusively demonstrated the role of bacteria in pulpal disease using gnotobiotic animals. Exposure of the pulp to the oral environment in germ-free animals elicited minimal inflammation. Pulpal necrosis and abscesses occurred only after exposure to bacteria.

Periapical infections have been examined microbiologically for (1) identification of microorganisms as etiologic agents for root canal infections, and (2) sterility testing of the root canal system as an end point for therapy prior to obturation (filling the root canal space).

Early studies of root canal infections enumerated only the aerobic and facultative anaerobic bacteria. In the 1970s, the advent of strict anaerobic culturing techniques led to the isolation of a significantly greater percentage of the flora in necrotic canals. Prior to this, many dental abscesses were reported to be sterile when they probably contained obligate anaerobic bacteria.

Table 30–1 ■ Aerobic versus anaerobic bacteria in periapical infections

Root Canal Specimen	No. of Cases	Anaerobic and Other Bacteria (%)	Anaerobic Bacteria Exclusively (%)	Facultative Bacteria Exclusively (%)
Necrotic teeth with periapical lesions	94	91 (97%)	38 (40%)	4 (4%)
Residual periapical lesions post–root canal treatment	6	5 (83%)	5 (83%)	1 (17%)

MICROORGANISMS ASSOCIATED WITH ROOT CANAL INFECTIONS

It is now clear that periapical infections are mixed infections with many species isolated from infected root canal systems. These infections are predominantly anaerobic, with gram-negative anaerobic bacilli the most common. Facultative anaerobes and aerobic bacteria are also isolated. Table 30–1 summarizes six reports on the incidence of anaerobes. Anaerobic bacteria were isolated from approximately 97 per cent of the cases and were exclusively isolated in 40 per cent of the cases. Among the anaerobic bacteria, *Bacteroides* species occur in 4 to 67 per cent of necrotic canals (Table 30–2) and 14 to 90 per cent of periapical abscesses (Table 30–3). Anaerobic bacteria isolated included *Actinomyces, Bacteroides corrodens, B. fragilis, B. melaninogenicus, B. oralis, Eubacterium, Fusobacterium nucleatum,* anaerobic *Lactobacillus, Peptococcus, Peptostreptococcus, Propionibacterium,* and *Veillonella.*

Bacteroides species, particularly *B. endodontalis,* have been singled out as potentially important pathogens in periapical infections. The *Bacteroides* possess potent lipopolysaccharides or endotoxins; a bacterial capsule that can inhibit their phagocytosis; enzymes such as collagenase, hyaluronidase, and fibrinolysin, which can affect the connective tissue stroma; and antigens capable of inducing cellular and humoral immune responses.

Recently, many *Bacteroides melaninogenicus* subspecies *asacharolyticus* isolated from infected root canals and odontogenic abscesses have been reclassified as the new species, *Bacteroides endodontalis* mentioned earlier. DNA homology, serology, and some biochemical tests have shown that *B. endodontalis* differs from other oral black-pigmenting *Bacteroides,* mainly in its capsular antigens (see Chapter 16). Three serotypes of *B. endodontalis* have been described with possible differences in pathogenicity and virulence. *B. endodontalis* shares some antigens with *B. asaccharolyticus* but not with *B. gingivalis.*

In acute endodontic lesions, large numbers of obligate anaerobic bacteria are present. These include *Bacteroides, Veillonella parvula, Actinomyces,* and *Peptostreptococcus.* Black-pigmented *Bacteroides* are more frequent in acute abscesses than in asymptomatic cases. *B. gingivalis* and *B. endodontalis,* in particular, are exclusively isolated from acute infections characterized by tenderness, swelling, and exudation. This association suggests an important role for these bacteria in the pathogenesis of acute infections. In contrast, *B. denticola* is mainly isolated from asymptomatic infections. In some acute periapical abscesses in children, *B. melaninogenicus* and *B. oralis* that produce beta-lactamase were found. These organisms could be resistant to penicillin.

Periapical infections can extend beyond the alveolar bone into the contiguous soft tissue,

Table 30–2 ■ Bacteroides in necrotic root canals

	Incidence
Positive culture	60–80%
Bacteroides species	4–67%
B. endodontalis	1–16%
B. gingivalis	5–11%
B. intermedius	5–28%
B. melaninogenicus	4–50%

Table 30–3 ■ Bacteroides in periapical abscesses

	Incidence
Positive culture	89–100%
Bacteroides species	14–100%
B. denticola	38%
B. endodontalis	2–69%
B. gingivalis	5–10%
B. intermedius	8–20%
B. melaninogenicus	30–50%

creating an orofacial infection. The incidence of bacteria in 50 cases of dentoalveolar abscesses is summarized in Table 30–4. *Streptococcus milleri*, *Peptostreptococcus* species, *Peptococcus* species, and *Bacteroides* species were most commonly isolated. Anaerobic gram-negative rods, particularly *Bacteroides* and fusobacteria, are more common in severe orofacial infections, whereas gram-positive cocci and rods are more frequent in mild infections. *F. nucleatum* appeared to be most closely associated with the severe infections.

BACTERIAL ROLE IN PERIAPICAL LESIONS

Experimentally, bacteria isolated from periapical infections have been shown to directly cause tissue damage. Combinations of isolates from infected root canals can induce purulent "mixed infections" including either transmissible, subcutaneous abscesses or experimental apical periodontitis with periapical bone loss. Pure cultures of single isolates usually were incapable of producing such lesions. *Bacteroides asaccharolyticus* (possibly *endodontalis*) in combination with *Peptostreptococcus micros* appeared to be necessary components of this mixed infection.

Microorganisms in necrotic root canal systems, as in subgingival plaque, can produce inflammatory disease. These microorganisms have the capacity for invasion, production of enzymes that cause adverse tissue reactions, and toxins that can directly and indirectly damage the tissue. The cell wall lipopolysaccharides or endotoxins of gram-negative bacteria are directly toxic for a variety of host cell types including fibroblasts. Endotoxin has been measured in infected root canal systems and periapical lesions of teeth with necrotic pulps. Higher concentrations of endotoxin can be detected in symptomatic pulpless teeth than in asymptomatic pulpless teeth. These substances also can cause osteoclastic bone loss and activate complement via the alternate pathway. Complement activation leads to the generation of chemotactic peptides, accumulation of leukocytes, and an inflammatory reaction (see Chapter 2).

Table 30–4 ■ Incidence of bacteria isolated from periapical abscesses

	% Isolates*
Facultative Anaerobes	
Streptococcus millereri	15
Streptococcus mitior	2
Streptococcus sanguis	2
Streptococcus mutans	1
Lactobacillus fermentum	1
Lactobacillus salivarius	1
Actinomyces odontolyticus	1
Actinomyces naeslundii	1
Actinomyces meyeri	1
Arachnia proprionica	1
Haemophilus parainfluenzae	1
Capnocytophaga ochracea	1
Eikinella corrodens	1
Strict Anaerobes	
Peptostreptococcus spp.	8
Peptococcus spp.	19
Streptococcus intermedius	2
Streptococcus constellatus	1
Propionibacterium acnes	1
Eubacterium lentum	1
Veillonella parvula	2
Bacteroides oralis	12
Bacteroides gingivalis†	8
Bacteroides melaninogenicus	7
Bacteroides intermedius	3
Other Bacteroides spp.	6
Fusobacterium nucleatum	4
Fusobacterium mortiferum	1

(Adapted from Lewis et al., 1986.)
*Percent isolates out of 166 isolates.
†Probably *B. endodontalis*.

MICROBIOLOGIC CULTURES IN TREATMENT OF ROOT CANAL INFECTIONS

With the identification of microorganisms in the etiology of periapical lesions, culture techniques were introduced as part of clinical therapy in the 1960s and 1970s. The root canal system was sampled and cultured prior to and during endodontic therapy as a means of determining the end point of therapy. Until a negative culture was achieved, indicating that no viable microorganisms could be cultured from root canal samples, the root canal system was not filled or obturated. Careful appraisal of the culture procedure suggested numerous false-positive and false-negative cultures. These resulted from inadvertent contamination of paper points used for collection, residual disinfectant used to medicate the canals being transferred to the paper point, inadequate chairside culture techniques particularly for anaerobes, and inappropriate culture media. As a consequence, the use of bacterial culture in endodontic therapy declined. Today, proper sampling, cultivation, characterization, and antimicrobial susceptibility permit the acquisition of clinically important and useful information.

Immunology

As in other soft tissues, the pulp and periapical tissues develop host responses to bacterial infections. Although such responses may be beneficial by eliminating, preventing, or minimizing the spread of bacteria, they may sometimes be harmful by inducing hypersensitivity reactions or excessive responses to the bacteria. A hypersensitivity reaction manifested as an inflammatory response in the confined root canal system may lead to further tissue destruction.

SENSITIZATION VIA THE PULP

Bacterial infection of the pulp leads to host sensitization to bacterial antigens. Experimental topical application of antigen to pulpal tissue of animals first sensitizes and then induces a local immune response. Once host sensitization occurs, severe pulpal inflammation and bone destruction result from topical exposure to the sensitizing antigen. The pulpal route of sensitization also induces serum antibodies to the antigen. In contrast, nonimmunized animals do not develop such inflammation.

Similarly, in an immunocompromised host, minimal inflammation may occur in pulpal infections. In one patient with an immunologic deficiency, extensive microbial invasion of the pulp failed to cause the usual cellular inflammatory infiltrate. As a consequence, there was almost no destruction of pulpal tissue.

IMMUNOPATHOLOGY OF PULPAL DISEASE

The pulpal and periapical tissues respond to the bacterial antigens by mounting a cellular and humoral response. Depending on the stage of disease, the tissues may be infiltrated by neutrophils, plasma cells (immunoglobulin containing cells), T-helper lymphocytes, T-suppressor lymphocytes, B lymphocytes, macrophages, and mast cells (Table 30–5). The T cells are more numerous than the B cells.

The neutrophils provide one of the first lines of defense against the bacteria by phagocytosing whole bacteria and their antigens. This phagocytosis is promoted by antibodies reacting with the bacteria. Sensitized T lymphocytes respond to the bacterial antigens by releasing soluble mediators or lymphokines, which not only can potentiate the protective host response but also can cause tissue destruction. Some of the lymphokines possibly important in periapical infections are chemotactic for macrophages, neutrophils, basophils, and eosinophils; inhibit migration of macrophages and leukocytes; activate macrophages; act as mitogens by inducing blast formation of nonsensitized lymphocytes; are cytotoxic for fibroblasts; and activate osteoclasts (osteoclast-activating factor, or OAF). Sensitized B lymphocytes also produce some lymphokines on exposure to the sensitizing antigen and evolve into plasma cells. The plasma cells elaborate immunoglobulins or antibodies, the effectors of humoral immunity. Antibody-antigen interactions, sometimes with activation of serum complement, may be either protective by lysing bacteria and promoting phagocytosis or destructive through immune complex disease and immediate hypersensitivity. Mast cells in the tissue contribute to immediate hypersensitivity reactions by release of histamines and other active substances upon reaction of antigens with mast cell IgE. Macrophages in the tissues play a role in processing of antigens for the lymphocytes and in phagocytosis.

Based on current knowledge, it is difficult to assess the contribution of immunity to the pathogenesis of periapical infections and whether it has a net protective or destructive

Table 30–5 ■ Immune components in pulpal and periapical tissues							
					Complement Components	Lymphocytes	
	IgG	IgE	IgA	IgM		*T*	*B*
Normal pulp	−	−	−	−	−	−	−
Inflamed pulp	+ + +	+ +	+ +	+	+ +	+	+ + +
Periapical lesions	+ + +	+ +	−	+	+ + +	+ + +	+

+ + + = Large numbers present; + + = Moderate numbers; + = Few; − = Not present.

result. It may be postulated that it plays more of a destructive than a protective role in most cases. This would occur because of the restricted environment imposed by the surrounding calcified structures, which leads to tissue necrosis when there is extensive inflammation and continuous exposure to large numbers of bacteria from carious lesions.

The elements necessary for immunopathology are present in inflamed pulp tissue, periapical granulomas, and periapical cysts. In the inflamed human dental pulp, plasma cells containing IgG, IgA, IgM, and IgE commonly occur, with 60 per cent of the cells containing IgG. The concentrations of IgG and IgA are elevated in inflamed pulps compared with normal pulps. The inflammatory response in periapical granulomas is characterized by lymphocytes, plasma cells, polymorphonuclear leukocytes, mast cells, and macrophages. Plasma cells containing IgG are most common, with IgA, IgM, and IgE plasma cells less frequently found. Immunoglobulins are also extracellular along with complement; C3c occurs within and adjacent to blood vessels.

The association of IgE with mast cells in periapical lesions also allows consideration of IgE hypersensitivity reactions within the lesions. Proposed sources of allergens have included not only the bacteria and their products but also denatured host tissues. Ultrastructurally, many of the mast cells demonstrate cell degranulation and discharge from the surface of granules suggesting histamine release as a result of immediate hypersensitivity reactions in periapical infections. This is consistent with elevated serum IgE levels in patients with acute apical abscesses.

Immune complex disease has been considered in the immunopathology of periapical lesions. Experimentally, immune complexes induce rapidly evolving periapical lesions characterized by bone loss, collagen breakdown, and leukocytic infiltration. In periapical infections, complement is frequently closely associated with IgG, IgA, and IgM, suggesting possible immune complexes of bacterial antigens with the immunoglobulins. Such reactivity could be protective and accelerate phagocytosis and bacterial lysis or could be destructive in the form of immune complex disease.

Cell-mediated immune reactions in periapical lesions have been suggested by the fact that macrophages and lymphocytes constitute a majority of the inflammatory infiltrate. Prostaglandin and other arachidonic acid metabolites, as well as OAF, a lymphokine involved in bone resorption, have also been identified in human periapical disease.

Treatment

Irreversible pulpitis with subsequent pulpal necrosis does not normally heal. As a result, endodontic therapy is directed toward removal or extirpation of the necrotic pulpal tissue, chemotherapy to reduce or eliminate the bacterial contamination, and filling the root canal system with an inert material such as gutta-percha to allow healing in the periapical area. When biologic principles are adhered to, endodontic therapy is a highly successful and dependable procedure for retaining teeth.

Successful endodontic therapy does not appear to depend on complete absence of all microorganisms but on significant reductions in their numbers and on complete seal of the canals, preventing further bacteria invasion. However, obligate anaerobic bacteria can sometimes be isolated from asymptomatic periapical lesions that previously had root canal therapy. Bacterial reduction is achieved by mechanical cleaning and shaping of the root canals with files and reamers, irrigation of the canals during treatment with solutions such as sodium hypochlorite, and antibacterial medicaments placed in the canals between treatments. Mechanical instrumentation and irrigation is thought to be the most important phase of therapy leading to significant reduction in bacterial counts. When persistent infections occur following root canal therapy, enterococci are frequently isolated.

Although some believe that leaving a tooth open for drainage will "contaminate" the root canal system and periapical tissues causing further problems, current research does not support this concept. Clinically, Pekruhn (1986) has demonstrated a lower failure rate (3 per cent) for teeth kept open for drainage than for those kept closed during treatment (9 per cent). This suggests that apical tissue can heal following treatment when the root canal system has been left open.

Effective antimicrobial therapy for periapical infections that have progressed into cellulitis is based upon awareness of the causative etiologic microorganism. Ideally, after a specimen is obtained for culture, the patient should begin receiving antibiotic therapy. If the patient fails to respond clinically to the initial drug, the dose can be increased or an alternative drug employed as a result of the culture report.

Penicillin or amoxicillin is the drug of choice for a serious periapical infection based upon clinical responses and their cost effectiveness. For patients who fail to respond to penicillin, or who are allergic to it, the drug of choice is clindamycin. It is estimated that close to 70,000 patients per year receive clindamycin for serious odontogenic infections. Recent studies have demonstrated that some bacteria, including *Bacteroides*, may be resistant to penicillin.

Summary

It is clear that the predominant bacteria in periapical infections are obligate anaerobic bacteria. Many cases are *exclusively* made up of obligate anaerobic bacteria, while very few cases are made up exclusively of facultative bacteria. Gram-negative rods such as *Bacteroides* and *Fusobacterium* seem to be the most common.

Treatment must be directed at the removal of the necrotic substrate, the establishment of drainage as atraumatically as possible, and the use of support of antimicrobial agents. Because bacterial resistance is frequent, therapy in the absence of culture/susceptibility testing is a questionable practice.

REFERENCES

Aderhold, L.: Bacteriology of dentogenous pyogenic infections. Oral Surg. 52:587, 1981.

Bergenholz, G.: Inflammatory response of the dental pulp to bacterial irritation. J. Endodont. 7:100, 1981.

Brook, I., Grimm, S., and Kielich, R. B.: Bacteriology of acute periapical abscesses in children. J. Endodontol. 7:378, 1981.

Chow, A. W., Roser, S. M., and Brady, F. A.: Orofacial odontogenic infections. Ann. Int. Med. 88:392, 1978.

Cymerman, J. J., Cymerman, D. H., Walters, J., and Nevins, A. J.: Human lymphocyte subpopulations in chronic periapical lesions. J. Endodontol. 10:9, 1984.

Fabricius, L., Dehlen, G., Holm, S. E., and Moller, A. J. R.: Influence of combinations of oral bacteria on periapical tissues of monkeys. Scand. J. Dent. Res. 90:200, 1982.

Goodman, A. D.: Isolation of anaerobic bacteria from the root canal systems of necrotic teeth by the use of a transport solution. Oral Surg. 43:766, 1977.

Goodman, A. D.: Antibiotics in endodontics, in Guide to Antibiotic Use in Dental Practice, M. G. Newman and A. D. Goodman eds. Quintessence Publishing Co., Chicago, 1984.

Haaspasalo, M., Ranta, H., Ranta, K., and Shah, H.: Black-pigmented *Bacteroides* spp. in human apical periodontitis. Infect. Immun. 53:149, 1986.

Heimdahl, A., von Konow, L., Satoh, T., and Nord, C. E.: Clinical appearance of orofacial infections of odontogenic origin in relation to microbial findings. J. Clin. Microbiol. 22:299, 1985.

Johannessen, A. C., Nilsen, R., and Skaug, N.: Deposits of immunoglobulins and complement factor C3 in human dental periapical inflammatory lesions. Scand. J. Dent. Res. 91:191, 1983.

Kakehashi, S., Stanley, H. R., and Fitzgerald, J. R.: The effects of surgical exposure of dental pulps in germfree and conventional laboratory rats. Oral Surg. 20:340, 1965.

Kantz, W. E., and Henry, C. A.: Isolation and classification of anaerobic bacteria from intact pulp chambers of non-vital teeth in man. Arch. Oral Biol. 19:91, 1974.

Kuntz, D. D., and Genco, R. J.: Localization of immunoglobulins and complement in persistent periapical lesions. J. Dent. Res. 53:215, 1974.

Lewis, M. A. O., MacFarlane, T. W., and McGowan, D. A.: Quantitative bacteriology of acute dento-alveolar abscesses. J. Med. Microbiol. 21:101, 1986.

Megran, D. W., Scheifele, D. W., and Chow, A. W.: Odontogenic infections. Pediatr. Infect. Dis. 3:257, 1984.

Morand, M., Schilder, H., Blondin, J., Stone, P., and Franzblair, C.: Collagenolytic and elastolytic activities from diseased human dental pulps. J. Endodontol. 7:156, 1981.

Morse, D. R.: The endodontic culture technique: An impractical and unnecessary procedure. Dent. Clin. North Am. 15:793, 1971.

Oguntebi, B., Slee, A. M., Tanzer, J. M., and Langeland, K.: Predominant microflora associated with human dental periapical abscesses. J. Clin. Microbiol. 15:964, 1982.

Pantera, E. A., Jr., Zambon, J. J., Reynolds, H. S., and Shih-Levine, M.: Identification of black-pigmented *Bacteroides* sp. in human dental pulp by indirect immunofluorescence microscopy. J. Dent. Res. 64 (Sp. Iss.):176, 1985.

Pekruhn, R. B.: The incidence of failure following single visit endodontic therapy. J. Endodontol. 12:68, 1986.

Perrini, N., and Fonzi, L.: Mast cells in human periapical lesions: ultrastructural aspects and their possible physiopathological implications. J. Endodontol. 11:197, 1985.

Pulver, W. H., Taubman, M. A., and Smith, D. J.: Immune components in normal and inflamed human dental pulp. Arch. Oral Biol. 22:103, 1977.

Schonfeld, S. E., Greening, A. B., Glick, D. H., Frank, A. L., Simon, J. H., and Herles, S. M.: Endotoxin activity in periapical lesions. J. Endodontol. 8:10, 1982.

Stabholz, A., and McArthur, W. P.: Cellular immune responses of patients with periapical pathosis to necrotic dental pulp antigens determined by the release of LIF. J. Endodontol. 4:282, 1978.

Sundqvist, G. K., Eckerbom, M. I., Larsson, A. P., and Sjogren, U. T.: Capacity of anaerobic bacteria from necrotic dental pulps to induce purulent infections. Infect. Immun. 25:685, 1979.

Torabinejad, M., Eby, W. C., and Naidorf, I. J.: Inflammatory and immunological aspects of the pathogenesis of human periapical lesions. J. Endodontol. 11:479, 1985.

Trenstad, L., Barnett, F., Flax, M., and Slots, J.: Anaerobic bacteria in periapical lesions of human teeth. J. Endodontol. 12:131, 1986.

Trowbridge, H., and Daniels, T.: Abnormal immune

response to the infection of the dental pulp. Oral Surg. 43:902, 1977.

van Winkelhoff, A. J., Kippuw, N., and de Graaff, J.: Serologic characterization of black-pigmented *Bacteroides endodontalis*. Infect. Immun. 51:972, 1986.

Williams, B. L., McCann, G. F., and Schoenknecht, F.

D.: Bacteriology of dental abscesses of endodontic origin. J. Clin. Microbiol. 18:770, 1983.

Zavistocki, J., Dzink, J., Onderdonk, A., and Bartlett, J. G.: Quantitative bacteriology of endodontic infections. Oral Surg. 49:171, 1980.

chapter 31

Medical infections of interest

Russell J. Nisengard, D.D.S., Ph.D. □ *Joseph Zambon, D.D.S., Ph.D.*
Michael G. Newman, D.D.S.

CHAPTER OUTLINE

- SYSTEMIC DISEASES CAUSED BY ORAL BACTERIA
- SYSTEMIC DISEASES WITH MULTIPLE ETIOLOGIES

Many systemic infections of medical importance have been described throughout this text. Two facets not adequately discussed elsewhere are systemic diseases caused by oral microorganisms and systemic diseases that can be caused by more than one pathogen.

Systemic Diseases Caused by Oral Bacteria

Many oral, indigenous bacteria have significant pathogenic capabilities. Infections and tissue destruction can result from (1) direct effects of bacteria on the tissues including bacterial cell surface constituents, enzymes, toxins, and invasive ability; and (2) indirect effects on the host immune system by microbial factors. When oral microorganisms gain access to other locations of the body, they no longer are held in check by the complex oral ecology and may produce disease. Among the more significant systemic diseases caused by the oral flora are subacute bacterial endocarditis, infections in joints, abscesses, and human bite infections.

SUBACUTE BACTERIAL ENDOCARDITIS

Subacute bacterial endocarditis (SBE) is a potentially life-threatening heart disease resulting from bacterial colonization of previously damaged heart tissues, particularly the valves. Conditions predisposing to SBE include rheumatic fever when there has been cardiac damage, congenital heart disease including ventricular septum defects, mitral valve prolapse when there is insufficiency, aortic stenosis and persistent ductus arteriosus, prosthetic heart valves, and previous endocarditis. Patients with vascular grafts are sometimes at risk as well.

The oral cavity is the most common source for the bacterial colonization of the heart in SBE. Bacteremias usually occur following dental procedures that cause bleeding, such as scaling and root planing, extractions, gum surgery, endodontic therapy, biopsies, and impressions for crowns and bridges. The relatively high numbers of bacteria that gain entrance to the alveolar blood and circulate throughout the body are usually eliminated by the host defenses. However, in patients with predisposing factors that have damaged the heart tissue, the bacteria can rapidly colonize, leading to SBE.

Bacteremias can also occur, although quantitatively less, following toothbrushing and chewing hard substances, particularly in patients with periodontal disease. While brushing and chewing have not been reported to cause SBE, the risk should be minimized by preventing and controlling periodontal disease in patients with predisposing factors for SBE.

Several microorganisms have been identified as causing SBE. These include the alpha-hemolytic streptococci or viridens group of streptococci (*Streptococcus mitior, Streptococcus sanguis* and *Streptococcus mutans*), *Staphylococcus epidermidis*, and *Actinobacillus actinomycetemcomitans*. *A. actinomycetemcomitans*, a known pathogen in periodontal disease, has only recently been identified as a causative agent in SBE. There are now more than 60 reported cases of SBE caused by this organism, including at least two cases in patients who were taking penicillin, the usual antibiotic for prevention of SBE. SBE caused by *Staphylococcus epidermidis* is more common in intravenous drug users.

Bacterial factors allow adherence to heart tissue with colonization and rapid growth. At times, bacterial aggregates or emboli break away from the colonized heart tissue and lodge in other organs, leading to further systemic complications. In SBE, death results from heart failure, hemorrhage, and emboli affecting other organs.

As in many other diseases, prevention of SBE is far easier and simpler than its treatment. Patients with predisposing factors for SBE should be prophylactically premedicated with an antibiotic prior to any dental treatment in which the gingival tissue is manipulated so that there may be some bleeding. The antibiotic of choice is penicillin and, in patients allergic to this drug, erythromycin (see Chapter 33).

Patients who have localized juvenile periodontitis (LJP), and others with *A. actinomycetemcomitans* infections, should be managed differently if they are at risk of developing SBE. These patients have two types of bacteria that are capable of causing SBE: gram-positive bacteria that are usually sensitive to penicillin and gram-negative bacteria that are usually resistant to penicillin. In these cases, it is recommended that patients first be given tetracycline for several weeks to suppress the *A. actinomycetemcomitans*. This is then followed by the usual prophylactic regimen of penicillin, starting 1 hour before the dental procedure.

INFECTIONS IN JOINT IMPLANTS FOLLOWING DENTAL PROCEDURES

Joint replacements, particularly of the hip, are increasingly common and must be considered prior to any dental treatment in which there may be bleeding leading to bacteremias. As with damaged heart tissue, joint replacement sites are prone to bacterial colonization, infection, and subsequent injury. Such infections are often difficult to treat and may lead to crippling.

Patients with hip replacements who will undergo dental procedures in which bacteremias may occur require prophylactic antibiotics to prevent joint infections. The current practice is to use the same antibiotic regimen employed for prevention of SBE.

ABSCESSES

Aspirating dental materials contaminated by the septic oral environment (including saliva and plaque) into the lungs can lead to lung abscesses. Pieces of fillings or crowns that are inadvertently aspirated can be responsible for severe, sometimes life-threatening, lung infections. These are often caused by the gram-negative, subgingival, anaerobic bacteria including *Bacteroides* species, *Actinobacillus actinomycetemcomitans*, *Actinomyces* species, and *Eikinella corrodens*.

Abscesses of this type are best prevented by exercising caution when performing dental procedures. At times, rubber dams and gauze can aid in blocking the posterior part of the oral pharynx. Usually, swallowing of dental materials is of no consequence. However, if aspiration of a crown or filling is suspected, the patient should immediately be referred to a hospital emergency room, where radiographs of the lungs should be taken to confirm the aspiration. If confirmed, antibiotics are usually immediately given as a prophylactic measure.

A. actinomycetemcomitans can cause other extraoral infections in addition to abscesses of the lungs, including thyroid gland abscesses, urinary tract infections, brain abscesses, and vertebral osteomyelitis. These extraoral infections occur as a result of both direct and hematogenous transmission of bacteria residing in the oral cavity.

INFECTIONS AS A RESULT OF HUMAN BITES

Infections of hands, fingers, and other tissues can result from exposure of cuts to the oral flora. Bites, particularly human bites, leading to puncture wounds, fights with blows to the mouth causing abrasions and cuts on hands, fingernail biting, and inadvertent oral exposure of previous cuts on the hands of dental practitioners during dental treatment can all cause infections.

The causative agents in these types of traumatic infections are generally considered to be anaerobic microorganisms. As expected with the complex flora in the mouth, many infections are mixed infections involving more than one organism. Anaerobes isolated include *Bacteroides, Clostridium, Fusobacterium, Arachnia,* and *Peptostreptococcus*; aerobes isolated include staphylococci, streptococci, and diphtheroids.

The pathogenicity of oral bacteria has been demonstrated in studies of periodontal disease. Human plaque subcutaneously injected into experimental animals can cause a transmissible, mixed anaerobic infection mainly involving gram-negative bacteria. These infections are sometimes fulminating, causing death.

Because of the pathogenicity of the oral flora, lesions resulting from bites and related trauma should be immediately treated. The area should be thoroughly washed and debrided and a topical antibiotic or antiseptic applied. Depending on the depth of the wound, a systemic antibiotic may also be considered. Preventive measures, particularly the use of gloves, should be employed by dental personnel with cuts on their hands.

Systemic Diseases with Multiple Etiologies

Many systemic diseases can be caused by more than one microorganism. The practitioner must recognize this in the differential diagnosis and ultimate treatment of a dis-

Table 31–1 ■ Microorganisms associated with venereal disease

Neisseria gonorrhoeae
Treponema pallidum
Chlamydia trachomatis
Haemophilus ducreyi
Herpesvirus type 2

Table 31–2 ■ Microorganisms associated with meningitis

Neisseria meningitidis
Haemophilus influenzae
Streptococcus pneumoniae
Group B streptococci
Escherichia coli

ease. This section focuses on five of the diseases with multiple etiologies: venereal disease, meningitis, food poisoning, pneumonia and osteomyelitis. The predominant organisms causing these diseases are listed, but it should be recognized that other bacteria have occasionally been associated with these diseases.

VENEREAL DISEASE

Venereal diseases are a group of diseases transmitted by direct genital-to-genital, genital-to-oral, or oral-to-oral routes. These include both bacterial and viral agents (Table 31–1). While not considered a venereal disease in the classic sense of transmission by contact with a lesion, the AIDS virus, or HTLV III, should be included.

MENINGITIS

Meningitis, a sometimes life-threatening disease of the nervous system, can also be caused by several microorganisms (Table 31–2). Commonly, meningitis follows pharyngitis or a sore throat.

FOOD POISONING

Food poisoning can occur immediately or several hours after ingestion of contaminated food containing high concentrations of bacterial toxins. Depending on the organism and degree of contamination, the disease may be

Table 31–3 ■ Microorganisms associated with food poisoning

Clostridium perfringens
Staphylococcus aureus
Vibrio cholerae
Escherichia coli
Vibrio parahaemolyticus
Bacillus cereus

relatively mild with nausea and vomiting, or it may lead to death. Several bacteria are associated with food poisoning (Table 31–3). The most common form of food poisoning occurs following ingestion of poorly refrigerated foods leading to bacterial growth. An example would be food containing dairy products that has been left in the sun for several hours. More recently, raw or incompletely cooked meat and fish or improperly canned foods have been implicated.

PNEUMONIA

A large number of bacteria, including some oral bacteria, can cause pneumonia (Table 31–4). Because both gram-positive and gram-negative organisms may be involved, cultural identification is necessary prior to effective treatment.

Table 31–4 ■ Microorganisms associated with pneumonia

Streptococcus pneumoniae
Staphylococcus aureus
Klebsiella pneumoniae
Proteus spp.
Pseudomonas aeruginosa
Escherichia coli
Serratia spp.
Actinobacillus actinomycetemcomitans and other anaerobes

Table 31–5 ■ Microorganisms associated with osteomyelitis

Staphylococcus aureus
β-hemolytic streptococci
Haemophilus influenzae
Escherichia coli
Pseudomonas spp.

OSTEOMYELITIS

Osteomyelitis or infections of the bone can also be caused by several microorganisms (Table 31–5). This disease is particularly difficult to treat and often amputation is necessary. Many patients continue to harbor bacteria for months or years after clinical healing, which may eventually lead to reactivation of the infection. Patients with compromised resistance to infections, such as those with diabetes, are more prone to develop osteomyelitis.

REFERENCES

Ciancio, S. G., and Bourgault, P. C.: Clinical pharmacology for dental professionals. PSG Publishing, Littleton, MA, 1984, p. 361.
Finegold, A. M.: Anaerobic bacteria in human disease. Academic Press, New York, pp. 428–432, 1977.
O'Connell, C. J.: Microbiology in the practice of medicine. In Milgram, F., and Flanagan, T. D. (eds.): Medical Microbiology. Churchill-Livingstone, New York, 1982, pp. 697–716.

section V

Applied microbiology and immunology

V

chapter 32

Sterilization and asepsis

W. Eugene Rathbun, D.D.S., Ph.D.

All dental health care workers including dentists, hygienists, assistants, and laboratory personnel are frequently exposed to life-threatening microorganisms. Practicing the current methods of sterilization and asepsis in the dental office and laboratory will significantly decrease the risk of infectious disease for the patient, dentist, and staff.

It is worthwhile noting that concern about the transmission of disease has been expressed for thousands of years. Written guidelines for "disease control" are found in the Bible, especially in the books of Leviticus and Numbers. The Israelites were required to follow principles of heat sterilization, hand washing, and isolation. Early records indicated the use of chemicals for wound-cleansing hygiene and methods of food preservation.

More effective chemical disinfectants began to be used in the mid-19th century with the use of iodine as a wound dressing by Davies in 1839. Chlorine water was introduced by LeFerne in 1843 and used by Sammelweis, who in 1847 began using chlorinated lime to dramatically reduce the incidence of childbirth infections. Heat sterilization by using heated water in a pressurized vessel was first utilized in 1832 by William Henry.

The field of asepsis and sterilization has undergone considerable growth and development in the last 100 years with the discovery of numerous chemical and physical agents and barrier techniques to prevent the transmission of infective organisms from patient to patient or to the staff.

The major impetus for the current interest in the science and the art of asepsis has been the concern about hepatitis B beginning in the early 1970s and the AIDS and ARC epidemic in the 1980s. The public as well as the health professionals are now clearly aware of dangers of nosocomial infection, and patients are frequently demanding new standards of care for their protection.

The "standard of care" now includes the uniform wearing of gloves, instrument sterilization, and unprecedented needs for awareness and frequent educational updates in this critical area.

The goals of this chapter are to develop an awareness of diseases that may be transmitted in the dental environment and the present methods of sterilization, disinfection, and asepsis that will help students and practitioners develop a safe, efficient, and medico-legally acceptable clinical practice.

Infectious Diseases

Many infectious diseases may result from dental care. It is a goal of dental and medical practice to, first of all, do no harm. It is in the arena of "infection control" that we may prevent serious infections and even death that could result from less careful attention to the critical details of dental asepsis. Many sources of potential infection exist in the dental office (Fig. 32–1). Hands, saliva, nasal secretions, blood, dust, clothing, and hair as well as dental instruments and equipment all need to be studied in order to minimize the risk of disease to the patients, the doctor, and staff. Briefly, we must consider some common situations.

Contamination of the oral cavity or open wounds may be caused by organisms that are airborne, aerosol, respiratory secretion, splatter, and dustborne; and those found on contaminated hands, instruments, or dental supplies. The patient's microorganisms may be transmitted to the clinician and staff by aerosols; splatters or droplets; respiratory secretions; and plaque, calculus, tooth restorative materials, and debris. The patient's pathogenic oral flora may be transmitted to other tissues or organs ("**autogenous infection**") such as susceptible heart valves, artificial joints, and adjacent soft tissue or bone.

Prevention and Control of Autogenous Infections

HISTORY

Patients with a history of rheumatic heart disease, endocarditis, mitral valve prolapse, heart murmur, heart valve prosthesis, or joint prosthesis are especially susceptible to infection. Prophylactic antibiotics as recommended by the American Dental Association and the American Heart Association should be given in consultation with the patient's physician whenever the treatment will cause bleeding, especially prophylaxis and surgery. Although the risk of infective endocarditis or arthritis is minimized by using appropriate antibiotics, it is apparent that a wide range of bacteria and fungi may infect the damaged heart valve or joint, leading to infection. Patients should be carefully instructed to contact their dentist and physician should any change in their health occur following dental care. Topical antibacterial therapy is frequently recommended for these susceptible patients prior to dental treatment. These

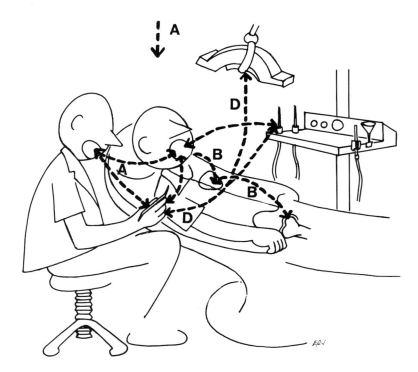

Figure 32–1 ■ Examples of sources of infection in the dental operatory. *A*, Airborne—aerosols, secretions; *B*, bloodborne—autogenous: to heart valves or joint prosthesis; *D*, direct contact—blood and saliva or hand pieces, instruments, charts, telephones, and so on.

may include plaque removal by the patient or staff, or both, and vigorous mouth rinsing with an antimicrobial such as chlorhexidine gluconate or an aqueous solution of povidone iodine. Before administering local anesthesia and before surgery the mucosa should be wiped with 0.12 percent chlorhexidine gluconate or 0.5 to 1 percent povidone iodine.

Patients with a history of diabetes or immunodeficiency should be treated after consultation with their physician to minimize their risk of infection.

Bacterial or fungal infections following dental therapy require careful diagnosis and therapy. Laboratory aerobic and anaerobic culture and antibiotic sensitivity determination are frequently necessary. In the case of infective endocarditis or infective arthritis, hospitalization and intense prolonged care are often required. The infected valve or joint may need to be replaced surgically. The diagnosis of endocarditis is often not made for several weeks to months after the infection begins, and the mortality approaches 30 percent.

Cross Infections

The dentist, staff, and patients are at significant risk of being exposed to pathogenic bacteria, viruses, and fungi as a consequence of dental treatment. Table 32–1 summarizes some of the principal pathogenic agents and the diseases that they may produce.

HEPATITIS B

The most serious pathogen of consequence to the practicing dentist is hepatitis B (see Chapter 22). Hepatitis B produces the most significant illness, practice disruption, and death of any of the pathogenic agents known to be transmitted in dentistry. Numerous surveys and studies have shown that the incidence of hepatitis B developing after accidental exposure by cuts with sharp instruments or needle stick from a hepatitis BsAg–positive patient is approximately 20 percent compared with an estimate of 0 to 1.65 percent following a similar exposure to the AIDS virus. There have been numerous reports on the prevalence of antibodies to hepatitis B among general dentists ranging from 12.9 percent in 1976 to 30 percent in 1984. The prevalence of HBV carrier states for dentists and dental students has been reported by numerous authors from 0.8 to 3.9 percent.

Studies indicate that for dentists the risk for acquiring hepatitis B is six times that of

Table 32–1 ■ Representative cross-infections in dentistry

Agent/Disease	Routes	Incubation Period	Estimated Survival at Room Temperature
Bacterial			
Mycobacterium tuberculosis	Saliva Sputum	To 6 mo	Months
Staphylococcus aureus Staphylococcal infections	Saliva Exudates Skin	4–10 days	Days
Streptococcus pyogenes Streptococcal Wound infections Endocarditis	Open wound Blood-borne	1 day–1 wk	Hours–days
Treponema pallidum Syphilis	Direct contact with lesions	1–10 wk	Seconds
Viral			
Respiratory viruses Flu, colds	Saliva Secretions	1–14 days	Hours
Hepatitis A virus Hepatitis A	Blood Feces Saliva	2–6 wk	Days
Hepatitis B virus Hepatitis B	Blood Saliva Semen	6 wk–6 mo	Months
HIV, formerly HTLV III/LAV AIDS, ARC	Blood, Semen Secretions	To 10 yr	Days
Herpes simplex I and II Recurrent herpes Whitlow Conjunctivitis	Saliva Secretions	2 wk	Minutes

(Adapted from Crawford, 1986, p. 23.)

the general population. That risk seems to be related to the frequency of contact with patients' blood. Dental hygienists show a slightly lower prevalence than general dentists, followed by laboratory technicians, dental assistants, and dental clerical workers.

There have been at least nine reported outbreaks of patients involving from 3 to 53 cases with hepatitis B following previous inoculation by hepatitis B carrier dentists. In one outbreak, 2 of 27 patients died of fulminating hepatitis and one patient was paralyzed. Most often the dentist was not aware of his or her hepatitis B exposure, illness, or carrier status. The potential loss for the dentist who is infected with hepatitis B is devastating in terms of the health, practice, and financial challenges that will have to be faced. The usual time lost from practice is 2 to 3 months.

Pre-exposure active immunization against hepatitis B is strongly recommended using Heptavax B (Merck, Sharp and Dohme). If possible, this should be accomplished at the beginning of professional education. Heptavax B immunization requires a series of three intramuscular injections in the arm, at 0 time, 30 days, and 180 days. It is recommended that immunized persons be tested after the series to determine that immunization has been effective. The vaccine has been proven to be very safe and is approximately 96 percent effective.

Summarized CDC guidelines for postexposure immunization against hepatitis B follow.

Inoculation from known HBsAg-positive patient ■ Immediately administer HBIG (hepatitis B immune globulin) and initiate active immunization (Heptavax B).

Inoculation from a "high-risk population" patient (Table 32–2) ■ Test the patient for HBsAg. If positive, administer HBIG as soon as possible, preferably within 2 days, and begin active immunization regimen.

Inoculation from a low-risk patient ■ Begin active immunization regimen.

Careful medical histories will usually reveal approximately 20 percent of individuals who have had hepatitis B. It is strongly suggested that all patients be presumed to be active hepatitis B carriers. The ethical, legal, and financial costs of a dentist developing hepatitis B are very serious, including transmission to spouses, vertical transmission to newborn offspring, as well as transmission to patients and staff. Reading and

Table 32–2 ■ Hepatitis B high-risk populations
Health care personnel
Dentists
Physicians and surgeons
Nurses
Paramedical personnel and custodial staff who may be exposed to the virus
Dental hygienists and dental assistants
Laboratory personnel handling blood, blood products, and other patient samples
Dental, medical, and nursing students
Dental laboratory technicians
Selected patients and patient contacts
Patients and staff in hemodialysis units and hematology-oncology units
Patients requiring frequent or large-volume blood transfusion or clotting-factor concentrates (for example, persons with hemophilia, thalassemia)
Clients (residents) and staff of institutions for the mentally handicapped
Classroom contacts or deinstitutionalized mentally handicapped persons with persistent hepatitis B antigenemia
Household and other intimate contacts of persons with persistent hepatitis B antigenemia
Newborns of HbsAg-carrier mothers
Populations with high incidence of the disease
Alaskan natives
Indo-Chinese refugees
Haitian refugees
Native Pacific Islanders
Sub-Saharan Africans
Certain military personnel
Morticians and embalmers
Blood bank and plasma fractionation workers
Persons at increased risk of diseases because of sexual practices
Persons who repeatedly contract sexually transmitted diseases
Female prostitutes
Prisoners
Users of illicit injectable drugs
International travelers

(From Cottone, J., 1986, p. 12, with permission.)

heeding the frequent recommendations from the CDC and the ADA will be very helpful in avoiding disastrous medical and legal complications. Please note the recommendations of the CDC in Table 32–3.

HERPES

Herpes simplex viruses I and II are frequently in the mouth of dental patients and may lead to serious infection for the dentist or staff. (See Chapter 22.) The most serious infection, "ocular herpes," may lead to blindness. Another troublesome herpes infection is a viral whitlow of the operator's finger

Table 32–3 ■ Recommendations for hepatitis B surface antigen-positive health care personnel not known to have transmitted hepatitis B

Understand the modes of transmission of hepatitis B

Wash (but do not scrub) hands before direct contact with patients

Wear gloves
1. For all patient procedures involving trauma to skin or mucosal surfaces
2. For all direct contact with open wounds
3. For all patient contact if any dermatitis, wounds, or other skin lesions are present on the hands

Retest for hepatitis B surface antigen and hepatitis B e antigen-antibody every 6 to 12 mo

Wear gloves and exercise extreme care in handling sharp instruments for all surgical procedures

Informed consent or surveillance activities are generally not required

If a contaminative incident occurs, exposed patient should be given hepatitis B immune globulin (0.06 ml/kg IM)

Investigation by state health department if any apparent transmission to patient occurs

(From Cottone, J., 1986, pp. 16, with permission.)

causing severe pain on pressure and inability to practice dentistry.

There was one report of 20 patients with herpes gingivostomatitis having been infected by a dental hygienist with herpes simplex virus I infection on her fingers. Most of these patients developed serious illnesses, and each lost several days of work or school.

AIDS

Infection by human immunodeficiency virus (HIV), formerly HTLV III/LAV, is extremely serious (see Chapter 22) and for those individuals who develop AIDS it is uniformly fatal. The AIDS "epidemic" has generated a great deal of research, politics, and interest in "dental asepsis." Since 1985 large numbers of dentists have rethought and updated their asepsis programs to protect their patients, themselves, and their practices. Even the best informed and conscientious practitioners are challenged by the fact that hepatitis B and AIDS follow very long incubation periods and most infected individuals are not identifiable. In the several studies underway and reported to date the incidence of infection following needle stick or cut with HIV-infected blood or serum is 0 to 1.65 percent. The fact that many AIDS and ARC (AIDS-related complex) patients have oral symptoms and diseases make it manda-

tory that the whole dental profession be prepared technically and emotionally to serve those individuals. It is estimated by the CDC that by the end of 1991 in the United States alone there may be up to 270,000 patients who have suffered from AIDS; this is compared with approximately 48,139 as of December 30, 1987. Although at present 90 percent of AIDS victims are from the highest risk groups of homosexual/bisexual men and intravenous drug users, it is feared that increasing heterosexual contacts will change the percentages to increase the number affected in the general United States population. Although the number of HIV viruses per milliliter of infected blood is 10,000 to 1 million times less than in hepatitis B, there will be great distress among those dentists who puncture themselves while treating any AIDS patient or who refuse to wear gloves during treatment and later discover that their patient had AIDS.

The ADA and CDC as of May 1986 recommended the following infection control procedures be used routinely to minimize the risk of transmitting AIDS and other infectious diseases from patients to dental personnel or from patient to patient through the dental office:

1. Gloves should be worn in treating all patients.

2. Masks should be worn to protect oral and nasal mucosa from splatter of blood and saliva.

3. Eyes should be protected with some type of covering to protect from splatter of blood and saliva.

4. Sterilization methods known to kill all life forms should be used on dental instruments. These include steam autoclave, dry heat oven, chemical vapor sterilizers, and chemical sterilants.

5. Attention should be given to clean-up of instruments and surfaces in the operatory. This includes scrubbing with detergent solutions and wiping down surfaces with iodine or chlorine (diluted household bleach) solutions.

6. Contaminated disposable material should be handled carefully and discarded in plastic bags to minimize human contact. Sharp items such as needles and scalpel blades should be contained in puncture-resistant containers prior to disposal in the plastic bags.

The definitions in Table 32–4 will be useful in understanding the material that follows.

Table 32–4 ■ Definitions

Antiseptics:	Agents that prevent the growth or action of microorganisms on living tissue.
Asepsis:	(1) The opposite of sepsis, i.e., freedom from infection. (2) The prevention of contact with pathogens. In dentistry this includes the techniques of barrier protection, sterilization, and disinfection.
Cold sterilization:	Sterilization at room temperature usually with an aqueous solution of a chemical. This type of sterilization is subject to serious drawbacks including dilution, cutting short the required exposure time, organic contamination, or inactivation.
Cross infections:	The transmission of pathogenic microorganisms from one patient to another.
Disinfectants:	Chemicals capable of killing pathogenic organisms when applied to inanimate objects. Frequently, the range of activity, directions for use, and conditions are cited by the manufacturer on the label.
Disinfection:	The destruction of pathogenic agents by directly applied chemical or physical means.
Nosocomial:	Office or hospital-acquired infections.
Sepsis:	The presence of pathogens in the blood or other tissues.
Sterilization:	The destruction of all life. Practically, sterilization denotes the use of physical or chemical agents to eliminate all viable microorganisms, including bacteria, fungi, viruses, and spores.

Practical Asepsis

An outline of practical asepsis will include barrier techniques, sterilization, disinfection, and monitoring office procedures. In order to be effective the dentist must assume that all patients and dental staff are carriers of hepatitis B or AIDS.

Discussing the topic of environmental contamination more than 100 years ago, Joseph Lister remarked that "you must be able to see (the contamination) with your mental eye as distinctly as with the corporeal eye." No asepsis program will reach its maximal effectiveness without the exercise of this ability.

Many have found it helpful to practice their disinfection procedures by pretending that saliva is red. By touching all instruments, charts, chairs, equipment, cabinets, telephones, pens, and other objects that would normally be handled when working on a patient, with a "harmless" red poster paint one can gain an appreciation of the extent of the need for disinfection. Many dental schools have slides or videotapes of this type of procedure that are available for loan.

PERSONAL ASEPSIS

Hands

The major route of transmission of respiratory and oral microorganisms is by the hands. It is recommended that nails be kept short and that all rings and bracelets be removed prior to patient contact. Before the first patient contact clean hands thoroughly with a brush and hand cleaning "soap." Lather and rinse a total of three times using cool water, and dry with disposable paper towels. Each hand scrubbing should take at least 10 seconds.

Sinks are now available that have either foot-operated or "electronic eye"–operated faucets to break the cycle of contaminating the faucet when turning the water on and off (Fig. 32–2). As an alternative, a paper towel may be used to adjust or to turn off the flow of water.

Hand cleansers are available containing a number of antimicrobial agents and other ingredients. Iodophors (about 1 percent iodine), chlorhexidine gluconate (4 percent), parachlorometa-xylenol (PCMX) (0.5 to 3 percent), and alcohols (i.e., 70 percent isopropyl alcohol foam) are ingredients in available preparations.

Several of the commercially available products should be tried to determine which combination is practical and acceptable for each office situation. One might choose a broad-spectrum antiseptic such as one containing Chlorhexidine iodophor for the first scrub of the day, before and after lunch, before leaving for the day, and when treating a high-risk patient. A less effective hand soap may be used between regular patient visits.

The ADA and CDC recommend that "for protection of personnel and patients, gloves must always be worn when touching blood, saliva, or mucous membranes. Gloves must be worn by dental health care workers (DHCWs) when touching blood-soiled items, body fluids, or secretions, as well as surfaces contaminated by them. Gloves must be worn when examining all oral lesions. All work

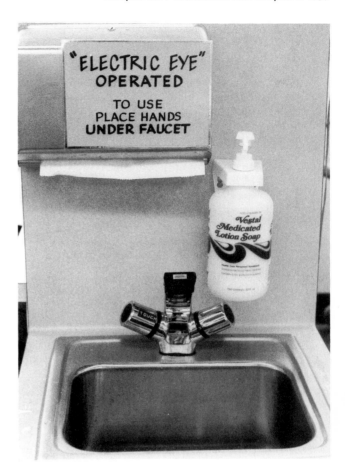

Figure 32–2 ■ "Electronic eye"–operated faucet.

must be completed on one patient, when possible, and the hands must be washed and regloved before performing procedures on another patient (Fig. 32–3). Repeated use of a single pair of gloves is *not* recommended, since such use is likely to produce defects in the glove material, which will diminish its value as an effective barrier."

Most individuals are able to use latex gloves of the many different available sizes and brands. Hypoallergenic gloves and various plastic gloves are available for those who develop allergies to the typical latex gloves.

It is further recommended that heavier utility gloves be used when disinfecting the operatory or when handling infected instru-

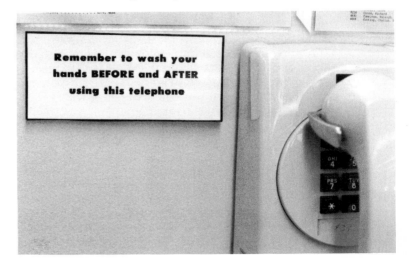

Figure 32–3 ■ Wash hands before and after using the telephone.

ments or debris. Remember to wash your hands with a broad-spectrum cleanser before leaving for lunch or before going home at the end of the day. Hands should be washed after removing gloves between patients to cleanse the hands of skin bacteria and possible contamination if the gloves were cut or punctured during treatment. The bacteria that entered the defect may multiply rapidly and will need to be removed before putting on a new pair of gloves for the next patient.

Dental health care workers who have exudative lesions or weeping dermatitis should refrain from all direct patient care and from handling dental patient-care equipment until the condition resolves.

Facial Protection

Protect your face using surgical masks and protective eyewear or chin-length plastic shields when splashing or splattering of blood or other body fluids is possible. This would include during rinsing, polishing, scaling, the use of ultrasonic or sonic scaling, and the use of rotary burs or stones with either high- or low-speed handpieces. Masks should also be worn whenever the operator or patient has a respiratory infection. Masks should be discarded when wet or after approximately 1 hour of use.

Either tied or formed masks are effective at reducing the risks of aerosol or splatter. There are significant differences between brands and types as to fit and comfort. Choose a style and brand that feels good to your face. It is a good idea to wash your glasses or protective eyewear frequently and at least before leaving the office to decrease the likelihood of taking pathogens home to your friends or family.

The use of high-velocity evacuation greatly decreases the amount of aerosols and splatter. These may be further reduced by using a rubber dam whenever possible. Contamination will be further reduced if patients thoroughly remove their plaque with a brush and floss and then rinse with a broad-spectrum mouthwash such as chlorhexidine gluconate (0.12 percent) or povidone iodine (0.5 to 1 percent).

Clothing and Hair

Reusable and disposable gowns, laboratory coats, or uniforms must be worn when clothing may be soiled with blood of other body fluids such as saliva. If reusable gowns are worn, they should be washed in hot water with a detergent and chlorine bleach. Gowns should be changed at least daily or when visibly soiled with blood. Contaminated office clothing should not be worn at home; wearing infected clothing is especially hazardous to children and other family members. Hair should be kept away from the treatment field. A hair covering protects the hair from splatter and aerosols. It is a good idea to wash your face before going to lunch and to wash your face and hair before bed. Pathogenic bacteria and some viruses, particularly hepatitis B virus, can survive for days to weeks on clothing.

OPERATORY ASEPSIS

The general rule to follow in operatory asepsis is: What you do not contaminate does not need to be disinfected or sterilized.

During the course of treatment many objects, surfaces, instruments, and equipment become contaminated either directly by hands or via splatter and aerosols. Remember "if saliva were red." Decide as a staff what objects are necessary in the operatory or treatment room and then decide which can be (a) covered, (b) sterilized, and what must be (c) disinfected (the poorest choice). Have a plan as to when floors and other horizontal flat surfaces need to be cleaned and disinfected, whether daily or weekly. Horizontal surfaces at or below the operatory field are subject to considerably more contamination than are vertical surfaces.

Coverings

The most useful and simple coverings are paper, plastic, and foil that has been cut into the desired shape before use and stored where they will remain clean. Covers eliminate contaminating surfaces that then have to be disinfected. A new cover is used for each patient. Some useful covers are as follows:

1. Cover the instrument tray with a plastic backed patient bib, or with plastic film to reduce contamination of the tray and cart or table. Place a paper tray cover, if desired, over the bib. Arrange the instruments and supplies. After the procedure the instruments can be removed to the "clean-up" area wrapped in the bib or plastic cover.

2. Cover x-ray cone and head with plastic wrap or paper secured with tape.

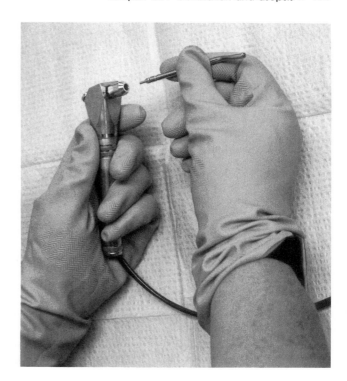

Figure 32–4 ■ Replaceable triplex syringe tips.

3. Cover switches and controls, when possible, with plastic secured by double-faced type or with small pieces of aluminum foil.

4. Cover the headrest with plastic or paper covers or bags to reduce transfer of bacteria, viruses, fungi, mites, and so on.

5. Triplex (air/water) syringes may be covered with small (2-inch by 6-inch) plastic bags to save a great deal of cleaning time. This is especially helpful when using cements and impression materials. Replaceable, sterilizable triplex syringe tips are available for most syringes (Fig. 32–4).

6. High-velocity vacuum valves and hose can be covered with a 2-inch by 6-inch (or larger) plastic bag slit in the end for insertion of the vacuum tip (Fig. 32–5).

7. Lamp handles can be covered with foil, paper, or 4-inch by 4-inch gauze sponges. Sterilizable lamp handles are available for some units (Fig. 32–6).

8. Light "guns" for curing composite restorations can be covered by wrapping the tip with plastic wrap secured with masking tape. Similarly, the handle and control trigger can be covered with plastic wrap (Fig. 32–7).

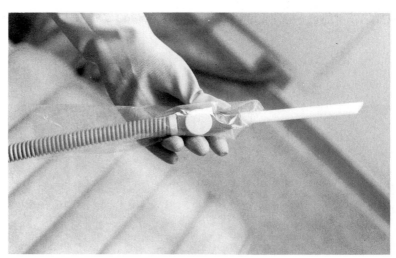

Figure 32–5 ■ Cover difficult to clean high-velocity vacuum valve.

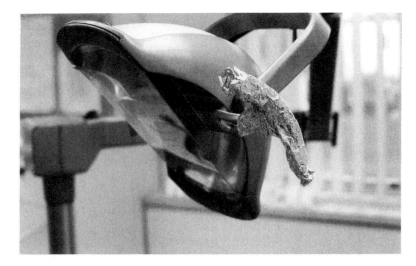

Figure 32–6 ■ Cover light handles with foil.

9. For high-risk patients, cabinet surfaces may be covered with paper or plastic sheeting and the unit and chair individually wrapped in large clear bags with only the necessary handpieces and syringes open to contamination.

What you do not cover or remove will have to be disinfected or sterilized. Make it easier on your staff! With proper planning and covers, an operatory can be disinfected in less than 5 minutes.

SURFACE DISINFECTION

Disinfectants are chemicals capable of destroying pathogens on inanimate objects. It is frequently useful to separate the disinfectants according to their efficacy in killing certain groups of organisms: "high-level" disinfectants being synonymous with sterilization; "intermediate-level" meaning capable of destroying all forms of life except bacterial spores; and "low level" destroying such viruses as influenza and herpes but not polio, hepatitis B, or *Mycobacterium tuberculosis* (Table 32–5).

For surface disinfection of operatory surfaces, three disinfectants are commonly used. Each is an effective intermediate level disinfectant when surfaces are kept wet for 5 to 10 minutes.

1. Iodophors may be diluted according to manufacturers' directions. They should be diluted fresh daily in soft or distilled water. Only an iodophor registered as a surface disinfectant by the EPA should be used. These are not to be confused with surgical handscrubs regulated by the FDA and used undiluted. Iodophors (such as Wescodyne

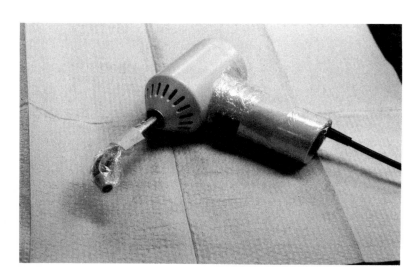

Figure 32–7 ■ Cover composite light-curing "gun" with plastic wrap.

Table 32–5 ■ A comparison of three levels of disinfection and test groups of organisms

| | Bacteria | | | | | Viruses | |
	Gram-positive	Gram-negative	Mycobacterium Tuberculosis	Spores	Fungi	Lipid	Nonlipid
High	+	+	+	+	+	+	+
Intermediate	+	+	+	−	+	+	+
Low	+	+	−	−	±	+	−

(From Crawford, J., 1986, p. 28, with permission.)

and Biocide) are loose complexes of iodine bound to synthetic carriers, such as povidone. In their "tamed" and diluted form, they are still effective disinfectants but are much less liable to stain cloth or plastic.

2. Phenolic derivatives (O-phenyl phenol 9 percent, and O-benzyl-P-chlorophenol 1 percent) as in Dentaseptic, Multicide, and Omni II are diluted 1:32, and at least one product is stable after dilution for 60 days. Other claimed advantages are residual phenolic effect and lack of discoloration of instrumentation or hard surfaces.

3. Sodium hypochlorite (laundry bleach) diluted fresh daily 1:10 to 1:100 is inexpensive and is very effective. It is the recommended surface disinfectant by the CDC for hepatitis B and HIV. Caution should be exercised during use because sodium hypochlorite is corrosive to some metals, particularly aluminum. Sodium hypochlorite has the additional disadvantage of bleaching fabrics and making the office smell like an indoor swimming pool.

Suggested Steps for Surface Disinfection

Scrub items thoroughly and rinse them clean. At best this would utilize a sink, scrub brush, and running water. Otherwise, one may elect to use 4-inch by 4-inch sponges and paper towels.

Wet items or surfaces to be disinfected with the chosen disinfectant, for the time specified by the manufacturer, usually about 10 minutes.

Specific techniques ■ There are two methods to disinfect and prepare the dental unit. *Technique I* (Dr. James Crawford, UNC 1986) utilizes paper towels and a fine-mist spray bottle. Paper towels are cheaper, larger, and faster to use than gauze sponges.

First, put on utility gloves. Remove instruments, tip of air-water syringe, and so forth. Discard any used covers. Wash the gloves.

Second, disinfect smooth surfaces and controls. (Most control switches should not be sprayed directly because excess fluid may cause short circuits.) To do this, moisten a paper towel with disinfectant spray and scrub smooth surfaces and controls. Wipe each item clean. Spray another paper towel and wipe them again, leaving them moist so the disinfectant will continue to act.

Third, hoses and attached instrumentation must be disinfected.

1. Hold a paper towel behind items in the forked holders to catch excess spray. Spray both sides of the items with disinfectant; for example, suction hose ends, air-water syringe handle, any handpieces that cannot be removed and sterilized (Fig. 32–8).

2. Use a clean brush to scrub each item with irregular surfaces, and lay it across the support or empty instrument tray.

3. Spray supports and wipe them clean with a paper towel.

4. Spray another towel and wipe each hose end and attached instrumentation. Wipe each hose along its most accessible length; place it back in its support.

5. When all items are replaced, hold a paper towel behind them to catch excess spray. Spray and leave them wet until they are ready to use. Ten minutes is specified on most labels. (That usually allows enough time for disinfection.) Any items still wet can be dried with a paper towel before use.

6. Moisten a paper towel with disinfectant and wipe the chair, controls, and arms. Leave the chair to dry for the patient.

Fourth, disinfect trays and lamp handles. To do this, wipe trays clean and dry and cover with film backed covers. Place foil or film covers on the lamp handles. (There is no need to disinfect anything that has been covered.) Spray and clean outside, then inside of cuspidor. Wash gloves, disinfect faucet handles, remove gloves, and wash hands.

The final step to remember is, after each appointment, put on utility gloves; remove instruments, tip of air-water syringe, and so on; discard any used covers; wash gloves;

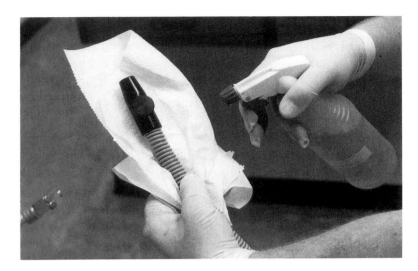

Figure 32–8 ■ Example of surface disinfection of suction hose end using spray mist technique.

and clean the unit as described. Do *not* replace covers when vacating the unit.

In *Technique II* three-by-three-inch or four-by-four-inch gauze sponges wet with disinfectant solution are used. Gauze sponges can be soaked ahead in solution of Omni II but not iodophor (Wescodyne-D or Biocide). Put on "heavy-duty" utility gloves, and remove instruments, tip of air-water syringe, and other such items. Discard any used covers; wash gloves. Next, moisten each item and surface to be disinfected, and scrub or brush to remove all debris. Remove each syringe, handpiece, and the vacuum hose from its holder to clean forks (Fig. 32–9). Then, with a second four-by-four-inch soaked sponge, thoroughly wet the items and leave wet for the required time. Some clinicians like to wrap gauze around the item to be disinfected until needed for the next patient. After each

appointment, put on utility gloves, remove instruments, tip of air-water syringe, and so on. Discard any used covers, wash gloves, and clean the unit as described earlier. Do not replace the covers when vacating the unit.

Handpieces and air-water syringe tips are subject to heavy contamination. The preferred method for decontaminating the handpiece and the air-water syringe tip is sterilization. When purchasing equipment, especially hand pieces, choose heat sterilizable units. All handpiece manufacturers in the United States market handpieces that can be sterilized by either an autoclave 121°C or a chemiclave 132°C, but not usually in dry heat, 160°C.

Units, controls, and hoses of smooth material are much easier to disinfect than those with knurled knobs, recesses, and corruga-

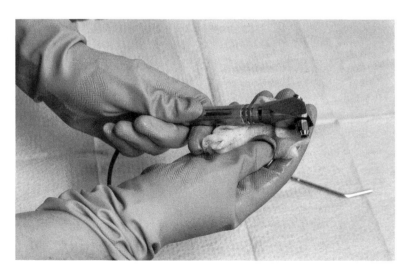

Figure 32–9 ■ Surface disinfection using 4 × 4 sponge to clean and disinfect triplex syringe. *Note* heavy gloves.

tions. Operatory floors of seamless vinyl or a similar product are relatively easy to clean and disinfect, whereas carpet is impossible to clean or disinfect. Dental water systems frequently grow *Pseudomonas aerogenosa* overnight. To reduce their numbers many clinicians flush the water syringe and high-speed handpiece for at least 30 seconds prior to patient contact.

IMPRESSIONS

Laboratory technicians and other patients are frequently exposed to pathogens from dental impressions, stone casts, and appliances. Several recent articles have reported the results of studies on disinfection of various impression materials. One must keep up with the current literature, especially the *Journal of the American Dental Association*, because changes in this area will be frequent.

Table 32–6 describes the effect of disinfectant treatment on cast dimensions. Their results indicate that disinfection of dental impressions by 30-minute immersion in 0.5 percent or 1 percent sodium hypochlorite does not significantly affect the dimensional accuracy of the resultant cases. Other disinfectants such as the gluteraldehydes, povidone iodine, or halogenated phenol had no apparent effect on rubber impression materials. The findings of other authors suggest that such disinfectant is also suitable for rubber-based and vinyl polysiloxane impressions for cast restorations. An alternative to impression disinfection is to sterilize the stone cast in any ethylene oxide sterilizer. At the minimum, impressions should be rinsed carefully of saliva and debris and then immersed for 10 minutes in an approved disinfectant, such as diluted iodophor.

APPLIANCES

Prosthodontic and orthodontic appliances should be disinfected prior to delivery and before and after any laboratory adjustments. The simplest techniques utilize a disposable plastic drinking cup or zip-lock baggie. The appliance is scrubbed free of debris and then immersed in the chosen disinfectant for a minimum of 10 minutes. Ultrasonic cleaning for 3 to 5 minutes will greatly aid the removal of debris of heavily contaminated appliances.

Freshly diluted povidone iodine is the disinfectant most widely recommended. The clinician must be careful to rinse the appliance thoroughly with water prior to delivery.

Rag wheels, felt wheels, points, and bristle brushes can be easily sterilized with the steam autoclave or chemiclave. One should use fresh pumice delivered in a disposable paper or plastic tray and moistened with a disinfectant. After adjustment and polishing the appliances are disinfected, rinsed carefully, and delivered to the patient.

Recommendations for the commercial laboratory are very similar to those for the dental office and are addressed in guidelines published by the ADA in June 1985.

| | Impression Material | | | |
Disinfectant	Alginate (Jeltrate)	Polysulfide (Permalastic)	Polysiloxane (Reflect)	Polyether (Impregum)
0.5% Sodium hypochlorite (Clorox)	NS*	NS	NS	NS
1% Sodium hypochlorite (Clorox)	NS	NS	NS	NS
0.5% Povidone-iodine (Betadine)	Significant difference†	NS	NS	NS
0.13% Neutral glutaraldehyde (Sporicidin)	NS	NS	NS	NS
2% Neutral glutaraldehyde (Glutarex)	Significant difference	NS	NS	NS
0.16% Halogenated phenol (CD-100)	Significant difference	NS	NS	NE*

Table 32–6 ■ Effect of disinfectant treatment on cast dimensions as compared with room temperature controls

*NS denotes no significant difference ($P > .05$), and NE denotes not evaluated.
†Significant differences ($P < .05$) only in the anteroposterior dimensions as compared with room temperature controls.
(From Herrara and Merchant, 1986, with permission.)

Sterilization

All instruments that contract saliva or blood should be sterilized, using ADA-accepted methods of sterilization, before storage or subsequent patient use (Table 32–7). Since 1974, and certainly since the 1985 AIDS "epidemic," the standard of care in the United States is for sterilization according to the ADA/CDC guidelines rather than disinfection. It is considered unethical to ignore the recommendations of the ADA and the CDC; in addition, ignoring those guidelines would leave the practitioner defenseless in court regarding post-treatment infections.

CLEANING

The first requirement for instrument sterilization is the removal of most organic debris, blood, and saliva. Instruments and other reusable items from the operatory are removed to a central cleaning and sterilizing area, where the assistant wears heavy-duty rubber gloves to discard the disposable items and then either to cleanse or to submerge the instruments in a holding disinfecting solution to prevent drying of organic debris before cleaning. Holding for a short period of time (30 to 60 minutes) can be accomplished using iodophors or 70 percent isopropyl alcohol. For longer periods (more than 60 minutes) of time, gluteraldehydes or the newer phenols would be the agents of choice owing to their antirust and disinfectant properties.

Regardless of the decision on holding solutions, thorough cleaning requires the operator to wear heavy rubber gloves and brush visible debris from instruments under running water. Continue cleaning with an ultrasonic cleaner with detergent specifically designed for these cleaners. Ultrasonic cleaning is generally thought to be much safer, efficient, and more effective than handscrubbing (Fig. 32–10). Operate the ultrasonic cleaner with closed cover for at least 5 minutes. Following cleaning, the instruments are rinsed under running water and dried before sterilizing.

The cleansing action of ultrasonic cleaners frequently decreases with time, so it is useful to test its action periodically. Recommended user testing requires filling the ultrasonic cleaner with detergent solution and running the cleaner until it is warmed up. A piece of regular-strength aluminum foil is one-half immersed by holding it vertically into the solution for exactly 20 seconds. It is then inspected for the evidence of minute bubbles and holes in the immersed half of the foil by holding it up to a light. If there are holes or bubbles, the ultrasonic cleaner is still operating efficiently; if not, it needs to be repaired or replaced.

Table 32–7 ■ A comparison of ADA-approved sterilization methods

Method	Steam	Formalin-alcohol Vapor	Dry Heat	Ethylene Oxide	Glutaraldehyde
ACTIVITY	Protein denaturation	Alkylation and protein denaturation	Oxidation	Alkylation	Alkylation
CONDITIONS	121° C (250° F) 15 min; 132° C (270° F) 3–7 min	132° C (270° F) 20 min	160° C (320° F) 30 min	Ambient 36 hr 49° C (120° F) 2–3 hr	20 min ultrasonic to ambient 10 hr depending on product
LIMITATIONS	Rust, corrosion; heat damage to plastics	Heat damage to plastics	Moderately slow; heat damage to plastics	Very slow; porous plastics, etc., require aeration for 1 day or more before use	Postexposure rinsing and handling required; not suitable for packs and cloth goods
ADVANTAGES	Penetrates cloth and surgical packs best	Penetrates paper-wrapped packs, but does not penetrate multicloth drape packs and cloth-wrapped surgical packs	Low price, large capacity	No heat damage to rubber goods	Lack of heat protects plastic goods, fiber optics

(From Crawford, J., 1986, p. 44, with permission.)

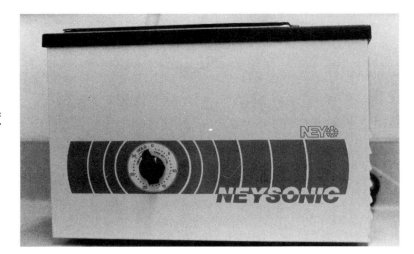

Figure 32–10 ■ Use ultrasonic cleaners to clean instruments prior to sterilizing.

Drying instruments before sterilization is important for proper sterilization function and for rust inhibition.

PACKAGING

Packaging of instruments prior to sterilization depends on the method chosen for sterilization and will be discussed with each methodology. Generally, packaging instruments prior to sterilization is preferred because handling and storage after sterilization is simplified and chances of contamination are minimized. There are numerous systems of instrument packaging including trays and cassettes that fit specific sterilizers and simplify packaging and reuse. Several manufacturers make sterilizing bags and wraps from a variety of materials. Packaging guidelines from the ADA and the sterilizer manufacturers should be followed. The following is a summary of ADA-approved sterilization methods (Table 32–8), from James Crawford's text, *Clinical Asepsis in Dentistry*.

STORAGE

Storing sterilized instruments in packages or packed on trays has several advantages over "loose" storage. The safest, most efficient handling of storage is to use separate packs of instruments for each anticipated procedure. These packs are stored after sterilization in closed cabinets and opened just prior to the procedure. Obtaining and handling of "loose," or cabinet-stored, instruments requires sterile pick-up forceps or two-by-two-inch gauze sponge or paper towel,

being careful not to contaminate doors or drawers.

Disposable items are best stored in covered containers and dispensed in appropriate numbers anticipated for the immediate procedure.

AUTOCLAVE STERILIZATION

The word "autoclave" means self-locking and is used to denote an apparatus that sterilizes by the use of steam under pressure. Autoclaves operate on the same principle as pressure cookers (Fig. 32–11). Saturated steam is a much more efficient means of destroying microorganisms than either boiling water or dry heat. At 100°C there is at least seven times as much available heat from saturated steam as from boiling water. Thus, the presence of air in packages hinders the penetration of steam and delays or prevents sterilization. The following section summarizes the different holding times required for sterilization (Fig. 32–12).

Parameters

The parameters are 121°C (250°F), for 15 minutes, at 15 psi; or 132°C (270°F), for 3 to 7 minutes, at 30 psi for unwrapped instruments. Add 5 minutes for moderately wrapped packs.

Recommended Packaging

The instruments should be packaged either "loose" or wrapped in muslin cloth, paper, nylon, aluminum foil, steam permeable plastic; there should be no impermeable closed containers.

Table 32–8 ■ Guide to chemical agents for disinfection and/or sterilization

Accepted Products	Chemical Classification	Disinfectant Level	Disinfectant	Sterilant	Comments
Wescodyne-D Biocide	Iodophors, 1% Available iodine	Intermediate to high	Diluted according to manufacturer's instructions, 10 min	—	May stain some plastics (fresh daily)
Household Bleach	Sodium hypochlorite	Full strength-high diluted-intermediate	Diluted 1:5 to 1:100 10 to 30 min	—	Chlorine odor (fresh daily) Corrosive—full strength
Dentaseptic Multicide Omni II	0-phenylphenol 9.0% and 0-benzyl p-chlorophenol, 1.0%	Intermediate	Diluted 1:32 10 min at room temperature	—	Mild irritant 60 days diluted self-life
Sporicidin	Glutaraldehyde 2% alkaline with phenolic buffer	Full strength-high diluted intermediate	Diluted 1:16, 10 min at 20° C (68° F)	Full strength 6¾ hr at 20° C (68° F)	Irritating to skin, nose Full strength less so—diluted
Glutarex	Glutaraldehyde 2% neutral	High	Full strength, 10 min at room temperature	Full strength 10 hr at room temperature	Irritating to skin, nose, eyes
Banicide Sterall Wavicide 01	Glutaraldehyde 2% acidic potentiated with nonionic ethoxylates of linear alcohols	Full strength-high diluted-intermediate	Diluted 1:2, 10 min at 25° C (77° F)	Full-strength, 1 hr at 60° C 4 hr at 40 to 50° C, 10 hr at 25° C (77° F)	Irritating to skin, nose, and eyes
Exspor	Chlorine dioxide	High	2 min at room temperature	6 hr at room temperature	Chlorine odor May corrode on long contact
Centra 28, Cidex 7, CoeCide, Germ-X K-Cide 10, Maxicide, Omnicide, Orthocide, Procide, Protec-top Saslow, Sporex, Steril-Ize, Vitacide	Glutaraldehyde 2% alkaline	High	Full strength, 10 min at room temperature	Full strength, 10 hr at room temperature	Irritating to nose, eyes, skin

(From Soloman, A. L., 1986, with permission.)

Advantages

Autoclaving provides the most efficient and reliable sterilization available. Autoclaves are usually quite simple to operate and are relatively inexpensive. Most dental instruments and devices can be safely autoclaved (Table 32–9). Flexibility of packaging, loading and cycles for liquids, and cloth goods are advantageous.

Disadvantages

Nonstainless metal instruments may oxidize (rust) unless protected by a reducing agent or "emulsion" dip prior to packaging and autoclaving. One to 2 percent sodium nitrite is an effective rust inhibitor. (See the ADA's *Accepted Dental Therapeutics*). Low-melting plastics and rubber cups may melt or distort. Items that retain moisture take time to dry, thus extending the cycle time.

Monitoring Autoclave Sterilization

Biologic indicators such as spore strips and glass ampules are available. Process and dosage indicators are also available to indicate processing or gross errors in technique.

DRY HEAT STERILIZATION

When used properly dry heat is an effective and accepted method of instrument ster-

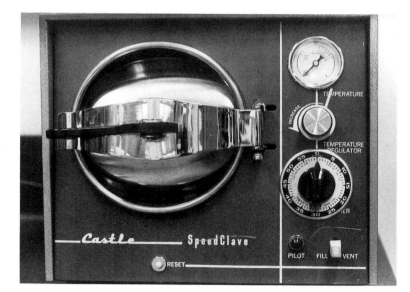

Figure 32–11 ■ Steam autoclave.

ilization. This method requires more time to sterilize owing to warm-up time of the instrument load of from 10 to 90 minutes per cycle.

Ovens are manufactured specifically for medical and dental use (Fig. 32–13). However, a number of commercial, home, laboratory, and industrial ovens will be suitable. Mechanical convection ovens, usually available, provide more even and rapid heating.

The efficiency of dry heat ovens depends mainly on the power available per cubic foot of the chamber. The minimum for a 30-minute warm-up time is 550 watts per cubic foot.

An accurate pyrometer, thermocouple, or thermometer is needed to verify the actual temperatures for determining cycle time.

Parameters

The parameters are as follows: 170°C (340°F) for 60 minutes cycle time, 160°C (320°F) for 120 minutes, and 150°C (300°F) for 150 minutes.

Recommended Packaging and Loading

Instruments should be packaged "loose" (or bare); lightly wrapped with paper or aluminum foil, thus increasing time 45 to 60 minutes; or loaded a finger's space apart for minimum warm-up time.

Advantages

The advantages of this method include large volume capacity, low-cost equipment

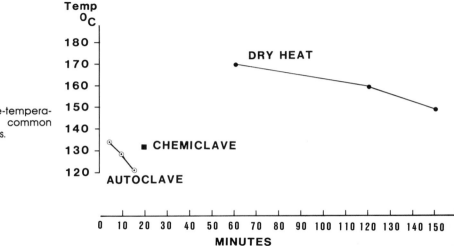

Figure 32–12 ■ Time-temperature comparison of common sterilization techniques.

Table 32–9 ■ Sterilization and disinfection of dental instruments, materials, and commonly used items

	Steam Auto-	Dry Heat	Chemical Vapor	Ethylene Oxide	Chemical Disinfect/ Sterilize	Comments
Angle attachments	2	2	2	1	2	Confirm with manufacturer
Burs						
Carbon steel	3	1	1	1	3	
Steel	2	1	1	1	2	
Tungs-carbide	2	1	2	1	2	
Endo instruments						
Stainless steel handles	1	1	1	1	2	
Nonstainless metal handles	4	1	1	1	4	
Stainless plastic handles	3	3	3	1	2	
Fluoride gel trays						
Heat-resistant plastic	1	4	3	1	3	
Non-heat resistant	4	4	3	1	3	Discard
Hand Instruments						
Carbon steel	3	1	1	1	3	
Stainless steel	1	1	1	1	2	
Handpieces						
Autoclavable	1	3	3	1	4	
Contra-angle	3	3	3	1	2	
Non-autclavable	3	3	3	1	2	Indophor, phenols
Prophy angle	2	2	2	2	2	
Impression trays						
Aluminum metal-chrome plated	1	1	1	1	2	
Custom acrylic	4	4	4	1	2	Discard
Plastic	4	4	4	4	2	
Instrument packs	1	2 (small)	1	1 (small)	4	
Instrument trays	2	2	2	1	4	
Needles disposable	Discard—do not reuse					
Polishing wheels/disks						
Garnet & cuttle	4	3	3	1	4	
Rag	1	3	2	1	4	
Rubber	2	3	3	1	2	Chlorine solution iodophor
Prostheses removable	3	3	3	2	2	
General items by material						
Stainless steel	1	1	1	1	2	
Rubber	2	3	3	1	2	
Plastic	3	3	3	1	2	
Carbon steel	3	1	1	1	3	

Code: 1 = Effective method and preferred method
      2 = Effective and acceptable method
      3 = Effective method, but risk of damage to instruments
      4 = Ineffective method—risk of damage to instruments
(Adapted from Accepted Dental Therapeutics and Dentists' Desk Reference, with permission.)

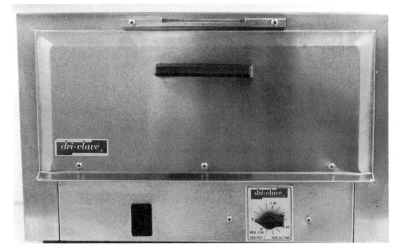

Figure 32–13 ▪ Dry heat (Dri-clave) sterilizer.

and operation, and no rusting or dulling of dry instruments.

Disadvantages

The disadvantages are as follows:
1. Careful loading, packaging, and temperature monitoring are essential.
2. Temperatures above 175°C (350°F) may melt solders in instruments and impression trays.
3. Dry heat is not suitable for rubbers, plastics, and high-speed handpieces.
4. Longer long-cycle times compared with autoclave.

Sterilization Monitoring

Spore strips are used as a biologic indicator. Color change strip labels and bags are available as process indicators. Stick-on labels are available as dosage indicators.

UNSATURATED CHEMICAL VAPOR

A mixture of formaldehyde, alcohol, ketone, water, and acetone heated under pressure forms a gas that can sterilize instruments. The Chemiclave requires the use of a solution, "Vapo-steril." The Chemiclave is in widespread effective use in offices and clinics at present (Fig. 32–14).

Parameters

For this method, heat at 270°F (132°C), at 20 to 40 psi for 20 minutes. The unit must be preheated before use.

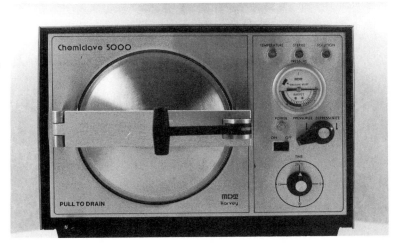
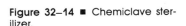

Figure 32–14 ▪ Chemiclave sterilizer.

Recommended Packaging

Pack instruments bare or in muslin, paper, steam-permeable plastic, or nylon. Avoid paper or tape with a high sulfur content due to blackening of the interior of the chamber and possible damage to the valve.

Advantages

The advantages of this method are rapid efficient cycle time, lack of rust and corrosion, and the availability of very good instructions and services.

Disadvantages

Unsaturated chemical vapor does not penetrate heavily wrapped packages as well as steam. The high temperature necessary may melt some plastics and rubber goods. Chemiclave may not be safe to sterilize some autoclavable handpieces. Consult the handpiece manufacturer.

Monitoring Sterilization

Biologic indicators—spore strips—must be used to determine sterilization. Instrument bags are available that include a process indicator. The process indicator's color change does not ensure sterilization has occurred.

ETHYLENE OXIDE STERILIZERS

Gas sterilization with ethylene oxide at ambient temperatures is useful for sterilizing virtually any material including plastics, rubber, handpieces, casts, and appliances (Fig. 32–15). Ethylene oxide gas is toxic to all bacteria, fungi, viruses, and spores at room temperature.

Parameters

Heat at 120°F for 2 to 3 hours for sterilization. At room temperature, sterilization time is 12 hours. Aeration of permeable materials, plastics, rubber, or cloth requires 12 to 24 hours. Adequate humidity is required for sterilization. Ventilation to the outdoors is required.

Advantage

This method sterilizes virtually anything, except liquids, at room temperature.

Disadvantages

The EPA and OSHA are very careful to monitor the use or misuse of ethylene oxide sterilizers since the gas is potentially mutagenic and carcinogenic and is directly toxic to skin. Ethylene oxide should be used only by exactly following the manufacturer's instructions including venting to the outside by a hood and blower device (Fig. 32–16). Total cycle times vary from 2½ to 36 hours.

Monitoring Sterilization

Spore strips and ampules are available for biologic monitoring. Tape and labels are available for process indicators. Glass ampules and paper strips are available for dosage indicators.

GLUTERALDEHYDE STERILIZATION

Several gluteraldehyde solutions are available that are approved by the ADA for sterilization. Depending on their use, gluteraldehydes are effective up to 28 days after activation. Products are available in alkaline,

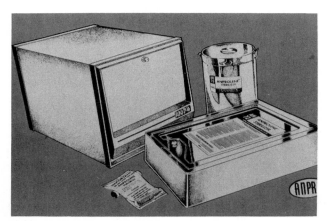

Figure 32–15 ■ Ethylene oxide gas sterilizer.

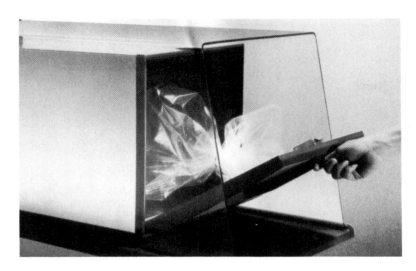

Figure 32–16 ■ Ethylene oxide gas sterilizer in exhaust hood.

neutral, and acidic pH ranges with at least 17 products awarded ADA approval as of April 1986 (see Table 32–6). Gluteraldehydes are useful as immersion solutions for instrument and product sterilization.

Parameters

For this method, 6¾ to 10 hours are required for sterilization at room temperature. Some products require 1 hour at 60°C or 4 hours at 40° to 50°C. Dilution by water limits the useful life to 14 days or less in most examples.

Advantages

Heat sensitive plastics, rubbers, and fiber optics can be safely sterilized. No expensive equipment is required. The cost for use is relatively low.

Disadvantages

Postexposure rinsing and handling are required. Skin and mucous membrane toxicity requires gloves while handling. Dilution is difficult to detect except by test kits or indicator strips that monitor the concentration of gluteraldehyde.

Monitoring Sterilization

Monitoring sterilization is very difficult because there are no biologic monitors available to the user. Concentration test strips and indicator solutions are now available to monitor gluteraldehyde concentration. Solution should be discarded below 1 percent gluteraldehyde.

Other sterilization methods are being studied and evaluated for possible dental use. They include microwave irradiation, chlorine gas generators, acid chlorite/chlorine family of liquid sterilants, and chlorine dioxide liquid sterilant. (See Table 32–9 for a summary of sterilization and disinfection methods and materials.)

Sterilization Assurance

It is very important to know and record that sterilization has occurred. Surveys using biologic indicators (spore strips) have shown that from 30 to 40 percent of sterilizers in private practices fail to sterilize when tested with standard spore strips.

Theoretically, sterilizers function properly when used according to the manufacturer's directions. In clinical use there are many ways to reduce the effectiveness of sterilization function, including improper packaging and loading and lack of water in autoclaves (or solution in chemiclaves) resulting in normal temperature readings but no sterilization.

Sterility assurance requires the use of bacterial spores. These are required when setting up new or repaired equipment and at regular intervals. The ADA recommends weekly spore tests. Process or dosage indicators are used for each load to verify sterilizing conditions or to detect gross errors.

BIOLOGIC INDICATORS

Biologic monitors or spore tests use paper strips containing a measured number of heat-

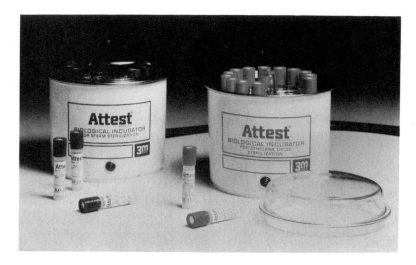

Figure 32–17 ■ Biologic indicator ampules and incubators.

resistant harmless bacterial spores. These strips are packaged in envelopes, capsules, or ampules (Fig. 32–17). Usually, two test strips and one control are needed for each testing procedure. The procedure should be performed in the following manner.

The test strips are placed in the sterilizing load in the center of the load or in a large pack. The control strip is left outside the sterilizer. The sterilizer is operated according to the manufacturer's instructions including times, temperatures, and solution required.

After the sterilizing cycle is completed, the test monitor strips are removed and, with the control strip, are cultured and incubated for growth. This may be done in the office, by the manufacturer, or at a clinical or university laboratory (Fig. 32–18). The results of each test are recorded and maintained for future reference.

If the results indicate that sterilization has not occurred, the unit should be retested immediately and instruments should be sterilized by alternate methods until the results

of further testing indicate that sterilization has occurred. If the second test fails, the sterilizer needs to be repaired by qualified service personnel.

Advantage ■ The results are proof of sterilizing conditions at time of test.

Disadvantage ■ The results are not available for several days to a week after culturing.

Process Indicators

Process indicators are used to indicate sterilizer processing for each load cycled. They do not prove sterilization but are very useful for indicating processing and gross handling problems or sterilizer failure to heat.

Process indicators are found on bags, tags, and strips, as well as the familiar "autoclave tape," and indicate processing by color change. The results of process indicator tests should be recorded and saved for future reference.

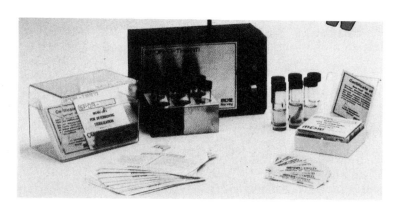

Figure 32–18 ■ Biologic monitors and incubator using spore strips.

Advantages ■ The advantages to process indicators include that they afford "instant" results and can be used for each load.

Disadvantage ■ The disadvantage is that process indicators do not monitor sterilization, only processing.

Dosage Indicators

Dosage indicators indicate heat or gas penetration into packs or instrument loads but do not indicate precise conditions of sterilization. Stick-on labels, paper strips, or glass ampules are supplied for various techniques. The results of dosage indicators should be retained for reference.

Advantages ■ Dosage indicators can be read immediately and provide more useful information than process indicators.

Disadvantages ■ These indicators are not a biologic monitor of sterilization and are not considered an acceptable substitute for spore strips.

Conclusions

As dentists or other health care workers, we seek first the best for our patients. We certainly would not want to be the source of serious illness among our patients, coworkers, or family. However, it is difficult to make significant changes in the way we approach everyday asepsis in the office. The technology is now available to decrease to a large degree the risk of infection for the patient and the dental staff.

First, and perhaps most importantly, steps should be taken to wash the hands carefully and to wear gloves whenever there is any contact between the hands and saliva. Second, sterilization methods known to kill all life forms should be used on dental instruments. Third, surfaces, units, and controls should be cleaned and disinfected.

REFERENCES

Block, S. S.: Disinfection, sterilization and preservation, ed. 3. Lea and Febiger, Philadelphia, 1983.

CDC: Current Trends—Recommended Infection—Control Practices for Dentistry. MMWR 35:237, 1986.

CDC: Hepatitis B Among Dental Patients in Indiana. Epidemiologic Notes and Reports. MMWR 34:73, 1985.

CDC: Preventing the Transmission of Hepatitis B, AIDS, and Herpes in Dentistry. Atlanta, 1986.

CDC: Recommendation for prevention of HIV transmission in health-care settings. MMWR (Suppl.)36:25, 1987.

Control: The Infectious Newsletter. Infection Control Publications, 850 N. Highway 91, Suite 7-K, P.O. Box 541, North Salt Lake, UT 84054.

Cottone, J.: Hepatitis B. Transmission and Epidemiology in the Dental Profession. Proceedings of National Conference on Infection Control in Dentistry, U.S. Dept. of Health Care and Human Services. Atlanta, GA, 1986, pp. 12, 13, 16.

Council on Dental Therapeutics: Accepted Dental Therapeutics, ed. 40. American Dental Association, Chicago, 1984.

Council on Dental Therapeutics: Dentist's Desk Reference, ed. 2. American Dental Association, Chicago, 1983.

Council on Dental Therapeutics and Council on Prosthetic Services and Dental Laboratory Relations: Guidelines for Infection Control in the Dental Office and the Commercial Dental Laboratory. J.A.D.A. 110:969, 1985.

Crawford, J.: Clinical Asepsis in Dentistry, ed. 3. R. A. Kolstad, Mesquite, TX, 1986.

Herrara, S. P., and Merchant, V. A.: Dimensional stability of dental impressions after immersion disinfection. J.A.D.A. 113:419, 1986.

Manella, J. P., et al.: An outbreak of herpes simplex virus type I gingivostometitis in a dental hygiene practice. J.A.M.A. 252:2019, 1984.

McCray, E.: Special report, occupational risk of the acquired immunodeficiency syndrome among health care workers. N. Engl. J. Med. 314:1131, 1986.

Runnels, R.: Infection control in the wet finger environment. Publishers Press, Salt Lake, UT, 1984.

Russell, A. D., Hugo, W. B., and Ayliffe, G.A.J.: Principles and Practice of Sterilization. Blackwell Scientific Publications, Oxford, 1982, pp. 3–6.

Schafer, M. E.: Practical Infection Control in the Dental Office. Henry Scheiss, Port Washington, NY, 1985.

Soloman, A. L.: Facts about AIDS for the Dental Team. American Dental Association, Chicago, 1986.

Whitaker, R. J., Robins, S. K., Williams, B. L., and Crawford, J. J.: Dental Asepsis. Stoma Press, Seattle, 1979.

chapter *33*

Antimicrobials and antibiotics

Sebastian C. Ciancio

CHAPTER OUTLINE

- **ANTIBIOTICS—BASIC PRINCIPLES**
- **ANTIBIOTICS USED IN DENTISTRY**
- **SULFONAMIDES**

- **ANTIBIOTIC MANAGEMENT OF THE PATIENT WITH VARIOUS CARDIAC PROBLEMS**

Antimicrobial agents either suppress the growth of microorganisms or destroy them. They are divided into three categories: antibiotics, sulfonamides, and antiseptics. In dentistry, antibiotics are the most frequently used; however, the introduction of strong nonantibiotic antibacterial agents will result in their increased use.

Antimicrobial drugs were first used by Paul Ehrlich, who treated syphilis with salvarsan, an organic chemical. Much later, in 1936, sulfonamides were introduced. Antibiotics became available in 1941 with the clinical introduction of penicillin. Since then, numerous antibiotics have been introduced and new ones are constantly being evaluated. Topical "antiseptics" were considered as early as the 1800s, but with the introduction of chlorhexidine in the 1960s in Europe and in 1986 in the United States, considerable dental interest has been stimulated in antiseptic agents.

This chapter focuses on antimicrobial agents of clinical importance in dentistry because of their use in treatment of oral disease. Other antimicrobials are discussed elsewhere in this book.

Antibiotics—Basic Principles

Antibiotics are substances originally isolated from microorganisms that either retard the growth of microorganisms or kill them. Today many antibiotics are chemically synthesized. The properties of an ideal antibiotic are summarized in Table 33–1.

Depending on the antibiotic, there are several mechanisms of action, including inhibi-

---

Table 33–1 ■ Properties of an ideal antibiotic

1. Selective and effective against microorganisms without injuring the host
2. Destroy microorganisms (bactericidal action) rather than retard their growth (bacteriostatic action)
3. Not become ineffective as a result of bacterial resistance
4. Not be inactivated by enzymes, plasma proteins, or body fluids
5. Quickly reach bactericidal levels throughout the body and be maintained for long periods of time
6. Have minimal adverse effects

---

tion of bacterial cell wall synthesis, alteration of bacterial cell membrane permeability, alteration in the bacterial synthesis of cellular components, and inhibition of bacterial cell metabolism.

GENERAL CONCEPTS

Certain terms and concepts are necessary for understanding the pharmacology of antibiotics.

Resistance

Microorganisms are sometimes resistant or unaffected by an antibiotic. Resistance can be (1) natural (present before contact with the antibiotic) or (2) acquired, developing during exposure to the drug. Acquired resistance via a plasmid is a result of a change in the microorganism's DNA, which is genetically inherited by subsequent generations. Therefore, once resistance develops, a new antibiotic must be found to control the resistant bacteria.

Microorganisms resistant to one antimicrobial agent frequently are resistant to other chemically related drugs. This is referred to as cross-resistance. Occasionally, cross-resistance to two chemically dissimilar drugs occurs. Resistance usually results from antibiotic inactivation by bacterial enzymes, development of alternate bacterial metabolic pathways unaffected by antibiotics, or biochemical alterations in the bacteria preventing uptake or binding of the antibiotic.

Antibiotic ineffectiveness results not only from resistance but also from inadequate therapy that does not control the large numbers of microorganisms. At other times, low doses of an antibiotic only destroy the more susceptible microorganisms and allow the more resistant to survive and multiply. This phenomenon is called *selective pressure*. The process of selecting increasingly less susceptible or resistant microorganisms occurs in a stepwise manner over a period of time. Therefore, it is imperative that the initial antibiotic dose is sufficient and given long enough for successful therapy. Finally, antibiotics can also be ineffective if they are antagonized by interacting with other drugs.

Spectrum of Activity

No antibiotic is effective against all microorganisms. Instead, they have a certain spectrum of activity. Antibiotics may affect only a few microorganisms and have a very limited spectrum of activity or affect a wide variety and have a broad spectrum of activity. Broad-spectrum antibiotics are only necessary if an infection is caused by a mixed flora. Often, an infection caused by one microorganism will respond more readily to a limited-spectrum antibiotic directed toward that microorganism. Because of the limited range of activity of antibiotics, it is important to select one that would be effective against the infecting microorganism. The ideal method is to isolate the microorganism from the lesion or infected site and culture it to determine its susceptibility to different antibiotics (culture and sensitivity). At times, selection of an antibiotic is based on clinical experience, a procedure sometimes leading to mistakes.

Superinfections

Suppression of one group of microorganisms by an antibiotic may permit the growth of another group that is normally present but usually does not cause disease. In large numbers, however, a "superinfection" can result.

Type of Action

Antibiotics are either bacteriostatic or bactericidal. Bacteriostatic antibiotics inhibit the growth and multiplication of microorganisms, permitting the host defenses to deal with their removal. Bactericidal antibiotics directly kill or destroy microorganisms. In general, bacteriostatic antibiotics alter metabolic pathways or synthesis of cellular components that do not destroy the cell. In contrast, bactericidal drugs cause cell death by interfering with the synthesis or function of the cell wall, the cell membrane, or both.

When two bactericidal antibiotics are given together, they may exert a greater effect than when given separately. This is called antibiotic synergism. Sometimes, however, when a bacteriostatic and a bactericidal antibiotic are given together, their effectiveness is negated or reduced. This is called antibiotic antagonism.

Antibiotics Used in Dentistry

The antibiotics currently used in dentistry are summarized in Table 33–2.

Table 33–2 ■ Antibiotics of use in dentistry

Antibiotic	Action	
	Bacteriostatic	Bactericidal
Penicillin V		✓
Penicillin G		✓
Ampicillin		✓
Erythromycins	✓	
Tetracyclines	✓	
Oxacillin, nafcillin		✓
Cephalosporins		✓
Metronidazole		
Nystatin	✓	
Bacitracin		✓
Lincomycin	✓	
Vancomycin		✓
Streptomycin		✓

(From Ciancio and Bourgault, Clinical Pharmacology for Dental Professionals, 1984, p. 52, with permission.)

PENICILLIN

Penicillin, derived from a mold, *Penicillium notatum*, was the first antibiotic used in humans. Although the effects of penicillin were discovered in 1928, therapeutic trials did not take place until 1941. Research in the United States has since resulted in quantity production not only by biosynthetic *Penicillium* but also by semisynthetic methods.

Types of Penicillin

The first penicillin, penicillin G, is still the most effective penicillin against susceptible microorganisms that do not produce penicillinase. Penicillinase, an enzyme produced mainly by staphylococci, breaks down penicillin and renders it inactive. Newer semisynthetic penicillins are not inactivated by penicillinase and are therefore effective against penicillinase-producing bacteria.

Mechanism of Action

Penicillin is a bactericidal drug that inhibits the synthesis of cell walls of some bacteria. This leads to high osmotic pressure with swelling, membrane disruption, and subsequent cell death. Because penicillin acts during the synthesis of cell walls, it is most effective against multiplying bacteria.

Once absorbed, penicillin is widely distributed throughout the body including, in small amounts, saliva and gingival crevicular fluid. It crosses the placenta but does not pass the blood-brain barrier in healthy individuals,

although it does so in those with meningitis. Penicillin is rapidly eliminated from plasma by the kidneys.

Penicillins are excreted in breast milk in low concentrations. Although significant problems have not been documented, the risk-benefit ratio must be considered before their use by nursing mothers, which could lead to sensitization, diarrhea, and candidiasis.

Adverse Effects

Penicillin toxicity is extremely low and, except for allergic reactions, is one of the safest drugs known.

The incidence of allergic reactions to penicillin has been estimated at 1 to 5 per cent. Topical and aerosol preparations of penicillin are more likely to lead to allergic reactions. The oral route is the least likely to cause penicillin allergy.

Patients allergic to one penicillin are likely to be allergic to all other penicillins. Also, those with a history of hypersensitivity to cephalosporins, griseofulvin, or penicillamine may also be allergic to penicillin.

Various procedures have been attempted to determine if a person is allergic to penicillin. The most promising is a skin test with a small amount of penicillin combined with various penicillin derivatives. However, 5 per cent of patients with a negative reaction to this skin test still had allergic reactions to penicillin.

CEPHALOSPORINS

These antibiotics are semisynthetically derived from a mold, *Cephalosporium acremonium*, and are structurally related to penicillin.

Types of Cephalosporins

The cephalosporins of dental interest are summarized in Table 33–3. Usually, the one advantage of using these antibiotics rather than other antibiotics for treating dental infections is that they may be safe for patients with penicillin allergies. However, there have been reports of cross-hypersensitivity between cephalosporins and penicillin.

Mode of Action

Cephalosporins are bactericidal and inhibit bacterial cell wall synthesis in a manner sim-

Table 33–3 ■ The cephalosporins

Name				
Generic	Trade	Adult dose	Maximum adult dose	Administration route
Cefadroxil	Duricef Ultracef	1–2 g every 12 h	4 g	po
Cephadrine	Anspor, Velosef	0.5–1.0 g every 6 h	8 g	po, IM, IV
Cephalexin	Keflex	0.25–0.5 g every 6 h	4 g	po
Cephalothin	Keflin	0.5–3 g every 6 h	12 g	IM, IV
Cephapirin	Cefadyl	0.5–1 g every 6 h	12 g	IM, IV
Cephazolin	Ancef, Kefzol	0.25–0.5 g every 8 h	8 g	IM, IV
Cefamandole	Mandol	0.5–1 g every 6 h	8 g	IM, IV
Cefaclor	Ceclor	0.25 g every 8 h	4 g	po

(From Ciancio and Bourgault, Clinical Pharmacology for Dental Professionals, 1984, p. 55, with permission.)

ilar to penicillin. They also inhibit cell division and growth so that lysis of some bacteria occurs. Cephalosporins are broad-spectrum antibiotics and are effective against most gram-negative microorganisms, including staphylococci. They are also effective against *Proteus mirabilis, Escherichia coli, Klebsiella*, and *Enterobacter*.

The cephalosporins are recognized as the first drug of choice for non–hospital acquired *Klebsiella* infections and secondly as a substitute for penicillin.

Some bacteria produce cephalosporinases, which inactivate cephalosporins, rendering the bacteria resistant to them.

Metabolism

Most cephalosporins are widely distributed throughout the body. However, they do not easily cross into the cerebrospinal fluid and are therefore not indicated in meningitis. Most of the administered dose is excreted unchanged in the urine within 4 to 6 hours after administration.

These antibiotics occur in low concentrations in breast milk and do cross the placenta.

Adverse Effects

The incidence of allergic reactions is almost as high as with penicillin. Although patients allergic to penicillin may not be allergic to the cephalosporins, the possibility of an allergic reaction to cephalosporins is higher in these patients than in others. Also, cephalosporins can cause erythrocyte hemolysis. Because of this, tests for hemolysis should be performed. On occasion, renal damage has occurred as well as local pain and tissue sloughing at the site of injection. Oral moniliasis has been reported in patients on long-term therapy. Other side effects include rash, urticaria, fever, gastrointestinal disorders, glossitis, neutropenia, and superinfections (especially with *Pseudomonas* and *Enterobacter*).

ERYTHROMYCIN

These drugs are classified as macrolide antibiotics. They are one of the safer antibiotics in use today and often are a satisfactory alternate for penicillin, particularly in patients who are allergic to penicillin. They are derived from *Streptomyces*.

Mechanism of Action

Erythromycins are bacteriostatic or bactericidal, depending on the dose and microorganism. They produce their antibacterial effect by inhibiting the synthesis of bacterial protein. Usually with dental infections, low doses are bacteriostatic and high doses are bactericidal.

Spectrum of Activity

Erythromycin is effective against most gram-positive microorganisms sensitive to penicillin G. It is also effective against *Staphylococcus aureus* but not as effective as the "antistaphylococcal penicillins." In general, its antibacterial spectrum lies between those of penicillin and the tetracyclines.

Bacterial resistance appears relatively early in patients taking erythromycin for prolonged periods of time.

Metabolism

Erythromycin rapidly diffuses throughout the body, and the brain contains higher concentrations than are found in plasma. As with penicillin, it passes into cerebrospinal fluid in patients with meningitis.

This antibiotic is concentrated in the liver and is excreted in bile, urine, and feces. Although the kidneys remove erythromycin from the body, nonrenal mechanisms are more important. A large amount can be found in bile and only about 15 percent in urine. During pregnancy erythromycin passes the placental barrier but does not appear to harm the fetus.

Adverse Effects

Following oral administration, gastrointestinal irritation occurs including nausea, vomiting, and abdominal pain. This can be minimized if erythromycin is taken with food. Tablets with acid-resistant coatings (enteric coated) are available and should be prescribed if taken with food to prevent inactivation by stomach acids. Cholestatic hepatitis has also been associated with the use of the estolate form. Symptoms of this disorder include nausea, vomiting, and abdominal pain followed by jaundice, fever, and a disturbance in white blood cells. Because of this, the estolate form should be avoided in patients with a history of liver disease.

The incidence of allergic reactions to erythromycin is low and is manifested as fever, eosinophilia, and skin eruptions.

TETRACYCLINE

The tetracyclines are a group of broad-spectrum antibiotics initially obtained from soil microorganisms. They are useful in a number of dental infections and are often used in place of penicillin or erythromycin. However, they are not acceptable substitutes for the prophylaxis of patients with a history of rheumatic fever.

Types of Tetracyclines

Seven basic types of tetracyclines are currently in use. They are all similar chemically, possess similar antibacterial spectra, and have cross-hypersensitivity. When resistance or hypersensitivity to one tetracycline occurs, it also occurs to all. The types of tetracyclines are summarized in Table 33–4. Although topical sensitization is theoretically possible, this has not been widely reported for tetracyclines.

While all tetracyclines have a similar spectrum of activity, minocycline is the most effective in treatment of meningococcal infections. Most of the tetracyclines—but doxycycline and minocycline to a lesser extent—are bound to metal ions. Dairy products and antacids that contain calcium limit the gastrointestinal absorption of tetracycline so that minimal therapeutic benefits can be expected. A similar interaction has been reported with products containing iron, magnesium, and aluminum. Therefore, patients should be told to refrain from these products for at least 1.5 hours prior to or following administration of oral tetracycline (Fig. 33–1).

Mechanism of Action

The tetracyclines are bacteriostatic and inhibit protein synthesis in susceptible bacteria.

Table 33–4 ■ Various Tetracyclines

Generic name	Trade name	Route of administration	Affected by metal ions
Chlortetracycline HCl	Aureomycin	po, IV	+
Demeclocycline HCl	Declomycin	po	+
Doxycycline and salts	Vibramycin	po, IV	−
Methacycline HCl	Rondomycin	po	+
Minocycline HCl	Minocin	po, IV	−
Oxytetracycline and salts	Tetramycin	po, IM, IV	+
Tetracycline and salts	Achromycin V, Cyclopar, Panmycin, Robitet, SK-Tetracycline, Tetracyn, Sumycin, Tetrex	po, IM, IV	+

(From Ciancio and Bourgault, Clinical Pharmacology for Dental Professionals, 1984, p. 58, with permission.)

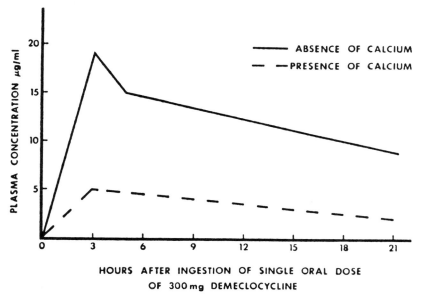

Figure 33–1 ■ Alteration of absorption of a tetracycline by calcium. (From Ciancio and Bourgault, 1984. Clinical Pharmacology for Dental Professionals, with permission.)

Since they all have the same mechanism of action, resistance to one implies resistance to all tetracyclines.

Tetracyclines can block the antibacterial effect of penicillin. Penicillin is most effective on multiplying, growing bacteria, while tetracyclines slow down the rate of bacterial growth and multiplication. Therefore, concomitant administration of these drugs is contraindicated.

Spectrum of Activity

The tetracyclines are broad-spectrum antibiotics that are effective against a number of gram-negative and gram-positive bacteria. They are also effective against a few viruses, treponemata, mycoplasma, chlamydia, and rickettsia. Minocycline may also be effective against staphylococci not affected by other tetracyclines.

Metabolism

These antibiotics pass into most body fluids and tissues. They also pass through the placenta and occur in low doses in milk of lactating mothers. However, no adverse effects on the newborn have been reported when the child receives low doses in the mother's milk. This antibiotic also concentrates in gingival crevicular fluid and is therefore in intimate contact with plaque in the gingival crevice.

They have an affinity for and occur in higher concentrations in rapidly growing and metabolizing tissue such as liver, tumors, bone, and developing teeth.

Tetracyclines are excreted mainly by the kidneys and can be recovered from the urine in the unchanged form.

Adverse Effects

Treatment with tetracyclines can adversely alter the normal oral and intestinal flora, resulting in gastrointestinal problems including diarrhea. Some patients have also developed monilial infections of the gastrointestinal tract, the oral cavity, and the vagina due to alterations in the flora.

The side effects associated with tetracycline therapy are varied. A number of side effects have resulted from the use of outdated tetracyclines. Side effects are also more common in pregnant patients (in addition to the tooth-staining problem). Therefore, these drugs are contraindicated during pregnancy.

Although the incidence of allergy is low, allergy to one tetracycline usually means allergy to all other forms.

Another side effect is the discoloration of the dentin of teeth during their formation. The stain is permanent and is only correctable by covering the tooth with a restorative material. This is another reason that tetracycline should be avoided during pregnancy.

Primary Indications for Nondental Conditions

Since their introduction in 1948, tetracyclines have been widely used, particularly for the treatment of acne. This widespread use has led to frequent antibiotic resistance, decreasing the effectiveness of the tetracyclines.

Several species of *E. coli*, beta-hemolytic streptococci, *S. pneumoniae*, *N. gonorrhoeae*, *Bacteroides*, *Shigella*, and *S. aureus* are resistant to the tetracyclines. Since there is evidence that resistance develops in direct proportion to usage, the prevalence of these resistant strains may increase in the future. However, tetracyclines remain the drug of choice for a variety of rarely occurring infections.

Indications for Dental Conditions

Tetracyclines have been suggested for treatment of various oral conditions including their use as an adjunct for periodontal therapy, in prevention of some forms of subacute bacterial endocarditis, for treatment of acute necrotizing ulcerative gingivitis (ANUG), and for treatment of periodontal abscesses. Their use for treating ANUG and periodontal abscesses, however, has not been substantiated.

Adjunct to periodontal therapy ■ Tetracyclines improve the healing after periodontal surgery and minimize postsurgical discomfort and infection. Clinical studies on humans indicate that tetracycline enhances bone formation and possibly reattachment. In addition, animal studies demonstrate early crestal bone repair and reversal of a periodontal disease in the rice rat. Part of the effectiveness of tetracyclines following oral administration results from their occurrence in gingival crevicular fluid in higher concentrations than in serum.

Prevention of subacute bacterial endocarditis ■ Tetracyclines are not drugs of choice for prevention of subacute bacterial endocarditis (SBE). As early as 1962, McCormick and colleagues showed that 15 to 19 percent of group A streptococci are resistant to tetracyclines, whereas none were resistant to penicillin or erythromycin. Because of studies such as this, the American Heart Association and the American Dental Association recommend that the drug of choice for the prevention of subacute bacterial endocarditis is penicillin, and the second drug of choice is erythromycin.

Recent reports have indicated that non-streptococcal subacute bacterial endocarditis is often caused by *Actinobacillus actinomycetemcomitans*, an organism strongly associated with localized juvenile periodontitis (LJP). This bacterium is only weakly susceptible to penicillin or erythromycin. For this reason, therapy of patients with LJP who are predisposed to subacute bacterial endocarditis may consist of 2 to 3 weeks' therapy with 1 g daily of a tetracycline (to eliminate *A. actinomycetemcomitans* prior to dental treatment) followed by the penicillin or erythromycin therapy to control the streptococci (Table 33–5). Therapy with either penicillin or erythromycin cannot be simultaneous with tetracyclines, as these drugs are antagonistic to each other.

METRONIDAZOLE

Metronidazole, a systemic trichomonacide, is highly effective in the treatment of *Trichomonas vaginalis* infections. The drug is biologically active in semen and urine and, therefore, is active against trichomonads in extravaginal as well as vaginal foci. However, it is ineffective against *Candida albicans* and other yeasts or bacteria that cause vaginitis. It is also recommended by some investigators as an adjunct to periodontal therapy, because it is active against plaque bacteria, including anaerobes and spirochetes.

Adverse Effects

This drug should be used with caution, as it is carcinogenic in mice and possibly also in rats. It is also mutagenic to some bacteria in concentrations found in individuals receiving therapeutic doses of the drug. Because the drug has not also been shown to be carcinogenic in hamsters, other animal species so far studied, or in humans, other authorities believe that the risk of using the drug is justified.

The incidence of adverse effects with metronidazole is low and no serious reactions have been reported clinically. The most frequent reaction is nausea. Diarrhea occurs less commonly.

Temporary leukopenia can occur following metronidazole therapy; therefore, total and differential white cell counts should be performed once a week if the drug is given for longer than 7 days, especially in very young, very old, and debilitated patients or if a second course of therapy is necessary because of relapse or reinfection. Metronidazole

Table 33–5 ■ Recommended antibiotic regimens for prevention of bacterial endocarditis*

	Dosage for adults	Dosage for children
DENTAL AND UPPER RESPIRATORY PROCEDURES†		
Oral administration‡:		
Penicillin V	2 g 1 hr before procedure and 1 g 6 hr later	>60 lb: adult dosage <60 lb: half the adult dose 1 hr before procedure and 6 hr later
Penicillin allergy: Erythromycin	1 g 1 hr before procedure and 500 mg 6 hr later	20 mg/kg 1 hr before procedure and 10 mg/kg 6 hr later
Parenteral administration‡: Ampicillin	1–2 g IM or IV 30 min to 1 hr before procedure and 1.5 mg/kg	50 mg/kg IM or IV 30 min to 1 hr before procedure and repeat once 8 hr later 1.5 mg/kg
Plus gentamicin	1.5 mg/kg IM or IV 30 min to 1 hr before procedure and repeat once 8 hr later or orally 1 g of penicillin V	2.0 mg/kg IM or IV 30 min to 1 hr before procedure and repeat once 8 hr later (or orally 1 g of Penicillin V)
Penicillin allergy: Vancomycin	1 g IV infused over 1 hr beginning 1 hr before procedure	20 mg/kg IV infused over 1 hr beginning 1 hr before procedure

*For patients with valvular heart disease, prosthetic heart valves, most forms of congenital heart disease (but not uncomplicated secundum atrial septal defect), idiopathic hypertrophic subaortic stenosis, and mitral valve prolapse.

†Data are limited on the risk of endocarditis with a particular procedure. For a review of the risk of bacteremia with various procedures, see Everett, ED, Hirschmann JV: *Medicine* 1977;56:61.

‡An oral regimen is safer and is preferred for most patients. Parenteral regimens are more likely to be effective; they are recommended especially for patients with prosthetic valves, those who have had endocarditis previously, or those taking continuous oral penicillin for rheumatic fever prophylaxis.

(From Ciancio and Bourgault, Clinical Pharmacology for Dental Professionals, 1984, p. 362, with permission.)

should be used with caution in individuals who have or are prone to blood dyscrasias, since it has a potential for depressing bone marrow activity. Similarly, it should be used cautiously in individuals with any pronounced central nervous system disorder. No adverse reactions affecting the fetus have been reported. There is evidence, however, that the drug readily crosses the placenta, and it may be the only known drug not used for cancer chemotherapy that has mutagenic activity against certain bacteria at concentrations readily obtainable in body fluids following therapeutic doses. Therefore, metronidazole should definitely *not* be used during the first trimester of pregnancy and should be avoided throughout pregnancy. Metronidazole is excreted in breast milk, but no adverse effects have been observed in nursing infants. It is also found in crevicular fluid in levels slightly below those found in serum.

LINCOMYCIN AND CLINDAMYCIN

These antibiotics were discovered in 1962 in soil samples from Lincoln, Nebraska. Their use should be reserved for patients who cannot take penicillin or erythromycin. Since their adverse effects can be severe, they are seldom used in dental patients.

Types of Antibiotics

Lincomycin (Lincocin) and its semisynthetic derivatives, clindamycin hydrochloride (Cleocin) and other salts, have similar spectra of activity. Clindamycin is better absorbed and more potent than lincomycin but has more frequent adverse effects. These antibiotics inhibit bacterial protein synthesis and are usually bacteriostatic, but in high doses they are bactericidal.

Spectrum of Activity

Their antibacterial spectra are similar to those of the erythromycins. Because of their ability to penetrate bone, however, they are particularly useful in treating osteomyelitis involving alveolar bone. They are also the drugs of choice for serious infections caused by anaerobic microorganisms. Their use is primarily for microorganisms resistant to penicillin and erythromycin or for patients who cannot tolerate other antibacterial agents.

Metabolism

Lincomycin is only partially absorbed from the gastrointestinal tract, while clindamycin is almost completely absorbed. These drugs are excreted in feces, urine, and bile, with the biliary route being the most important.

Both drugs are widely distributed in body tissues, including bone. They also cross the placental barrier. Although lincomycin will pass through inflamed meninges as in meningitis, clindamycin does not.

Adverse Effects

The incidence of diarrhea with these drugs is high. However, a more serious problem is the development of a severe, sometimes fatal, hemorrhagic colitis. This has been termed antibiotic-associated colitis (AAC). This severe diarrhea has sometimes been successfully treated by the restoration of fluid and electrolyte balance and vancomycin (500 mg every 6 hours). In view of this side effect, serious consideration should be given before using this drug. Other side effects include glossitis, stomatitis, nausea, vomiting, skin rashes, vaginitis, and changes in blood cells. The incidence of hypersensitivity reactions to these drugs is low.

VANCOMYCIN

Vancomycin, discovered in 1956, is a glycopeptide with an unknown chemical structure. It is useful in both preventing and treating bacterial endocarditis. The only commercially available derivative is Vancocin.

Mechanism of Action

Vancomycin is bactericidal and exerts its effect by inhibiting cell wall synthesis.

Spectrum of Activity

This drug is bactericidal for gram-positive bacteria. Cross-resistance with other antibiotics has not been reported.

Metabolism

It is poorly absorbed following oral administration. Therefore, the intravenous route is preferred. It penetrates most body fluids, including cerebrospinal fluid, when the meninges are inflamed. Its main route of excretion is via the kidney. The drug is poorly absorbed through oral mucosa, and some studies have reported improvement in gingivitis following topical application.

Adverse Effects

Side effects are severe. Therefore, it should be restricted to bacterial endocarditis prophylaxis and gram-positive infections in which no other antibiotic is effective.

The untoward effects include phlebitis and pain at the injection site, deafness, toxic changes in the kidney, anaphylaxis, skin rashes, and fever. No adverse effects have been reported from the topical route of administration.

NYSTATIN

Nystatin (Candex, Mycostatin, Nilstat, O-V Statin), a polyene antibiotic, was discovered in 1954 and is an excellent antibiotic for the treatment of fungal infections.

It is most useful for the treatment of both oral and vaginal candidiasis (thrush).

Metabolism

This drug can be given orally but is poorly absorbed from the gastrointestinal tract. Also, it is not absorbed from skin and mucous membranes. When taken orally, large amounts are found in feces. It exerts its main effect via the topical route in most cases.

Adverse Effects

Adverse effects are rare and include nausea, vomiting, and diarrhea following ingestion. However, no adverse effects have been reported via the topical route. Neither hypersensitivity reactions nor resistance have occurred.

KETOCONAZOLE

Ketoconazole (Nizoral) is one of the newest drugs approved for oral treatment of systemic fungal infections. It is also useful for the treatment of oral candidiasis (thrush).

Ketoconazole interferes with the synthesis of chemicals needed to form the plasma membrane of fungi, resulting in disorganization of the membrane.

Metabolism

Its absorption from the gastrointestinal tract is better than that of nystatin. It is metabolized in the liver, and only small amounts are found in urine and feces. Since data are lacking for use in pregnancy, it is not recommended at that time. It does appear in maternal milk.

Adverse Effects

The most common adverse effects are nausea and pruritus. Headache, dizziness, gastrointestinal problems, nervousness, and liver dysfunction have occurred less frequently.

STREPTOMYCIN

Streptomycin, discovered in 1949, is an antibiotic useful to dentistry only in the prophylaxis of certain patients with a history of complications from rheumatic fever and will be discussed only in this respect. It is also used in the treatment of tuberculosis and bacterial endocarditis. Because of its severe toxicity, the drug has limited usefulness.

Streptomycin is bactericidal, inhibiting bacterial protein synthesis.

Spectrum of Activity

It is effective against gram-positive, gram-negative, and acid-fast microorganisms. Unfortunately, bacterial resistance develops rapidly, thus limiting its usefulness.

Metabolism

Since it is not absorbed from the intestinal tract, the injectable form must be used. It distributes throughout plasma and all extracellular fluids before being excreted mainly unchanged by the kidneys.

Adverse Effects

Severe eighth nerve damage is common, causing loss of both balance and hearing. Its use can also cause blood disorders and severe kidney damage. Allergic reactions may occur, ranging from rashes to shock.

BACITRACIN

Bacitracin, discovered in 1943, is sometimes used topically for dental infections. It is effective against gram-positive cocci and bacilli, *Actinomyces*, and *Fusobacterium*. Rarely, hypersensitivity reactions have been reported after topical application. It is available as an ointment containing 500 units per gram for topical use and often is combined with other topical antibiotics such as neomycin and polymyxin, which have some broad-spectrum properties. It has been placed in some periodontal dressings, but its value was questionable. It is not used parenterally, since kidney damage is common following such usage.

Sulfonamides

The first sulfonamide was synthesized in 1908 as para-aminobenzoicsulphonamide but was not used as an antibacterial agent until 1936. Since that time many sulfonamides have been synthesized. Although they are effective in some infections of dental origin, antibiotics are more effective and safe. Therefore, sulfonamides are indicated for infections of dental origin in which antibiotics cannot be used. The sulfonamides are contraindicated for topical application on oral mucosa because they are highly allergenic. However, they are sometimes used topically for minor eye infections and over burn areas.

The sulfonamides are bacteriostatic. Since the sulfonamides are structurally similar to para-aminobenzoic acid, they interfere with its uptake by bacteria. Para-aminobenzoic acid is important to bacterial metabolism because bacteria use it to make folic acid, which is essential to the vitality of most microorganisms.

Spectrum of Activity

The sulfonamides are effective against many gram-positive and some gram-negative bacteria. They are also effective against some large viruses of trachoma and lymphogranuloma venereum. They are mainly used to treat lower urinary tract infections.

Metabolism

Once sulfonamides enter plasma, they are rapidly concentrated in urine. Some are excreted unchanged, while others are metabolized in the liver. The sulfonamides can be classified as short-, intermediate-, and long-acting on the basis of duration of effect in the body.

Many bacteria develop a high degree of resistance to sulfonamides during therapy. Once resistance to one sulfonamide develops, resistance to all others also occurs. Because the sulfonamides concentrate in urine, crystals may form in the urinary tract as a complication of therapy. Therefore, sulfonamides are usually administered with large amounts of fluid and in combination with other sulfonamides to decrease the concentration of any one agent.

Adverse Effects

A number of adverse effects are associated with sulfonamide therapy, the most common being allergic reactions. The most frequent allergic reactions include urticaria, rash, fever, pruritus, dermatitis, and photosensitivity. Less frequent allergic reactions include Stevens-Johnson syndrome, erythema nodosum, and exfoliative dermatitis. Sensitivity to one sulfonamide usually indicates sensitivity to all sulfonamides.

Other adverse effects include nausea, vomiting, diarrhea, headache, dizziness, vertigo, tinnitus, and mental depression.

Sulfonamide therapy may result in toxic effects in the urinary tract owing to the formation of sulfonamide crystals in urine. Adequate urinary volume is important to minimize this effect. Also, since some sulfonamides are not soluble in alkaline media, agents such as sodium bicarbonate are given concurrently to make urine more alkaline.

Blood dyscrasias have also occurred with sulfonamide therapy. Clinical signs associated with these are sore throat, fever, pallor, or jaundice. These symptoms should be watched for in patients on long-term therapy, and periodic blood counts are indicated during such therapy. These drugs cross the placenta and are excreted in milk. Therefore, since sulfonamides can cause problems in infants, they should not be given to pregnant or lactating females.

Antibiotic Management of the Patient with Various Cardiac Problems

Patients may have histories of cardiovascular problems such as those associated with rheumatic fever that require antibiotic prophylaxis prior to dental therapy that produces bleeding from oral tissues.

The occurrence and extent of bacteremias following dental procedures vary with the extent of the procedure and the amount of trauma and health of the gingival tissues. Prophylactic antibiotic therapy is recommended for dental procedures that are likely to cause gingival bleeding to minimize the risk of bacteremias leading to subacute bacterial endocarditis. *Streptococcus viridans*, a microorganism found in the gingival crevice, has an affinity for diseased heart valves or weakened cardiac tissues. This microorganism can lodge in heart tissues and produce bacterial endocarditis, a life-threatening disease. Therefore, these patients must be premedicated with antibiotics, as outlined in Table 33–5. The question of prophylactic antibiotics in a patient who has a history of rheumatic fever but no signs of cardiac damage is left to the judgment of the dentist. If the dentist is certain that a physician has examined the patient with such a history and has found no sign of cardiac damage, prophylactic therapy should not be necessary. *Actinobacillus (Haemophilus) actinomycetemcomitans*, a microorganism often found in patients with localized juvenile periodontitis, also has an affinity for diseased heart valves or weakened cardiac tissue. No definite therapeutic regimen has been developed, but a number of clinicians premedicate these patients with tetracyclines followed by the prophylactic regimen shown in Table 33–5.

Acknowledgment

This chapter has been partially adapted from *Clinical Pharmacology for Dental Professionals*, Second Edition, by Sebastian G. Ciancio and Priscilla C. Bourgault, copyright 1984 by PSG Publishing Company, Littleton, Massachusetts, used with permission.

REFERENCES

Archard, H. O., and Roberts, W. C.: Bacterial endocarditis after dental procedures in patients with aortic valve prosthesis. J.A.D.A. 72:648, 1966.

Ariaudo, A. A.: The efficacy of antibiotics in periodontal surgery: A controlled study with Lincomycin and placebo in sixty-eight patients. J. Periodontol. 40:150, 1969.

Baer, P. N., Sumner, C. F., and Miller, G.: Periodontal dressings. Dent. Clin. North Am. 13:181, 1969.

Breloff, J. P., and Caffesse, R.: Effect of achromycin ointment on healing following periodontal surgery. J. Periodontol. 54:368, 1983.

Cianco, S. G., Mather, M. L., McMullen, J. A.: An evaluation of minocycline in patients with periodontal disease. J. Periodontol. 54:530, 1980.

Ciancio, S. G.: Tetracyclines and periodontal therapy. J. Periodontol. 43:155, 1976.

Ciancio, S. G., Slots, J., Reynolds, H. S., Zambon, J., and McKenna, J.: The effect of short term administration of minocycline HCl on gingival inflammation and subgingival microflora. J. Periodontol. 53:557, 1982.

Cunha, R. A., and Stucca, A. M.: Third generation cephalosporins. Med. Clin. North Am. 66:283, 1982.

Kannangara, D. W., Thadepalli, H., and McQuirter, J. L.: Bacteriology and treatment of dental infections. J. Clin. Pharmacol. 50:103, 1980.

Sabbath, L. D.: Drug resistance in bacteria. N. Engl. J. Med. 280:291, 1969.

Slots, J., Rosling, B., and Genco, R.: Suppression of penicillin-resistant oral *Actinobacillus actinomycetemcomitans* with tetracycline: Considerations in endocarditis prophylaxis. J. Periodontol. 54:193, 1983.

Stahl, S. S.: The healing of a gingival wound in protein-deprived, antibiotic-supplement adult rats. Oral Surg. 17:443, 1964.

Tedesco, F. J., Barton, R. W., and Alpers, D. H.: Clindamycin associated colitis. Ann. Intern. Med. 81:429, 1974.

Walker, C. B., Gordon, J. M., McQuikin, S. J., Niebloom, T. A., and Socransky, S. S.: Tetracycline: Levels achievable in gingival crevice fluid and in vitro effect on subgingival organisms. J. Periodontol. 52:613, 1981.

Weinstein, L.: Antimicrobial agents, penicillins, and cephalosporins. In Goodman, L. S., and Gilman, A. (eds.): The Pharmacological Basis of Therapeutics. New York, MacMillan, 1975.

chapter 34

Diagnostic microbiology and immunology

Michael G. Newman, D.D.S. □ *Russell J. Nisengard, D.D.S., Ph.D.*

CHAPTER OUTLINE

- **IDENTIFICATION OF BACTERIA**
- **IDENTIFICATION OF ANTIBODIES**

- **OTHER DIAGNOSTIC TESTS**

Numerous microbiologic and immunologic tests are currently available, with new assays continually being introduced. This chapter focuses on diagnostic tests of value in dentistry that are currently offered by clinical laboratories, as well as tests used in dental research and practice.

The fields of microbiology and immunology have been rapidly expanding with a virtual explosion in two diverse types of diagnostic tests: (1) those dependent on increasingly sophisticated techniques and instrumentation requiring highly trained personnel, which are available in clinical laboratories; and (2) those employing relatively simple procedures and requiring less skill to perform, which lend themselves to a clinician's office. The greatest growth in the next decade will be in diagnostic tests designed for office use. Currently, a large number are available for use in physicians' offices.

Identification of Bacteria

In dentistry, many oral infections are successfully treated empirically without identification of the specific etiologic agent. For example, most abscesses respond to penicillin and many types of periodontal diseases are alleviated to some degree by tetracycline therapy. This empirical approach is not always successful, as antibiotic resistance can occur and the antibiotics may be erroneously selected based on incorrectly identifying the putative infectious agent. As in all medical microbiology, the best approach is first to identify the etiologic microorganism and then to select the appropriate therapy. Several methods of identifying bacteria have been used in dental research (Table 34–1).

DIRECT EXAMINATION

Many clinical specimens are directly examined under light, phase contrast, or dark-field microscopy, preferably as soon as they are collected from the patient. This provides a rapid assessment of the relative morphotypes and numbers of bacteria. Culture requires at least a 24-hour incubation, and currently many oral bacteria, including most spirochetes, can be identified.

Table 34–1 ■ Identification of bacteria
Direct Examination—Microscopy
Culture and Sensitivity Assays
Culture techniques—aerobic and anaerobic
Speciation techniques—GLC, DNA homology, and so on
Antimicrobial susceptibility—requirements and interpretation
Immunologic Assays
Immunofluorescence
Latex Agglutination
Immunodot/blot
Flow cytometry
Other Assays
DNA Probes

If the oral sample is very concentrated, as is the case with plaque, it must be diluted in sterile culture media or physiologic saline before microscopic examination.

Bacterial samples can be examined microscopically as either stained or unstained preparations. A variety of stains have been developed to aid in the differentiation of different bacteria.

Phase Contrast and Darkfield Microscopy

Fresh, unstained, wet oral samples are frequently examined by either phase contrast or darkfield microscopy. These "wet mount" techniques allow evaluation of the relative numbers of bacterial morphotypes and bacterial motility. Spirochetes, other motile bacteria, and trophozoites or parasites can be identified by these techniques.

Both phase and darkfield microscopy require special microscope condensers, which alter the way the light is reflected or refracted off the cell surface. The outline of the bacteria is black against a light background in phase contrast microscopy and light against a black background in darkfield microscopy.

Gram Stain

The Gram stain, first developed by Hans Christian Gram in the late 19th century, is one of the most important procedures in the diagnostic laboratory. While it does not allow species identification, it is usually the first step in identification of unknown bacteria. The Gram stain is a differential stain that divides all bacteria into two groups: gram-positive bacteria, which stain blue-violet, and gram-negative bacteria, which stain pink-red.

Method ■ The Gram stain consists of a sequential application of four reagents: (1) crystal violet as the primary stain; (2) iodine to chemically bind the alkaline crystal violet to the cell wall; (3) alcohol as a decolorizer that increases the permeability of the cell wall, allowing the crystal violet stain to be washed out of gram-negative bacteria and those gram-positive bacteria that have lost cell wall integrity from antibiotics or autolysis; and (4) safranin as a counterstain to allow visualization of gram-negative bacteria as red to pink in color.

Acid-Fast Stain

This stain primarily identifies tubercle bacilli. Cells of some bacteria and parasites contain long-chain fatty acids, which resist destaining of basic dyes by acid alcohol. These microorganisms are thus called "acid-fast." Mycobacteria such as *M. tuberculosis* and *M. marinum* are characterized by their acid-fast stain.

Method ■ The bacteria are stained with hot carbol-fuchsin, decolorized with acid alcohol, and counterstained with methylene blue. Acid-fast bacteria maintain the initial red color of carbol-fuchsin, while non–acid fast bacteria stain blue from the methylene blue counterstain.

CULTURE AND SUSCEPTIBILITY

A specimen is usually sent to the microbiology laboratory to *culture* and identify the organism(s), as well as to determine its susceptibility and resistance to various antimicrobial agents.

Although future trends in clinical microbiology point to the rapid, non–growth dependent methods for detecting infectious agents, the isolation and identification of viable pathogens is still the current "gold standard." The major advantages of culturing are the elucidation of all major microorganisms and determination of the antimicrobial susceptibility of pathogens.

Guidelines

Microbial sampling from orofacial infections is often necessary for effective patient management. The dental clinician should be aware that each infection has specific sampling and processing requirements and laboratory procedures are constantly updated.

Methods of specimen collection and transport are important because many diagnostic tests for infectious diseases depend upon the selection, timing, and method of specimen collection. These factors are often more critical for microbiologic specimens than for chemical or hematologic laboratory tests.

The following general rules apply to all specimens:

1. A sufficient quantity of specimen must be provided to permit thorough study.

2. The sample should be representative of the infectious process.

3. Only sterile equipment and aseptic techniques should be used to prevent specimen contamination.

4. The specimen must be transported to the laboratory and examined promptly. Special transport media may be helpful or required (i.e., anaerobes).

5. The specimen should be accompanied by a request form indicating the genera suspected. Separate samples must be submitted for aerobic and anaerobic cultures. Depending on the laboratory, duplicate request forms may be required for the aerobic and anaerobic laboratory if they are processed in separate locations.

TYPES OF SPECIMENS

Mucosal Surfaces

Since bacterial infections of mucosal surfaces are often aerobic or facultative, only aerobic culturing may be necessary.

Blood Samples

Blood specimens are rarely collected by the dentist. Such samples are taken to determine the causative agent of a septicemia.

Periodontal Pockets

With increased understanding about specific bacteria associated with different types and stages of periodontal disease, culture of periodontal pathogens is becoming more common.

Sampling methods ■ The most common sampling devices for periodontal pockets are periodontal curettes (that are normally used for scaling and root planing) and paper points (that are normally used for endodontic therapy) (Table 34–2). Paper points are being increasingly used but may selectively remove the loosely adherent tissue-associated, gram-negative microorganisms and leave the tooth-adherent, gram-positive microorganisms in the pocket. Samples can also be taken with

Table 34–2 ■ Subgingival plaque sampling methods
1. Calcium alginate wrapped barbed broach/syringe
2. Nickle-plated curette-scaler
3. Paper points
4. Irrigation
5. Surgical

a barbed broach, an endodontic instrument, that is modified by soldering a long wire wrapped with calcium alginate fibers on the tip. A wash of a pocket obtained with an irrigating device has also been used for dark-field microscopic analysis. By this technique, a predetermined volume of liquid is introduced into the sulcus, and then part of it is removed for analysis.

Processing Plaque Specimens

To identify plaque microorganisms, it is imperative that proper transport and processing of the specimens takes place. Important parameters are

1. *Anaerobiosis.* Since plaque—especially subgingival plaque—contains many anaerobic bacteria, it is important to provide an anaerobic transport medium.

2. *Viability during transport.* The transport medium must preserve the microbial viability until the specimen is processed at the laboratory. At the same time, it should not allow selective growth of species, leading to distorted results.

3. *Dispersion.* Because clumping of bacteria in plaque is common, the plaque must be dispersed prior to culturing in order to obtain representative results. This is usually accomplished by sonification, stirring with glass beads, or vigorous agitation.

4. *Dilution.* Since the numbers of microorganisms in plaque samples are usually quite high (ranging from 10^4 to 10^8), the specimen must be diluted before culturing on solid media to allow accurate colony counts.

5. *Incubation.* Most oral isolates are anaerobic and must be incubated in an anaerobic environment. If aerobic or microaerophilic microorganisms are suspected, however, the specimen must be cultured in one of these environments.

CULTURAL MICROBIOLOGY

Atmosphere of Culture

Organisms are (1) *aerobic*, utilizing oxygen as a terminal electron acceptor, and growing very well at normal room atmosphere; (2) *anaerobic*, growing in the absence of oxygen; (3) *microaerophilic*, growing best in an atmosphere of reduced oxygen; or (4) **facultative anaerobic**, growing in an aerobic or anaerobic environment. Most clinically significant "aerobic" organisms are actually facultative anaerobes. Strict aerobes include *Pseudomonas* species, members of the *Neisseriaceae* family, *Brucella* species, *Bordatella* species, *Francisella* species, *Mycobacterium*, and filamentous fungi. Organisms that require greater concentrations of carbon dioxide are "**capnophilic**." An example is *Actinobacillus actinomycetemcomitans*.

Artificial Media

Many ingredients necessary for the growth of pathogens can be supplied by (1) human or animal hosts, (2) cell or tissue culture, and (3) synthetic or semisynthetic media in the form of dehydrated media powder and prepared media, which are commercially available. A combination of enriched, supportive, nonselective, selective, and differential media is used for the isolation and presumptive identification of bacteria from clinical material.

1. *Enriched* media encourage the growth of organisms found in large numbers in normal flora.

2. *Supportive* media allow growth of most nonfastidious organisms at their natural rates without permitting a growth advantage for any organism.

3. *Nonselective* media permit the growth of most oral microorganisms without specific inhibitory agents (Table 34–3).

4. *Selective* media contain dyes and antibiotics that are inhibitory to all organisms except those being sought. Many selective media are available (Table 34–4).

Table 34–3 ■ Typical non-selective media

1. Trypticase soy agar
   5% sheep blood
2. Brain heart infusion agar
3. Trypticase soy agar
   5% sheep blood supplemented with hemin and menadione
4. Columbia base agar
5. Trypticase soy agar
   5% rabbit blood supplemented with hemin and menadione

---

5. *Differential* media allow selective morphologic identification of certain microbial colonies.

The most supportive, differential media is blood agar, which allows growth of many microorganisms and separation on the basis of red cell hemolysis, colony morphology, and production of pigment. Because of this, most specimens sent to a clinical laboratory are plated onto media containing blood and a source of protein such as tryptones or soybean-protein digest. Bacteria produce extracellular enzymes that cause complete red blood cell lysis (*beta hemolysis*), a greenish discoloration around the colony (*alpha hemolysis*), or no hemolysis (sometimes called *gamma hemolysis*). Hemolysis is controlled by many environmental factors, including pH and atmosphere of incubation.

The colony morphology and type of hemolysis are initial screening tests to determine further steps in identification of an isolate. In some cases, rabbit blood rather than sheep blood is selected for enhancement of organisms of black-pigmented *Bacteroides*.

Anaerobic Culture Techniques

Several techniques are available for the anaerobic growth of microorganisms.

Jar techniques ■ Anaerobic jars are used to control the atmosphere with two methods that yield comparable numbers of anaerobes.

One common method utilizes commercially available H_2- and CO_2-generator envelopes. An envelope is placed in the jar with the inoculated agar plates, water is added, and the jar is sealed. Along with the gas mixture generated, residual oxygen is removed to establish anaerobiosis by catalytic reaction with hydrogen to form water. A catalyst composed of palladium-coated aluminum pellets within a wire mesh container is preferred, as it is convenient and there is no explosion hazard. Reduced anaerobic conditions as demonstrated by an indicator of methylene blue or resazurin are achieved in 1 to 2 hours.

The second technique is an evacuation-replacement system whereby air within the jar is removed by vacuum followed by replacement with an oxygen-free gas containing 80 to 90 percent N_2, 5 to 10 percent H_2, and 5 to 10 percent CO_2. Flushing with this anaerobic gas is repeated twice.

Bio-bag technique ■ This technique utilizes a clear, gas-impermeable bag into which

Table 34–4 ■ Selective media for periodontal bacteria

Bacteria	Media (main ingredients)	References
1. Black-pigmented *Bacteroides*	a. Tryptic soy agar, 5% rabbit blood	Zambon et al., 1981
	b. BPBSM (brucella agar + 10% rabbit blood)	Sasaki and Takazoe, 1982
2. *Bacteroides gingivalis*	BGA media (Columbia agar base + 5% sheep blood)	Hunt et al., 1986
3. *Fusobacterium*	a. CVE (trypticase agar + 5% sheep blood)	Walker et al., 1979
	b. FEA (brucella agar + 2.5% egg yolk)	Morgenstein et al., 1981
4. *Actinobacillus actinomycetemcomitans*	a. TSBV (tryptic soy agar, 10% serum)	Slots et al., 1982
	b. Modified MGB (tryptic soy agar, 5% sheep blood)	Mandell et al., 1986
5. *Capnocytophaga*	a. TBBP (tryptic soy agar, 5% sheep blood)	Mashimo et al., 1977
	b. CAP (G-C agar, 10% hemoglobin)	Rummeus et al., 1985
6. *Eikenella corrodens*	Todd-Hewitt agar	Slee and Tanzer, 1978
7. *Actinomyces*	a. GMC	Kornman and Loesche, 1978
	b. CFAT (trypticase soy agar, 5% sheep blood)	Zylber and Jordan, 1985
8. *Streptococcus*	Mitis salivarius agar	Difco Laboratories, Detroit, MI
9. *Spirochetes*	Brain-heart infusion broth and ingredients	Fiehn and Frandsen, 1984

is placed an ampule containing resazurin as an anerobic indicator, and a gas generator ampule. One or two plates are placed inside the bag (Bio-bag type A), which is then sealed with a heat sealer. Reduced conditions are achieved in one-half hour. The viability of organisms can be maintained within the bag for up to 1 week. These bags are particularly convenient for incubation of primary plates and whenever only a few plates are used.

Prereduced anaerobically sterilized (PRAS) roll tubes ■ PRAS tubes are prepared by dissolving the medium constituents, boiling the medium to remove dissolved air, and then flushing with oxygen-free gas. The tubes can be inoculated by either closed or open methods. The closed or Hungate method utilizes a syringe and needle to inoculate the medium through a seal. By the open method, the tube is opened, a cannula or blunt needle is inserted into the tube, and the medium is constantly flushed through the cannula with oxygen-free gas until the medium is inoculated and the tube is capped. Platinum wires and loops should be used for inoculation, since tungsten wire may oxidize the PRAS medium.

Anaerobic chamber techniques ■ Rigid gas-tight cabinets or flexible, gas-impermea-ble plastic bags are used as anaerobic chambers. All materials used in the chamber are introduced through a series of air locks and access to perform culture procedures in the box is through sealed gloves. Anaerobiosis is initially achieved by flushing with 5 to 10 percent H_2, 5 to 10 percent CO_2, and 80 to 90 percent N_2 in the presence of an active palladium catalyst and maintained by use of a palladium catalyst and 3 to 10 percent H_2.

Gas-Liquid Chromatography

Anaerobic bacteria produce a variety of metabolic end products that are often unique enough to serve as markers for identification (Table 34–5). Because the nutritional composition of the medium, particularly the carbohydrate-to-peptide ratio, affects the metabolic products, the medium for determining end points must be standardized. Although different species produce a variety of end products, the majority form acetic and succinic acids. The gram-positive bacilli produce large amounts of proprionic acid. *Actinomyces* produces succinic acid, and *Fusobacterium* produces butyric acid.

The fatty acid end products are measured by different detectors in the gas chromato-

Table 34–5 ■ Metabolic end products of commonly encountered anaerobes

Gram-positive cocci	
Peptostreptococcus anaerobius	Acetic acid, isobutyric acid, isovaleric acid, isocaproic acid
Streptococcus	Lactic acid
Peptostreptococcus micros	Acetic acid
Gram-negative cocci	
Veillonella	Acetic acid, propionic acid
Gram-positive bacilli	
Actinomyces	Acetic acid, succinic acid, lactic acid
Lactobacillus	Lactic acid
Eubacterium	Acetic acid, isobutyric acid, butyric acid, isovaleric acid, valeric acid, caproic acid
Gram-negative bacilli	
Fusobacterium	Acetic acid, butyric acid, lactic acid
Bacteroides	Acetic acid, propionic acid, isobutyric acid, butyric acid, isovaleric acid, lactic acid, succinic acid

graph. Thermal conductivity (TC) and flame ionization detectors (FID) require helium as a carrier gas and can measure both volatile and nonvolatile end products. The separation of fatty acids is achieved by injecting the prepared samples through a siphon into a column in a heated oven. The high temperature volatizes the sample, and the flow of the carrier gas moves the sample down the length of the column, separating the fatty acids according to molecular weight and polarity. When a fatty acid reaches a detector, it causes an electrical response, which creates a peak on a chart. The more fatty acid present, the larger the height and width of the peak. The retention line (the length of the line from the injection of the sample to the detection of the peak) determines the identity of the peak as compared with a standard of known fatty acid composition.

DNA-DNA Hybridization

This method, which determines the similarity between two different bacterial clones, is based on the ability of single-stranded DNA to bind complementary sequences. Clones from a single colony of a known bacterium are grown in a medium containing radiolabeled substrates that are incorporated into the bacterial DNA during growth. The bacteria are then lysed and the released DNA

cleaved into small fragments with endonucleases. The fragments dissociate into single-stranded DNA after heating or chemical treatment.

The unknown or test bacteria are cultured in unlabeled media, attached to a filter matrix, and treated to dissociate their double-stranded DNA into single strands. The labeled single-stranded DNA of the known bacteria are reacted with the DNA of the unknown strain on the filter matrix. The filter is then washed to remove unbound DNA. Labeled DNA pieces will only bind (hybridize) to complementary DNA so the amount of label remaining on the filter after washing indicates the relatedness of the known and unknown bacteria. Bacteria with similar morphologic and biochemical characteristics exhibit approximately 70 percent genetic relatedness.

ANTIMICROBIAL SUSCEPTIBILITY

Cultivation and isolation of clinically important anaerobic bacteria are relatively slow requiring at least 2 to 4 days. Susceptibility tests are necessary for isolates from patients with serious infections and infections that persist or recur despite appropriate empiric antimicrobial therapy. The susceptibility to antimicrobial agents cannot always be predicted, and testing of the isolated pathogen is required. The effects of antibiotics or chemotherapeutic agents against pathogenic or potentially pathogenic microorganisms can be measured qualitatively, semiquantitatively, or quantitatively.

There are three degrees of susceptibility:

1. A microorganism is *susceptible* if it is inhibited by the concentration of an antimicrobial agent that can be achieved in the blood or tissues of patients taking the recommended doses.

2. A microorganism is *resistant* if the concentration of antimicrobial agent required for inhibition is greater than that obtained in the blood or tissues during therapy. A particular strain is considered resistant if it can tolerate considerably higher concentrations of antimicrobial agents than other strains of the same species.

3. A microorganism is *intermediate* in susceptibility if the inhibitory concentration is equal to or slightly higher than normally obtained in the blood. Only a small group of organisms are intermediate.

Antimicrobial susceptibility is determined

as either the **minimum *inhibitory* concentration (MIC)** or the **minimum *bactericidal* concentration (MBC)**. The MIC is the lowest chemotherapeutic concentration that inhibits microbial growth in broth as defined by lack of visual turbidity. The MBC is the lowest concentration of the antimicrobial agent that allows less than 0.1 percent microbial survival.

Broth Dilution Tests

Broth dilution tests allow determination of the bactericidal and bacteriostatic activity of a drug. Bactericidal end points are determined by streaking 0.1 ml sample from each diluted broth culture onto agar plates. Microdilution tests are a miniaturized version of the broth dilution procedure. Various manual, semiautomated, and automated devices are available that improve the economy and speed of the tests. The automated systems do not lend themselves to testing of oral bacteria because of these organisms' fastidious nature.

Broth Disk Test

Disks with various concentrations of antimicrobial agents are placed in broth, which is then inoculated with 0.1 ml of an actively growing culture and incubated for 18 to 24 hours. A tube without the chemotherapeutic agent serves as a positive control.

Bacterial Disk Diffusion Test

Several methods have been developed for evaluating susceptibility to multiple antimicrobial agents. The most important is the bacterial disk method of Bauer and colleagues (1966), which has been standardized and correlated with MICs. First, the test organism is inoculated onto the surface of agar, and then disks impregnated with different agents are placed on the surface. The antimicrobial agents diffuse into the agar, creating concentration gradients with the highest concentrations closest to the disks. The zone of growth inhibition around the disk indicates the relative susceptibility to the chemotherapeutic agent. The degree of susceptibility (susceptible, intermediate, or resistant) is determined according to a chart published by the National Committee for Clinical Laboratory Standards (NCCLS). Proper interpretation of this test is influenced by factors such as (1) agar depth, pH, cation content, and media

supplements; (2) age and turbidity of the bacterial inoculum; (3) method of inoculating onto the agar; (4) atmosphere of growth; (5) time of incubation; and (6) antimicrobial content of the disks, as well as their age and method of storage.

Rapid Test for Antimicrobial Susceptibility

Certain bacteria such as gonococci, *Staphylococcus aureus*, and *Bacteroides* may be resistant to the beta-lactam antibiotics such as penicillin and cephalosporin due to production of the enzyme beta-lactamase. This enzyme binds antibiotics possessing a beta-lactam ring and usually opens the ring leading to inactivation of the antibiotic.

The most sensitive method for detection of this enzyme is to test the microorganism on a chromogenic cephalosporin, which turns red when its beta-lactam ring is broken. This cephalosporin called nitrocefin is commercially available in impregnated filter paper disks and strips. The disks or strips are moistened with sterile water, smeared with isolated colonies, and incubated for 5 to 10 minutes. A positive reaction is indicated by a color change from yellow to red.

IMMUNOLOGIC ASSAYS

Several immunologic assays have been used clinically as "stains" to identify microorganisms in clinical specimens. These include immunofluorescence and enzyme immunoassays.

Immunofluorescence

Immunofluorescence combines the sensitivity and specificity of an immunologic assay with that of microscopic localization. This permits the identification of specific bacteria in bacterial smears such as subgingival plaque samples. Two types of immunofluorescence assays have been employed for the identification of specific bacteria in clinical samples: direct and indirect immunofluorescence (Fig. 34–1*A* and *B*).

By **direct** immunofluorescence, antisera to a microorganism is conjugated to a fluorescent dye such as fluorescein. When this conjugate is incubated on a clinical smear containing the organism and then washed off, the antibodies attach to their corresponding bacterial antigen and the organism is visualized by its fluorescent outline when viewed

DIRECT IMMUNOFLUORESCENCE

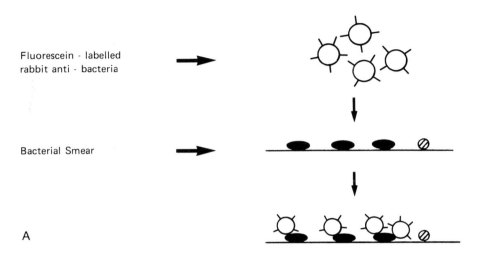

Fluorescein - labelled
rabbit anti - bacteria

Bacterial Smear

A

INDIRECT IMMUNOFLUORESCENCE

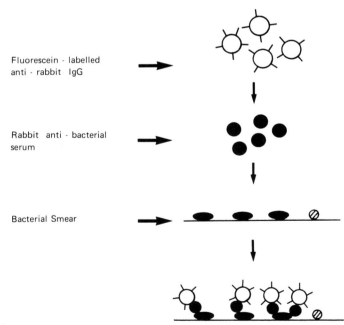

Fluorescein - labelled
anti - rabbit IgG

Rabbit anti - bacterial
serum

Bacterial Smear

B

Figure 34–1 ■ Direct immunofluorescence *(A)* and indirect immunofluorescence *(B)* for identification of bacteria in clinical samples.

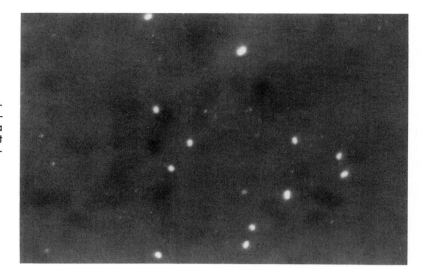

Figure 34–2 ■ Indirect immunofluorescence for *Actinobacillus actinomycetemcomitans* in a subgingival sample from a first molar site in a patient with localized juvenile periodontitis.

with a microscope equipped with special filters and light source (Fig. 34–2). If that organism is not present, the conjugated antibodies will not attach to any bacteria and will be removed by washing so that the smear will appear dark with no fluorescence.

Indirect immunofluorescence is similar to direct immunofluorescence but is a two-step test rather than a one-step test. In an indirect immunofluorescence test, antiserum to a microorganism is incubated on the clinical smear and washed off, and then a conjugate of a fluorescent dye and an antiserum to the first antiserum are incubated on the smear and then washed off. For example, rabbit antisera to *B. gingivalis* would be first incubated on a clinical smear followed by fluorescein-labeled, goat antirabbit IgG.

Direct and indirect immunofluorescence assays have proven to be useful laboratory tests for the diagnosis of specific bacterial pathogens. Studies of periodontopathogens have demonstrated the advantages of identifying the percentage of the pathogen in the plaque smears. These have been determined by dividing the total specific fluorescent bacteria by the total number of bacteria counted with phase contrast microscopy or counterstain.

Enzyme Immunoassays

Horseradish peroxidase, a small enzyme, is conjugated to specific bacterial antibodies in this assay and incubated on bacterial smears. An orange-brown color is developed by incubation with a substrate for the peroxidase. This can be visualized by examination with a regular light microscope. Such tests are commonly available for detection of *cytomegalovirus* and other viruses and bacteria.

Latex Agglutination

Latex agglutination is an immunologic assay with moderate sensitivity that is based on the binding of protein to latex and its agglutination or clumping on exposure to its specific antigen or antibody.

Latex agglutination tests are commercially available for identifying antigens or antibodies in clinical specimens. Because of its simplicity and speed, it is one of the most rapidly growing areas of diagnostic microbiology. Examples of some of the diagnostic kits currently available are summarized in Table 34–6. They have been particularly useful in detection of bacteria but have also been used in tests for viruses and antibodies to bacteria or tissue. The sensitivity level of these tests is similar to those of traditional culture tech-

---

Table 34–6 ■ Examples of commercial latex agglutination tests

I. Detection of antigen
    Group A, B, C, D, F, and G streptococci
    H. influenzae
    S. pneumoniae
    N. influenzae
    C. difficile
    Thyroglobulin
    Antinuclear antibodies
II. Detection of Antibody
    Cytomegalovirus (CMV)
    Rheumatoid factor

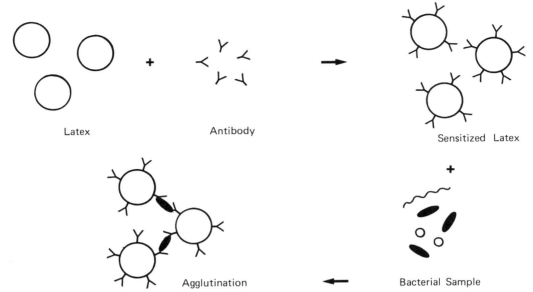

Figure 34–3 ■ Principle of the latex agglutination test.

niques for microorganisms, but the results are available in minutes rather than hours or days. The latex tests are considered to be qualitative or semiquantitative.

The two major types of latex agglutination tests are the indirect (passive) assay and the inhibition assay. The indirect assay is illustrated in Figure 34–3. The **indirect assay** is the most common latex agglutination test for bacteria. Either bacterial antigens or antibodies to bacterial antigens can be determined.

In the indirect test, antibody is either passively or covalently bound to latex for detection of bacterial antigens. In performing the tests, a suspension of the sample is mixed with the sensitized latex and gently agitated for 3 to 5 minutes. The test is then examined

for clumping or agglutination indicative of a positive test for the bacteria being tested for in Figure 34–4.

The latex **inhibition assay** is based on the principle of inhibiting the expected agglutination reaction between known antigen and known antibody as a result of competition. For example, known antibody is mixed with a sample thought to contain bacteria (antigen). The mixture is then reacted with latex coated with antibody to bacteria. If the clinical sample contains the organism, then the antibody will be bound, preventing the expected agglutination. If it is absent from the clinical sample, the antibody would bind with the antigen on the latex, leading to agglutination. Thus, the occurrence of agglu-

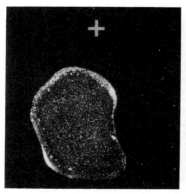 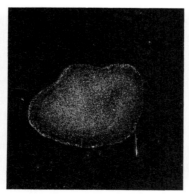 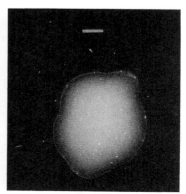

Figure 34–4 ■ Latex agglutination test for *Actinobacillus actinomycetemcomitans*. The square on the *right* is the positive control and the square on the *left* is the negative control. The *middle* well with the clinical sample is positive, indicating the presence of the organism.

tination indicates that the clinical sample does not contain the bacteria tested for, and lack of agglutination indicates that the organism is present.

Flow Cytometry

Flow cytometry, or fluorescence-activated flow cytometry, is a newer technique that permits identification and quantification of cell populations. It has been applied to lymphocyte subsets and to bacteria. Cells in suspension are reacted with monoclonal antibodies to a cell-surface constituent(s) that is labeled with one or more fluorescent dyes such as fluorescein. After incubation, the cells are passed through a focused beam of laser or lamp arc light. The cells scatter the light at low and wide angles, which is then measured. Each type of cell generally has a characteristic volume and scatter pattern. "Gating" allows the selection of a single scatter parameter permitting identification of a limited population of cells.

Flow cytometry techniques have recently been applied to identification of oral bacteria. However, many technical questions must be solved to demonstrate the efficacy of this technique for identification of specific bacteria in plaque.

Enzyme-Linked Immunosorbent Assay (ELISA)

ELISA is similar in principle to radioimmunoassays but an enzymatically derived color reaction is substituted as the label in place of a radioisotope. The assay is very sensitive and relatively economical to run. ELISA assays detect either antigens or antibodies. Similar to immunofluorescence, both direct and indirect techniques can be employed for detection of bacteria. Tests for serum antibodies usually employ an indirect assay, as illustrated in Figure 34–5. Bacterial antigens are assayed in a similar fashion. Antigen is incubated in wells in a plastic plate (or occasionally in test tubes) to allow absorption or coating by the material. After washing to remove free antigen, the plates are ready for tests. Samples containing suspected antibodies and controls are then incubated in separate wells to allow antibodies to bind to the antigen on the surface of the wells. After washing to remove unbound serum components, antisera to the immunoglobulin (for example, goat antihuman IgG) conjugated to either alkaline phosphatase or horseradish peroxidase is then incubated in the wells. A positive reaction is visualized by the addition of a chromogen, which changes from a colorless to a colored

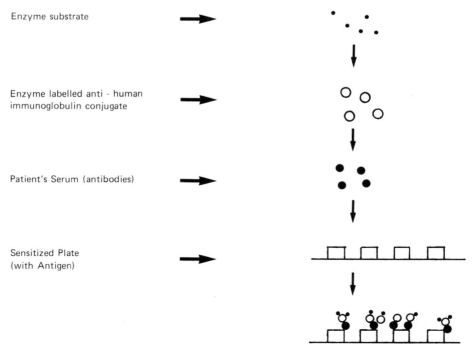

Enzyme substrate

Enzyme labelled anti - human immunoglobulin conjugate

Patient's Serum (antibodies)

Sensitized Plate (with Antigen)

Figure 34–5 ■ Principle of the ELISA assay.

solution. The intensity depends on the concentration of reactants. Tests are usually read photometrically for optimal quantitation. Sensitivity of the assays has frequently been improved by the use of the avidin-biotin system.

ELISA assays have been used primarily as research tools in dentistry. They are most commonly used for determination of serum antibodies to periodontopathogens. Preliminary studies have also examined use of ELISA assays for identification of *Bacteroides* in periodontal pocket samples.

OTHER ASSAYS FOR BACTERIAL IDENTIFICATION

DNA Probes

In recent years, DNA probe technology has progressed from a research technique to a practical clinical laboratory assay. Although few DNA probes are now available, it is expected that the use of this methodology will greatly expand because of its exquisite specificity and sensitivity. Potential uses for these probes include identification of (1) bacteria and antibiotic resistance of bacteria, (2) viruses, (3) specific cancer, (4) genetic diseases, (5) tissue typing, and (6) susceptibility to disease. Clinical assays for periodontopathogens are now available in dentistry.

DNA probe technology developed as an offshoot of genetic engineering. Assays with DNA probes are based on the ability of DNA to hybridize or bind to complementary strands of DNA or RNA having exactly the same base sequence. A portion of DNA from a bacterium, virus, cancer, and so on, is isolated with the aid of restriction endonucleases, enzymes that cut the DNA molecule at specific locations. The DNA plasmid is then spliced into a bacterial plasmid and propagated in large volumes in bacteria such as *E. coli*. The desired cloned DNA fragment is isolated from the bacterial genome with the aid of restriction endonucleases and then dissociated into single strands. The single-strand DNA fragments serve as the probe for complementary sequences in the assay. To identify a complementary fragment, the DNA probe is labeled with a radioactive isotope or an avidin-biotin enzyme system. Depending on the assay, DNA or RNA in the clinical sample is denatured to form single strands and then incubated on a membrane such as nitrocellulose to allow binding.

The labeled DNA probe is incubated on the membrane to allow hybridization and then washed. If the specimen contains complementary DNA or RNA, hybridization or binding of the two single strands occurs, which is visualized via the label on the probe.

Identification of Antibodies

Antibodies to bacteria and other antigens can be measured in serum, saliva, and crevicular fluid. Antibody determinations for oral bacteria are primarily a research tool. Serum tests for viruses are of practical clinical significance but rarely are ordered by dentists. Tests for autoantibodies (discussed separately further on) are also clinically relevant and are requested by dentists whenever autoimmune disease is suspected.

The main antibody assays in dentistry are the ELISA, immunofluorescence, and precipitation assays. The ELISA and immunofluorescence assays have been described earlier in this chapter for detection of bacterial antigen. Substitution of antigen for antibody in the assays allows determination of antibody titers or units of antibody.

Other Diagnostic Tests

ALLERGY TESTING

Various allergy tests are used for the diagnosis of dental patients with suspected allergies (Table 34–7).

Immediate Hypersensitivity

A major concern in dentistry is an allergic reaction to a drug or dental medicament. An anaphylactic reaction occurs very rapidly within minutes and could be life-threatening. This type of hypersensitivity is called immediate hypersensitivity, anaphylactic reactions, reagenic allergy, and IgE-mediated reactions.

The immediate hypersensitivity reactions occur within minutes after contact in a sen-

Table 34–7 ■ Allergy Tests in Dentistry
Patch tests
Skin tests
Serum tests
RAST test
Histamine release

sitized individual and frequently occur in response to chemicals, drugs, dust, pollens, and so on. In a person with an allergy, IgE antibodies specific for the allergen or antigen are formed. (See Chapter 2.) These homocytophilic antibodies fix to or sensitize mast cells and basophils through the Fc portion of the antibody (the end not involved in reaction with the antigen). Subsequent antigenic exposure to the allergen forms complexes of the antigen with two antibody molecules and results in the degranulation of the mast cell or basophil with release of biochemically active mediators including histamine, slow-reacting substance of anaphylaxis, prostaglandins, and eosinophil chemotactic factor. These mediators cause smooth muscle contraction, edema resulting from increased capillary permeability, constriction of small venules, platelet aggregation, and mobilization of phagocytes.

The assays for immediate hypersensitivity reactions include skin tests, assays for histamine release from basophils, and assays for the concentration of IgE specific for an allergen. Skin tests are office procedures usually performed by an allergist. The histamine-release assay is performed on freshly drawn blood and the assay for specific IgE antibodies on serum; both assays must be performed by a laboratory.

Skin tests ■ The two types of skin tests are the intradermal skin test, in which small volumes of the test material are injected into the skin, and the prick test, in which a drop of the test material is applied to the surface of the skin and then a needle is used to prick the area. Both are performed with dilute solutions of antigen, usually on the skin of the arm or back. After 15 to 20 minutes, the site is examined for a wheal (localized, circumscribed area of edema) and flare (irregular, often poorly defined erythema) indicative of a positive reaction. Often positive reaction sites itch because of the localized histamine release. Multiple tests can be performed simultaneously. Frequently, several dilutions of the test material are also tested. Usually, positive immediate skin test reactions are indicative of an allergy to the test substance. However, false-positive and false-negative reactions can occur. Because of the possibility of an anaphylactic reaction which can be life-threatening and the complexity of interpretation, skin testing should be performed by an allergist. A practical consideration in dentistry is a patient with a suspected allergy to

penicillin. This will be discussed in greater detail further on.

Histamine release from peripheral blood basophils ■ The measurement of histamine released by basophils in peripheral blood upon challenge or exposure to an antigen is an in vitro assay for immediate hypersensitivity. Basophils sensitized with IgE antibodies on their surfaces are stimulated to secrete histamine upon challenge with complementary antigen. The amount of histamine released is directly proportional to the extent of antigen-IgE antibody concentration and can be quantitated as to the percentage of histamine release relative to the total cellular histamine content. The concentration of blocking antibody or antigen-neutralizing antibody developed by desensitization can also be measured by this method. Blocking antibodies are a measure of protection against a specific allergen.

Radioallergosorbent Test (RAST)

The RAST test is a solid phase immunoassay that provides quantitative data on the concentration of IgE in serum specific for an allergen or antigen (Fig. 34–6). The antigen is first coupled with an insoluble particle. The serum to be tested is then incubated, with the particle allowing the specific antibody to bind to the antigen. After washing to remove the unbound serum components, the particles are reacted with radiolabeled or enzyme-labeled anti-IgE. The amount of radioactivity or enzyme-generated color is directly proportional to the concentration of specific IgE antibodies. Because the RAST test takes 24 to 48 hours to obtain results, compared with the 15 to 20 minutes for the skin test, the skin test is often preferred.

The common occurrence of penicillin allergies and the frequent use of penicillin in the treatment of oral diseases necessitates a consideration of allergy testing for penicillin. An allergy to penicillin is primarily an IgE-mediated response and is detected by means of a skin test. Early studies using penicillin alone as a skin test reagent frequently yielded false-negative results. It now appears that the reason many patients with penicillin allergies had negative reactions when tested with penicillin was that the penicillin acted as a hapten. Allergic reaction to this low molecular weight substance only resulted when the molecule covalently bound in vivo to larger carrier proteins to form penicilloyl-

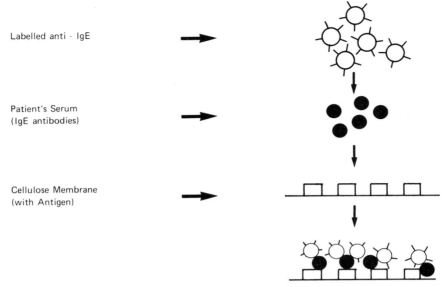

Labelled anti - IgE

Patient's Serum
(IgE antibodies)

Cellulose Membrane
(with Antigen)

Figure 34–6 ■ Principle of the RAST test.

protein complexes or was partially metabolized. Two types of skin test reagents are now available to detect the major and minor antigenic determinants. A reagent composed of penicillin linked to a polylysine chain to form penicilloyl polylysine detects the major antigenic determinant, and a reagent composed of penicillin and one or more of its highly reactive metabolites detects the minor antigenic metabolites. Skin testing may be used in patients with a suspected penicillin allergy, particularly in a life-threatening situation in which penicillin is the drug of choice, and in patients with a suspected but uncertain reaction during penicillin therapy.

Delayed Hypersensitivity

Delayed or cell-mediated hypersensitivity is also important in dentistry. This type of hypersensitivity reaction occurs when sensitized small lymphocytes are exposed to the sensitizing antigen with the release of lymphokines. The major assays for this are the skin test (intradermal and patch tests), lymphocyte proliferation, and lymphokine production assay. The skin test is an in vivo assay, whereas the latter two are in vitro assays. The two in vivo assays are primarily used for research purposes.

Skin tests ■ The skin tests are performed either as an intradermal injection (e.g., tuberculin test) or as a topical application of the suspected allergen (patch test) held in contact by a bandage. The sites are examined in 24 to 48 hours. Positive intradermal injections exhibit induration (hardness) and edema. Positive patch test results exhibit eczematous reddened areas and are compared with areas to which just a bandage was applied. In dentistry, a patch test would be indicated for suspected allergies to metals, medicaments, and so on, and could be performed by the dentist. The skin tests are usually used for the diagnosis of a systemic disease such as mycobacterial infections and are usually performed by a physician.

TESTS FOR ORAL AUTOIMMUNE DISEASES

Several autoimmune diseases have oral manifestations. These include pemphigus, pemphigoid, systemic lupus erythematosus (SLE), discoid lupus erythematosus (DLE), and some forms of desquamative gingivitis. The most common clinical immunologic tests for these include direct immunofluorescence for in vivo deposits of immune reacts in biopsy specimens, indirect immunofluorescence for tissue reactive antibodies in serum, and gel precipitation tests for serum antibodies to tissue components.

Direct Immunofluorescence (Fig. 34–7)

Immunoglobulins, complement, and fibrin are localized in biopsy specimens by direct

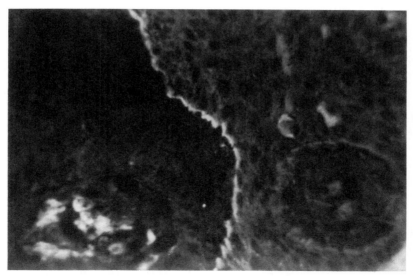

Figure 34–7 ■ Example of a direct immunofluorescence test for the third component of complement (C3) on oral mucosa. Identification of the C3 along the basement membrane is diagnostic for cicatricial pemphigoid.

immunofluorescence. Biopsy specimens are either placed in a special holding solution for transport to the laboratory or quick frozen in liquid nitrogen and transported on dry ice. Frozen sections 2 to 4 microns thick are cut with a cryostat and stored frozen until tested. Sequential sections are incubated with fluorescein-labeled IgG, IgA, IgM, C3, or fibrin. After washing off the specimens to remove the unreacted antisera, the slides are examined with a microscope equipped with a special light source and fluorescent filters. A green fluorescence indicative of the antigen in the tissue is interpreted as to tissue location and pattern of staining.

Indirect Immunofluorescence
(see Fig. 34–1A)

Antibodies in serum to tissue components are determined by indirect immunofluorescence. Frozen sections of tissue, depending on the antibody to be detected, are prepared (e.g., monkey esophagus for pemphigus and pemphigoid antibodies and mouse kidney for antinuclear antibodies associated with connective tissue disease). Dilutions of the sample serum are incubated on sections and then washed off. Fluorescein-labeled anti-human IgG is then incubated on the sections and washed off. Antibodies in the sample serum to a specific tissue constituent are then microscopically visualized as a green fluorescence.

Gel Precipitation

Double diffusion gel precipitation tests are employed to identify serum antibodies to nuclear constituents, which are of significance in systemic lupus erythematosus. Partially purified nuclear antigens are placed in wells and allowed to diffuse toward wells containing serum. Precipitation lines are indicative of an antigen-antibody reaction.

TESTS FOR IMMUNOGLOBULINS AND COMPLEMENT

Several methods are currently employed for quantitation of serum proteins. These are divided into two major groups: (1) assays that measure the physical properties of the immune complexes formed when antisera specific for the serum protein react with the protein (precipitation in gel, turbidimitry, and light scattering); and (2) assays that measure the amount of labeled antibody bound to the antigen. The two most common clinical methods are radial immunodiffusion (RID) and rate nephelometry.

In the **RID assay**, antibodies specific for the protein to be quantitated are incorporated into a gel. Serum or other fluid samples to be assayed are added to wells in the gel and allowed to incubate. A ring of precipitation forms as the antigen diffuses into the gel and reacts with the antibodies. The ring is directly proportional in size to the concentration of

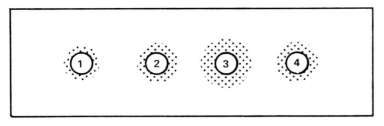

Wells No. 1 - 3: known concentrations of antigen
Wells No. 4: unknown sample

Figure 34–8 ■ Principle of the RID assay. The diameter of precipitation is proportional to the antigen concentration. The concentration of the unknown sample is extrapolated from the line formed by graphing the three diameters of the three known concentrations.

Gel Containing Antibody

antigen. The protein concentration of the sample is determined from a line formed by graphing the ring diameters against protein concentrations of three controls with different protein concentrations (Fig. 34–8).

Rate nephelometry is based on the principle that soluble immune complexes formed by the reaction of antibody with antigen scatters incident light. Since the antibody is constant, the amount of scatter is proportional to the antigen concentration. The concentration in samples are calculated from a dose response curve generated with reference control sera.

The quantitation of immunoglobulins and complement in serum, saliva, and crevicular fluid has been a research tool in dentistry for some time, particularly for studies of periodontal disease and caries. It is also of clinical relevance in such diseases as systemic lupus erythematosus, in which decreased C3 levels correlate with disease activity.

The authors wish to thank Sushma Nachnani for her contributions to this chapter.

REFERENCES

Adkinson, N. F., Jr.: Tests for immunological drug reactions. In Rose, N. R., Friedman, H., and Fahey, J. L.: Manual of Clinical Immunology, ed. 3. Washington, D.C., American Society of Microbiology, 1986, p. 692.

Adkinson, N. F., Jr.: Measurement of total serum immunoglobulin E and allergen-specific immunoglobulin E antibody. In Rose, N. R., Friedman, H., and Fahey, J. L.: Manual of Clinical Immunology, ed. 3. Washington, D.C., American Society of Microbiology, 1986, p. 664.

Anonymous: Products of microbiology: technical manual. Madison, Wisconsin: GIBCO Laboratories, 1983.

Appelbaum, P. C., Kaufman, C. S., Keifer, J. C., and Venbrux, M. J.: Comparison of three methods for anaerobic identification. J. Clin. Microbiol. 18:614, 1984.

Aranki, A., Syed, S. A., Kenney, E. B., and Freter, R.: Isolation of anaerobic bacteria from human gingiva and mouse cecum by means of a simplified glove box procedure. Appl. Microbiol. 17:568, 1969.

Bauer, A. W., Kirby, W. N. M., Sherris, J. C., and Torck, M.: Antibiotic susceptibility testing by a single disc method. Am. J. Clin. Pathol. 45:493, 1966.

Bonta, Y., Zambon, J. J., Genco, R. J., and Neiders, M. E.: Rapid identification of periodontal pathogens in subgingival plaque: comparison of indirect immunofluorescence microscopy with bacterial culture for detection of *Actinobacillus actinomycetemcomitans*. J. Dent. Res. 64:793, 1985.

Carlone, C. M., Valadez, M.J., and Pickett, M. J.: Methods for distinguishing gram-positive from gram-negative anaerobic bacteria. J. Clin. Microbiol. 13:444, 1983.

Check, I. J., and Piper, M.: Quantitation of immunoglobulins. In Rose, N. R., Friedman, H., and Fahey, J. L.: Manual of Clinical Immunology, ed. 3. Washington, D.C., American Society of Microbiology, 1986, p. 138.

D'Amato, R. F., McLaughlin, J. C., and Ferraro, M. J.: Rapid manual and mechanized/automated methods for detection and identification of bacteria and yeasts. In Lennette, E. J., Balows, A., Hausler, W. J., Jr., and Shadomy, H. J. (eds.): Manual of Clinical Microbiology, ed. 4. Washington, D.C., American Society of Microbiology, 1985.

Dowell, V. R., Jr., and Lombard, G. L.: Reactions of anaerobic bacteria in differential agar media. U.S. Dept. of Health and Human Services, Public Health Service, Centers for Disease Control, Atlanta, GA, 1981.

Dzink, J. L., Socransky, S. S., Ebersole, J. L., and Frey, D. E.: ELISA and conventional techniques for identification of black-pigmented Bacteroides isolated from periodontal pockets. J. Periodontal Res. 18:369, 1983.

Holdeman, L. V., Cato, E. P., and Moore, W. E. C.: Anaerobe Laboratory Manual, ed. 4. Anaerobe Laboratory, Virginia Polytechnic Institute and State University, Blacksburg, VA, 1977.

Jackson, A. L., and Warner, N. L.: Preparation, staining, and analysis by flow cytometry of peripheral blood leukocytes. In Rose, N. R., Friedman, H., and Fahey, J. L.: Manual of Clinical Immunology, ed. 3. Washington, D.C., American Society of Microbiology, 1986, p. 226.

Kornman, K. S., Patters, M., Kiehl, R., and Marucha, P.: Detection and quantitation of *Bacteroides gingivalis* in bacterial mixtures by means of flow cytometry. J. Periodontal Res. 19:570, 1984.

MacFaddin, J. F.: Media for isolation—cultivation identification. In Maintenance of Medical Bacteria, Vol. 1. Baltimore, Williams and Wilkins, 1985.

Mulcahy, L.: DNA probes: an overview. Am. Clin. Prod. Rev. 5:14, 1986.

Norman, P. S.: Skin testing. In Rose, N. R., Friedman, H., and Fahey, J. L.: Manual of Clinical Immunology, ed. 3. Washington, D.C., American Society of Microbiology, 1986, p. 660.

Nichols, W. S., and Nakamura, R. M.: Agglutination and agglutination inhibition assays. In Rose, N. R., Friedman, H., and Fahey, J. L.: Manual of Clinical Immunology, ed. 3. Washington, D.C., American Society of Microbiology, 1986, n 49.

Nisengard, R. J., and Neiders, M.: Desquamative lesions of the gingiva. J. Periodontol. 52:500, 1981.

Roit, I., Brostöff, J., and Male, D.: Immunology. St. Louis. C.V. Mosby, 1985, p. 191.

Smith, R. F.: Microscopy and Photomicrography: A Practical Guide. Appleton-Century-Crofts, New York, 1982.

Sutter, V. L., Citron, D. M., Edelstein, M. A. C., and Finegold, S. M.: Wadsworth Anaerobic Bacteriology Manual, ed. 4. Star Publishing, Belmont, CA 1985.

INDEX

Note: Numbers in *italics* refer to illustrations; numbers followed by *t* indicate tables.

515